P9-DFX-385

Pharmacy Practice

for Technicians

Fifth Edition

Don A. Ballington, MS
Robert J. Anderson, PharmD

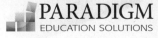

PARADIGM
EDUCATION SOLUTIONS

St. Paul

Managing Editor	Brenda M. Palo
Developmental Editor	Nancy Papsin
Production Editors	Sarah Kearin and Lori Michelle Ryan
Editor/Proofreader	Thomas McNellis
Copy Editor	Kristin Melendez
Cover and Text Designer	Jaana Bykonich
Photo Researchers	Thomas McNellis, Nancy Papsin, and Lindsay Ryan
Permissions Coordinators	Nancy Papsin and Lindsay Ryan
Illustrators	Cohographics; Rolin Graphics, Inc.; S4Carlisle Publishing Services (page 144)
Indexer	Terry Casey
Cover Images	Shutterstock/Lisa F. Young (top left), George Brainard (top right), iStockphoto/stevecoleimages (bottom left)

Care has been taken to verify the accuracy of information presented in this book. However, the authors, editors, and publisher cannot accept responsibility for Web, e-mail, newsgroup, or chat room subject matter or content, or for consequences from application of the information in this book, and make no warranty, expressed or implied, with respect to its content.

Trademarks: Some of the product names and company names included in this book have been used for identification purposes only and may be trademarks or registered trade names of their respective manufacturers and sellers. The authors, editors, and publisher disclaim any affiliation, association, or connection with, or sponsorship or endorsement by, such owners.

Photo Credits: Following the index.

We have made every effort to trace the ownership of all copyrighted material and to secure permission from copyright holders. In the event of any question arising as to the use of any material, we will be pleased to make the necessary corrections in future printings. Thanks are due to the authors, publishers, and agents listed in the Photo Credits for permission to use the materials therein indicated.

ISBN 978-0-76385-223-8 (Text)
ISBN 978-0-76385-226-9 (Text and Study Partner CD)
ISBN 978-0-76385-225-2 (eBook)

© 2014 by Paradigm Publishing, Inc., a division of EMC Publishing, LLC
875 Montreal Way
St. Paul, MN 55102
E-mail: educate@emcp.com
Web site: www.emcp.com

All rights reserved. No part of this publication may be adapted, reproduced, stored in a retrieval system, or transmitted in any form or by any means, electronic, mechanical, photocopying, recording, or otherwise, without prior written permission from the publisher.

Printed in the United States of America

22 21 20 19 18 17 16 15   4 5 6 7 8 9 10

Brief Contents

Contents

Chapter 4
Routes of Drug Administration and Dosage Formulations 107

Chapter 7
The Business of Community Pharmacy 253

Chapter 8
Nonsterile Pharmaceutical Compounding................. 309

Unit 3
Institutional Pharmacy 355

Chapter 9
Hospital Pharmacy Practice 357

Chapter 10
Infection Control 399

Unit 4
Professionalism in the
Pharmacy 483

Chapter 12
Medication Safety 485

Chapter 13
Human Relations and Communications............. 525

Chapter 14
Your Future in Pharmacy Practice....561

Preface

Pharmacy Practice for Technicians, Fifth Edition provides students with a comprehensive body of knowledge on the roles and responsibilities of pharmacy technicians in both community and institutional pharmacy practices. The text focuses on teaching the techniques and procedures to prepare and dispense medications, including the interpretation of prescriptions and medication orders; the maintenance of the patient profile; the counting, measuring, and compounding of nonsterile and sterile preparations; and the preparation, packaging, and labeling of medications. In addition, the text supports practical skills related to billing and inventory management and addresses the soft skills of professionalism, effective communication, cultural awareness, and ethical behavior in the workplace. Lastly, the text offers important chapter features that provide students with the knowledge, skills, and confidence to provide safe and effective care for the patients they serve.

Chapter Features: A Visual Walk-Through

Chapter features are designed to help students learn all facets of current pharmacy practice, including knowledge of community and institutional facilities and their equipment, an understanding of the duties of technicians in the daily operation of these facilities, and insights into effective communication with patients and other healthcare team members.

1

LEARNING OBJECTIVES establish clear goals for pharmacy technician students as they begin their chapter study.

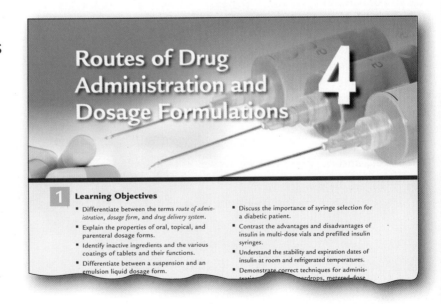

Routes of Drug Administration and Dosage Formulations — 4

1 **Learning Objectives**

- Differentiate between the terms *route of administration*, *dosage form*, and *drug delivery system*.
- Explain the properties of oral, topical, and parenteral dosage forms.
- Identify inactive ingredients and the various coatings of tablets and their functions.
- Differentiate between a suspension and an emulsion liquid dosage form.
- Discuss the importance of syringe selection for a diabetic patient.
- Contrast the advantages and disadvantages of insulin in multi-dose vials and prefilled insulin syringes.
- Understand the stability and expiration dates of insulin at room and refrigerated temperatures.
- Demonstrate correct techniques for administering eardrops, metered-dose

2

KEY TERMS are highlighted using boldface type and are defined both in context as well as in a separate Key Terms section at the end of each chapter. Students are encouraged to preview the chapter's key terms on the Study Partner CD before beginning their chapter study.

2

• Explain the advantages and disadvantages of oral, topical, and parenteral dosage formulations.

Preview chapter terms and definitions.

2 Healthcare providers have numerous pharmacological agents at their disposal and a wide variety of dosage forms with which to customize patient treatment. Before selecting the appropriate medications for their patients, however, providers must have a good understanding of two scientific areas in addition to pharmacology: pharmaceutics and pharmacokinetics. **Pharmaceutics** is the study of the release characteristics of various dosage forms or drug formulations. As you know, medications can be taken orally, inhaled, injected, inserted, or spread on the skin, and each of these routes affects the drugs' onset and duration of action. The characteristics of the drug formulation itself also impact the pharmacological action of any given drug. For example, a tablet or capsule may be formulated to release the drug immediately or slowly over a period of 8-12 hours, or even more slowly over a 24-hour period. **Pharmacokinetics** is the study of how drugs are absorbed into the bloodstream (absorption), circulated to tissues throughout the body (distribution), inactivated (metabolized), and eliminated from the body (excretion). Pharmacokinetic processes affect the medications' effectiveness, dosing schedule, and use.

2

107

2 Key Terms

aerosol a pressurized container with a pro-pellant that is used to administer a drug

controlled-release (CR) formulation a dos-age form that is formulated to release medi-

ar

bu

multiple compression tablet (MCT) a tablet formulation on top of a tablet or a tablet within a tablet, produced by multiple com-pressions in manufacturing

nebulizer a device used to deliver medication in a fine-mist form to the lungs; often used in treating asthma

needle a thin, hollow transfer device used with a syringe to inject drugs into the body or withdraw fluids such as blood from the body

ocular route of administration the place-ment of sterile ophthalmic medications into

patient-controlled analgesia (PCA) infusion device a device controlled by a patient to deliver small doses of medication for chronic pain relief

pharmaceutics the study of the release char-acteristics of various dosage forms or drug formulations

2

pharmacokinetics the study of how drugs are absorbed into the bloodstream, circulated in tissues throughout the body, inactivated, and eliminated from the body

phlebitis an inflammation of the vein from

3

TIMELY TOPICS in pharmacy practice are introduced in this revised edition, including innovative drug delivery systems, medication therapy management services, pharmacy automation, e-prescribing, medication safety initiatives, and healthcare reform.

New!

3 **Targeted Drug Delivery Systems** In the near future, **targeted drug delivery systems** will become increasingly available. In this system, a drug is "carried" by a liposome, a biocompatible and biodegradable substance, and released at a targeted organ site (see Figure 4.10). Several chemotherapeutic agents are formulated for this drug delivery system, targeting only the cancerous organ. Employing this method avoids the adverse effects associated with chemotherapy, including decreased blood counts, alopecia (hair loss), and severe GI disturbances that occur when the toxic chemotherapeutic agent is distributed throughout other body systems.

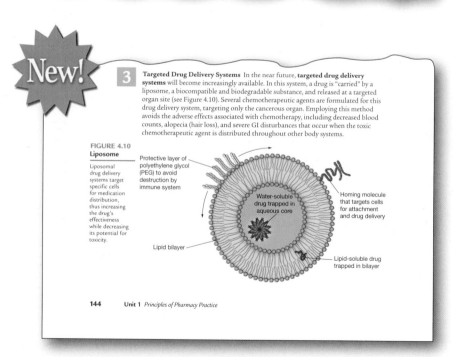

FIGURE 4.10
Liposome

Liposomal drug delivery systems target specific cells for medication distribution, thus increasing the drug's effectiveness while decreasing its potential for toxicity.

Protective layer of polyethylene glycol (PEG) to avoid destruction by immune system

Water-soluble drug trapped in aqueous core

Homing molecule that targets cells for attachment and drug delivery

Lipid bilayer

Lipid-soluble drug trapped in bilayer

144 Unit 1 *Principles of Pharmacy Practice*

4

SAFETY NOTES are included in the page margins to alert students to important safety reminders that must be heeded to provide safe and effective patient care.

5

PRACTICE TIPS appear in the margins of the pages and highlight best practice guidelines for pharmacy technicians to follow in the workplace.

6

PHOTOGRAPHS reinforce the text and help students to visualize pharmacy procedures, medication dosage forms, pharmacy supplies and equipment, and real-world patient interactions.

4

Safety Note

Sublingual nitroglycerin tablets are sensitive to air and light and, consequently, will lose potency over a certain period. These tablets should be kept in their original container and replaced every six months.

Sublingual Medications Nitroglycerin, a common sublingual medication, has specific storage requirements to safeguard the potency of the tablets. Because this medication is a relatively unstable drug, pharmacy technicians must instruct patients to store the nitroglycerin tablets in their original brown bottle (and not in a pillbox) to shield the medication from sunlight, which degrades its potency. Technicians should also remind patients to tightly secure the lid of the nitroglycerin container to avoid the introduction of air—another factor that lessens the medication's potency. Physicians usually advise patients to refill their nitroglycerin with a fresh bottle every three to six months.

Buccal Medications For buccally administered medications, it is important that the patient understand the difference between the technique for chewing regular gum and the technique for chewing nicotine gum. If the nicotine gum is chewed vigorously like chewing gum, then too much nicotine will be released, causing unpleasant side effects such as nausea and vomiting. Proper administration allows the gum to release the nicotine slowly, decreasing cravings. Counseling on the proper technique for administration of the nicotine gum is provided in Table 4.3.

4

Safety Note

If nicotine gum is chewed vigorously, too much nicotine can be released, causing

Technique is also critical for oral transmucosal fentanyl citrate (OTFC), a narcotic analgesic lozenge. OTFC is available in multiple dosage strengths and is used in adults for relief of severe breakthrough pain. The lollipop is placed between the gums and the lining of the cheek, the so-called buccal pouch; it is then sucked to slowly

---

New!

5

Practice Tip

Remember that the larger the gauge number of a needle, the smaller the lumen and, consequently, the smaller the hole that the needle makes. Conversely, the smaller the gauge number of a needle, the larger the lumen, and, consequently, the larger the hole that the needle makes.

A **needle** is attached to the tip of a syringe and is used to either draw fluid into the syringe or push fluid out of the syringe. Needles come in various lengths and sizes. Needle length and size depend on the route of administration, patient factors such as body size, and drug formulation characteristics. Needles commonly range from 18 gauge to 32 gauge. The size of the gauge corresponds conversely to the size of the lumen (inner core) of the needle: the larger

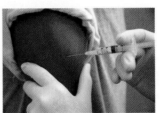

Disposable syringes and needles are used to administer drugs by injection. Different sizes are available depending on the type of medication and injection needed.

number... lumen of the... learn more about needle

---

administered. For these patients, the sublingual route provides a rapid onset of action, which is critical in this health crisis.

Buccal Medications In the **buccal route of administration**, a drug is absorbed by the blood vessels in the lining of the mouth. Common examples of drugs that are administered via this route are OTC nicotine gum (for nicotine addiction) or a lollipop-like lozenge such as oral transmucosal fentanyl citrate (OTFC), a narcotic. A **lozenge**, also known as a *troche*, is a solid dosage form containing active ingredients and flavorings, such as sweeteners, that are dissolved in the mouth. Lozenges generally have local therapeutic effects. Using proper technique when chewing nicotine gum or sucking on a lozenge is very important for appropriate drug release.

Commercial OTC lozenges for relief of sore throats are quite common, although many other drugs, including such prescription drugs as nystatin or clotrimazole, are also available in a lozenge form. Compounding pharmacies may prepare lozenge formulations for specific indications in special needs pediatric or geriatric patients.

A pharmacy technician working in a compounding pharmacy may prepare lozenge formulations by pouring compounded solution into a lozenge mold.

Ophthalmics, Otics, and Nasal Sprays/Solutions Ophthalmics, otics, and nasal products can all be delivered to a specific site with a minimum of systemic side effects. An **irrigating solution**, or a solution for cleansing or bathing an area of the body, can be used both topically in the ear (for example, acetic acid) as well as instilled in the eye (for example, normal saline).

7

FIGURES in the form of illustrations feature helpful captions and callouts that simplify important concepts technicians need to understand to meet the needs of patients in a pharmacy setting.

8

FIGURES in the form of grouped photographs provide additional detail and visual reinforcement of chapter topics.

9

TABLES encapsulate pertinent information related to the chapter topics and serve as a study aid for students.

---

7 FIGURE 4.6
Intramuscular Injection

Intramuscular (IM) injections are administered at a 90-degree angle.

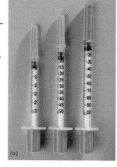

epidermis

dermis

subcutaneous tissue

muscle

90°

large muscle on either side of the buttocks. Another common site, especially for children, is the deltoid muscles beneath the shoulders. Figure 4.6 shows the needle angle and injection depth for an IM injection.

Subcutaneous Route Subcutaneous injections are typically administered on the outside of the upper arm, the top of the thigh, or the lower portion of each side of the abdomen. These injections should not be made into grossly adipose, hardened, inflamed, or swollen tissue. For the subcutaneous administration of insulin, the patient should be instructed by the pharmacist to carefully administer the medication while following a routine plan for site rotation. The site of insulin administration must be ...d from the abd... ...ach leg (upper th... ...hen to the arm to avoid or

---

cian, are encouraged to use the abbreviation for milliliters (mL) instead.

...an... the syringe... ...an hypoderm... ...ject parenteral drugs into the body or to remove blood from the body (see Figure 4.4). These syringes may be glass or—more commonly—disposable plastic with clear demarcations for accurate dosing. Hypodermic syringes (without a needle) are often used to more easily administer oral liquids to infants, children, and pets.

8 FIGURE 4.4
Common Types of Syringes

(a) Insulin syringes in 30 unit, 50 unit, and 100 unit sizes
(b) Tuberculin syringes marked with metric measures
(c) Hypodermic syringes in 6 mL and 3 mL sizes

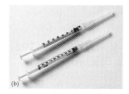

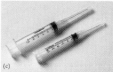

(a)

(b)

(c)

---

a reduced dosing schedule. Consequently, this tablet form improves patient compliance and, therefore, patient outcomes. DR tablets also have several disadvantages: They cannot be split or crushed, have a slower onset of action, have prolonged side effects, and are more expensive (higher co-pays) due to patent protection (see Table 4.2).

A patient can take one tablet, several tablets, or a portion of a tablet, as the prescribed dose requires. Many tablets are *scored* once or twice to facilitate breakage of the

9 TABLE 4.2 **Common Delayed-Release Tablets and Capsules That Cannot Be Split**

Adderall XR	Ditropan XL	oxycodone XR
Allegra-D 12/24	Effexor XR	potassium chloride
Alprazolam XR	GlipiZIDE XL	propranolol LA
Ambien CR	Glucotrol XL	SEROquel XR
Augmentin XR	indomethacin SR	Taztia XT
Avinza	Lamictal XR	theophylline XR
Budeprion XL/SR	metformin ER	verapamil XR
carbidopa/levodopa ER	methylphenidate LA	Voltaren XR
Concerta ER	Metoprolol ER	Wellbutrin XL
Depakote ER	MS Contin	
Diltia XT/diltiazem XL/ER	Niacin SR	
Divalproex ER/DR	nifedipine XL/CC	

10

CHAPTER SUMMARY provides an overview of the key points of the chapter.

11

CHECKING YOUR UNDERSTANDING provides 15 multiple-choice questions that cover important concepts from the chapter.

12

REINFORCING YOUR LEARNING offers three to five enrichment activities that reinforce chapter concepts.

New!

13

THINKING ON YOUR FEET presents real-world scenarios to help pharmacy technician students gain practice in handling challenging situations in the workplace.

New!

10

Chapter Summary

- Drugs are administered in many dosage forms. Factors influencing the decision on route of administration include ease of administration; site, onset, and duration of action; quantity to be administered; drug

- The inhalation or intrarespiratory route of administration allows medication to be inhaled through the oral respiratory route.
- Aerosols and sprays are common inhalation dosage forms and offer a rapid onset of

---

11

Chapter Review

 Additional Quiz Questions

Checking Your Understanding

To check your comprehension of this chapter's key concepts, read the following multiple-choice questions and then record your answers on a separate sheet of paper. Write your answers as modeled in these examples: 1d; 2c; 3b; etc.

1. The most common drug dosage form is a(n)
   a. compression tablet.
   b. extended-release capsule.
   c. enteric-coated tablet.
   d. inhalation aerosol.

2. Which of the following medications is
   disadvantage of insulin pens?
   a. less accurate dosing
   b. inconvenience during travel
   c. cost
   d. increased injection pain

14. Opened vials of insulin kept at room temperature should be replaced every
   a. 7 days.
   b. 14 days.
   c. 30 days.
   d. 6 months.

7. An example of a water-in-oil emulsion is
   a. mupirocin ointment.
   b. hydrocortisone cream.
   c. clobetasol lotion.
   d. Aveeno oatmeal.

8. Which of the following topical medications
   formulations will have the longest onset
   of action?
   a. delayed-release formulations
   b. enteric-coated formulations
   c. controlled-release formulations
   d. sustained-release formulations

12

Reinforcing Your Learning

To build on your understanding of the topics in this chapter, complete the following enrichment activities.

1. Nitroglycerin is an example of a drug that comes in a wide variety of dosage forms appropriate for a wide variety of routes of administration. Research the different dosage forms, routes of administration, and advantages and disadvantages of nitroglycerin. To gather your information, refer to Internet sites or reference works, as well as ask healthcare professionals. Then fill in the following table with your findings.

2. Demonstrate in class the correct technique for the administration of:
   a. eyedrops
   b. eardrops
   c. a metered-dose inhaler (with and without a spacer device)
   d. an IM injection
   e. a subcutaneous injection

[TDR] for the following inform... reconstituted antibiotic suspensions for these drugs: amoxicillin, amoxicillin/clavulanate, azithromycin, and cefdinir. How should each of these medications be stored? What expiration date is recommended after reconstitution at room temperature and under refrigeration? What auxiliary labels are needed for each?

Crestor... cholesterol. If a patient asks you to get authorization from his prescriber for a new prescription for the 40 mg strength in order to split the tablets, would you be able to follow through on the patient's request? Does 40 mg Crestor meet FDA criteria for tablet splitting? What are the advantages and disadvantages of tablet splitting?

13

Thinking on Your Feet

To gain practice in handling challenging situations in the workplace, consider the following real-world scenarios and then use the guiding questions to help you formulate your responses.

1. A prescription has been brought in for a steroid cream (0.25%) to be applied to an infant's eczema on the cheeks. The mother states that she has a similar drug at home in an ointment formulation (1%) and wants to know whether she can use what she has at home because the drug is expensive. Creams and ointments are very different, and, in this case, the strength (and maybe the drug) is different as well. How should the pharmacy technician respond to this question? What should the pharmacist tell this mother about the differences between the two products?

2. A young man has come in to pick up some

3. An older man has just picked up two prescriptions for nitroglycerin: One prescription is for sublingual tablets, and the other prescription is for transdermal patches. When the patient asks why he has been prescribed two different formulations of the same drug, how would you respond?

4. A patient has come in to pick up some prescriptions for fertility drugs. Some of the medications are given subcutaneously and others are given IM. The pharmacist has selected the appropriate syringes for each of these routes.
   a. Which needle is appropriate for the IM in... and which needle is

14

ACQUIRING FIELD KNOWLEDGE allows students to expand their knowledge of pharmacy practice by exploring Web-based projects.

14

5. An elderly patient with Type II diabetes has recently been placed on Humalog and Lantus insulin to control his blood glucose levels. The Humalog dose is 8 units before breakfast, 12 units before lunch, and 20 units before dinner. The Lantus dose is 40 units at bedtime. How soon before breakfast should the patient administer the Humalog insulin? What size insulin syringes are needed for the Humalog? the Lantus?

6. It is Saturday night and an out-of-town patient visits your pharmacy and requests a box of insulin syringes. What questions would you ask him or her? Can insulin syringes be legally dispensed without a prescription in your state? Check your response with a local pharmacist.

Acquiring Field Knowledge

To expand your knowledge of pharmacy practice, explore the following online activities that focus on research and information retrieval.

Reminder: As you navigate the Internet, remember to exercise caution and good judgment when evaluating information. A thoughtful review of online text should take into consideration the following factors: the creator and sponsors of the website, the intended audience, the credentials of the authors and contributors, the reliability and validity of the posted information, the frequency of updates to the site, and the ease of navigation for a range of user skill levels.

1. Visit a drug information site, such as www.paradigmcollege.net/pharmpractice5e/drugs or www.paradigmcollege.net/pharmpractice5e/rxlist, and research the drugs listed below. For each drug, write down the various dosage forms available and the route by which each dosage formulation is administered. (Each drug is available in at least two dosage forms.) Why are different routes of administration available?
   a. sumatriptan   d. morphine
   b. promethazine   e. triamcinolone
   c. diazepam   f. albuterol

associated with a decrease in the risk of breast cancer.

4. TV media is actively promoting the Zostavax (or shingles) vaccine. Conduct an online search to find answers to the following questions: Who are candidates for this vaccine? What storage conditions are required for this vaccine? How stable is the drug once it is reconstituted? What is the recommended route of administration? What is the cash price of the vaccine?

5. Bupropion is available in three dosage formulations: immediate-release, SR, and

---

15

SAMPLING THE CERTIFICATION EXAM provides students with 10 practice problems that model the test format of the certification exams.

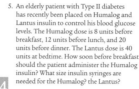

15

Sampling the Certification Exam

To provide you with practice for the Certification Exam, read the following questions that have been patterned after the test format and then record your answers on a separate sheet of paper. Write your answers as modeled in these examples: 1d; 2c; 3b; etc.

1. Which of the following dosage forms will deliver nitroglycerin (NTG) over a continuous 24-hour period?
   a. ointment
   b. sublingual tablets
   c. aerosol
   d. transdermal patch

2. The route of administration with the fastest onset of action is
   a. sublingual.
   b. subcutaneous.
   c. intramuscular.
   d. intravenous.

3. In a patient with severe nausea and vomiting, the most appropriate dosage form would be a
   a. liquid suspension.
   b. caplet.
   c. rectal suppository.
   d. magma.

4. A patient is administering 30 units of Novolin R insulin before each meal. Which of the following insulin syringes

   b. syrup.
   c. emulsion.
   d. tincture.

7. You receive a prescription for an infant for Ranitidine in the dose of 0.8 mL po bid. To deliver the most accurate dosing, what measuring device should accompany the medication?
   a. 1 mL tuberculin syringe (without the needle)
   b. measuring cup
   c. dropper
   d. 5 mL oral syringe (without the needle)

8. A patient is prescribed an ophthalmic solution and ointment. How should they be administered?
   a. The solution and the ointment can be administered simultaneously.
   b. The ointment should be administered first; the solution should be administered 10 minutes later.
   c. The solution should be administered first; the ointment should be

Resources for the Student

To support their study of the textbook, students have access to additional print and electronic resources that enhance the development of pharmacy technician skills and address different learning styles.

Appendices

Three appendices provide important reference material for pharmacy technician students:

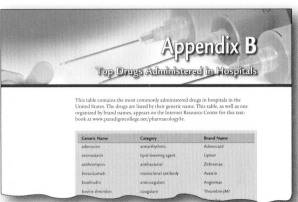

- **Appendix A:**
  Most Commonly Prescribed Drugs
- **Appendix B:**
  Top Drugs Administered in Hospitals
- **Appendix C:**
  Common Pharmacy Abbreviations and Acronyms

Study Partner CD

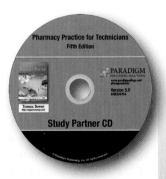

The Study Partner CD included with each textbook offers the following tools to support student learning:

- **Key Terms and Flash Cards**—to help students learn pharmacy terminology
- **Matching Activities**—to provide students with a fun, interactive way to learn chapter content
- **Quizzes**—to test students' understanding of important chapter concepts in both practice and reported modes
- **Link to Internet Resource Center**—to allow students access to additional course-related resources

Student Internet Resource Center

The Internet Resource Center for this title at www.paradigmcollege.net/pharmpractice5e provides additional reference information and resources for students. One of these resources is the *Canadian Pharmacy Technician Supplement*. This supplement presents general information about the Canadian healthcare system, including drug regulation, the top 100 dispensed drugs in Canada, and the role of the pharmacy technician in the practice setting. For students who may have the option to work in Canada, this supplement provides valuable insights into the differences between the U.S. and Canadian healthcare systems.

eBook

For students who prefer studying with an eBook, this text is available in an electronic form. The Web-based, password-protected eBook features dynamic navigation tools, including bookmarking, a linked table of contents, and the ability to jump to a specific page. The eBook format also supports helpful study tools, such as highlighting and note taking.

Resources for the Instructor

Pharmacy Practice for Technicians, Fifth Edition is supported by several tools to help instructors plan their courses and assess student learning.

Instructor's Guide with Instructor Resources CD

In addition to course planning tools and syllabus models, the *Instructor's Guide* provides chapter-specific teaching hints and answers for all end-of-chapter exercises. The *Instructor's Guide* also offers ready-to-use chapter tests and midterm and final examinations. Included in the package is the Instructor Resources CD, which offers PowerPoint® presentations as well as the **Exam***View*® Assessment Suite. **Exam***View*® is a full-featured, computerized test generator that provides both print and online tests and the option for instructors to create customized tests using the chapter item banks.

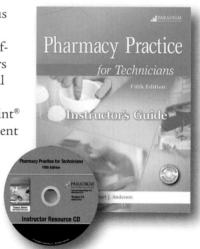

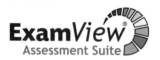

Instructor Internet Resource Center

Many of the features that appear in the printed *Instructor's Guide* also are available on the password-protected instructor section of the Internet Resource Center for this title at www.paradigmcollege.net/pharmpractice5e. An additional posted resource to be aware of is the *Canadian Pharmacy Technician Supplement*. This supplement presents general information about the Canadian healthcare system, including drug regulation, the top 100 dispensed drugs in Canada, and the role of the pharmacy technician in the practice setting. For students who may have the option to work in Canada, this supplement provides valuable insights into the differences between the U.S. and Canadian healthcare systems.

Distance Learning Cartridges

Distance learning cartridges are available for this program.

Textbooks in the Pharmacy Technician Series

In addition to *Pharmacy Practice for Technicians, Fifth Edition*, Paradigm Publishing, Inc. offers other titles designed specifically for the pharmacy technician curriculum:

- *Pharmacology for Technicians, Fifth Edition*
- *Pharmacology for Technicians Workbook, Fifth Edition*
- *Pharmacy Labs for Technicians, Second Edition*
- *Pharmacy Calculations for Technicians, Fifth Edition*
- *Certification Exam Review for Pharmacy Technicians, Third Edition*
- *Sterile Compounding and Aseptic Technique*
- *Pharmacology Essentials for Technicians*

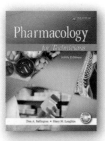 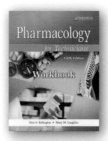 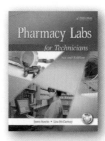 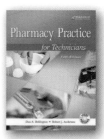

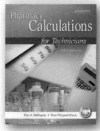 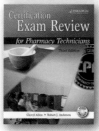 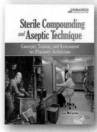 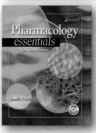

About the Authors

Don A. Ballington, MS, served as program coordinator of the pharmacy technician training program at Midlands Technical College in Columbia, South Carolina, for 27 years. He has also served as president of the Pharmacy Technician Educators Council and in 2005 received the Council's Educator of the Year award. Mr. Ballington has conducted site visits for pharmacy technician accreditation and helped develop the American Society of Health-System Pharmacists' Model Curriculum. He has also been a consulting editor for the *Journal of Pharmacy Technology*. Over the course of his career at Midlands Technical College, he developed a set of high-quality training materials for pharmacy technicians. These materials became the foundation for Paradigm's Pharmacy Technician series.

Robert J. Anderson, PharmD, has more than 40 years of experience in academia and pharmacy practice, having worked in both independent and chain community pharmacies. Dr. Anderson is professor emeritus at the Southern School of Pharmacy at Mercer University in Atlanta, Georgia, and is currently a part-time community pharmacist. He is also president of RJA Consultants, LLC for legal consulting. He has been a guest lecturer in clinical pharmacology at several state nurse practitioner programs, as well as a clinical pharmacy specialist at Kaiser Permanente, Southeast Region, in Atlanta. Dr. Anderson has served as an associate director for the Department of Pharmaceutical Services at the University of Nebraska Medical Center in Omaha, Nebraska, and is a past member of the United States Pharmacopeia (USP) Expert Committee. He is co-author on the third, fourth, and fifth editions of *Pharmacy Practice for Technicians*, as well as the second and third editions of *Certification Exam Review for Pharmacy Technicians*. In addition, he has written chapters in *Clinical Pharmacology and Therapeutics* and *Handbook of Nonprescription Drugs* and has served on the editorial boards of *Family Practice Recertification* and *American Journal of Managed Care Pharmacy*.

Author's Acknowledgments

I would like to offer a special thank-you to the staff at Walgreens Pharmacy in Jasper, Georgia—Kelly Nettleton, Meagan Mills, Andy Saul, Shannon Bell, and Jessica Walker—for their ongoing efforts and support in educating me on the business of retail pharmacy and providing suggestions on content additions. I would also like to recognize Jeff Richardson and his staff at Ball Ground Pharmacy for giving me valuable insights into the practice of independent community pharmacy over the past few years. I thank Dale Coker and his staff at Cherokee Custom Scripts—especially Kathy Sheffey and Kelly Jackson—for their time and patience in making me understand the day-to-day operations of an accredited compounding pharmacy. I would like to give special thanks and recognition to Marcus Dennis, CPhT, for his reviews, contributions, and insights into modern-day hospital pharmacy practice in Unit 3. I would also like to recognize the valuable assistance from David Anderson—my brother—who provided a nursing perspective on pharmacy operations and the most common drugs prescribed in a hospital. I would be remiss to not thank Jason Sparks for always being there to answer and address our questions on the up-to-date responsibilities and impending national issues on curriculum development that impact pharmacy technician certification. I certainly want to thank Nancy Papsin and Brenda Palo for their almost daily guidance and support throughout this ambitious project to make the Fifth Edition the very best yet. Personally, I would like to thank my wife, Peggy, for having the patience and understanding over the past year to see me through this review process.

Robert J. Anderson

Acknowledgments

The quality of this body of work is a testament to the feedback we have received from the many contributors and reviewers who participated in *Pharmacy Practice for Technicians, Fifth Edition.*

Robert W. Aanonsen, CPhT
Platt College
Tulsa, Oklahoma

Harold S. Bender, PharmD, RPh
National College of Business
  and Technology
Spring Hill, Tennessee

Diana Vasquez Broome, BS, CPhT, PhTR
Lone Star College
Tomball, Texas

Christina Cox, BS, CPhT
Heald College
Honolulu, Hawaii

Erika D'Arezzo, BS, CPhT
Sanford-Brown
Cranston, Rhode Island

Marcus Dennis, CPhT
Northside-Forsyth Hospital
Forsyth, Georgia

Elizabeth Garcia, AA, CPhT
San Joaquin Valley College
Visalia, California

Aldo Gatti, BSc Pharm, RPh
Centennial College
Toronto, Ontario, Canada

Joseph P. Gee, PharmD
Cosumnes River College
Sacramento, California

Mary Good, AA, CPhT
National College
Harrisonburg, Virginia

Jeff Gricar, MEd, CPhT, PhTR
HCC Coleman College
Houston, Texas

Lisa Homburg, RPh
College of the Mainland
Texas City, Texas

Susan Howell, BS, CPhT
Ivy Tech Community College
Muncie, Indiana

Philip E. Johnston, BS, RPh
Austin Community College
Austin, Texas

Kent LaFary, CPhT

Michelle C. Ma, MAT, BS, CPhT
Heald College
Milpitas, CA

Belva J. Matherly, BA, BA, CPhT
National College
Salem, Virginia

Lisa McCartney, BAAS, CPhT, PhTR
Austin Community College
Austin, Texas

Shawn McPartland, MD, JD
Harrison College
Indianapolis, Indiana

Lynda Melendez, AS, CPhT, PhTR
Texas State Technical College
Waco, Texas

Mary Stende Miller, BS, RPh
Minnesota State Community &
  Technical College
Wadena, Minnesota

Michael T. Mockler, MBA, RPh
Heald College
Portland, Oregon

Jody Myhre-Oechsle, MS, CPhT
Chippewa Valley Technical College
Eau Claire, Wisconsin

Elina Pierce, MS, CPhT
Southeast Community College
Beatrice, Nebraska

Vickey L. Rose, CPhT

Becky Schonscheck, BS
Maricopa, Arizona

Julia B. Sherwood, AA, CPhT
Spartanburg Community College
Spartanburg, South Carolina

Shahriar Siddiq, MBBS (MD), DNM
Algonquin Careers Academy
Ottawa, Ontario, Canada

Jacqueline T. Smith, RN, CPhT
National College
Princeton, West Virginia

Jason P. Sparks, MEd, CPhT, PhTR
Consultant and Instructional Designer
Austin, Texas

Maureen Simmons Sparks, CPhT
Clover Park Technical College
Lakewood, Washington

Bobbi Steelman, MEd, CPhT
Daymar College
Bowling Green, Kentucky

Cynthia J. Steffen, MS, RPh
Milwaukee Area Technical College
Milwaukee, Wisconsin

Dawn M. Tesner, DHEd, MSHA, CPhT
Mid Michigan Community College
Mt. Pleasant, Michigan

Sandi Tschritter, MEd, CPhT
Spokane Community College
Spokane, Washington

Terry Walker, RN (retired)
Selkirk College
Castlegar, British Columbia, Canada

Margaret L. Wallace, PharmD, BCACP
University of Wisconsin

Jeremy Watson, BS, CPhT, RT
National College
Knoxville, Tennessee

Elaine Young, MEd, CPhT
Angelina College
Lufkin, Texas

We offer a special thank-you to Jason Sparks, Lisa McCartney, Phil Johnston, and Marcus Dennis for their valuable input on chapter content; Dr. Shahriar Siddiq for his creation of the online *Canadian Pharmacy Technician Supplement* that addresses topics specific to Canadian pharmacy technicians; and Diana Vasquez Broome, Michelle Ma, and Maggie Wallace for their expert chapter reviews. We would also like to thank Judy Johnson for her writing of the ExamView test banks and Andrea Redman for her creation of the PowerPoint presentations.

The authors and editorial staff invite your feedback on the text and its supplements. Please reach us by clicking the "Contact us" button at www.emcp.com.

Unit

1

Principles of
Pharmacy Practice

The Profession of Pharmacy

1

Learning Objectives

- Describe the various cultural origins of pharmacy and their impact on the profession today.
- Discuss the four stages of development of the pharmacy profession in the twentieth century.
- Differentiate the major roles and responsibilities of the pharmacist and the pharmacy technician.

- Understand the educational and licensing requirements for today's pharmacist and pharmacy technician.
- Differentiate among various workplace environments such as community and institutional pharmacies.

STUDY PARTNER

Preview chapter terms and definitions.

Over the past several centuries, the profession of pharmacy has undergone significant change. What began as an ancient art combining nature's elements with a dose of spiritualism or magic has now become a scientific pursuit involving the compounding and dispensing of prescriptions and the dissemination of drug information. In the wake of this paradigm shift from an art to a science, pharmacy practice has moved from the backrooms of village apothecary shops to modern workplaces that cater to specific patient populations and healthcare needs. Pharmacy practitioners have also evolved, from ancient healers and alchemists whose methods were largely based on trial and error, to educated and trained **pharmacists** and **pharmacy technicians** who rely on quality assurance and safety standards to ensure the well-being of the patient population. To provide a better understanding of these evolutionary changes, this chapter discusses the origins of pharmacy practice, the specialized pharmacy workplaces, the general roles and responsibilities of the pharmacist and the pharmacy technician, and the education and licensing requirements for these pharmacy professionals.

The Origins of Pharmacy Practice

In early civilizations, sickness or disease was thought to be a form of punishment or curse placed on individuals by demons or evil spirits. To rid the victim of ill health, relatives would call upon a priest, sorcerer, or medicinal healer to identify the evil spirit and then determine the appropriate remedy. Predictably, early recipes for drug preparations were freely mixed with prayers, chants, incantations, rituals, and magic.

The use of drugs in the healing arts by all cultures is as old as civilization itself. Modern archaeologists, exploring the 5,000-year-old remains of the ancient city-states of Mesopotamia (near modern-day Iraq and Iran), have unearthed clay tablets listing hundreds of medicinal preparations from various sources, including plants, animals, and minerals. These early inhabitants used the trial-and-error method to compile lists of drugs known as **pharmacopeias**, or *dispensatories*. In fact, the concept of modern-day **formularies** is based on these drug lists. The most famous formulary was the Ebers Papyrus, which was a collection of medicinal recipes written around 1500 BCE. This list marked the early beginnings of a more empirical and rational approach to medicine.

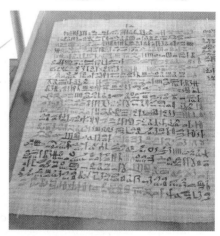

The 110-page Ebers Papyrus contains more than 700 prescriptions for ailments that affected early Egyptian cultures.

Emergence of Traditional Eastern and Western Medicine

In the Far East, a similar mixture of natural sources of medicine and magic existed. These early cultures relied mainly on the healing properties of plants and herbs to treat common ailments and restore harmony to the body. The use of botanicals as a healing modality became the basis of **traditional Eastern medicine**, a practice that continues today in China and India. Many of these herbal treatments from the Far East are widely used in Western culture today—for example, ginseng for energy.

The ancient Greeks were the first culture to shift medical practice from a spiritual-based approach to a more logical, scientific-based approach. Famous Greek physician Hippocrates (ca. 460–370 BCE) believed that illness had a rational and physical explanation and was not the result of possession by evil spirits or disfavor with the gods. He believed that the four humors of the body (blood, phlegm, yellow bile, and black bile) must be in the correct balance to maintain optimal health. His hypothesis formed the origins of the **traditional Western medicine** practiced today. During his lifetime, Hippocrates published more than 70 medical texts that scientifically categorized diseases, their signs and symptoms, and their treatments. He is also credited with establishing a lexicon for the medical terminology that healthcare professionals continue to use in their practices. In fact, the word *pharmacy* comes from the ancient Greek word *pharmakon*, meaning "drug or remedy." Because of his many contributions to the practice of Western medicine, Hippocrates is known as the "Father of Modern Medicine," and the Hippocratic Oath—an oath taken by medical practitioners to uphold the highest standards of medical ethics—is named after him.

Another early Greek physician, Dioscorides, is credited with writing one of the world's greatest pharmaceutical texts: *De Materia Medica (On Medical Matters)*. Written in the first century CE, Dioscorides' text included descriptions of herbal remedies and

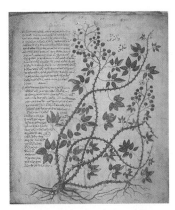

De Materia Medica (On Medical Matters), written by Dioscorides, describes natural medicinal agents and their curative properties.

their usage, side effects, quantities, dosages, and storage guidelines. Dioscorides gathered his knowledge of medicinal herbs and minerals as a soldier serving in the Roman army during the rule of Nero. As he traveled across the European continent, he collected samples of herbs, which he later studied and tested for potential medicinal properties. All told, Dioscorides catalogued more than 1,000 substances—mainly botanicals—that had medicinal value. For 15 centuries, *De Materia Medica* served as the standard reference text for drugs and is considered the forerunner of such modern-day references as the *United States Pharmacopeia (USP)* and the *Physician's Desk Reference (PDR)*.

Like Dioscorides, Galen (129–216 CE) was another notable Greek physician who fought in the Roman army. Galen's theory that the human body contained two circulatory systems was accepted by physicians for centuries, until William Harvey disproved his theory in 1616. Galen also studied the effects of herbal medicine on the body, which led to the coining of the term *galenical pharmacy*, or the process of creating extracts of active medicinals from plants. His legacy to the medical world, however, was his systematic classification of six centuries of medical and pharmaceutical knowledge, including the treatments for various pathologies—a classification that went unchallenged for nearly a century. For his extensive body of work in pharmaceutical sciences, Galen is considered to be "The Father of Pharmacy."

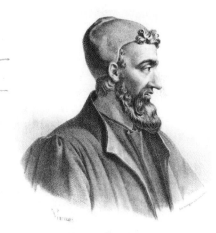

Galen is considered "The Father of Pharmacy" for extracting, identifying, and classifying active ingredients from natural sources.

Roots of the Pharmacy Profession

At the beginning of the Middle Ages, the profession of pharmacy was evolving in both the Persian and European empires. Early Arabic civilizations were some of the first cultures to develop a list of drugs introducing various dosage formulations (pills, syrups, extracts) and to identify the pharmacist as a qualified and licensed healthcare professional. Modeled after ancient Greek and Arabic cultures, the **apothecary** (or pharmacy) concept developed in western Europe in the eleventh and twelfth centuries, along with the creation of professional guilds. The guilds existed primarily to maintain a monopoly over the training and length of apprenticeships of chemists and pharmacists. The establishment of these guilds led to the rise of formalized universities and professional organizations devoted to the pharmaceutical sciences. Thus, state boards of pharmacy are considered the offspring of these ancient professional guilds.

The Greek, Roman, and Arabic influences on the development of the profession of pharmacy were questioned in Europe during the Renaissance (1350–1650 CE). This period saw the rise of alchemy and a regression of the scientific principles championed by the Greeks. **Alchemy** combined elements of chemistry, metallurgy, physics, and medicine with astrology, mysticism, and spiritualism in order to turn something ordinary into something special. In one common example of the application of their trade, alchemists would attempt to change base metals—such as iron, nickel, or lead—into silver or gold.

The Renaissance also experienced the emergence of hospitals and pharmacies run by religious orders. These monastic facilities served the larger communities by providing free health care and medicines to the poor, thus serving as the archetypes of today's community healthcare clinics, public health departments, and charity hospitals.

In the seventeenth century, the publishing of scientific and medical research led to advances in pharmacy practice. At the beginning of the Scientific Revolution, most scholars in western Europe were deeply learned in the Greek and Latin classics, and so it is not surprising that, when inventing new terms to describe their discoveries and observations, they borrowed word parts from these ancient languages. This lexicon—based on Greek and Latin root words, prefixes, and suffixes—remains at the heart of the scientific naming of many medical terms today.

Herbal Medicine and Apothecaries

With the arrival of exotic plants and spices brought back by European explorers to the New World, the list of medicinal agents grew. The import of these new species of plants required pharmacists to be skilled not only in chemistry but in **botany**, as they created medicinal agents from these natural substances. Rudimentary research to determine the efficacy of botanical drugs was initiated—a process that served as the catalyst for the scientific fields of pharmacology and pharmacognosy.

During the 1800s, pharmacists were becoming increasingly recognized as providers of health care, although many apothecary shops in Europe were still being operated by physicians. Each major city in Europe published its own pharmacopeia or drug list, which later was officially adopted as the standard for the individual country. One of those drug lists, *Martindale: The Extra Pharmacopoeia*, was created in Great Britain in 1883 and is still considered a well-respected and useful pharmacy reference.

In the United States, during the early period of colonization, **herbal medicine** was commonly practiced by both Native Americans and settlers. For Native Americans, the time-honored tradition of using medicinal plants to treat illness and disease was often accompanied by prayers, chants, and rituals seeking spiritual intervention for those who were sick. Herbs such as echinacea (used to prevent infection), ginger (used to treat a stomachache), and saw palmetto (used to treat prostate problems) were common natural remedies for restoring harmony to the body, mind, and spirit. These herbs continue to be sought-after cures today as more individuals embrace the practice of holistic and natural medicine.

Extracts from the echinacea plant are still used today to build up immunity and prevent infection.

Roles of Early Pharmacy Practitioners

Among the early colonists of the United States, there were very few pharmacists. Predictably, the profession followed the European model, albeit at a much slower pace. Pharmacists in the colonies were doctors, druggists, merchants, or storekeepers. Until the nineteenth century, it was commonplace for a physician to own the dispensary that distributed drugs to patients. However, gradually the professions separated, and the pharmacy or apothecary shop became an independent entity that was owned and operated by the pharmacist.

By 1820, the United States developed its own formulary of drug standards called the *United States Pharmacopeia (USP)*. A revision of this early formulary exists today and is written by the United States Pharmacopeia, an independent, nonprofit organization that sets quality standards for prescription medications and over-the-counter (OTC) drugs and dietary supplements. The current *USP* provides guidelines for the compounding of sterile and nonsterile products by pharmacists and pharmacy technicians. The publication also sets national drug standards for all pharmaceutical manufacturers of brand and generic drugs, both domestic and foreign.

In 1852, the American Pharmacists Association (APhA) was organized to address the **adulteration** of imported drugs—an issue that continues to plague U.S. pharmacy practices. The founding principles of the APhA were based on pharmacy's roots in science—an approach that is maintained by the organization to this day. Other pharmacy organizations—such as the National Association of Retail Druggists (NARD) founded in 1898 (now known as the National Community Pharmacists Association)—have focused more on the business side of the profession. The purposes of these two organizations reflect the schism of pharmacy: Is pharmacy primarily a business or a profession?

Community pharmacy practice in the United States in the late 1800s involved the compounding of many herbs and chemicals for medicinal use. Pharmacists often experimented by compounding refreshing drinks served at a soda fountain, a mainstay of local pharmacies at that time. For example, in 1886, John Pemberton, a pharmacist by trade in Atlanta, Georgia, began to sell a compounded tonic called Coca-Cola. Its name was derived from one of its ingredients: cocaine. For more than two decades, the Coca-Cola formula contained this plant alkaloid, until growing concerns over the effects of cocaine forced its manufacturer to substitute caffeine for the cocaine. Another pharmacist, Caleb Bradham, created a similar carbonated drink, later called Pepsi-Cola, in 1893 in North Carolina. These pharmacist-created fountain drinks continue to be popular beverages, though the soda fountain pharmacy setting faded away in the 1960s.

By the beginning of the twentieth century, pharmaceutical manufacturing began to take hold. Although many pharmacists continued to rely on plants as ingredients in their compounded preparations, they now incorporated mass-manufactured ingredients as well. Pharmacists formulated their own liquids and powders and rolled their own pills. By the middle of the century, the traditional compounding tasks of pharmacists became less common, and the practice of pharmacy gained more of a scientific and technical framework. Consequently, the education and training of pharmacists focused on their changing roles—a topic that is discussed more in depth in the section titled "The Pharmacist."

The American Society of Hospital Pharmacists was formed in 1942 initially to address the interests of hospital pharmacists but broadened its scope to advance the pharmacy profession. The organization is now known as the American Society of Health-System Pharmacists, or ASHP, and is credited with many innovations in practice and training programs, including setting standards for pharmacy technicians.

Modern-Day Pharmacy Practice

In the past 50 years, with the explosion of scientific research and the accessibility of drug information, new synthetic drugs have been introduced, allowing the pharmacy profession to keep pace with medical advances. Although modern pharmaceutical science still relies on a combined understanding of botany and chemistry to discover and synthesize these new medications, compounding practices have evolved over the centuries from a trial-and-error process to an exact science. Today's pharmacists and pharmacy technicians work in tandem to fill more than four billion prescriptions each year—a number that will continue to rise in the coming years as the population ages. In light of that statistic, a number of new pharmacy schools have opened in the past decade to address these expected pharmacist shortages. With these increasing demands for pharmacists, and the predicted expansion of their roles and responsibilities, pharmacy technicians will be increasingly called upon to assist in providing essential pharmacy services in a variety of practice settings.

The Pharmacy Workplace of Today

Pharmacy technicians are employed in most of the same practice settings as pharmacists, including community pharmacies (i.e., drugstores), hospital pharmacies, home healthcare systems, and long-term care facilities. These work environments must be clean, well-lit, and well-ventilated in order for pharmacists and pharmacy technicians to effectively fulfill their job duties. For the most part, their work requires standing, often for long hours. Because patients' healthcare needs continue beyond the traditional workday, both pharmacists and pharmacy technicians may be on call or may work days, nights, weekends, and holidays. At any time, 24 hours a day, some number of the estimated 334,400 pharmacy technicians in the United States are practicing in a pharmacy workplace.

Community Pharmacies

Most pharmacists and technicians work in a **community pharmacy**, also called a *retail pharmacy*. The staff of a typical community pharmacy consists of several pharmacists with bachelor of science (BS) or doctor of pharmacy (PharmD) degrees and several pharmacy technicians including those who have passed the certification examination.

Prescription drugs and select OTC drugs must be stored in a locked and secured area with a pharmacist always on duty.

Some pharmacists will have additional education, training, and experiences in business and clinical practice. The ratio of pharmacy technicians allowed to practice with pharmacists differs in each state and is under the auspices of that state's board of pharmacy.

Most community pharmacies are divided into a restricted and secure prescription area offering prescription merchandise and related items and a front-end area offering OTC drugs, dietary supplements, medical supplies, and other merchandise. There are many types of community pharmacies. Some of these facilities are independently owned small businesses; others are part of large retail chains; and still others are smaller franchise operations. However, the recent trend is toward fewer independent pharmacies, especially in metropolitan areas, because these small pharmacies have difficulty competing with the large-scale operations of chain pharmacies.

Independent Pharmacies An **independent pharmacy** is a community pharmacy that is owned and usually operated by one pharmacist or a group of pharmacists. Consequently, the pharmacist-owner makes his or her own decisions regarding the practice of pharmacy, with more attention and time spent on improving customer service. An independent pharmacy prides itself on getting to know its customers. Most compounding of prescribed medications is also done in this type of pharmacy, in addition to the dispensing of prescriptions. Some independent pharmacies have evolved into "compounding only" pharmacies. A **compounding pharmacy** specializes in the preparation of nonsterile (and sometimes sterile) preparations that are not commercially available.

Chain Pharmacies A **chain pharmacy** may be national or regional and may be found in department stores (for example, Wal-Mart, Target), grocery stores (for example, Kroger, Publix), or typical corner drugstores (for example, Walgreens, CVS, Rite-Aid). Most chain pharmacies are strategically located in metropolitan areas to allow for large-volume dispensing, with heavy use of both pharmacy technicians and automation. Unlike an independent pharmacy, a chain pharmacy is owned by a corporation, with many of the administrative decisions made at the corporate level. Some chains have established walk-in clinics staffed by nurse practitioners, specialty pharmacies for HIV/AIDS, or specialty services such as diabetes education.

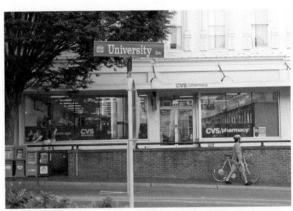

Many metropolitan areas have one or more community pharmacies that provide pharmacy services 24 hours a day, 7 days a week.

Franchise Pharmacies A **franchise pharmacy** combines characteristics of an independent business and a large retail chain. Franchise agreements vary but typically grant the franchisor exclusive use of the company name and rights to market and sell company products to an owner/operator of a drugstore, the franchisee. Franchise pharmacies are sometimes called *apothecaries* and sell only medication and health-related products and services such as health screenings.

One example of a franchise operation is Medicine Shoppe International (MSI), which was purchased by Cardinal Health Company in 1995. MSI purchased the Medicap franchise in 2003. It is the largest franchisor of independent community pharmacies in the United States. Franchise pharmacies attempt to provide more personalized health care than their competition. Due to its size and focus, a franchise pharmacy typically has one pharmacist-owner and one pharmacy technician.

Mail-Order Pharmacies One of the fastest-growing types of pharmacies, which is also somewhat related to retail pharmacy, is the **mail-order pharmacy**. A mail-order pharmacy is run as a centralized operation using extensive automation and a number of pharmacy technicians to dispense and mail large volumes of prescriptions every day. Unlike other community pharmacies, this type of pharmacy involves no direct patient contact or customer transaction for pharmacy personnel. Because of economies of scale, mail-order pharmacies, like chain stores, can acquire drugs at lower cost and pass on some of the savings to insurers. Some common mail-order pharmacies include Medco, Express Scripts, Tricare (military), CVS Caremark, and Walgreens Mail Service Pharmacy.

Studies of mail-order pharmacies have not confirmed a significant cost savings for patients. For example, a patient with a chronic disease who uses a mail-order pharmacy typically must order a three-month supply of his or her prescribed medication. If the patient experiences a side effect or adverse reaction from the medication or if the prescriber changes the medication, then the patient's potential drug savings could be offset by drug wastage. Another trade-off for the supposedly lower cost of using a mail-order pharmacy is that medication counseling is limited to reading a printout or calling a toll-free number. Concerns also exist about the time delay patients experience when waiting for chronic disease medications, which typically should be taken on a regular basis. Also, there are safety, storage, and legal issues of delivering medications through the mail.

However, despite these limitations, more patients each year are filling their prescriptions using mail-order pharmacies—many of which are located out of state. In fact, many health insurance companies encourage or even require enrollees to use mail-order pharmacies, ostensibly to save money. These pharmacies are regulated by each state's board of pharmacy; many of these state boards require that the mail-order pharmacy not only be licensed but be physically housed within the state's borders.

Trends in Community Pharmacies The U.S. prescription market share for dispensed prescriptions varies considerably (see Figure 1.1). The trends suggest a gradual increase in chain and mail-order pharmacies at the expense of independent community pharmacies. Also, long-term care and home healthcare pharmacies are expected to increase concurrently with the aging U.S. population.

FIGURE 1.1
U.S. Prescription Market Share by Type of Pharmacy

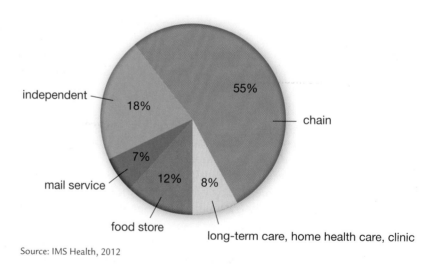

independent — 18%
chain — 55%
mail service — 7%
food store — 12%
8% — long-term care, home health care, clinic

Source: IMS Health, 2012

Institutional Pharmacies

Broadly defined, an **institutional pharmacy** is a pharmacy associated with any organized healthcare delivery system. Traditionally, a **hospital pharmacy** is the most common example. However, long-term care facilities, home healthcare systems, managed-care organizations, and nuclear pharmacies are more recent examples of places where institutional pharmacies can be found.

The staff of an institutional pharmacy is typically comprised of pharmacists who have a variety of educational and training backgrounds. Some of these individuals hold a BS degree; others have a PharmD degree; still others hold a master of business administration (MBA) degree. More pharmacists will have postgraduate residencies in a specialty area of practice such as parenteral nutrition, pharmacokinetics, drug information, infectious disease, geriatrics, nuclear pharmacy, and so on. Pharmacy technicians who work in an institutional pharmacy must typically be certified and have experience.

Hospital Pharmacies Approximately one-fourth of all pharmacists work in a hospital setting. The hospital pharmacists and pharmacy technicians prepare, or supervise the preparation of, a unit-dosage system (or a 24–72 hour supply of medication for a patient), sterile intravenous (IV) medications, and an extensive floor stock inventory. Hospital pharmacy personnel perform these tasks under the guidance of a detailed Policy and Procedure (P&P) manual. (For more information on hospital pharmacy practice, see Chapter 9 of this textbook.)

The pharmacy provides an important service to the hospital. Here, a pharmacist reviews a patient's medication administration record (MAR).

Many pharmacy technicians in the hospital (and some in a compounding retail pharmacy) work in a "clean room" environment. In that setting, the technicians are required to don sterile gowns, masks, hair covers, bootees, and gloves to prevent the spread of infection. Clean room personnel must also prepare sterile preparations and hazardous drugs under specialized ventilation cabinets called laminar airflow hoods. To work in a clean room environment, pharmacy technicians must undergo specialized education, training, and certification. (For more information on the topics of infection control and the preparation of sterile and hazardous products, see Chapters 10 and 11, respectively.)

Long-Term Care Facilities A **long-term care facility** may be at two different levels of care. An extended-care facility (ECF) or nursing home provides institutional services predominantly to older adults or disabled residents who can no longer provide for routine or medical care for themselves (called activities of daily living or ADLs), including adults who suffer from chronic diseases or such debilitating disorders as stroke or Alzheimer's disease. Both medical care and residential care are provided to meet the residents' needs.

The second level of care is called a skilled-care facility (SCF) and is limited to patients requiring more round-the-clock nursing care (such as IV infusions) or recovery after a recent hospitalization. Most patients are discharged from an SCF to home or to an ECF when they have adequately recovered. An SCF or an ECF generally provides a higher level of nursing care than home health care. Medicare insurance generally covers some SCF costs but not ECF costs, which are covered with optional long-term care insurance plans.

Some long-term care facilities have an in-house pharmacy on their premises, whereas others either contract with a community pharmacy or allow each resident (or the resident's family) to choose his or her pharmacy. In-house pharmacies typically provide a seven-day supply of medication for the long-term care residents in specially packaged blister packs. Community pharmacies that provide medications to nursing homes will generally fill medication carts or trays with a 30-day supply of medication because medication orders infrequently change in this environment.

Other examples of long-term care facilities include facilities that treat patients with acute or chronic psychiatric disorders or rehabilitation facilities for those with serious traumatic brain or spinal cord injuries. These types of facilities provide medical care for a specific period, which is determined by each patient's needs.

Home Healthcare Systems **Home health care** is the delivery of medical, nursing, and pharmacy services as well as medical supplies to patients who remain at home. Treating patients at home is generally less costly than round-the-clock care in the hospital or in an SCF. In light of that, many patients are discharged as soon as possible from these care facilities to continue their medication regimen and recovery at home. As the population ages in the coming years, the home healthcare system is predicted to continue to grow.

Pharmacists and pharmacy technicians working in a **home healthcare pharmacy** provide IV and oral medications and often must be available on a 24/7 basis for emergencies. The pharmacy technician prepares medications that are checked and verified by the pharmacist and then delivered to the patient's home. A pharmacist or nurse is responsible for educating the patient or the patient's caregiver on the appropriate and safe use of these medications and, if necessary, any medical devices.

A form of home health care is called **hospice care**. Hospice nurses take care of patients (and their families) who are terminally ill from cancer, HIV/AIDS, or other debilitating medical conditions. Hospice works with local pharmacies to provide round-the-clock pain medications to keep these patients as comfortable as possible. Several long-term care insurance policies cover many of the costs associated with home health or hospice care.

Pharmacists and pharmacy technicians work with nurses to provide medications for nursing home, hospice, and homebound patients.

Managed-Care Pharmacy Services **Managed care** has grown dramatically over the past 40 years. Kaiser Permanente, a nonprofit private venture started in California in the 1930s, was an early managed-care or **health maintenance organization (HMO)**. Most HMOs are outpatient clinics, but some may own hospitals. An HMO is an organization that provides health insurance for medical and pharmacy services using a managed-care model. The philosophy guiding the care provided by an HMO is that keeping patients of all ages healthy, or their chronic illnesses controlled, decreases hospitalizations and emergency room visits and therefore lowers expenses to the healthcare system.

HMOs encourage their patients to take an active role in their own health care by eating right, exercising often, and avoiding negative lifestyle choices such as smoking and alcohol abuse. HMOs also urge patients to have annual checkups, to get all their immunizations on schedule, and to get necessary laboratory tests (such as a cholesterol or blood glucose test) and screening tests (such as a Pap smear or mammogram) to detect early diseases, which may be promptly treated through medication or surgical intervention.

Most HMOs are centralized primary-care clinics, which means they serve adult, pediatric, and obstetric/gynecology (ob/gyn) patients and offer pharmacy, X-ray, and laboratory services on-site. HMOs have their own staff physicians who are salaried; some private-practice physicians may have a contractual agreement with an HMO. If patients would like to see a specialist, they often are required to first get a referral from their HMO primary-care physician in order to control access and costs. The primary-care physician serves as the "gatekeeper" to health care.

An HMO, like a hospital, usually has an approved drug list or formulary that has been recommended by a pharmacist and approved by the medical staff. The formulary—plus the use of low-cost generic drugs—allows the organization to purchase select drugs at greater volumes, which lowers operational and patient costs. HMOs have been *generally* successful in slowing the pace of the inflationary increases in the costs of health care without compromising the quality of care. As a result, many employers now include an HMO option in their health plans.

After the patient sees the physician, the patient may go to the HMO pharmacy to fill a prescription. As with many community pharmacies, patients seeking refills of prescription medication may call an automated telephone number to expedite processing and reduce waiting times. Many refills are filled in an off-site warehouse similar to a small mail-order pharmacy and delivered to the clinic for patient pickup. Besides reducing waiting time by the patient, this call-in system also allows the pharmacist to spend more time reviewing the computerized medication profile, which is an important part of the prescription preparation process. An HMO pharmacy generally has a lower inventory of brand name drugs than a community pharmacy due to the presence of a more restricted drug formulary. A decrease in drug inventory results in less overhead costs and more savings. There generally is little to no cash or insurance transactions in an HMO pharmacy, which is considerably different from the operations of a community pharmacy. The responsibility of a pharmacy technician in an HMO pharmacy is similar to that of a technician working in a community pharmacy. With the effective use of pharmacy technicians, the pharmacist has more time to provide personalized counseling to patients. This additional time in reviewing profiles and counseling patients should result in fewer medication errors and lower costs.

Nuclear Pharmacies A **nuclear pharmacy** is a highly specialized practice that compounds and dispenses sterile radioactive pharmaceuticals for more than 100 diagnostic or therapeutic uses. These pharmacies are typically located off-site and managed by one of several specialty pharmaceutical manufacturers.

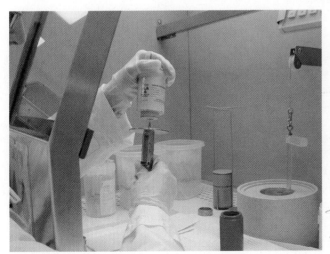

A pharmacy technician with a specialized certification in nuclear pharmacy prepares a sterile, radioactive medication using special equipment and protective shields.

Because of their specialized equipment and inherent hazards, nuclear pharmacies are staffed by pharmacists and pharmacy technicians with advanced training and certification in radiation safety. To work in this environment, pharmacy personnel must *always* wear badges that monitor their levels of radiation exposure.

The Pharmacist

The role of the pharmacist is to safeguard the health of the patients whom he or she serves. This tenet has not changed since the beginnings of the profession. What has changed is the complexity of this task. Today, with the vast number of medications on the market, pharmacists need to draw upon their education and training and exercise their professional judgment to meet the individual needs of their patients while protecting their patients' health and well-being. To fulfill these responsibilities, the pharmacist must be vigilant in detecting an error in the dosing of a medication; a problematic combination of drugs; a dangerous use of a drug, such as the use of a cancer-causing drug by a pregnant patient; and any interactions of a medication with food, drink, or environmental elements. He or she must also be watchful for any adverse reactions that are reported by patients.

To gain a better understanding of the current role and responsibilities of the pharmacist, you need to go back to the beginning of the twentieth century, when the modern-day pharmacist prototype first emerged on the scene.

Evolution of the Pharmacist's Role

During the twentieth century, the role of the pharmacist changed dramatically to keep pace with the advances in medicine and science that occurred during this period. This time frame can be broken down into four distinct eras or stages: the Traditional Era, the Scientific Era, the Clinical Era, and the Pharmaceutical Care Era.

Traditional Era At the beginning of the twentieth century, pharmacists—like their nineteenth-century predecessors—formulated and then compounded medications from natural sources such as plants. They would use their knowledge of botany and chemistry to produce drugs that targeted specific illnesses or diseases; subsequently, they would package and label the drugs in containers and then dispense the medications to their patients. Prescriptions at this time were compounded by hand, using a mortar and pestle, and ingredients and dosages were tailored to individual patients. This practice continued well into the 1920s, when more than 80% of all prescriptions were compounded individually by the pharmacist. Today, pharmacy compounding is nearly a lost art: Of all prescriptions written, less than 1% requires compounding by a pharmacist.

During this era, pharmacists-in-training would spend the majority of their time serving as apprentices in pharmacies rather than sitting in

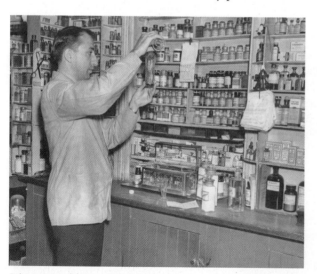

Prior to World War II, many pharmacists compounded their own preparations from natural sources.

university classrooms. Serving apprenticeships at this time was not unusual for learning a trade. The limited formal education for pharmacists focused on galenical pharmacy (as defined earlier) and the study of **pharmacognosy**, or the knowledge of the medicinal functions of natural products from animal, plant, or mineral origins.

Scientific Era The emergence of the pharmaceutical industry in the middle of the twentieth century had a significant impact on the pharmacy profession. During the post–World War II period, pharmaceutical manufacturers such as Eli Lilly, Merck, and Pfizer scientifically tested and developed many new drugs (antibiotics, hormones, and vaccines) and dosage forms (tablets and capsules). These medications were synthesized, developed, and mass-produced more economically and with better quality than by the individual pharmacist.

As the manufacturing of drugs moved from the apothecary shop to the assembly lines of the pharmaceutical manufacturers, the pharmacist increasingly became more of a retail merchant selling premanufactured products. To counter this trend and keep up with the many scientific advances, educational institutions increased the emphasis on the sciences and expanded the pharmacy curriculum. In addition to physics, medicinal chemistry, and anatomy and physiology, pharmacists were required to complete several courses in pharmacognosy and **pharmacology**, or the scientific study of drugs and their mechanisms of action and side effects. By 1960, a five-year BS degree (including two years of pre-pharmacy course work) was required.

Clinical Era The clinical era began in the early to mid-1960s and combined the traditional role of the pharmacist with a new role as dispenser of drug information to the patient and physician. Additional basic science courses were developed and added to the pharmacy curriculum, including **pharmaceutics**, or the study of how drugs are introduced to the body (for example, oral dosage forms, inhalation, injection, and so on). By this time, many pharmacy students and practitioners began to feel that their training had shifted too far in the direction of basic scientific knowledge and, consequently, away from the actual practice of pharmacy. Although pharmacists at this time were highly educated, scientifically trained professionals with a vast knowledge of drugs, they were often underutilized. They devoted the bulk of their energies to completing routine tasks, running a business, and dispensing drugs rather than sharing information on drugs and interacting with patients and other professionals. In fact, up until 1969, it was *not ethical* for a pharmacist to label the medication vials with the drug name or discuss the potential side effects of the medication with the patient.

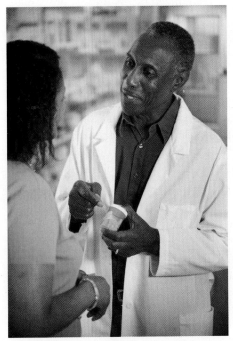

The pharmacist, with the support of the pharmacy technician, works to ensure positive outcomes for drug therapy through careful medication monitoring and patient counseling.

In 1973, the American Association of Colleges of Pharmacy (AACP) established a study commission under Dr. John S. Millis to reevaluate the mission of the pharmacy profession. The 1975 Millis Commission report, titled *Pharmacists for the Future*, defined pharmacy as a primarily knowledge-based profession and emphasized the *clinical* role of pharmacists in sharing their knowledge about drug use. The Millis Commission report led to a new emphasis in the profession called *clinical-* or *patient-oriented pharmacy*. Pharmacy curriculum was again changed, and more colleges of pharmacy eventually adopted a six-year PharmD degree program. New courses were developed, such as **pharmacokinetics** (individualizing doses of drugs based on absorption, distribution, metabolism, and excretion from the body), biochemistry (applying chemistry to biological processes), therapeutics, and pathophysiology. **Therapeutics** is the study of applying pharmacology to the treatment of illness and disease states, whereas **pathophysiology** is the study of disease and illnesses affecting the normal function of the body. In addition, laboratories were moved from the university to more patient-oriented pharmacy practice settings, especially in hospitals. Interdisciplinary experiences with physicians, residents, and interns in the university hospital also became a standard component of pharmacists' course work.

Pharmaceutical Care Era In 1990, Dr. Charles Hepler and Dr. Linda Strand built on the Millis Commission report with a new framework defined as **pharmaceutical care**, which further expanded the mission statement of the profession to include responsibility for ensuring positive outcomes for drug therapy. The mission statements of many pharmacy organizations now reflect this new philosophy. At the beginning of this current era, the patient-oriented focus in the hospital began to move more to the community pharmacy and ambulatory clinic setting. Patient counseling and medication monitoring and management by the pharmacist were becoming more accepted by physicians and consumers.

Today, pharmacy education has continued to evolve and better prepare the pharmacist for his or her role in "ensuring positive outcomes for drug therapy." This philosophy of practice is called "medication therapy management," or MTM, and has become a core component of a pharmacy student's four-year professional curriculum. MTM practices may include recommending a less costly drug to a physician, identifying a potential serious drug-drug interaction or adverse reaction, or counseling a patient on the importance of adhering to a prescribed drug therapy to better control his or her disease. These MTM practices are being recognized by insurance companies, which are providing additional reimbursement for these pharmacist interventions.

Current Role and Responsibilities of a Pharmacist

Today's pharmacist has a broader scope of practice that includes not only dispensing drugs for existing disease but also creating patient care initiatives to prevent or identify future disease. The advanced education and training of pharmacists have better prepared them to assume more patient care responsibilities and subsequently more liability. Although the pharmacist still compounds and dispenses drugs or supervises these processes, he or she increasingly spends more time doing the following tasks:

- gathering information and inquiring about the medical, medication, and allergy histories of patients
- checking age-appropriate dosing for medications and avoiding duplications of therapy
- counseling patients on possible side effects and adverse reactions of their medications
- screening patients for chronic diseases such as hypertension, heart disease, and diabetes by checking blood pressure, cholesterol levels, and blood glucose laboratory tests, respectively
- educating patients on how to better self-manage chronic diseases such as diabetes, heart disease, asthma, and other disorders
- checking computer monitors for warnings of drug interactions with other prescription drugs, OTC drugs, and dietary supplements
- screening patients for minor illnesses that can be safely self-medicated

- assisting and supporting motivated patients to quit smoking
- providing patients with information and recommendations about OTC medications, as well as vitamins, minerals, herbs, and dietary supplements
- providing drug information to physicians, physician assistants, nurse practitioners, and nurses
- dispensing advice about home healthcare supplies (for example, home test kits, insulin needles, support hose) and medical equipment (for example, blood glucose monitors, wheelchairs, crutches, walkers, canes)
- monitoring drug response in patients with chronic diseases such as hypertension, diabetes, hyperlipidemia, and asthma
- monitoring the safe use of controlled substances such as narcotics
- vaccinating high-risk adults for influenza, pneumonia, shingles, and other disorders

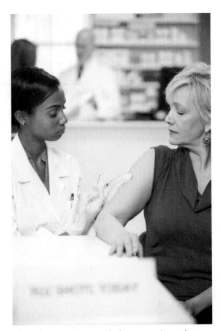

The pharmacist's role has continued to evolve, and now many pharmacists provide services to promote public health. For example, many pharmacists administer flu, pneumonia, and shingles vaccines.

Additional Responsibilities A pharmacist may have additional responsibilities that are specific to particular pharmacy settings. These additional responsibilities would not be possible without the assistance of certified pharmacy technicians.

Community Pharmacies The community pharmacist may also be responsible for preparing both nonsterile and sterile medications in a compounding pharmacy for ambulatory or home healthcare patients. The pharmacist may also dispense and send prescribed medications in special packaging to nursing homes. In an independent pharmacy, the pharmacist takes on the added responsibilities of being a businessperson and entrepreneur, offering needed but as yet unmet services to the community. He or she typically hires and supervises employees, evaluates insurance contracts, reconciles unpaid insurance claims, maintains and orders sufficient inventory, sells merchandise not directly related to health, and manages the overall retail operation.

Institutional Pharmacies In a hospital setting, typical responsibilities of a pharmacist may include entering physicians' orders into the computer database, preparing medications and IVs, providing drug information, recommending drug formulary changes, educating nurses, developing departmental policies and procedures, dispensing investigational and hazardous drugs, purchasing drugs and medical supplies, monitoring narcotic and antibiotic use, and providing medications to each unit of the hospital, including medication carts (crash carts) to be used in medical emergency situations. In larger university hospitals, pharmacists with advanced training in such areas as pediatrics, neonatal care, internal medicine, critical care, cancer, transplant, nutrition, and surgery often accompany physicians on their morning rounds, advise them on appropriate medication use, and monitor patients for adverse effects or drug interactions. These pharmacists are often responsible for educating and counseling patients about their drugs and diseases when they are discharged from the hospital.

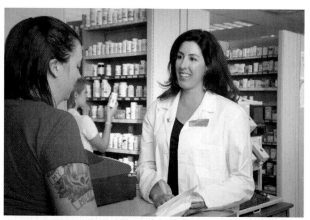
The pharmacist plays an important role in dispensing medications, as well as instructing patients about side effects of medications, food and drug interactions, and dosing schedules.

Similar to a hospital pharmacist, a home healthcare pharmacist often prepares medications and IVs, including parenteral nutrition and antibiotics, for home use for patients of all ages, as well as chemotherapy and pain medications for cancer patients. A consulting pharmacist who practices in a long-term care facility or nursing home has some unique duties as well, including the review of patients' medical and medication records in several nursing homes on a monthly basis.

In addition to dispensing prescriptions in an HMO pharmacy, a managed-care pharmacist who has advanced training may work closely with primary-care physicians to better control chronic disease by educating, monitoring, and—if necessary—ordering lab tests and adjusting the dosages of medications per physician-approved protocols. A managed-care pharmacist may also be more involved in monitoring and adjusting the drug therapy for patients with chronic diseases such as hypertension, diabetes, asthma, hyperlipidemia, and clotting disorders.

Educational Requirements of a Pharmacist

To fulfill the roles and responsibilities for modern-day pharmacy work, a pharmacist must be highly educated and trained. This rigorous preparation was not always the case but rather has evolved over the last century. The education of a pharmacist has transformed from an apprenticeship in the pharmacy to full-time study of the sciences in an academic setting to a combination of formal courses and supervised and structured internships.

In the early 1800s, the Philadelphia College of Pharmacy became the first school to offer courses in the pharmaceutical sciences and to grant pharmacy-specific diplomas. By 1868, land-grant universities, beginning with the University of Michigan, offered formal education and degree programs in pharmacy. As the number of formalized pharmacy programs increased, so did the need for practice standards. In the late 1800s, the APhA encouraged state governments to regulate the pharmacy profession by requiring pharmacists to pass formal certification examinations to obtain licensure to practice. Still, up until 1920, formal educational requirements were *not* required in order to take an examination to become a pharmacist. As long as applicants completed a three- or four-year apprenticeship in a pharmacy, they were eligible to take the examination.

With the advancement of the sciences in the twentieth century, the training of pharmacy students moved from apprenticeships under the guidance of practicing pharmacists to a two-year, formalized higher-education program. On-the-job internships became a component of these academic programs, and students were trained by practitioners who were products of the old apprenticeship program.

In the past 80 years, the rising professional status of pharmacy, plus the explosive marketing of new drugs, demanded more education and training for prospective pharmacists, and educational requirements for pharmacy programs expanded from two years to six years. Today, all colleges of pharmacy offer a PharmD degree, which typically is a six-year program. This program consists of two years of pre-pharmacy course work, including calculus, chemistry, physics, microbiology, and biology. Then,

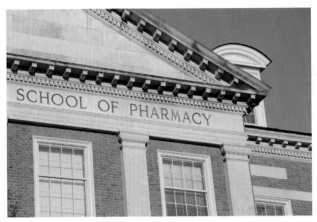

All U.S. schools of pharmacy now offer the equivalent of a four-year professional program of coursework and experiential training.

for many colleges, pharmacy students must apply for pharmacy school by taking the Pharmacy College Admission Test (PCAT) and scheduling an on-site interview. Acceptance into a pharmacy school has become extremely competitive in recent years. The typical successful applicant has a prior degree (typically in biology or chemistry), a grade point average (GPA) of 3.5–4.0, good scores on the PCAT (>80), experience in pharmacy and community service projects, excellent communication skills, and self-motivation. Many pharmacy students started out working as pharmacy technicians in a community or hospital pharmacy, gaining valuable experience that helped shape their career goals.

Once accepted at a university, pharmacy students find that the course work is extremely challenging. Basic science courses include anatomy and physiology, pathophysiology of disease, biochemistry, immunology, pharmaceutics, pharmacokinetics, pharmacology, and therapeutics. Practice or internship time in community and hospital pharmacies is interspersed throughout the curriculum. The last year in the PharmD program is spent in various practice settings such as hospitals, clinics, community pharmacies, home health care, and nursing homes to better prepare students for pharmacy practice in different workplace environments. At graduation, it is tradition for all graduates to recite the Oath of a Pharmacist (see Figure 1.2).

Many graduates will find employment in the community or hospital pharmacy setting; others will enter specialty fields such as managed care or work in mail-order pharmacies, home health care, long-term care, or nuclear pharmacy. Still others will choose careers in pharmaceutical sales, marketing, or research. Some pharmacy graduates will go on to pursue further education and specialization with higher degrees (MBA, PhD), residencies, or fellowships and pursue a career in academia, government, or the pharmaceutical or insurance industry.

FIGURE 1.2
Oath of a Pharmacist

At this time, I vow to devote my professional life to the service of all humankind through the profession of pharmacy.

I will consider the welfare of humanity and relief of human suffering my primary concerns.

I will apply my knowledge, experience, and skills to the best of my ability to assure optimal drug therapy outcomes for the patients I serve.

I will keep abreast of developments and maintain professional competency in my profession of pharmacy.

I will maintain the highest principles of moral, ethical, and legal conduct.

I will embrace and advocate change in the profession of pharmacy that improves patient care.

I take these vows voluntarily with the full realization of the responsibility with which I am entrusted by the public.

Source: Courtesy of the American Association of Colleges of Pharmacy

Licensing Requirements of a Pharmacist

In the United States, all states require pharmacists to be licensed. Obtaining a license involves graduating from an accredited college of pharmacy, passing a state board certification examination, and serving an internship under a licensed pharmacist either during and/or after formal schooling. In addition, in most states, pharmacists must meet specified continuing education requirements to renew their licenses. Most states have reciprocal agreements recognizing licenses granted to pharmacists in other states. Pharmacists who work in a government facility such as a Veterans Administration (VA) hospital are only required to have a valid license in one state, regardless of which state they practice in. Licensing and professional oversight are carried out by individual state boards of pharmacy.

The Pharmacy Technician

The modern-day role of the pharmacist would not be possible without the assistance of well-trained, educated, and certified pharmacy technicians. The pharmacy technician can assume routine functions that allow the pharmacist to spend more time reviewing computerized patient profiles, counseling patients, or communicating with prescribers. Without pharmacy technicians, the risk of preventable and costly medication errors would most certainly increase.

Regardless of practice setting, the pharmacy technician can assist with workload by entering patient and prescription information into the computer, preparing the medication to be dispensed, and providing customer service. The pharmacist oversees the work of the technician by always providing the final verification check of the original prescription with the medication label prior to counseling the patient. In addition, the pharmacist must verify the preparation of all medication prior to its transfer to a patient care unit of a hospital.

Evolution of the Pharmacy Technician's Role

The role of the pharmacy technician has evolved throughout history. In the early twentieth century, registered "pharmacy assistants"—the predecessors of pharmacy technicians—were commonly employed as apprentices. With no formal education, these individuals received their training under seasoned pharmacy professionals. Many early pharmacy technicians were also trained as military medics and, after fulfilling the terms of their service, returned to their country and used their skills in hospitals. In particular, these technicians were trained to participate in drug delivery systems and in the compounding of sterile IV and cancer chemotherapy preparations.

In more recent times, the role of the pharmacy technician in the community pharmacy has slowly evolved, gaining recognition both within and outside the pharmacy profession. At one time, the position was more of a part-time floor stocking clerk, part-time cashier. Now, the pharmacy technician is an invaluable assistant to the pharmacist in all practice settings.

Current Role and Responsibilities of a Pharmacy Technician

A central defining feature of the pharmacy technician's job is accountability to the pharmacist for the quality and accuracy of his or her work. Although the technician carries out many of the duties traditionally performed by pharmacists, the pharmacist must always check the technician's work. Medication errors such as entering incorrect data from the prescription or selecting the wrong drug, dose, or dosage form can cause serious and sometimes life-threatening reactions if not detected. The pharmacist, then, takes final responsibility (and liability) for the pharmacy technician's actions.

Nearly everywhere a pharmacist practices, he or she will be surrounded by one or more pharmacy technicians to lend assistance. However, the responsibilities of the technicians may vary, according to the needs of the pharmacy workplace.

In a community pharmacy, technicians perform many tasks, including:

- meeting and greeting patients presenting or picking up prescriptions
- entering patient demographic and prescription information into a computerized patient database
- assisting the pharmacist in the filling, labeling, and recording of prescriptions
- operating and assuming responsibility for the pharmacy cash register and credit card/check transactions
- stocking and inventorying prescription and OTC medications as well as necessary supplies
- billing and resolving online insurance claims

Safety Note

Rather than working independently, the pharmacy technician works under the direction of the supervising pharmacist.

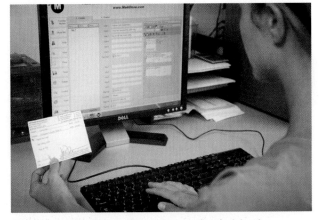

An important function of the pharmacy technician is to accurately input prescribed medications into the computer database.

For more information on the duties of a community pharmacy technician, refer to Unit 2.

The pharmacy technician in a hospital setting may perform similar tasks to that of a community pharmacist but may also be responsible for the preparation of sterile and sometimes hazardous products. Other tasks of a hospital pharmacy technician may include delivering, stocking, or inventorying medications anywhere in the hospital and operating manual or computerized robotic dispensing machinery. Unit 3 contains an expanded discussion on the role and responsibilities of the hospital pharmacy technician.

In a long-term care or nursing home setting, the responsibilities of the pharmacy technician parallel those of the community and hospital technician. However, a long-term pharmacy technician may, under the supervision of a pharmacist, repackage drugs in unit doses labeled for each patient, deliver medications to the nursing home or patient residence, and conduct regularly scheduled inspections of drugs in inventory and in nursing stations to remove expired or recalled medications.

Regardless of practice setting, a pharmacy technician must possess certain personal characteristics to successfully contribute to patient care in a pharmacy. These characteristics include good communication and interpersonal skills; a strong mathematical background; a methodical, detail-oriented approach to tasks; and a high standard of ethical conduct. The importance of communication skills and professional attitudes and behaviors is discussed in greater detail in Chapter 13.

Although the specific duties of pharmacy technicians vary according to the needs of the pharmacy workplace, all technicians must function in strict accordance with state and federal pharmacy laws and standard written procedures and guidelines.

These laws, as well as the P&P guidelines of the individual facilities, clearly delineate the responsibilities of the pharmacist and the pharmacy technician. Technicians must keep in mind that the following tasks are solely the responsibility of the pharmacist: patient counseling on prescription and nonprescription drugs, reviewing computer profiles for drug interactions, and discussing therapy doses, allergies, and alternative therapies. It is important to note that the essential differences in the duties of a pharmacist and a technician involve accountability and making decisions about patients' health care.

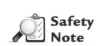 **Safety Note**

Pharmacy technicians play a valuable role in reducing the risk of medication errors.

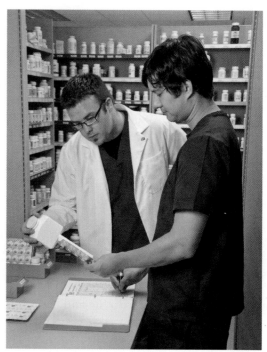

The pharmacist is ultimately responsible and liable for the pharmacy technician's work. All prescriptions and medication orders must be checked by the pharmacist.

Educational Requirements of a Pharmacy Technician

In the past, on-the-job training was sufficient for any "clerk" working in a community pharmacy. Responsibilities for these pharmacy assistants were often limited to answering the telephone, stocking the inventory, and operating the cash register. But, as the role of the pharmacist expanded, so did the role of pharmacy assistants. In response to these changes, formal pharmacy technician training programs were developed to better train technicians to assist the pharmacist. Initially, these training programs were conducted in hospitals to educate their staff in the necessary functions of the hospital pharmacy. Today, the ASHP has developed a model curriculum as a guide to meet the needs of pharmacy technicians primarily in the hospital setting.

Currently, some technician training programs remain hospital-based, but many more are being developed in community colleges and technical schools to meet the projected increased staffing needs for pharmacy technicians in both community and hospital pharmacy settings. Academic-based programs vary in accreditation status, curriculum, and length. The National Association of Boards of Pharmacy (NABP) is working with each state to develop standards in the educational curriculum for pharmacy technicians.

The course work required to complete a pharmacy technician training program varies with the program and state but commonly includes:

- introduction to practice
- medical terminology
- pharmacology (a working knowledge of drug names, usual doses, common indications)
- inpatient and outpatient dispensing procedures and record keeping
- sterile compounding and aseptic technique
- pharmacy laws and regulations
- pharmacy calculations
- communications and customer service

The student then completes some degree of experiential training in either the community or hospital pharmacy or, possibly, both settings.

The goal of all training programs is to better prepare the student to pass a pharmacy technician certification examination and start a challenging career as a certified pharmacy technician. (For more information on certification, refer to Chapter 14 of this textbook.) Since 1995, more than 400,000 pharmacy technicians nationwide have been certified by taking the Pharmacy Technician Certification Exam offered by the Pharmacy Technician Certification Board (PTCB). Many hospital and community pharmacies require that pharmacy technicians be initially certified or become certified within a specified period. In fact, some facilities encourage technicians to become certified by paying for the certification exam and giving salary increases to those who successfully pass it.

In a specialized area of practice such as sterile compounding, nonsterile compounding, or nuclear pharmacy, the pharmacy technician must have additional training and certifications. For sterile compounding, it is considered best practice that personnel complete a training program in sterile product preparation and aseptic technique from the Accreditation Council for Pharmacy Education (ACPE). In addition, sterile compounding technicians typically complete a minimum of 40 hours of hands-on training in a laboratory setting, along with classroom instruction, written examinations, and process validation procedures, to work in IV rooms. To be certified as a nonsterile compounding technician, the technician must successfully complete a training program from the Professional Compounding Centers of America (PCCA). To receive certification as a nuclear pharmacy technician (NPT), the technician must complete a rigorous 300 hours of online self-study and supervised instruction in addition to experiential training with nuclear pharmacists serving as preceptors. The PCCA offers didactic courses and laboratories in which pharmacy technicians learn the latest innovations in compounding unique dosage forms in hospital and community pharmacies. With additional training, certifications, and responsibilities, pharmacy technicians can also expect an increase in salary.

State Board Requirements of a Pharmacy Technician

All state boards of pharmacy now recognize the importance of the pharmacy technician in protecting the health and safety of patients. According to the NABP's 2012 Survey of Pharmacy Law, 41 state jurisdictions require licensure, registration, or certification of pharmacy technicians. To be licensed or registered, a technician must have earned a high school diploma or GED, passed a criminal background check, and completed a formal training program.

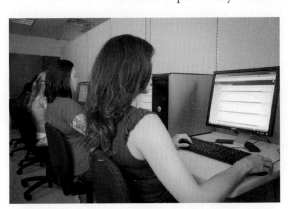

Certification exams for pharmacy technicians can now be taken online with near immediate scoring.

In nine states, technicians must be certified in order to practice. Certification requires the successful completion of a standardized national pharmacy technician examination approved by the state board of pharmacy. To maintain certification status, a technician must attend annual or biannual continuing education programs. Due to variances from state to state, pharmacy technicians who choose to practice in a different state must check the state board of pharmacy of their new residence to verify the state's requirements (certification, registration, or license).

The APhA supports state regulation of technicians by either registration or licensure. Most state boards of pharmacy regulate the activities and even the ratio of pharmacy technicians to pharmacists within a pharmacy. In many states, technicians—similar to pharmacists—are required to attend seminars to keep their knowledge and skills current for continuing certifications and/or licensure.

Healthcare Team

Optimal patient health care is a collaborative effort among prescribers (physicians, nurse practitioners, dentists, veterinarians), nurses, and pharmacists. Physician assistants, dental assistants and hygienists, veterinary assistants, licensed practical nurses (LPNs), and pharmacy technicians all, to some degree, assist professionals in the performance of routine but necessary tasks. The use of these paraprofessionals allows more patients to be seen each day in clinics, hospitals, and pharmacies and helps to tamp down the rising cost of health care in this country.

In the pharmacy workplace, pharmacy technicians assist pharmacists by filling prescriptions and medication orders, which allows pharmacists more time to review patient and allergy profiles; consult with prescribers on less costly drugs of choice and optimal dosages based on age, weight, and liver or renal function; screen for drug interactions; provide patient education on chronic illnesses; vaccinate patients; and counsel patients on the appropriate use of OTC drugs and the importance of adherence to prescribed therapy.

With the valuable assistance of pharmacy technicians and other members of the healthcare team, pharmacists can meet the mission of the profession: to ensure positive outcomes for drug therapy in the patient population.

To provide quality and affordable health care today requires the combined efforts of all members of the healthcare team.

Chapter Summary

- The profession of pharmacy has ancient roots, dating to the use of drugs for magical and curative purposes.
- Pharmacy has evolved over the past 50 years, from preparing natural medications to dispensing synthetic medications.
- The primary mission of pharmacy is to safeguard the public and help patients achieve favorable outcomes with their prescribed medications.
- Today, pharmacists are highly educated professionals who are licensed to practice in a wide variety of settings.
- The pharmacist is responsible for dispensing medications to patients, as well as the necessary information to appropriately use the products.

- Pharmacists in all settings provide a readily available resource to healthcare professionals on information related to drug therapy.
- The pharmacy technician is a paraprofessional who, under the direct supervision of a pharmacist, carries out a wide range of duties in order for the pharmacist to effectively carry out his or her professional responsibilities.
- Formal educational training programs and opportunities to become a certified pharmacy technician are becoming more important in all practice settings.
- Because of our aging population and the subsequent need for prescription medications required for many people to live longer and better lives, pharmacists and pharmacy technicians are in great demand.

Key Terms

adulteration the process of corrupting or tainting drug products by the addition of foreign, impure, or inferior substances that may be toxic

alchemy the European practice during the Middle Ages that combined elements of chemistry, metallurgy, physics, and medicine with astrology, mysticism, and spiritualism to turn a common item into something special or extraordinary; an example would be the transmutation of a base metal into silver or gold

apothecary a shop in which medicines were compounded by skilled artisans using herbs and other natural ingredients

botany a branch of biology dealing with plant life

chain pharmacy a community pharmacy that consists of several similar pharmacies in the region (or nation) that are corporately owned

community pharmacy any independent, chain, or franchise pharmacy that dispenses prescription medications to outpatients; also called a *retail pharmacy*

compounding pharmacy a pharmacy that specializes in the compounding of nonsterile (and sometimes sterile) preparations that are not commercially available

formulary a list of drugs that has been preapproved for use by a committee of healthcare professionals; used in hospitals, in managed care, and by many insurance providers; also called a *pharmacopeia* or *dispensatory*

franchise pharmacy a pharmacy that is part of a small chain of professional community pharmacies that dispense and prepare medications but are independently owned; sometimes called an *apothecary*

health maintenance organization (HMO) an organization that provides health insurance using a managed-care model

herbal medicine the use of natural plant products to maintain health by preventing or curing certain illnesses

home health care the delivery of medical, nursing, and pharmaceutical services and supplies to patients at home

home healthcare pharmacy a pharmacy that prepares and dispenses drugs and medical supplies directly to the home of the patient

hospice care home healthcare services typically involving pain management of a terminally ill patient

hospital pharmacy an institutional pharmacy that dispenses and prepares drugs and provides clinical services in a hospital setting

independent pharmacy a community pharmacy that is privately owned by a pharmacist

institutional pharmacy a pharmacy that is organized under a corporate structure, following specific rules and regulations for accreditation

long-term care facility an institution that provides care for geriatric and disabled patients; includes extended-care facility (ECF) and skilled-care facility (SCF)

mail-order pharmacy a large-volume, centralized pharmacy operation that uses automation to fill and mail prescriptions to a patient

managed care a type of health insurance system that emphasizes keeping the patient healthy or diseases controlled to reduce healthcare costs

nuclear pharmacy a specialized practice that compounds and dispenses sterile radioactive pharmaceuticals to diagnose or treat disease

pathophysiology the study of disease and illnesses affecting the normal function of the body

pharmaceutical care a philosophy of care that expanded the pharmacist's role to include appropriate medication use to achieve positive outcomes with prescribed drug therapy

pharmaceutics the study of the release characteristics of specific drug dosage forms

pharmacist one who is licensed to prepare and dispense medications, counsel patients, and monitor outcomes pursuant to a prescription from a licensed healthcare professional

pharmacognosy the study of medicinal functions of natural products of animal, plant, or mineral origins

pharmacokinetics individualized doses of drugs based on absorption, distribution, metabolism, and excretion

pharmacology the scientific study of drugs and their mechanisms of action

pharmacopeia a listing of drugs; also called a *formulary* or *dispensatory*

pharmacy technician an individual working in a pharmacy who, under the supervision of a licensed pharmacist, assists in activities not requiring the professional judgment of a pharmacist; also called the *pharmacy tech* or *tech*

therapeutics the study of applying pharmacology to the treatment of illness and disease states

traditional Eastern medicine herbal-based treatments based on ancient East Indian or Asian philosophies that blend various healing modalities to bring balance and harmony to the body

traditional Western medicine medical treatment by a licensed professional who identifies the cause of an illness by physical examination and then treats the illness with various natural and synthetic medicinal products or drugs

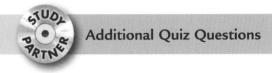
Checking Your Understanding

To check your comprehension of this chapter's key concepts, read the following multiple-choice questions and then record your answers on a separate sheet of paper. Write your answers as modeled in these examples: 1d; 2c; 3b; *etc.*

1. Modern-day formularies had their origins in
   a. Greece.
   b. Italy.
   c. China.
   d. Mesopotamia.

2. What country was the forerunner in developing a logical, scientific-based approach to medical practice?
   a. Greece
   b. Italy
   c. China
   d. Egypt

3. Another name for a community pharmacy is a
   a. home healthcare pharmacy.
   b. long-term care facility.
   c. retail pharmacy.
   d. health maintenance organization (HMO).

4. Which of the following is *not* considered an institutional pharmacy?
   a. mail-order pharmacy
   b. hospital pharmacy
   c. long-term care pharmacy
   d. managed-care pharmacy

5. A laminar airflow hood would most likely be found in a
   a. long-term care pharmacy.
   b. hospital pharmacy.
   c. chain pharmacy.
   d. managed-care pharmacy.

6. Knowledge of the medicinal functions of natural products from animal, plant, or mineral origins is known as
   a. pharmacognosy.
   b. pharmacology.
   c. nuclear pharmacy.
   d. clinical pharmacy.

7. The emergence of the pharmaceutical industry threatened to reduce the role of the pharmacist to that of a
   a. compounder of medications.
   b. pharmaceutical scientist.
   c. drugstore operator.
   d. toxicologist.

8. The work that heralded the emergence of modern clinical pharmacy was the
   a. Ebers report.
   b. Millis Commission report.
   c. Report of the President's Commission on Controlled Substances.
   d. Kefauver-Harris Amendment to the Food, Drug, and Cosmetic (FD&C) Act of 1938.

9. The primary role of a clinical pharmacist is to
   a. dispense medications.
   b. compound medications.
   c. develop a drug formulary.
   d. share knowledge about drug use.

10. Medication therapy management, or MTM, is best defined as
    a. ensuring positive outcomes for drug therapy.
    b. authorizing pharmacists to prescribe selected drugs.
    c. allowing reimbursement for pharmacists checking patients' blood pressures.
    d. empowering certified pharmacy technicians to counsel patients on over-the-counter (OTC) medications.

11. Which of the following items is *not* a recommendation for admission to a doctor of pharmacy educational program?
    a. a GPA of 3.5–4.0
    b. experience in pharmacy and community service
    c. a prior bachelor of science (BS) degree, typically in chemistry or biology
    d. two years of pre-pharmacy course work

12. Licensing and professional oversight of pharmacists and pharmacy technicians are tasks carried out by the
    a. colleges of pharmacy.
    b. American Pharmacists Association (APhA).
    c. state boards of pharmacy.
    d. United States Pharmacopeia (USP).

13. What professional pharmacy organization established a model curriculum for pharmacy technicians?
    a. Philadelphia College of Pharmacy
    b. American Society of Health-System Pharmacists (ASHP)

    c. American Pharmacists Association (APhA)
    d. United States Pharmacopeia (USP)

14. A pharmacy technician can do all the following *except*
    a. enter information into the computer.
    b. counsel a patient.
    c. prepare a label.
    d. return drug stock to the shelf.

15. The final responsibility for the accuracy of the pharmacy technician's work is
    a. the pharmacy technician himself/herself.
    b. another pharmacy technician.
    c. the supervising pharmacist.
    d. the store manager.

Reinforcing Your Learning

To build on your understanding of the topics in this chapter, complete the following enrichment activities.

1. Obtain a copy of the latest edition of the federal government's *Occupational Outlook Handbook* by searching online or in your local library. Using information from this handbook, prepare a short report on the work conditions, duties, training, salaries, and job outlook for pharmacy technicians.

2. Call a local community pharmacy and hospital pharmacy and arrange to interview pharmacy technicians in each practice setting about their job duties. Compare the information you gleaned from your interviews with your research findings from the previous activity. Prepare a report that summarizes the data and present your findings to the class.

3. Make a set of flash cards that focuses on various pharmacist and pharmacy technician responsibilities. On one side of the card, record a task that is performed in the pharmacy. On the other side of the card, designate which pharmacy staff member can perform that task: a pharmacist, a pharmacy technician, or both a pharmacist and pharmacy technician. Using the completed cards, check your own understanding of these chapter concepts, or find a partner and put his or her skills to the test.

4. Work in pairs to create a possible interview scenario between a hiring pharmacist and a prospective pharmacy technician who just graduated from a training program at a local community college. Prepare possible questions that the pharmacist might ask and appropriate responses that a pharmacy technician might say. Role-play the scenario for other class members to get their feedback.

5. Explain why you think it is important for patients to play an active role in their own health care. How can the pharmacist's role be adapted to meet this need? How can the pharmacy technician's role be adapted to meet this need? Record your answers using complete sentences and making sure that your answers are thorough and thoughtful.

Thinking on Your Feet

To gain practice in handling challenging situations in the workplace, consider the following real-world scenarios and then use the guiding questions to help you formulate your responses.

1. A mother approaches you at the pharmacy counter and requests the Plan B One-Step (or the "morning-after" pill) for her underage daughter. The law states that anyone over age 17 can purchase the medication without a prescription; if under age 17, a prescription from a prescriber is required. How would you handle this scenario?

2. Three different patients from another town request the purchase of the maximum quantity of pseudoephedrine decongestant tablets. As you know, this drug must be sold behind the pharmacy counter due to diversion for methamphetamine manufacture. With that in mind, you question whether this request is for a legitimate medical use. What course of action should you take?

3. An out-of-town patient ran out of insulin syringes but has no prescription. Your state allows the sale of insulin syringes without a prescription. Because syringe use is also associated with narcotic abuse, you proceed with caution. What questions might you ask the patient that might help you determine if the syringes are intended for legitimate medical use? Explain your approach in handling this situation.

Acquiring Field Knowledge

To expand your knowledge of pharmacy practice, explore the following online activities that focus on research and information retrieval.

Reminder: As you navigate the Internet, remember to exercise caution and good judgment when evaluating information. A thoughtful review of online text should take into consideration the following factors: the creator and sponsors of the website, the intended audience, the credentials of the authors and contributors, the reliability and validity of the posted information, the frequency of updates to the site, and the ease of navigation for a range of user skill levels.

1. Visit one of the many online news services such as Microsoft Network (MSN); Cable News Network (CNN); American Broadcasting Company (ABC); Reuters; or medical online news services such as Medscape, WebMD, or Mayo Clinic. Search these sites and find at least three recent news items about a medical treatment or a new drug. Read and summarize the articles; then present your summaries to the class.

2. Select a healthcare organization (such as the American Heart Association, the American Cancer Society, the American Diabetes Association, and so on) and visit the organization's website. Search for information on lifestyle changes that individuals can make to prevent the disease or minimize their risk of acquiring the disease. Make a list of tips and use your notes to create an informational brochure.

3. Visit www.paradigmcollege.net/ pharmpractice5e/techprofiles and read three featured pharmacy technician profiles. Report to class on the technicians' likes and dislikes about their role and responsibilities.

4. Search online for a copy of a curriculum from another pharmacy technician training program in your state. Compare and contrast this curriculum—including content, credit hours, and experiential training—with your current program. Discuss with classmates the pros and cons of accreditation of all pharmacy technician training programs.

5. Visit the website of the Pharmacy Technician Certification Board (PTCB) at www.paradigmcollege.net/ pharmpractice5e/ptcb. Compare and contrast the status of pharmacy technicians in your state and in a bordering state in the areas of regulation, certification, and, specifically, PTCB certification. Discuss in class whether all pharmacy technicians should be certified to practice. For extra credit, search your state board of pharmacy's regulations and note if pharmacy technicians have requirements for continuing education, a defined pharmacist/pharmacy technician ratio, and stated job responsibilities.

6. Search online for the results of the 2011 Gallup Trust Survey, an annual survey of the public's attitudes toward the honesty and ethics of different professions. The survey showed that pharmacists ranked second in terms of public trust. (Nurses often rank at or near the top of the survey.) Make a list of five things that you have noticed about the profession of pharmacy and/or a particular pharmacist that make you feel the trust is warranted.

Sampling the Certification Exam

To provide you with practice for the Certification Exam Review, read the following questions that have been patterned after the test format and then record your answers on a separate sheet of paper. Write your answers as modeled in these examples: 1d; 2c; 3b; etc.

1. The profession of pharmacy exists today to
   a. distribute prescription drugs to the public.
   b. control narcotic drug use by the public.
   c. provide necessary OTC and herbal medications to the public.
   d. safeguard the health of the public.

2. What is an advantage of using technology in the pharmacy?
   a. less need for technical help
   b. increased efficiency
   c. decreased need for pharmacist verification
   d. increased expense

3. Which of the following tasks is a pharmacy technician *not* allowed to do?
   a. counsel a patient about a prescription
   b. offer pharmacist counseling to a patient about his or her prescription

   c. receive a written prescription from a patient
   d. update a patient profile on the computer

4. An asthmatic patient comes in to the pharmacy and asks the technician to refill his prescription for his albuterol inhaler. He states that he is having more shortness of breath than usual and has been using his inhaler more than usual. The technician notices on his profile that he takes a diuretic for congestive heart failure, as well as asthma. What should the technician do?
   a. fill the prescription for the inhaler
   b. call the patient's physician to report an early refill of the inhaler
   c. suggest that the patient take more of his diuretic to help his breathing
   d. suggest that the patient talk to the pharmacist but prepare the inhaler anyway

5. A patient comes to the pharmacy counter and complains to a pharmacy technician that the pharmacy incorrectly filled her prescription. She was supposed to get medicine to treat her high blood pressure and instead was given the same medicine her friend takes for migraine headaches. What should the tech tell her?
   a. "Your friend has the wrong medicine, not you, and your friend should contact her pharmacy."
   b. "This pharmacy never makes mistakes; you are wrong."
   c. "Many medications have more than one use, and this medication may be one that does. Let me get the pharmacist."
   d. "Call your physician. He made the mistake."

6. Which of the following duties may be done by a pharmacy technician?
   a. checking and verifying finished prescriptions
   b. receiving verbal prescriptions in person or by telephone
   c. receiving written prescriptions
   d. verifying that weighing and measuring is done properly

7. A physician calls and asks a technician what the dose of a drug is. How should the technician respond?
   a. tell the physician the dose
   b. look up the dose and inform the physician
   c. ask another technician for help
   d. place the physician on hold and call the pharmacist

8. Which of the following tasks is a pharmacy technician allowed to do?
   a. counsel a patient about an OTC drug
   b. sell a product containing pseudoephedrine
   c. enter an e-prescription from a prescriber into the computer
   d. administer a flu vaccine to a patient

9. A pharmacy technician cannot read the prescriber's writing on the prescription. The pharmacist is also not sure of the directions after reviewing the prescription. What should the technician do?
   a. return the prescription to the patient
   b. call the doctor's office for clarification
   c. tell the nurse to have the doctor fax over a new, more legible prescription
   d. transfer the prescription to another pharmacy

10. An out-of-state patient comes into a pharmacy on a weekend to purchase some insulin syringes. How should the pharmacy technician handle this request?
    a. sell the syringes to the patient
    b. request a prescription before dispensing the syringes
    c. deny the request due to lack of familiarity with the patient and with the patient's legitimate need for syringes
    d. refer the patient to the pharmacist to make a professional judgment

Pharmacy Law, Regulations, and Standards

2

Learning Objectives

- Differentiate the meanings of the terms *laws, regulations, professional standards*, and *ethics*.

- List and describe the major effects on the profession of pharmacy by significant pieces of statutory federal drug law in the twentieth century.

- Discuss the impact of various provisions of the Patient Protection and Affordable Care Act of 2010 on health care and the practice of pharmacy.

- Discuss the roles of government regulatory agencies such as the Food and Drug Administration, the Drug Enforcement Administration, the Occupational Safety and Health Administration, and the national and state boards of pharmacy.

- Differentiate the meanings of the terms *licensure, registration*, and *certification* for pharmacy technicians.

- Enumerate the duties that may legally be performed by pharmacy technicians in most states.

- Define the term *standard of care* and its legal impact on the responsibilities of the pharmacy technician.

- Explain the potential for tort actions on a pharmacy technician related to negligence, malpractice, or the law of agency and contracts.

- Discuss the importance of drug and professional standards.

Preview chapter terms and definitions.

A variety of mechanisms control the practice of pharmacy, including common, statutory, and regulatory laws passed by federal, state, and local government entities. These laws are put into place to allow pharmaceutical manufacturers to bring safe products to market, and pharmacy personnel to provide safe and effective care for the patients they serve. In addition to these statutes, pharmacy professional organizations have established a set of standards that guide pharmacy professionals in their practice. Being aware of this complex system of interrelated laws, regulations, and standards is not enough for today's pharmacy practitioners. Pharmacists and pharmacy technicians must have a thorough understanding of their legal and ethical responsibilities to ensure that the marketing and dispensing of medications is carried out safely and in the public interest. They must also understand that any violations of pharmacy laws and standards may lead to patient consequences such as medication errors, injury, or death, and personal consequences such as legal action and loss of employment. In light of that, this chapter provides pharmacy technicians with an overview of pharmacy law, regulations, and standards as well as the important resources pertinent to their practice.

The Need for Drug Control

In the United States, the laws related to drug approvals and pharmacy practice are generally stricter than those in other countries. For example, in some countries you may be able to get many medications, including antibiotics, without a prescription. To pharmacy personnel in the United States, such lax drug control seems astonishing in light of the distinct possibility of inappropriate use, adverse reactions, and interactions with other drugs. Issues related to our stringent drug laws and regulations continue to be debated publicly because of the ongoing illegal importation of drugs from Canada and Mexico by many individuals. However, the need for tight drug controls in the United States has safeguarded the health of its citizens for many decades.

Due to the importance of drugs to our healthcare system, drug control and the profession of pharmacy are governed by both state and federal laws, regulations, and professional standards within the industry. Various groups and organizations exercise controls on the contemporary practice of pharmacy, including:

- federal, state, and local legislative bodies such as the U.S. Congress, state legislatures, and municipal governing councils
- federal and state regulatory agencies, including the:
  - Food and Drug Administration (FDA)
  - Drug Enforcement Administration (DEA)
  - Occupational Safety and Health Administration (OSHA)
  - Federal Trade Commission (FTC), with authority over business practices including direct-to-consumer drug advertising
  - Health Care Financing Administration (HCFA) of the Department of Health & Human Services (HHS) and Center for Medicare Services (CMS), with authority over reimbursement under the Medicare and Medicaid government drug insurance programs
  - state health and welfare agencies who budget for the provision of drugs needed by low-income or disabled individuals
- court system
- United States Pharmacopeia (USP)
- Joint Commission
- professional organizations
  - National Association of Boards of Pharmacy (NABP)
  - individual state boards of pharmacy
  - American Pharmacists Association (APhA)
  - American Society of Health-System Pharmacists (ASHP)
- individual institutions such as community pharmacies, hospitals, long-term care facilities, and home healthcare organizations

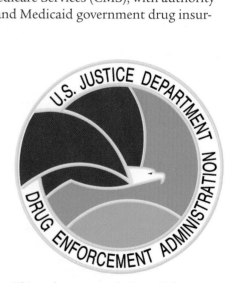

This seal represents the Drug Enforcement Administration, the federal regulatory organization that enforces the Controlled Substances Act.

Laws

A **law** is a rule that is passed and enforced by the legislative branch of government. Combined, laws are a system of rules that reflects the society and culture out of which they arise. The law offers a *minimum* level of acceptable standards. The legislature represents consumers in the passage and enforcement of laws that are designed to protect the public. Violations in laws may result in damages, fines, probation, loss of licensure, or incarceration in extreme cases.

Regulations

A **regulation** is a written rule and procedure that exists to carry out a law of the federal or state government. For example, the FDA, a federal government agency, has published regulations on the drug approval process, generic drug substitution, patient counseling, and adverse reaction reporting systems. Another federal government agency, the DEA, has rules regulating the distribution, storage, documentation, and filling of controlled substances. The federal programs of Medicare and Medicaid also have regulations put in place that pharmacists and pharmacy technicians must follow when dispensing and billing prescriptions for elderly, low-income, and disabled patients.

Aside from federal regulations, state governments also have established regulations that affect pharmacy practice. Each state's board of pharmacy has regulations that must be followed with regard to the practice of pharmacy within that state. Licensure, registration, and certification requirements for pharmacists and pharmacy technicians vary among states. When there is a conflict between a state and a federal law or regulation, the more stringent law or regulation *always* applies.

Standards

A **standard** is a set of criteria to measure product quality or professional performance against a norm. Standards exist for both drug products and individual professional behavior. For example, the USP, with input from scientists, sets standards or criteria for drug quality that must be met by pharmaceutical companies before their new products are submitted to the FDA. The USP also sets national standards for all pharmacies preparing sterile and nonsterile preparations.

The **Joint Commission** provides a higher standard of care in hospitals and other healthcare facilities through a rigorous inspection in its accreditation process. Receiving accreditation from the Joint Commission is the healthcare equivalent of getting the *Good Housekeeping* Seal of Approval. Although accreditation is voluntary under the law, many insurance carriers require it for reimbursement when providing services for its members.

Ethics

Whereas laws represent a minimum level of standards, ethics provide for the standards of personal conduct within a profession. **Ethics** are standards of behavior that pharmacists and technicians are encouraged to follow. Pharmacy personnel are legally and ethically required to provide safe, effective patient care. If a legal challenge is made, the behavior of the professional is compared with the standards of other professionals practicing in the community. This "standard of care" concept, discussed in depth later in this chapter, holds healthcare professionals accountable for their decisions and actions in the workplace.

As you learned in Chapter 1, pharmacists recite an oath upon their graduation to uphold "the highest principles of moral, ethical, and legal conduct." Pharmacy technicians, as well, often recite an oath that affirms their commitment to these same principles. (For detailed information about ethical conduct of pharmacy technicians in the workplace, see Chapter 13.)

History of U.S. Statutory Pharmacy Law

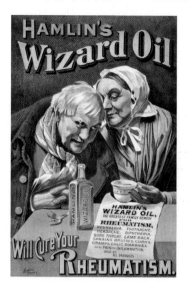

In the late 1800s, there was no control on the sale of pharmaceutical products. Thus, consumers were not protected.

During the nineteenth century, drugs in the United States were unregulated. Medicines did not have to be proven safe or effective in order to be marketed. Opium and many of its extracts—such as morphine, codeine, and heroin—found their way into medicines and were widely touted as cure-alls for a variety of ailments. These quack medicines were hawked by boisterous charlatans who would take their traveling medicine shows from town to town in the West to proclaim the latest "miracle cure." There were no regulations on labeling these so-called medicines and no research to support any of the claims. In addition to opium extracts, these potions contained a high content of alcohol that usually made the customer "feel better." Occasionally, some of these potions were not so innocuous and caused injury or death to those who consumed them.

By the advent of the twentieth century, there were also major concerns regarding the purity of drugs that were imported from other countries. As a result, statutory laws were established to protect the public from the dangers of unregulated drug manufacturing, marketing, and use. **Statutory laws** are laws passed by legislative bodies at the federal, state, and local levels. The following sections highlight, in chronological order, the major statutory laws impacting the profession of pharmacy.

Pure Food and Drug Act of 1906

To combat real-life abuses in drug formulation, labeling, and market claims, the U.S. Congress passed the first of a series of landmark twentieth-century laws to regulate the development, compounding, distribution, storage, and dispensing of drugs. The purpose of the Pure Food and Drug Act of 1906 was to prohibit the interstate transportation or sale of adulterated and misbranded food and drugs. This act required that the labels not contain false information about the drugs' strength and purity. In response to these mounting concerns, the manufacturer of Coca-Cola changed its product's key ingredient—from cocaine to caffeine—during the early developmental stages of this legislation. The act, although amended, proved unenforceable, and new legislation was later required.

Federal Food, Drug, and Cosmetic Act of 1938

With the realization that stronger legislation was needed to regulate the development and dispensing of manufactured drugs, lawmakers began to take a closer look at the pharmaceutical industry. Tragically, the catalyst for change was a poisoning incident that occurred in 1937. More than 100 individuals died as the result of poisoning by a sulfa drug product that contained diethylene glycol, a toxic chemical used in antifreeze. Its manufacturer, the S. E. Massengill Company, was unaware of diethylene glycol's poisonous nature, and the drug was marketed without being tested on animals. Because of this tragedy, the Federal Food, Drug, and Cosmetic (FD&C) Act of 1938 became one of the most important pieces of legislation in pharmaceutical history. This legislation created the FDA and required pharmaceutical manufacturers to file a **new drug application (NDA)** with each new drug in order to obtain FDA approval before marketing. Manufacturers needed to prove that the product was *safe for use by humans*. Unfortunately, this act required only that drugs be safe for human consumption, not that they be effective or useful for the purpose for which they were sold.

Pharmaceutical manufacturers were required to conduct and submit the results of toxicological studies on animals (to determine degree of toxicity) and clinical trials with humans (to determine drug effect). The NDA was then filed, detailing the chemical composition of the drug and the processes used to manufacture it. Under this act, the FDA also had the power to conduct inspections of manufacturing plants to ensure their compliance.

In addition, the FD&C Act of 1938 clarified the definitions of adulterated and misbranded drugs. An **adulterated product** is broadly defined as a product that differs in drug strength, quality, and purity. For example, an adulterated product may be a prescription drug, over-the-counter (OTC) drug, or dietary supplement contaminated with other drugs or chemicals that may or may not be harmful. A recent example of an adulterated product was a contaminated drug that was prepared in a compounding pharmacy and administered to patients, resulting in many deaths due to fungal meningitis. A **misbranded product**, on the other hand, is defined as a product whose label includes false statements about the identity or ingredients of the container's contents. Dietary supplements are commonly misbranded, with their labels making false claims or providing "less than stated" active ingredients.

Today, more than 80% of drug ingredients are manufactured overseas in a complex supply chain that is often beyond the jurisdiction of the FDA. Economically motivated adulteration includes the potential for contaminated, subpotent, or counterfeit medication to enter the supply chain at several levels, from the production of raw ingredients to the point of retail sale. In the recent past, adulterated samples of the blood thinner heparin were imported from China and resulted in many deaths in the United States. Adulterated cough medicines containing a toxin (interestingly, diethylene glycol again) were distributed in Panama and resulted in many deaths. Subpotent counterfeit medications have occasionally been discovered in the United States as well, adversely affecting patient health.

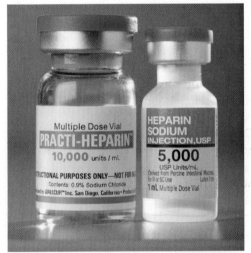

In 2008, vials of adulterated and counterfeit "heparin" were imported from China. Unlike the sterile vials shown here, these adulterated products contained chondroitin sulfate, a contaminant, and resulted in adverse reactions when administered to patients.

Pharmaceutical manufacturers have been found guilty and paid hefty fines for promoting the "off-label" marketing of approved prescription drugs. For example, a drug may be FDA approved for a high blood pressure indication, but representatives of the company may promote and market its use for Alzheimer's disease to physicians, even though there is little or no scientific evidence to support that indication. The FDA is as busy today as in 1938 in addressing the many challenges of adulteration and misbranding.

Durham-Humphrey Amendment of 1951

The FD&C Act of 1938 was amended in 1951. The Durham-Humphrey Amendment stated that stock drug containers do not have to include "adequate directions for use" as long as they contained the legend "Caution: Federal Law Prohibits Dispensing without a Prescription." The dispensing of the drug by a pharmacist with a label giving adequate directions for use from the prescriber met the law's requirements. The amendment thus established the distinction between so-called **legend drugs** (or prescription drugs) and **patent drugs** (OTC, or nonprescription drugs). (These types of drugs will be explained in more detail in Chapter 3 of this textbook.) The amendment also authorized the taking of prescriptions verbally over the telephone, rather than in writing, and set guidelines as to which prescriptions can or cannot be refilled. However, the refilling of prescriptions subject to abuse was limited. Under the amendment, prescriptions for such substances could not be refilled without the expressed consent of the prescriber.

Kefauver-Harris Amendment of 1962

The Kefauver-Harris Amendment of 1962 was passed in response to the birth of thousands of infants—mostly in Europe—with severe congenital abnormalities whose mothers had taken a new tranquilizer called *thalidomide*. It extended the FD&C Act of 1938 to require that drugs not only be safe for humans but also be *effective*. The amendment required drug manufacturers to file an investigational new drug application (INDA) with the FDA before initiating clinical trials in humans. Once the extensive trials were completed (typically 7–10 years) and the results proved that the product was both safe and effective, the manufacturer could then submit an NDA seeking approval to market the product. To compensate for innovation and research costs, the government issued "patent" protection for brand name products for a designated length of time.

Comprehensive Drug Abuse Prevention and Control Act of 1970

The Comprehensive Drug Abuse Prevention and Control Act of 1970, commonly referred to as the **Controlled Substances Act (CSA)**, was created to combat and control drug abuse and to supersede previous federal laws regarding drug abuse. The act classified drugs with potential for abuse as **controlled substances**, or drugs that have a risk for abuse and physical or psychological dependence. The controlled substances were then ranked into five categories, or **schedules** (see Table 2.1).

This controlled substance schedule continues to be used in pharmacy practice. Schedule I drugs are not commercially available or legally dispensed in the United States due to their high potential for abuse and addiction. Schedule II drugs are the most highly regulated drug category and have no refills. Schedule III, IV, and V drugs have less abuse and addiction potential than Schedule II drugs but have quantity and time limits on refills.

Often upon recommendation from the manufacturer and the FDA, the DEA classifies new drugs into a schedule and will even reevaluate drugs that have been on the market for some time to determine whether they warrant being changed to a "scheduled" drug. For example, there is current concern about the overuse of hydrocodone combination products such as Lortab, Vicodin, and Norco; consequently, the DEA is considering reclassifying this drug from Schedule III to Schedule II.

In addition to this controlled substances schedule, individual state boards of pharmacy have guidelines for the prescribing and dispensing of controlled substances. In fact, states have the authority to have a more stringent classification for certain drugs. For example, various butalbital products for migraine headaches may be more strictly regulated in some states.

The DEA—with the help of each state board of pharmacy and its agents—keeps a close watch on the prescribing and dispensing of all controlled substances in the United States. Any sudden increase in scheduled drug usage by a particular pharmacy (or in prescriptions by a particular physician) may trigger an investigation. Pharmacy personnel, therefore, must be diligent in their handling and record keeping of controlled substances as the misuse of these drugs has become a growing problem.

TABLE 2.1 Drug Schedules under the Controlled Substances Act of 1970

Schedule	Manufacturer's Label	Abuse Potential	Accepted Medical Use	Examples
I	C–I	highest potential for abuse	for research only; must have license to obtain; no accepted medical use in the United States	heroin, lysergic acid diethylamide (LSD)
II	C–II	high possibility of abuse, which can lead to severe psychological or physical dependence	dispensing severely restricted; cannot be prescribed by telephone except in an emergency; no refills on prescriptions	morphine; oxycodone; meperidine; hydromorphone; hydrocodone combination products (hydrocodone combined with acetaminophen, aspirin, or ibuprofen); fentanyl; methylphenidate; dextroamphetamine
III	C–III	less potential for abuse and addiction than C–II	prescriptions can be refilled up to five times within six months if authorized by physician	codeine combination products (codeine combined with acetaminophen, aspirin, or ibuprofen); ketamines; anabolic steroids
IV	C–IV	lower abuse potential than C–II and C–III; associated with limited physical or psychological dependence	same as for Schedule III	benzodiazepines, meprobamate, phenobarbital, carisoprodol
V	C–V	lowest abuse potential	some sold without a prescription, depending on state law; if so, purchaser must be over age 18 and is required to sign a log and present a photo ID	liquid codeine combination cough preparations, diphenoxylate/atropine

[handwritten annotations: "No-refill" next to Schedule II; "5 refills 6 months" next to Schedule III]

Poison Prevention Packaging Act of 1970

To prevent accidental childhood poisonings from prescription and nonprescription products, the Poison Prevention Packaging Act was passed in 1970. This act, enforced by the Consumer Product Safety Commission, required that most OTC and prescription drugs be packaged in a **child-resistant container** that cannot be opened by 80% of children under age 5 but can be opened by 90% of adults. The law also stipulated that a pharmacist or pharmacy technician, upon request from a patient, may dispense a drug in a non-child-resistant container. In fact, the patient—not the prescriber—could make a blanket request that all drugs be dispensed to him or her in non-child-resistant containers.

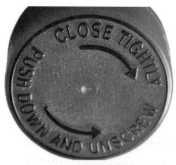

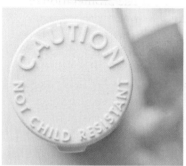

Unless specifically requested by the customer, medications are dispensed in child-resistant containers to prevent accidental poisoning.

Today, this blanket request is often made by older patients and those with severe rheumatoid arthritis and is typically documented in the patient database. Medications that are commonly dispensed in non-child-resistant containers include the antibiotic azithromycin (or Z-pak), Medrol Dosepak, birth control pills, sublingual nitroglycerin tablets, and metered-dose inhalers. For patients who request these containers, pharmacy personnel should remind them at medication pickup to place these non-child-resistant containers out of reach before young children visit their homes.

Drug Listing Act of 1972

The Drug Listing Act of 1972 gave the FDA the authority to compile a list of currently marketed drugs. Under the act, each new drug was assigned a unique and permanent product code, known as a **National Drug Code (NDC)**, consisting of 10 or 11 characters that identified the manufacturer or distributor, the drug formulation, and the size and type of its packaging, in that order.

Today, the FDA requests—but does not require—that the NDC appear on all drug labels, including labels of prescription containers. Using this code, the FDA is able to maintain a database of drugs by use, manufacturer, and active ingredients and of newly marketed, discontinued, and remarketed drugs. The bar-coded information is also widely used today to double-check the accuracy of prescriptions filled by automation. The NDC will be described more thoroughly in Chapters 3, 4, and 6.

Orphan Drug Act of 1983

An **orphan drug** is a drug that is intended for use in patients suffering from a rare disorder (defined as a condition that affects less than 200,000 people). Because developing and marketing such a drug would be prohibitively expensive, the Orphan Drug Act of 1983 encouraged the development of orphan drugs by providing tax incentives and allowing manufacturers to be granted a time for exclusive licenses to market such drugs.

Since 1983, orphan products have continued to receive expedited review and accelerated approval from the FDA due to their use in treating serious or life-threatening diseases. For example, one orphan drug, Cuprimine, was developed to treat Wilson disease, a progressive genetic disorder characterized by excess copper stored in various body tissues. This disease is rare (affecting 1 in 30,000) and can lead to life-threatening complications, such as organ dysfunction, and premature death. However, with early diagnosis and treatment with medication, serious long-term disability and life-threatening complications can be prevented. Treatment is aimed at reducing the amount of copper that has accumulated in the body and maintaining normal copper levels thereafter. The research costs for developing treatments for such a rare disorder would be prohibitive to a pharmaceutical manufacturer without financial incentives, patent and legal protections, and accelerated approvals.

To date, more than 350 orphan drugs have been approved by the FDA for marketing. Most of these rare diseases involve a genetic defect. For example, cystic fibrosis (CF), a genetic disease of the lungs and sweat glands, often leads to premature death in those who have been diagnosed with the disorder. With the development of orphan drugs such as tobramycin and Pulmozyme, patients with CF now have both an improved quality of life and a longer life span. Another group of orphan drugs—statins—were developed in 1985 in response to a rare genetic defect known as homozygous familial hypercholesterolemia. Today, statins are commonly prescribed medications for patients with high cholesterol levels.

Drug Price Competition and Patent-Term Restoration Act of 1984

Prior to the 1980s, drugs that had been given proprietary names, or **brand names**, by their manufacturers were primarily prescribed and dispensed. The proliferation of these brand name drugs was the result of the enactment of many anti-substitution laws passed by the states due to "counterfeit" generic drugs on the market.

However, by 1984, mounting pressure by lawmakers and pharmacists to reduce healthcare costs led to the passing of the Drug Price Competition and Patent-Term Restoration Act. This legislation, also known as the Waxman-Hatch Act, encouraged the development of drugs with nonproprietary names, or **generic names**. Generic drugs are comparable to their brand name counterparts in dosage form, strength, route of administration, quality, performance, safety, and intended use. Although generic drugs do not go through the same rigorous scientific review on safety and effectiveness as brand name drugs, they still must demonstrate bioequivalence to the brand name product. (The concept of *bioequivalence* will be discussed in detail in Chapter 3.)

To encourage generic drug development, the Waxman-Hatch Act also streamlined the process for generic drug approval and extended patent licenses as a function of the time required for the NDA approval process. The patent license was extended to allow the manufacturer of the brand name drug who completed the NDA to recoup research and development costs, as well as to provide an incentive to research new drugs for the marketplace. Once the original patent expires, any manufacturer is allowed to market a generic drug, an endeavor that is less costly than its brand name counterpart.

The rise in availability of cheaper, generic name drugs was due in part to the Drug Price Competition and Patent-Term Restoration Act of 1984.

The growth and expansion of generic manufacturers can be traced to this act. Today, more than 80% of prescriptions in community pharmacies are dispensed with generic drugs. In fact, generic drugs can be substituted (under regulations now existing in every state) for brand name drugs in prescriptions in every state unless the prescriber writes "brand only" or "do not substitute" on the prescription itself.

Because medications that are currently on the market are labeled by both their generic names and their brand names (and, at times, by their chemical names), pharmacy personnel must be familiar with the various names for the same medication. (See Table 2.2 for an example of the different names for the same medication.)

TABLE 2.2   Different Names for One Drug

Type of Name	Drug Name
chemical name	p-isobutylhydratropic acid
generic name	ibuprofen
brand name	Advil, Motrin, Motrin IB

Prescription Drug Marketing Act of 1987

Passed in response to concerns over safety and competition issues raised by secondary markets for drugs, the Prescription Drug Marketing Act of 1987 required that all drug wholesalers be licensed by the states. The act also prohibited the sale, trading, or distribution of drug samples, by mail or by common carrier, to persons other than those licensed to prescribe them. This action was taken in response to prescription drug samples being illegally diverted and distributed by a few unethical pharmaceutical sales representatives. This act also prohibited the reimportation of a drug into the United States by anyone except the manufacturer.

Today, the reimportation of drugs continues to be a major political and economic issue in the United States as many senior citizens travel across the Canadian border to fill their prescriptions or receive their prescriptions through the mail from Canadian drug wholesalers at presumed substantial savings. U.S. pharmaceutical manufacturers have threatened to reduce the supply of drugs to Canada if the practice of illegal reimportation continues. Canada, too, is concerned about the reimportation of drugs, fearing that the practice may create a shortage of medications for its own citizens. To address this issue, the United States has elected not to enforce the private contraband of individuals but to clearly discourage its practice. The Medicare Modernization Act of 2003 (discussed later in the chapter) has helped to mitigate but not eliminate the reimportation of drugs.

Anabolic Steroid Act of 1990

Anabolic steroids, or synthetic drugs that mimic the human hormone testosterone, have become a widely known class of drugs in the past few decades due to their abuse by professional athletes. These steroids are used to build muscle mass, enhancing the strength—and, ultimately, the performance—of the users. Many of these drugs are illegally manufactured, imported, and sold on the black market in the United States. Other anabolic drugs are contained in loosely regulated dietary supplements. Therefore, the potency, purity, and strength of the drugs are unregulated, making it virtually impossible for users to know how much medication they have ingested. In addition to dosage unknowns, anabolic steroids have a long list of serious adverse effects and can cause permanent damage to the body. Despite public warnings, the demand for black market steroids has risen.

In response to this increase in illicit traffic, Congress passed the Anabolic Steroid Act of 1990, which designated anabolic steroids as a Schedule III class of drugs and allowed the FDA to enforce the law for legal drugs as well as illegal imports. Because anabolic steroids are Schedule III drugs, prescriptions for anabolic steroids, such as AndroGel, Androderm, and Testim, and for testosterone injections can be refilled a maximum of five times or for up to six months from the date written, whichever comes first. This guideline is similar to prescriptions for many potent narcotic analgesics and sleep medications.

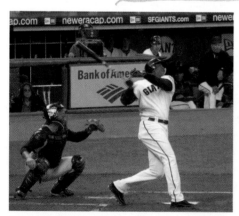

Barry Bonds, who hit more career home runs than any other baseball player, has been accused of using anabolic steroids to enhance his athletic performance.

Omnibus Budget Reconciliation Act of 1990

The Omnibus Budget Reconciliation Act of 1990 (OBRA-90) required that, as a condition of participating in the state Medicaid reimbursement program, states must establish standards of practice for drug utilization review (DUR) by the pharmacist. Among other provisions, the act required "a review of drug therapy before each prescription is filled or delivered to an individual . . . typically at the point of sale. . . . The review shall include screening for potential drug therapy problems due to therapeutic duplication, drug-disease contraindications, drug-drug interactions (including serious interactions with nonprescription OTC drugs), incorrect drug dosage or duration of treatment, drug-allergy interactions, and clinical abuse/misuse."

Today, the pharmacist reviews a computerized patient profile before filling each prescription. Following this law, a pharmacist—or a pharmacy technician acting on the pharmacist's behalf—must also offer pharmacist counseling services to the patient or customer. This offer is typically documented in print (in a book or registry that the patient or customer signs) or in an electronic format (such as an online computer notation or a message prompt at the cash register). The documentation also notes whether the offer for counseling was accepted or refused. If counseling was accepted, the pharmacist may counsel the individual in any of the following areas:

- name and description of medication
- dosage form
- dose
- route of administration
- duration of drug therapy
- action to take after a missed dose
- common severe side effects or adverse effects
- interactions and therapeutic contraindications, including preventive steps and actions to be taken if they occur
- methods for self-monitoring of the drug therapy
- prescription refill information
- proper storage of the drug
- special directions and precautions for preparation, administration, and use of drug by the patient

OBRA-90 enforces the clinical practice of screening prescriptions and counseling patients and caregivers by providing Medicaid reimbursements only to patients at pharmacies that adhere to this act. OBRA-90 also requires state boards of pharmacy or other state regulatory agencies to provide for the creation of DUR boards for prospective and retrospective review of drug therapies and educational programs for training physicians and pharmacists with regard to the use of medications.

In addition, the law requires that manufacturers rebate to state Medicaid programs the difference between the manufacturer's best price for a drug (typically, the wholesale price) and the average submitted cost. Most state boards of pharmacy now require counseling for all patients. Unfortunately, no additional reimbursement is provided for mandatory counseling. In fact, as states attempt to balance budgets in challenging economic times, reimbursements to pharmacists have not kept pace with inflation.

Dietary Supplement Health and Education Act of 1994

The Dietary Supplement Health and Education Act (better known as DSHEA) was passed in 1994 and provided definitions and guidelines on dietary supplements, including vitamins, minerals, herbs, and nutritional supplements. Because the use of dietary supplements was one area in which the FDA had limited oversight, this legislation stated that manufacturers of these supplements—unlike prescription and OTC

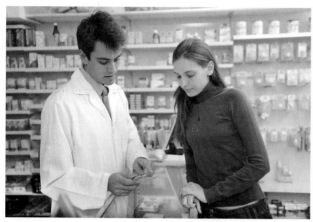

A patient may request the counseling of a pharmacist when purchasing a dietary supplement, since labeled information is quite limited.

drugs—were *not* required to prove efficacy or standardization to the FDA. The manufacturers simply had to prove the safety of the supplement and make truthful claims.

Today's dietary supplements are sold with nonprescription products, but many consumers are unaware of the subtle difference in their regulatory oversight. The FDA may only review "false claims" advertisements and monitor safety. Manufacturers of these dietary supplements are not permitted to make claims of curing or treating ailments; they may only state that the products are supplements to support health. If treatment claims or "miracle" cures are made, the FDA can then require manufacturers to provide scientific research and proof to back up those claims, similar to requirements for prescription and nonprescription drugs. Still, some manufacturers manage to tweak the verbiage of their dietary supplement labels to skirt this regulation—for example, using the tagline "for a healthy heart" rather than "to lower cholesterol."

 Safety Note

The FDA does not regulate dietary supplements.

If the FDA wants to remove a dietary supplement from the market for safety reasons, it may do so; however, it must then hold public hearings, and the burden of proof is shifted to the FDA to prove that the dietary supplement is unsafe. For example, the drug ephedra, or its herbal equivalent *ma huang*, was an ingredient in many weight-loss products. In 2004, the drug was removed from the market by the FDA as a result of multiple reports of serious adverse reactions and some deaths. The following year, the lower courts overruled the FDA's action but, in 2006, the Court of Appeals upheld the FDA action, thus removing all ephedra products from the market.

More recently, the FDA has warned consumers of fraudulent claims made for "all natural" weight loss supplements. Claims such as "magic pill," "melt your fat away," and "diet and exercise not required" should raise a red flag. Several of these products have been found to be tainted with off-the-market weight loss prescription drugs; thus, they are considered misbranded drugs by the FDA. Within the past 20 years, more than 40 weight-loss products have been withdrawn from the market.

Health Insurance Portability and Accountability Act of 1996

The **Health Insurance Portability and Accountability Act (HIPAA)** of 1996 had many provisions that have directly affected all healthcare facilities, including pharmacies. One provision was the "portability" of moving health insurance from one employer to another without denial or restrictions. In the past, an employer could refuse to provide a new employee with health insurance or restrict coverage. For example, if the employee had a preexisting medical condition such as diabetes, then the employer could exclude any expenses related to that condition for 6 months or more; pregnancy was considered a preexisting condition with medical expenses not covered for 12 months. In addition, if an employee leaves his or her current employment, then the former employer must offer COBRA (Consolidated Omnibus Budget Reconciliation Act of 1985) benefits. These benefits allow the employee to continue current medical coverage for up to 18 months but at his or her own expense.

HIPAA mostly affects the confidentiality of patient medical records including prescription records. With more and more electronic submission of prescription and personal data to healthcare professionals, insurance companies, and pharmaceutical manufacturers, HIPAA has placed safeguards to protect patient confidentiality. All healthcare facilities must provide a document to each patient that states the data privacy policy, and the facility must provide evidence that the document was given to the patient.

In pharmacy, this privacy policy may address the transmission of prescription data to anyone other than the patient and the healthcare professional, or it may indicate the existence of an area designed for private counseling. Every pharmacy must have a training program on patient data privacy for its employees, and this training must be renewed on an annual basis. Pharmacy personnel must, under penalty of law, not reveal any information on any patient outside the pharmacy workplace; failure to comply with this regulation is grounds for immediate termination. (For more information on the ramifications of HIPAA, see Chapter 13 of this textbook.)

Medicare Modernization Act of 2003

The Medicare Modernization Act (MMA), better known as Medicare Part D, was introduced into legislation in 2003 and became effective January 1, 2006, providing prescription drug coverage to patients eligible for Medicare benefits. This voluntary insurance program required patient co-payments but offered coverage for certain medications—especially for those patients with economic hardships or those needing high-cost medications. Patients were required to pay an extra premium, in addition to their Medicare premium, and might be subject to a deductible (depending on insurance selected) before benefits are realized. Patients might also be penalized if they elected not to join when they were eligible.

For patients taking high-cost medications or having certain health conditions, a pharmacist could provide—and get reimbursed for—medication management therapy services (MMTS), or an annual in-depth review of the patient's medication profile. The purpose of this review was to add a safety feature to prevent adverse reactions and drug interactions and to look at ways to reduce patient and insurance costs.

A lesser-known provision of the MMA included the development of health savings accounts (HSAs). This act provided a health insurance option for patients under age 65. Under an HSA, the patient (or his or her family) agreed to pay a monthly premium and carry a high deductible. In return, the premium was fully tax deductible, and whatever amount was not used during that calendar year carried over to the next year.

An HSA is an example of a consumer-driven health plan (CDHP) that is becoming more popular as health insurance costs skyrocket. The individual (rather than the insurance provider) decides which physician to see, which prescriptions to fill and where, and which surgical procedures to accept from his or her premiums. The CDHPs take advantage of lower negotiated medical expenses from their insurer in return for accepting more risk with a higher deductible. If a person should have a serious illness with catastrophic healthcare costs, then insurance would be provided after the deductible is met.

Today, pharmacy technicians are involved in educating patients on Medicare Part D as well as other drug insurance programs. Consequently, they must be knowledgeable about this important program. (For detailed information on the Medicare Part D insurance program, see Chapter 7.)

Food and Drug Administration Modernization Act of 2004

The Food and Drug Administration Modernization Act was passed to update the labeling on prescription medications. Products labeled with "Caution: Federal Law

Prohibits Dispensing without a Prescription" were changed to read "℞ only." As mentioned earlier, *legend* is the term formerly used to indicate whether a drug was available by prescription or over-the-counter (OTC). The new labeling requirements were implemented in 2004. The law also authorized fees, to be paid by the applicant drug manufacturer, to be added to an NDA to provide additional resources to the FDA to process and accelerate the review and approval of new drugs.

Combat Methamphetamine Epidemic Act of 2005

In response to the illegal manufacturing of methamphetamine—a highly addictive stimulant—from a common OTC ingredient, the Combat Methamphetamine Epidemic Act of 2005 was passed. This act was incorporated into the Patriot Act in 2006 and took effect in September 2006. The act reclassified all products containing the chemical pseudoephedrine (PSE) and restricted the amount that can be purchased at one time or in any 30-day period. In addition, all PSE products were required to be stored "behind the counter," and the purchaser had to present legal identification for purchase of the products. The legislation also dictated that a log must be kept of all sales of PSE products and that all pharmacy employees had to complete a training program for the handling of PSE products.

These regulations are currently in effect, with the DEA providing oversight for the enforcement of this act. (For additional information and procedures for the pharmacy technician to legally sell these OTC products, see Chapter 7.)

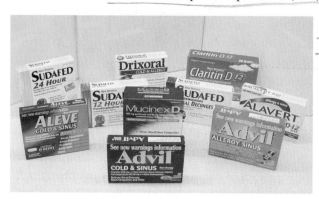

The Combat Methamphetamine Epidemic Act of 2005 was designed to reduce the availability of drugs used to illegally produce methamphetamine.

Patient Protection and Affordable Care Act of 2010

The passage of this controversial act, more commonly known as the Affordable Care Act (ACA), mandated universal healthcare coverage for all citizens of the United States by 2014 under threat of penalty. The ACA increased access to health care for more than 32 million uninsured citizens and for those individuals with preexisting medical conditions who were previously declared uninsurable. It also provided catastrophic insurance coverage for high-cost illnesses. In addition, this act addressed the unpopular "donut hole" in Medicare Part D drug insurance programs by putting into motion its gradual elimination by 2019 and promised long-term savings and extension of the financial viability of Medicare. (For more information on understanding prescription drug insurance and the "donut hole" of Medicare Part D, refer to Chapter 7 of this textbook.)

Recent studies have questioned the implications of this legislation—both the proposed cost savings as well as the final healthcare tab to taxpayers. The revenue needed for this program will come from lower reimbursements to healthcare providers and hospitals, a decrease in overpayments and subsidies to existing insurance programs, a decrease in fraud and waste, and higher taxes starting in 2013 for high-income taxpayers.

Regulatory Law—Role of National Oversight Agencies

The laws, acts, and amendments discussed in this chapter provide the minimum level of acceptable standards. The FDA and DEA have used the laws, acts, and amendments passed in the twentieth century to address a broad scope of issues and provide a basic structure for the safe use of drug products and for the practice of pharmacy. **Regulatory law** is the system of rules and regulations established by governmental bodies such as the FDA and state boards of pharmacy that exist to carry out the laws of the state or federal government. These national oversight agencies are discussed below.

Food and Drug Administration

The Office of Medical Products and Tobacco of the **Food and Drug Administration (FDA)** is under the U.S. Department of Health & Human Services (HHS) and consists of several organizations pertinent to the practice of pharmacy: the Center for Drug Evaluation and Research (CDER), the Office of Pediatric Therapeutics, the Center for Devices and Radiological Health, the Center for Biologics Evaluation (vaccinations), and the Office of Orphan Products Development. The profession of pharmacy is most impacted by the CDER. This center is primarily involved in the following tasks:

- new drug development and review
- generic drug review
- OTC drug review
- postdrug approval activities

Safety Note

The FDA regulates OTC labeling so it is understandable to a layperson.

The FDA has the primary responsibility and authority to enforce the law; however, the FDA has no legal authority over the practice of pharmacy in each state. This agency also has the ability to create and enforce regulations that will assist in providing the public with safe drug products. To that end, the FDA requires all manufacturers to file applications for investigational studies and approval of new drugs, provides guidelines for packaging and advertisement, and oversees the recall of products that are deemed dangerous to the public.

As a watchdog agency for public safety, the FDA enforces the packaging, labeling, advertising, and marketing guidelines for medications. For example, a manufacturer may not make speculative or false claims about the potential of the product, and it must also disclose the side effects, adverse reactions, and contraindications for each medication. The FDA has been known to ask a manufacturer to cancel advertising campaigns and even to instruct the manufacturer to present a new advertising campaign to clear up any misconceptions. OTC-marketed medications undergo this same level of scrutiny from the FDA. The labels of OTC products must conform to a preferred format to make all of the information "understandable and readable" to laypersons.

The FDA is also responsible for the annual publishing (available online) of *Approved Drug Products with Therapeutic Equivalence Evaluations*, better known as the *FDA Orange Book*. This reference identifies all drugs approved by the FDA based on both their safety and their effectiveness in compliance with the FD&C Act of 1938 and the Kefauver-Harris Amendment of 1962. This reference is used in the pharmacy primarily to make sure that generic products can be safely substituted for brand name products. The *FDA Orange Book* is discussed further in Chapter 3.

Drug Enforcement Administration

The **Drug Enforcement Administration (DEA)** is the primary agency responsible for enforcing the laws regarding both legal and illegal addictive substances. Although this agency directs most of its funds and personnel toward the illegal trafficking of drugs, it also has the responsibility to supervise the legal use of narcotics and other scheduled or controlled substances.

Inspection of all medical facilities, including pharmacies, is a function of the DEA and is usually limited to facilities where suspicious activity has been detected. The DEA works closely with the state drug and narcotic agencies that are responsible for annual physical inspections and local investigation of unsafe prescribing, dispensing, or forging of controlled drug prescriptions. The DEA has established an audit trail to allow the agency to track the flow of narcotics from manufacturer to warehouse to pharmacy to patient. Special forms and procedures must be completed and documented in all medical facilities for both the ordering and the disposal of narcotic drugs (see Chapter 7). Many pharmacies use a perpetual inventory record (or tablet-by-tablet records) for complete accountability of narcotic drugs. All prescriptions for Schedule II drugs must be filed separately and be available for inspection.

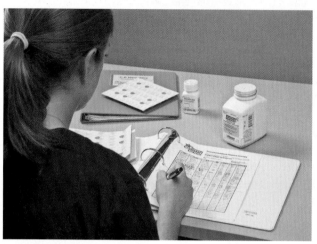

In many independent pharmacies, the pharmacist or pharmacy technician is responsible for maintaining a perpetual inventory record for Schedule II drugs.

Practice Tip

Remember that laws and regulations vary from state to state. When a conflict occurs between a state and a federal law or regulation, the more stringent law or regulation *always* applies.

Registration with the DEA Through the Controlled Substances Act (CSA), every individual, institution, or business involved with manufacturing, distribution, dispensing, research, instructional activities, detoxification programs, importing, exporting, or compounding of controlled substances must be registered with the DEA. The DEA issues a license to medical practitioners that enables them to write prescriptions for scheduled drugs (or controlled substances) and to each individual pharmacy to order scheduled drugs from wholesalers. A hospital will register with coverage for both inpatient and outpatient dispensing. Registrations will vary from one to three years in length. Most pharmacies are issued a three-year registration.

Pharmacy wholesalers who sell controlled substances to community pharmacies must also register with the DEA. In a much publicized case in 2012, the DEA suspended the license of a Florida wholesaler for two years, claiming that the company neglected its primary responsibility to prevent the diversion of controlled substance medications. Consequently, the wholesaler cannot sell or ship controlled substances to area pharmacies. The DEA also suspended the controlled substance license of two area chain pharmacies that purchased a majority of the controlled drugs from this wholesaler.

Prescribers of Controlled Substances The CSA defines who may prescribe controlled substances. The DEA can determine and monitor which practitioners prescribe scheduled drugs. These practitioners are authorized to prescribe controlled substances by the jurisdiction in which they are licensed. Examples of practitioners include physicians, nurse practitioners (advanced practice nurses, or APRNs), dentists, veterinarians, and podiatrists. Though state regulations and procedures may vary, if an APRN were to write prescriptions for Schedule III, IV, or V drugs, a written protocol signed by a delegating physician and approved by the state medical board would generally be required.

The prescription must be written for a legitimate medical purpose in the course of the practitioner's professional practice activities. For example, a dentist may write a narcotic prescription for dental pain but not for back or cancer-related pain. Physician assistants cannot sign for Schedule II prescriptions because they are not licensed with the DEA; in these cases, the physician must write, or at least sign, the prescription. A prescription for a controlled substance from a foreign physician (for example, a practicing physician in Canada or Mexico) cannot be filled in the United States because the prescriber must be licensed with the DEA.

With the exception of an emergency or use by a hospice patient, a prescription for a controlled substance must be written (no telephone or fax prescription orders) to minimize fraudulent use and to maintain a record-keeping system if necessary. The increasing adoption of electronic prescribing (e-prescribing) and electronic health records may minimize forged prescriptions for controlled drugs in the future.

Occupational Safety and Health Administration

The **Occupational Safety and Health Administration (OSHA)** is an agency of the Department of Labor. Its primary mission is to ensure the safety and health of America's workers by setting and enforcing regulations and standards; providing training, outreach, and education; establishing partnerships; and encouraging continual improvement in workplace safety and health. OSHA uses its resources effectively to stimulate management commitment and employee participation in comprehensive workplace safety and health programs. In the pharmacy workplace, OSHA is responsible for protecting healthcare personnel against inadvertent needle sticks and safe disposal of syringes to prevent the transmission of hepatitis and HIV. In hospitals, home health care, and compounding pharmacies that prepare hazardous substances, OSHA is responsible for overseeing policies and procedures to protect personnel from unnecessary drug exposures. (For detailed information on OSHA policies regarding hazardous agents, see Chapter 11.)

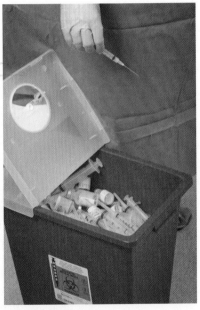

A sharps container is strongly recommended for pharmacy and home disposal of syringes and needles to prevent the transmission of infectious diseases.

National Association of Boards of Pharmacy

The **National Association of Boards of Pharmacy (NABP)** is the only professional organization that represents all 50 state boards of pharmacy. Unlike the FDA or DEA, the NABP has no regulatory authority. One of the primary roles of the NABP is to develop a national pharmacist examination for licensure that is administered by local state boards of pharmacy. The NABP also coordinates the reciprocation of pharmacists practicing in different states. **Reciprocation** is the administrative process of ensuring that pharmacists are eligible for relicensure to practice pharmacy in another state.

The NABP also provides guidance to the state boards of pharmacy by verifying the licensure legality of online pharmacies via its registered Verified Internet Pharmacy Practice Sites (VIPPS) program. Online pharmacies must also meet VIPPS criteria, which address such issues as the patient's right to privacy, authentication and security of prescription orders, adherence to a recognized quality assurance policy, and provision of meaningful consultation between patients and pharmacists.

In addition, NABP helps to coordinate the issuing of provider identification numbers administered by the National Council for Prescription Drug Programs (NCPDP); these numbers are called NCPDP Provider Identification Numbers. The NCPDP provides more than 70,000 pharmacies with a unique identifying number for interactions with the FDA, the DEA, and many third-party processors of prescription claims. The NCPDP has also established industry standards to facilitate online e-prescribing between pharmacies and medical offices.

Lastly, the NADP has put into place a model of pharmacy practice standards to help individual state boards of pharmacy build their own practice standards. This model, called the Model State Pharmacy Practice Act (MSPPA), gives states a common ground for regulations, thus streamlining many years of differing pharmacy laws that were enacted in individual states.

State Boards of Pharmacy

Each state has its own unique board of pharmacy organized under the NABP. These **state boards of pharmacy** consist of leaders from the pharmacy community and a consumer representative who are appointed by the governor. The pharmacists often represent community, hospital, and other areas of pharmacy practice within the state.

The state board reviews applications, administers examinations developed by the NABP, licenses qualified applicants, and regulates the practice of pharmacy personnel throughout the state. **Licensure** is defined as the process by which the state board grants permission to an individual to engage in a given occupation upon finding that the applicant has attained the minimum degree of necessary competency to safeguard the public. All pharmacists must obtain licensure in the state in which they practice. However, licensure for pharmacy technicians differs from state to state, with some state boards of pharmacy requiring licensure and certification and others requiring technicians to be registered.

Registration is defined as the process of being enrolled on a list created by the state board of pharmacy. This list is used to safeguard the public. Thus, if a pharmacy technician was summarily dismissed from a previous job due to documented problems (for example, drug pilfering), he or she would not be allowed to reregister in that state or any other state. A few states require neither licensure, registration, nor certification.

Each state board of pharmacy maintains a database of all active pharmacist licenses (and those of pharmacy technicians) and inspects all new pharmacies. This state agency is also responsible for developing and administering the pharmacy law exam for licensure or reciprocation of pharmacists from another state. The board has the authority to suspend or revoke the license or registration of a pharmacist or a pharmacy technician with evidence of violations of state or federal laws.

State boards of pharmacy also implement federal regulations regarding controlled substances. According to the CSA, medications categorized as Schedule III, IV, and V drugs are refillable for up to five times or six months from the date written. However, some states may enforce more stringent regulations than those established by the federal government. State boards of pharmacy may reclassify prescription drugs as scheduled drugs, or place a scheduled drug in a more restricted status in order to curb drug

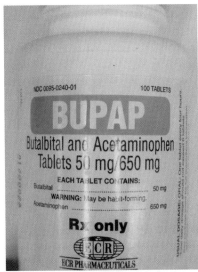

In several states, butalbital—an active ingredient in many headache medications—is classified as a Schedule III drug. Although the DEA does not consider butalbital as a controlled drug, the more stringent regulation of those states would take precedence.

abuse in their region. For example, federal law may classify butalbital, a migraine headache medication, as a nonscheduled drug. However, a state board of pharmacy may elect to make butalbital a Schedule III or Schedule IV controlled substance. Because the state law is more stringent than the federal law, the state law would override the federal law, and butalbital would be dispensed in that state according to the guidelines of a controlled substance.

Likewise, state boards of pharmacy may also place restrictions on Schedule II drugs. For example, some states may not recognize "emergency prescriptions" of Schedule II narcotics for nonhospice patients without a written prescription. Most states allow some mechanism to fill emergency narcotic pain-relieving medication for terminally ill hospice patients. Other states may have a time limitation on the dispensing of a Schedule II drug from the date it was originally written.

Another discrepancy among state boards of pharmacy lies with Schedule V drugs. Some states may require a prescription for Schedule V cough syrups; other states may allow the dispensing of this class of drugs without a prescription if certain conditions are met.

For nonscheduled medications, there are some variances in state regulations as well. Typically, a nonscheduled drug prescription written by a U.S. licensed prescriber is refillable for up to one year from the date written. In addition, the prescribing of a nonscheduled drug by a foreign physician (for example, a practicing physician in Canada or Mexico) is generally prohibited. However, some boards of pharmacy in states that are adjacent to the Canadian or Mexican border may allow dispensing if certain conditions are met. Even the dispensing of insulin syringes may be limited by state boards, with some boards requiring a prescription for the syringes and others limiting the accessibility of both insulin and hypodermic syringes to discourage illicit drug use.

Even with these state and federal guidelines in place, some community pharmacies may elect to enforce more stringent drug use control policies. For example, some pharmacies may implement a store policy requiring a written prescription from a licensed provider for the selling and dispensing of any Schedule V controlled drugs, especially in those areas that are vulnerable to drug abuse or diversion.

Due to the possibility of variances in regulations from state to state, pharmacy technicians need to have a good understanding of the state board regulations for the state in which they practice. They also need to have familiarity with their own facility's policies and procedures.

Legal Duties of Pharmacy Personnel

A statutory federal definition of the role of the pharmacy technician does not exist, and no uniform definition of the role and duties of the pharmacy technician has been adopted by all states. Rather, the job responsibilities of the technician are under constant review and change as pharmacists are called upon to perform more clinical functions. Because each state establishes its criteria for the education, training, and tasks of pharmacy technicians, a great deal of variance exists, and technicians must check with their own state board to understand the applicable statutes and regulations of the state in which they practice.

The following examples illustrate the differences that exist among states in the role and responsibilities of pharmacy technicians:

- Some states specifically authorize the scope of practice by technicians, whereas other states define what the technician may or may not do by detailing what the pharmacist must do. By default, duties not legally mandated to the pharmacist may be carried out by the technician.
- Many states limit the number of pharmacy technicians in all practice settings by specifying a ratio of technicians to pharmacists.
- Many states allow pharmacy technicians to compound solutions for intravenous (IV) infusion under the supervision of the pharmacist, whereas other states only allow pharmacy technicians with a special certification to prepare these solutions. Still, some states allow only pharmacists to prepare IV solutions.

In most states, the following duties can be legally performed by pharmacy technicians under the direct supervision of a licensed pharmacist:

- dispensing of medication
- keeping pharmacy medication records
- pricing/billing of medications
- preparing doses of premanufactured products
- compounding sterile and nonsterile medications per protocol
- performing customer service during the drop-off and pickup of prescriptions
- transporting medications to patient care units in the hospital
- checking and replenishing drug inventory

A detailed analysis of state laws and regulations that affect the practice of pharmacy technicians is beyond the scope of this book, but technicians in training are urged to contact knowledgeable professionals in training institutions and/or their state boards of pharmacy to learn about state-specific statutes and regulations, particularly those related to registration and/or certification by the state, as well as to the specification of those duties that the technician may lawfully undertake. Other references that are useful in comparing duties from state to state include the following:

- the *Pharmacy Law Digest*
- the annual NABP *Survey of Pharmacy Law*
- the Pharmacy Technician Certification Board website

Violation of Laws and Regulations

When certain violations occur under any level of law—local, state, or federal—a prosecutor or public representative may bring a case against the party who violated the law or regulation. Examples include tax evasion, driving under the influence of alcohol, and more serious cases such as manslaughter and murder. Such a crime or violation against the state (or federal government) is filed using terms such as *State vs. Emily Smith*, and it is the prosecutor's duty to see that society is protected from individuals who violate the law.

When cases are filed in court, the party or person filing the case is called the **plaintiff**, and the party being sued or that the case is against is called the **defendant**. The plaintiff is responsible for providing sufficient evidence to prove his or her case; this is referred to as **burden of proof**. The standard of proof in a case involving crimes

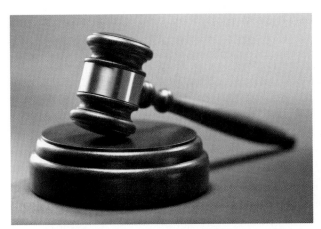
Serious violations of laws, regulations, or ethics may result in suspension or revocation of professional licenses.

against the local, state, or federal government is referred to as **reasonable doubt**. This means that the prosecutor or plaintiff must provide convincing evidence that the party committed the act, beyond any "reasonable" doubt of a normal person. If the party is found guilty, then the punishment may be monetary fines, probation, or incarceration.

If the defendant in a case is a licensed or registered healthcare provider (for example, a physician, nurse, pharmacist, technician), then the appropriate state board may examine the case and determine whether the defendant's license should be revoked or suspended. The license may be revoked on ethical grounds, or the board may have a specific regulation that allows it to revoke a license in the event the person is convicted of a felony. If evidence of alcohol or drug abuse is proven, the state board may require successful completion of a drug rehabilitation program before the license can be reinstated.

Civil Laws

Civil law is the term given to areas of the law that concern the citizens of the United States and the wrongs they may commit against one another but not generally against the local, state, or federal government and their respective laws and regulations. Civil law in the United States is derived from the precepts of common law used in England and brought here by the settlers. This law covers issues such as wrongs against one another and contracts. **Common law** is the system of precedents established by decisions in cases throughout legal history.

Occasionally, in a criminal case, a crime is committed in violation of a state or federal law, and the party is prosecuted. In these cases, the victim or his or her family may also sue the party in civil court for monetary damages. If this situation occurs, the person may be tried two times, facing two separate plaintiffs. In the criminal case, the defendant might face monetary fines, probation, or prison. The civil case might result in monetary awards to the plaintiff.

Torts

In the context of civil law, a **tort** refers to personal injuries. Torts relate to wrongs that one citizen commits against another. In the case of a tort, the injured party sues the party that caused the injury (e.g., *Edgar Gonzales v. Dave's Drugstore and Dave the Registered Pharmacist [RPh]*). The local, state, and federal governments do not take part in a lawsuit such as this one because the crime occurred between two citizens and not against the government and/or its laws and regulations.

Examples of torts include a broken contract, negligence, malpractice, slander (using spoken words to speak falsely of another), libel (using written words to falsely represent another), assault (threatening another with bodily harm), and battery (causing bodily harm to another). For example, if a pharmacist or pharmacy technician speaks unkindly to a customer about the professional competence of another healthcare professional, that pharmacist or technician may be found guilty of slander.

Negligence and Standard of Care The most common tort in the medical/pharmacy arena is **negligence**, or the failure to provide the minimum standard of care. **Standard of care** is the level of care expected to be provided by various healthcare providers in the local community. Standard of care, when used to judge the type of care provided to a patient, is based on (1) comparisons to the actions of other healthcare professionals in the same situation and geographic area; (2) compliance with existing written guidelines, protocols, or policies and procedures; and (3) expert testimony of healthcare professionals provided by the plaintiff or the defense. When the standard of care is not met and results in injury, a patient may sue the healthcare provider for **malpractice**, a form of negligence.

When considering standard of care, two criteria are always taken into account: the level of training of the healthcare provider and customary or standard practice for the geographic area in which the healthcare provider works. Only those healthcare providers who work in the same geographic area *and* have the same level of training would be compared. For example, a pharmacist in Denver would not be compared with a pharmacist in Boston because local practices and written protocols may differ by geographic area. He or she would, however, be compared with other pharmacists working in the Denver area. Likewise, the job performance of a pharmacist with advanced education and training who is practicing in Atlanta would be compared with a pharmacist with advanced education and training who is also working in the Atlanta area. Because of his or her advanced training, the Atlanta pharmacist would also be held to a higher standard in a court of law.

These criteria for standard of care apply to the role and responsibilities of pharmacy technicians as well. The behavior of a pharmacy technician in a particular situation would be compared with the behavior of a technician in the same geographic area. In the event of a serious medication error, a certified pharmacy technician would be held to a higher standard of care than a technician who is not certified.

Negligence and Burden of Proof When a case of negligence or malpractice is brought, the burden of proof is on the plaintiff to prove what is known as the **four Ds of negligence**: duty, dereliction, damages, and direct cause. The plaintiff must first prove the defendant had a duty to provide care or that there was a contract for care between the two parties. The plaintiff must then prove that the defendant was derelict in his or her duty, that this dereliction caused actual damages to the plaintiff, and that the damages were a direct cause of the defendant's dereliction.

The burden of proof in civil court is lower than the burden of proof in a criminal case. The plaintiff must prove his or her case by a "preponderance of the evidence," which means that it is more likely than not that the defendant is guilty of the accused act. If the defendant is found guilty, then he or she may be ordered to pay an award of money to the plaintiff. It is not possible for the defendant to be incarcerated because the crime was not committed against the state but rather against another citizen. All pharmacies, most practicing pharmacists, and some pharmacy technicians carry professional liability insurance to protect their business and personal assets from a civil lawsuit involving negligence or malpractice.

Legal Outcome of Negligence Investigation Several levels of negligence or malpractice may be determined during an investigation and subsequent trial. If two or more causes are a factor in the negligence and personal injury to the patient, then a case of contributory negligence may be determined. For example, if the physician and pharmacist were both responsible for the injury to a patient, then each may be found guilty. The award to the plaintiff may then be broken down according to the judge's or jury's assessment of the comparative negligence. If the physician was more responsible than the pharmacist, then the award may be broken down by a percentage, in which the physician must pay 70% of the damages award and the pharmacist must pay 30% of the damages award. Cases even exist in which the patient is found to have contributed to his or her own injury (for example, not taking medication as directed) and thus found to be comparatively negligent. In this type of case, the plaintiff's total award may be reduced by a certain percentage, depending on the judge's or jury's determination.

Law of Agency and Contracts

The **law of agency and contracts** is based on the Latin term *respondeat superior*, which translates to "let the master answer." This law is a general principle that applies to the employee–employer relationship. The employee is, in effect, an "agent" for his or her employer and may enter into contracts on the employer's behalf. This is an important agreement in the healthcare setting. For example, in a medical office, a nurse may act as an agent for a physician; in the pharmacy, a technician may act as an agent for a pharmacist or for the pharmacy. This principle means that not only does a contract exist in the healthcare setting but that the contract is just as valid as any verbal agreement or written contract drawn up by a physician or a pharmacist.

An example of how the contract is made in the pharmacy is simple: The exchange of a prescription between a patient and a pharmacy technician who agrees to fill the prescription is considered an implied contract. An implied contract means that the pharmacy and pharmacist are now obligated to provide the patient with a service. If a mistake is made, then the pharmacy and/or pharmacist may be held liable, even though the pharmacist was not the one who entered into the contract to provide the service. The pharmacist (or pharmacy, in the case of a chain) must therefore "answer" for all of the acts of his or her employees. However, a pharmacy technician can still be held liable if it can be proven that the technician overstepped the limitations of his or her position, such as dispensing a prescription drug without a check by the supervising pharmacist.

Invasion of privacy is another violation that may result in a lawsuit. Medical and prescription records, including those generated and filed in the pharmacy, are considered the physical property of the facility that generates them; however, the intellectual property contained in the medical record is the property of the patient. This information may not be divulged to another nonhealthcare provider or organization without the consent of the patient or by subpoena (a legal order). The pharmacy is held responsible for the actions of its personnel if a violation occurs. Privacy of medical information is now covered by federal law under HIPAA, as discussed earlier in the chapter. Violations of HIPAA may carry heavy personal fines and immediate termination of employment for the violator. Confidentiality of medical information is further discussed in Chapter 13.

Drug and Professional Standards

In addition to laws and regulations of the FDA, the DEA, and state boards of pharmacy, national standards for drug products and professional standards exist. **Professional standards** are guidelines of acceptable behavior and performance established by professional associations. National professional pharmacy organizations help advance the profession by setting high professional standards that are well above what is required by laws and regulations.

United States Pharmacopeia

The **United States Pharmacopeia (USP)** is an independent, nonprofit, scientific organization whose mission is to set public, quality standards for prescription drugs, OTC drugs, and dietary supplements legally marketed in the United States. The Federal Food, Drug, and Cosmetic Act provides an important role for *USP–NF* standards under that law's adulteration and misbranding provisions. This book of standards or compendium is called the **United States Pharmacopeia–National Formulary (USP–NF)**. All new drugs approved by the FDA must meet applicable *USP–NF* standards.

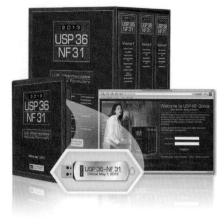

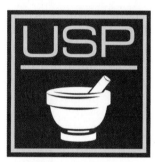

The *United States Pharmacopeia–National Formulary* is an important reference for pharmacists and pharmacy technicians.

In addition to setting quality standards for drugs, USP also has developed standards regarding the practice of pharmacy by pharmacists and pharmacy technicians. For example, **USP–NF General Chapters <795> and <797>** set standards that involve the storage, packaging, and preparation of nonsterile and sterile compounded preparations. These and other USP compendial standards are developed by various constituent committees of USP's Council of Experts. Specifically, General Chapter <795> addresses nonsterile compounding standards, and General Chapter <797> addresses sterile compounding standards. These standards can be found in the *USP–NF* (volume 1) as well as in an additional electronic publication: *USP on Compounding: A Guide for the Compounding Practitioner.* This resource offers compounding practitioners access to all compounding-related General Chapters from the *USP–NF* in a convenient PDF format.

USP–NF General Chapters <795> and <797> standards have been incorporated into the policies and procedures of compounding pharmacies and adopted by many accreditation organizations, including state boards of pharmacy and the Joint Commission. Adherence to these sterile and nonsterile compounding policies and procedures are reviewed upon physical inspections of the pharmacies. (General Chapters <795> and <797> are discussed in more detail in Chapters 8 and 10, respectively.)

National Professional Organizations

Various professional organizations advocate the establishment of high standards of practice in order to advance the pharmacy profession. Pharmacists and technicians who are members of professional organizations are generally assumed to support the mission statements and policies of those organizations. These mission statements provide a standard of care that is *above and beyond the minimum* of what is required by federal and state pharmacy laws and regulations. For example, the mission statement of the American Pharmacists Association is "to serve society as the profession responsible for the appropriate use of medications, devices, and services to achieve optimal therapeutic outcomes."

Aside from setting practice standards, these professional organizations also focus on the education and training of pharmacy personnel. For example, the American Pharmacists Association (APhA), the American Society of Health-System Pharmacists (ASHP), the National Association of Chain Drug Stores (NACDS), the American Association of Pharmacy Technicians (AAPT), and the Pharmacy Technician Educators Council (PTEC) collaboratively developed a model curriculum for pharmacy technicians based on task analysis. These national pharmacy organizations seek membership and input from pharmacy technicians.

Another focus of professional organizations is certification. **Certification** is defined as a voluntary process by which a nongovernmental organization recognizes an individual who has met predetermined qualifications specified by that organization. Twelve of these national professional organizations are members of the Council on Credentialing in Pharmacy (CCP), an organization that provides leadership and guidelines for the credentialing of pharmacists and the certification of pharmacy technicians in order to meet established professional standards. One of the founding members of the CCP is the Pharmacy Technician Certification Board (PTCB), an organization that has trained and certified more than 300,000 pharmacy technicians. Its mission is to develop, maintain, promote, and administer a high-quality certification and recertification program for pharmacy technicians across various practice settings. With certifications, pharmacy technicians are able to earn a higher salary and work more effectively with pharmacists to offer better patient care and service. (To learn more about the certification process, see Chapter 14.)

Lastly, one professional organization, ASHP—also a founding member of the CCP—has developed a national accreditation training program for pharmacy technicians. **Accreditation** is defined as the status achieved by a college or university that meets quality standards and fulfills the requirements designated by the accrediting organization. Currently, less than 30% of training programs for pharmacy technicians are accredited, allowing for wide variations in classroom content, experiential training, and length of program. As pharmacy professional organizations work to establish standards for the education, training, and certification of pharmacy technicians, accredited training programs will become the norm. In fact, future state boards of pharmacy may only recognize the certification of pharmacy technicians who have graduated from an accredited program.

Chapter Summary

- Governments and professional organizations have a right to exercise control over the manufacture, dispensing, and use of drugs to ensure quality and prevent harm to others because of the misuse or abuse of medications.
- Controls over the use of drugs are embodied in laws, regulations, and drug standards.
- Statutory laws and amendments passed by the U.S. Congress such as the Food, Drug, and Cosmetic (FD&C) Act, Durham-Humphrey Amendment, and Kefauver-Harris Amendment have improved public safety by classifying drugs and ensuring their safety and efficacy.
- The Comprehensive Drug Abuse Prevention and Control Act is another example of statutory law that established schedules for controlled substances with regulatory oversight provided by the Drug Enforcement Administration (DEA).
- The Medicare Modernization Act of 2003 provides a voluntary drug insurance program to patients eligible for Medicare benefits.
- The Affordable Care Act of 2010 mandates universal healthcare coverage for all citizens of the United States.
- The FDA regulates and enforces investigational and new drug applications to further protect the public.
- OSHA protects the employee from handling hazardous substances.
- State boards of pharmacy have regulations to license pharmacies, pharmacists, and technicians, and they have the power to take administrative actions against those that violate laws, regulations, and standards.
- The legal status of pharmacy technicians and their allowable duties vary from state to state, but technicians must *always* act under the direct supervision of licensed pharmacists.
- Pharmacy is affected by the potential for tort actions in common law because of negligence or other forms of malpractice.
- Violations of patient confidentiality by pharmacy personnel can result in both legal repercussions and immediate termination of employment.
- Standards for drugs and procedures for drug preparation are set by the United States Pharmacopeia (USP) in the *United States Pharmacopeia–National Formulary (USP–NF)*.
- Standards for the practice of pharmacy are set by state boards of pharmacy and by various professional organizations.
- National pharmacy organizations support the advanced training and skills necessary for pharmacy technicians to become certified.

Key Terms

accreditation the status achieved by a hospital, community college, college, or university that meets quality standards and fulfills the requirements designated by the accrediting organization

adulterated product a product that differs in drug strength, quality, and purity

anabolic steroid a synthetic, performance-enhancing drug that mimics the human hormone testosterone; because of abuse by athletes, this drug has been reclassified by the DEA as a controlled substance

brand name the name under which the manufacturer markets a drug; also known as the *trade name*

burden of proof the obligation of a person or party filing a lawsuit to provide evidence to prove a case

certification a voluntary process by which a nongovernmental organization recognizes an individual who has met predetermined qualifications specified by that organization; a pharmacy technician may become certified by the Pharmacy Technician Certification Board (PTCB)

child-resistant container a medication container with a special lid that cannot be opened by 80% of children under age 5 but can be opened by 90% of adults; a container designed to prevent child access to reduce the number of accidental poisonings

civil law the areas of the law that concern U.S. citizens and the crimes they commit against one another

common law the system of precedents established by decisions in cases throughout legal history

controlled substance a drug with potential for abuse; organized into five schedules that specify the way the drug must be stored, dispensed, recorded, and inventoried

Controlled Substances Act (CSA) laws created to combat and control drug abuse

defendant one who defends against accusations brought forward in a lawsuit

Drug Enforcement Administration (DEA) the branch of the U.S. Justice Department that is responsible for regulating the sale and use of drugs with abuse potential

ethics standards of behavior that all professionals are encouraged to follow

Food and Drug Administration (FDA) the agency of the federal government that is responsible for ensuring the safety and efficacy of food and drugs prepared for the market

four Ds of negligence four areas of negligence, which include duty, dereliction, damages, and direct cause; the plaintiff in a negligence or malpractice lawsuit must produce evidence that proves that the defendant committed a breach of responsibility and that this breach led to personal injury of the plaintiff

generic name a common name that is given to a drug regardless of brand name; sometimes denotes a drug that is not protected by a trademark; for example, acetaminophen is the generic drug name for Tylenol

Health Insurance Portability and Accountability Act (HIPAA) a law passed by Congress that primarily defines the confidentiality of patient medical records as well as prescription record

Joint Commission an independent governing body that sets standards for quality patient care and safety in hospitals and other healthcare facilities; this organization is responsible for the accreditation of hospitals

law a rule that is designed to protect the public and is usually enforced through local, state, or federal governments

law of agency and contracts the general principle that allows an employee to enter into contracts on the employer's behalf

legend drug a drug that requires a prescription; labeled "Rx only" on medication stock bottle

licensure the process by which a state board grants permission to an individual to engage in a given occupation upon finding that the applicant has attained the minimum degree of necessary competency to safeguard the public; all pharmacists must be licensed to practice by their state boards of pharmacy

malpractice a form of negligence in which the standard of care was not met and was a direct cause of injury

misbranded product a product whose label includes false statements about the identity or ingredients of the container's contents

National Association of Boards of Pharmacy (NABP) an organization that represents the practice of pharmacy in each state and develops pharmacist licensure exams

National Drug Code (NDC) a 10- or 11-character code that is assigned by the FDA to each drug product; each code is unique and identifies the manufacturer or distributor, the drug formulation, and the size and type of packaging

negligence a tort for not providing the minimum standard of care

new drug application (NDA) the process through which drug sponsors formally propose that the FDA approve a new pharmaceutical for sale and marketing in the United States

Occupational Safety and Health Administration (OSHA) an agency of the Department of Labor whose primary mission is to ensure the safety and health of U.S. workers by setting and enforcing regulations and standards

orphan drug a medication approved by the FDA to treat rare diseases

patent drug another name for an over-the-counter (OTC) medication

plaintiff one who files a lawsuit for the courts to decide

professional standards guidelines of acceptable behavior and performance established by professional associations

reasonable doubt the standard of proof or evidence that the plaintiff must provide in a case involving crimes against the local, state, or federal government

reciprocation the administrative process for relicensure of pharmacists in another state

registration the process of being enrolled on a list created by the state board of pharmacy; most state boards require pharmacy technicians to register with their state of practice

regulation a written rule and procedure that exists to carry out a law of the state or federal government

regulatory law the system of rules and regulations established by governmental bodies

schedule a listing of controlled substances categorized by the DEA according to their potential for abuse and physical or psychological dependence

standard a set of criteria to measure product quality or professional performance against a norm

standard of care the usual and customary level of practice in the community

state boards of pharmacy governing bodies responsible for the regulation of the practice of pharmacy within the states

statutory law a law passed by a legislative body at either the federal, state, or local level

tort the legal term for personal injuries that one citizen commits against another in a lawsuit

United States Pharmacopeia (USP) the independent, scientific organization responsible for setting official quality standards for all drugs sold in the United States as well as standards for practice

United States Pharmacopeia–National Formulary (USP–NF) a book that contains U.S. standards for medicines, dosage forms, drug substances, excipients or inactive substances, medical devices, and dietary supplements

USP–NF General Chapter <795> a chapter of the *United States Pharmacopeia* that contains national standards for pharmacies formulating nonsterile preparations

USP–NF General Chapter <797> a chapter of the *United States Pharmacopeia* that contains national standards for pharmacies formulating sterile preparations

Chapter Review

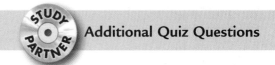

Checking Your Understanding

To check your comprehension of this chapter's key concepts, read the following multiple-choice questions and then record your answers on a separate sheet of paper. Write your answers as modeled in these examples: 1d; 2c; 3b; etc.

1. The Food, Drug, and Cosmetic (FD&C) Act of 1938 designated which agency to develop standards for all drugs marketed in the United States?
   a. DEA
   b. FDA
   c. NABP
   d. USP

2. The Kefauver-Harris Amendment of 1962 stated that all new drugs must be proven _____ before being marketed.
   a. safe for pediatric patients
   b. affordable
   c. effective
   d. safe for pregnant women

3. The Verified Internet Pharmacy Practice Sites (VIPPS) program is administered by the
   a. FDA.
   b. NABP.
   c. USP.
   d. DEA.

4. The first four numbers of the National Drug Code (NDC) found on a prescription or on an over-the-counter (OTC) medication represent the
   a. manufacturer.
   b. dosage of the drug.
   c. drug formulation (for example, tablet, capsule, suspension).
   d. packaging size of the stock drug container.

5. What organization is responsible for overseeing the policies and procedures of a pharmacy that prepares and dispenses hazardous drugs?
   a. OSHA
   b. DEA
   c. FDA
   d. CDC

6. The Omnibus Budget Reconciliation Act of 1990 (OBRA-90) requires the pharmacist or pharmacy technician to
   a. offer patient counseling regarding medications.
   b. fill prescriptions according to FDA guidelines.
   c. report all prescription drug errors to the FDA.
   d. provide the DEA with information regarding narcotics.

7. What agency is responsible for classifying controlled substances?
   a. CMS
   b. FDA
   c. DEA
   d. NABP

8. Which of the following controlled substances is classified as a Schedule III drug?
   a. amphetamine/dextroamphetamine
   b. anabolic steroids
   c. oxycodone
   d. zolpidem

9. The Dietary Supplement Health and Education Act (DSHEA) of 1994 limited the FDA's authority to regulate
   a. narcotic-prescribing habits of physicians.
   b. the manufacturing of orphan drugs.
   c. Medicaid payment for prescriptions.
   d. herbal, vitamin, and nutritional products.

10. Which organization was responsible for the development of the Model State Pharmacy Practice Act (MSPPA)?
    a. DEA
    b. FDA
    c. NABP
    d. Medicare

11. Which authority has the right to remove a pharmacist's or pharmacy technician's license or registration?
    a. state board of pharmacy
    b. FDA
    c. federal court judge
    d. DEA

12. If a patient sues a pharmacy, then which party is responsible for the burden of proof in the case?
    a. pharmacy
    b. pharmacist and pharmacy technician who filled the prescription
    c. patient
    d. state or local prosecutor

13. A pharmacist may be sued for _____ when he or she fails to meet a minimum standard of care.
    a. libel
    b. slander
    c. negligence
    d. malpractice

14. The *Orange Book* is published online by the
    a. FDA.
    b. DEA.
    c. OSHA.
    d. NADP.

15. To be approved as a generic drug, the pharmaceutical manufacturer must prove
    a. bioequivalence.
    b. safety.
    c. efficacy.
    d. affordability.

Reinforcing Your Learning

To build on your understanding of the topics in this chapter, complete the following enrichment activities.

1. A patient is suing a pharmacist and pharmacy technician for negligence. In his lawsuit, the patient (or plaintiff) claims that a medication error has caused him great psychological distress. Here are the facts surrounding his lawsuit:

   The plaintiff was given a prescription for trazodone to treat his insomnia and depression. When he went to the pharmacy to fill his prescription, the pharmacy technician inadvertently entered the drug tramadol (a medication used for pain relief) into the computer instead of the prescribed drug trazodone. The pharmacist failed to detect the error and verified that, indeed, tramadol was filled and dispensed to the plaintiff. After one month of taking the

   medication, the plaintiff experienced no relief of his insomnia or depression. When the plaintiff returned to the pharmacy to refill his prescription, another pharmacist detected the medication error and advised the plaintiff and his physician of the error. The correct medication was then dispensed.

   According to the law, the burden of proof rests with the plaintiff. To establish a valid case, what four claims must the patient prove, and to what degree must he prove them? Given the facts as stated, what arguments and/or evidence can the patient put forward to support each of these four claims? Record your answers using complete sentences and making sure that your answers are thorough and thoughtful.

2. In a legal case, the plaintiff, Baker, sued the pharmacy for negligence. In the lawsuit, the patient (or plaintiff) claimed that a failure in pharmacist review led to his subsequent stroke. Here are the facts surrounding his lawsuit:

Mr. Baker, the plaintiff, was taking the antidepressant drug tranylcypromine, under a prescription that he regularly filled at the pharmacy. The plaintiff went to a physician with a cold, and the physician—despite having records indicating that the plaintiff was taking tranylcypromine—prescribed a medication that contained the decongestant phenylpropanolamine. When Mr. Baker came to the pharmacy to have his prescription filled, the pharmacy's computer warned the pharmacist that a potential interaction existed between the new prescription and Baker's prescription for tranylcypromine that had been filled a few days earlier. The pharmacist overrode the computer warning and filled the prescription; the plaintiff was not offered counseling by the pharmacy technician and was unaware of the potential drug interaction. As a result of taking the phenylpropanolamine, Baker suffered a stroke. Baker sued the pharmacy and on appeal received a judgment against the pharmacy.

To address the legalities of this case, work with a partner to record answers to the following questions:
   a. Were both the pharmacist and the pharmacy technician guilty of negligence? Prior to formulating your response, consider all four criteria for negligence.
   b. In what ways did the physician, the pharmacy technician, and the pharmacist fail to carry out their duties properly?
   c. What requirement, under OBRA-90, was not met? What relevance does this case have to the expanded clinical role of the pharmacist?
   d. Under what legal principle did Baker sue the pharmacy for the actions of its employees—the pharmacist and the pharmacy technician?

   e. Under what legal principle could Baker not sue the manufacturer of the phenylpropanolamine product, given that the physician and the pharmacy had been warned of the dangerous drug interaction?
   f. In contemporary pharmacy, what role do computers play in helping pharmacists and pharmacy technicians meet the counseling requirements of OBRA-90?
   g. Is this a case in which a court could conceivably make a finding of contributory negligence or comparative negligence? Why? If you were on the jury and you awarded $500,000 in damages to the plaintiff, how would you split the negligence award among the physician, pharmacist, and pharmacy technician? Explain your reasoning.

3. In the course of her normal duties, a pharmacy technician employed by Hometown Drugs, Inc., discovers from a patient profile that the young man who is dating her daughter is taking a regular prescription for a powerful antipsychotic drug. The technician keeps this information to herself but, in response to the information, attempts to dissuade her daughter from dating the young man. Has the technician committed a breach of her ethical responsibilities? Address this question in a brief essay and be sure to provide evidence that supports your position.

4. Pharmacists and pharmacy technicians with alcohol or substance abuse problems sometimes fail to seek help for fear that a state board of pharmacy might take some disciplinary action should the problem become known. What might professional associations and state boards do, in your opinion, to combat this problem? Does your state board of pharmacy have a procedure in place to help those seeking to overcome their drug problem? Record your responses using complete sentences and making sure that your answers are thorough and thoughtful.

5. It is important to become familiar with using NDC numbers in filling prescriptions and minimizing medication errors. Visit a pharmacy and write down the NDC numbers of five different OTC medications such as ibuprofen, Motrin IB, and Advil. Compare the different manufacturers, different dosage forms (tablets, gelcaps, suspension), and package sizes. Notice the first four numbers of the NDC for the same manufacturer: Are they the same or different? Are the middle numbers of the NDC the same for ibuprofen suspension and ibuprofen tablets? Check two different size packages of Motrin IB or Advil: Are the last numbers of the NDC the same or different?

Thinking on Your Feet

To gain practice in handling challenging situations in the workplace, consider the following real-world scenarios and then use the guiding questions to help you formulate your responses.

1. A patient presents a prescription to your pharmacy for Valtrex, an antiviral medication often used in the treatment of herpes. In the exchange, you recognize that the patient is a former high school classmate and discuss the upcoming class reunion with him. The patient's expression immediately turns anxious, and he is clearly uncomfortable with your knowledge of his current health situation. How would you address his concerns? Which law protects patient confidentiality, and what are the ramifications if pharmacy personnel reveal health-related information?

2. An older patient complains of difficulty opening his medication vial. What procedures can the pharmacy technician take to legally assist this patient?

3. A parent presents three prescriptions for her son who is taking Adderall XR for his attention deficit hyperactivity disorder (ADHD). The prescriptions are accompanied by specific instructions from the boy's physician asking the pharmacy to refill this prescription every month for the next three months. You know that Adderall XR is a Schedule II drug with no refills. How would you handle this situation?

4. The spouse of a patient calls the pharmacy on a holiday weekend. Her husband has terminal cancer and is on around-the-clock morphine to alleviate his pain. The physician approved a dosage increase to provide better pain relief, but now more medication is needed and the prescription has no refills. How would you proceed to help this woman get the medication that she urgently needs for her husband? Does the fact that morphine is a Schedule II drug have any bearing on your actions?

5. A patient brings in a prescription for Synthroid with the box checked by the prescriber "dispense brand only." The patient has prescription drug insurance and requests that a lower-cost generic drug be dispensed. How would you handle this situation?

Acquiring Field Knowledge

To expand your knowledge of pharmacy practice, explore the following online activities that focus on research and information retrieval.

Reminder: As you navigate the Internet, remember to exercise caution and good judgment when evaluating information. A thoughtful review of online text should take into consideration the following factors: the creator and sponsors of the website, the intended audience, the credentials of the authors and contributors, the reliability and validity of the posted information, the frequency of updates to the site, and the ease of navigation for a range of user skill levels.

1. Plavix is an expensive brand name drug whose patent expired in 2012. To search for possible generic drug substitutions, go to www.paradigmcollege.net/pharmpractice5e/plavix and find the section designated "Approvals & Clearances." Then click on the title "Search Drug Approvals by Month Using Drugs @ FDA." Select two criteria: "All Approvals by Month" and then "May 2012." Search for the generic drug name for Plavix and check the website for the number of manufacturers that were approved on May 17, 2012. Record your findings. If possible, check a local pharmacy to compare the "cash" price of Plavix 75 mg #30 with a generic drug in stock.

2. A good friend of yours has a seven-year-old child who has been diagnosed with a rare form of cystic fibrosis (CF)—a G551D mutation of the CF gene. Research this disease online and write up a brief report on its cause, symptoms, treatment, and life expectancy. Then conduct an online search for a new drug called Kalydeco. What legislation made the production of this drug possible? Have orphan drugs improved the life expectancy of patients afflicted with this disease? Write a report that reflects your research findings.

3. Go to www.paradigmcollege.net/pharmpractice5e/dietsupprecalls and search for "recalls of diet supplements removed from the market." Use the following guiding questions to help you form a written response: Why were these drugs pulled from the market? Under what legislation are diet supplements regulated? Does the FDA have the authority to pull these drugs from the market?

4. To determine the legal requirements for dispensing Schedule V cough syrups and insulin syringes in your state, visit a retail pharmacy or visit the website of your state board of pharmacy. Write a brief paragraph that explains your state guidelines.

5. Go to the website of the Pharmacy Technician Certification Board at www.paradigmcollege.net/pharmpractice5e/ptcbcrestprogram and review the C.R.E.S.T. initiative. The steering committee of the initiative, comprised of 10 leaders in pharmacy practice, proposed a number of recommendations in certification and recertification for pharmacy technicians, as well as new certification programs. Do you agree or disagree with the committee's recommendations? Should all pharmacy technicians be certified? Should all pharmacy technician training programs be accredited? Thoughtfully consider these questions and then record your responses and corresponding rationales.

Sampling the Certification Exam

To provide you with practice for the Certification Exam Review, read the following questions that have been patterned after the test format and then record your answers on a separate sheet of paper. Write your answers as modeled in these examples: 1d; 2c; 3b; *etc.*

1. Which of the following drugs is a Schedule IV controlled substance?
   a. methadone
   b. testosterone cyprionate
   c. hydrocodone
   d. zolpidem

2. A pharmacy technician receives a prescription for amlodipine, and a review of the patient profile reveals a prescription for verapamil, a similar antihypertensive, which was filled a week ago. What should the pharmacy technician do?
   a. fill the prescription because it is not for the same drug
   b. notify the pharmacist of a potential duplication of therapy
   c. call the physician to discuss the duplication of therapy
   d. discontinue the verapamil prescription and fill the amlodipine

3. Which of the following concepts is the focus of the federal law known as OBRA-90?
   a. confidentiality
   b. compliance
   c. medication errors
   d. counseling

4. Which amendment to the Food, Drug, and Cosmetic (FD&C) Act of 1938 established prescription drugs and nonprescription drugs?
   a. Controlled Substance Act
   b. Durham-Humphrey Amendment
   c. Kefauver-Harris Amendment
   d. FDA Modernization Act

5. The *FDA Orange Book* is published online by the
   a. Drug Enforcement Administration (DEA).
   b. Food and Drug Administration (FDA).
   c. Department of Health and Human Services (DHHS).
   d. Consumer Product Safety Commission (CPSC).

6. The federal law that prohibits the reimportation of a drug into the United States by anyone except the manufacturer is the
   a. Prescription Drug Marketing Act of 1987.
   b. Drug Price Competition and Patent-Term Restoration Act of 1984.
   c. Omnibus Budget Reconciliation Act of 1990.
   d. Patient Protection and Affordable Care Act of 2010.

7. When a manufacturer of a new drug entity submits data to the Food and Drug Administration (FDA) for approval to market a new drug, the manufacturer must prove that the drug is safe and
   a. has greater potential benefit than previously marketed products.
   b. has no contraindications for use in humans.
   c. is effective for the intended indication.
   d. has no abuse potential.

8. What federal act established the National Drug Code (NDC)?
   a. Durham-Humphrey Amendment of 1951
   b. Drug Listing Act of 1972
   c. Prescription Drug Marketing Act of 1987
   d. Health Insurance Portability and Accountability Act of 1996

9. How many refills are allowed on a prescription for lisdexamfetamine (Vyvanse)?
   a. none
   b. 1
   c. 5, or six months from original date of prescription
   d. 11, or up to one year from original date of prescription

10. The federal government restricts the sale of _____, due to its/their use in making methamphetamine.
   a. pseudoephedrine
   b. syringes
   c. Plan B
   d. dextromethorphan

Drug Development

3

Learning Objectives

- Define the term *drug* and distinguish between active and inert ingredients.

- Identify several scientific discoveries of medications that improved individuals' quality of life and life span.

- Define the terms *drug tolerance*, *psychological dependence*, and *physical dependence*.

- Contrast the regulation and labeling requirements for over-the-counter drugs, homeopathic medications, and dietary supplements.

- Categorize drugs according to their various sources: natural, synthetic, synthesized, or semisynthetic.

- Define the term *pharmacogenomics* and its future impact on drug development and dosing.

- Understand the classifications that describe the various uses of drugs: therapeutic, pharmacodynamic, diagnostic, prophylactic, and destructive agents.

- Discuss the process and role of the Food and Drug Administration (FDA) and the United States Pharmacopeia in the marketing of new pharmaceutical products.

- Review statistics and costs of getting a new investigational drug to market.

- Understand the process for FDA approval for generic drugs, and define the terms *bioequivalence* and *therapeutic equivalence*.

- Explain the parts of a National Drug Code number and its use by the pharmacy technician.

- Identify the three classes of FDA drug recalls.

- Identify major sources of consumer and professional drug information.

- Understand postmarketing surveillance reporting programs for medication and product safety.

- List four drugs that are subject to risk evaluation and mitigation strategies, for their safe use.

- Identify the function of various commonly used pharmaceutical reference texts.

Preview chapter terms and definitions.

I n the past six decades, technological advances in the synthesis and delivery of pharmaceuticals have transformed people's lives, providing improved antibiotics, vaccines, and medications to better control chronic diseases such as hypertension, hyperlipidemia, and diabetes. The development of these drugs was built upon the scientific framework provided by earlier major research discoveries that have defined and shaped **pharmacology**, or the study of how drugs work inside the body. Along with the emergence of these lifesaving medications came improvements in the regulation of these drugs, including lengthy drug trials testing the efficacy and safety of medications before they are marketed. This chapter provides insight into pharmaceuticals by exploring the process of drug development, including the sources of drugs, their classifications and uses, and their approval by various regulatory agencies. More importantly, this chapter addresses the role that pharmacy personnel play in following the policies and procedures set forth by these regulatory agencies in order to safeguard the health and well-being of their patients.

What Is a Drug?

A **drug** is defined as any substance taken into or applied to the body for the purpose of altering the body's biochemical functions and thus its physiological processes. For early civilizations, many of these drugs were derived from plant sources and were compounded into powders, extracts, and tinctures by physicians or pharmacy practitioners. Although natural herbal remedies continue to be used today, scientific advances in several areas—including chemistry, anatomy and physiology, pathophysiology, and genetics—have led to the development of highly researched and standardized medications that are more potent and toxic than the natural remedies of the past. Therefore, a broader definition of a drug has emerged. Today's drugs include dietary supplements such as vitamins, minerals, and herbs; homeopathic remedies; over-the-counter (OTC) drugs; and prescription drugs. Many of these drugs are available as generic and/or brand name products, and some are classified as controlled substances, or drugs that are under tight legal and administrative controls.

A drug may contain one or more active ingredients that have many specific therapeutic uses. An **active ingredient** is the biochemically active component of the drug that exerts the desired **therapeutic effect**—for example, eradicating a bacterium or virus, lowering blood pressure or cholesterol, or controlling heart rate. Most drugs contain one or more active ingredients as well as several inactive or inert ingredients. An **inert ingredient** has little or no physiological effect on the body. Common inert ingredients include antimicrobial preservatives and flavorings. These inert ingredients are needed to stabilize the tablet, capsule, or liquid formulation; to provide the raw material for many topical creams and ointments; to ensure sterility of injectable products; or to assist in the masking of unpleasant oral medications for pediatric patients. Due to patient allergies and hypersensitivities, the Food and Drug Administration (FDA) requires manufacturers to list all inert ingredients on product package inserts and on bottles of OTC products. (For more information on the function of various inert ingredients, see Chapter 4 of this textbook.)

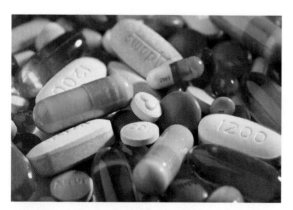

All tablets and capsules are composed of both active and inactive or inert ingredients; a patient may be allergic to either component.

Significant Drug Discoveries

As discussed in Chapter 1, the past 300 years saw pharmacy and medicine evolve from magic and superstition to well-organized, scientific exploration, but most individuals take for granted the current availability of medications used to maintain their health.

What would life be like without vaccines, insulin, penicillin, the birth control pill, or HIV medication? Significant changes in our longevity and quality of life are due in part to these drug discoveries, as well as many other important medications formulated since World War II. Pharmacy personnel should have an appreciation and understanding of these landmark drug advancements and their essential role in improving patient health care.

Smallpox—The First Vaccination

In the late 1700s, smallpox was a major cause of premature death, much like heart disease and cancer are today. In 1796, Dr. Edward Jenner performed the first experimental vaccination, an inoculation of cowpox to treat the dreaded smallpox infection. He observed that dairy workers who had previously been exposed to cowpox were immune to smallpox. This observation led to Jenner's realization that cowpox exposure produced antibodies that provided immunity to smallpox. An **antibody** is the part of the body's immune system that neutralizes antigens or foreign substances. Armed with this knowledge, Jenner proceeded to introduce bacteria from a cowpox lesion into a healthy individual and discovered that the individual did not contract smallpox despite exposure to the disease. Jenner called the inoculation procedure a *vaccination*, a term that comes from the Latin word *vacca*, meaning "cow." The substance introduced into the body in order to produce immunity to disease, therefore, is called a **vaccine**.

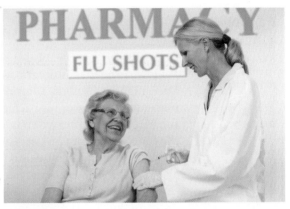

Due to Jenner's experiments with antibodies, many vaccines—such as the flu shot—have been developed to prevent serious illnesses in adults and children.

Safety Note

It is important for pharmacy technicians to be up-to-date on their vaccinations and to reassure patients that the benefits of vaccine protection outweigh the small risk of adverse reactions.

The vaccine was a success, and smallpox was the first disease in history to be eradicated. Despite this outcome, the use of early vaccinations had a high complication rate due to problems of purity and mass production. Today, however, drug consistency is virtually guaranteed, and vaccines are considered quite safe. With the assistance of pharmacy technicians, pharmacists in many community pharmacies can now administer vaccines against influenza, pneumonia, shingles, and many other potentially dangerous conditions.

Insulin—A Lifesaver!

Sir Frederick Banting was a Canadian scientist, doctor, and Nobel Laureate who—along with his assistant, Charles Best—discovered insulin in the 1920s while experimenting with beagles. Previous research demonstrated a link between the pancreas and diabetes, which at the time was referred to as "the sugar disease." Dogs with diabetes were kept alive with an extract from the pancreas, which Banting and Best called *isletin*. This extract was later isolated and purified and named *insulin* after the Latin word *island* (as in the islets of Langerhans, the area of the pancreas secreting insulin).

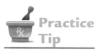
Practice Tip

Pharmacy technicians can assist diabetic patients by helping them select diabetic supplies—such as syringes, needles, lancets, and test strips—and by stressing the importance of insulin dosing and blood glucose monitoring.

The discovery of insulin was hailed as one of the most significant advances in medicine at the time. Prior to the discovery of insulin, people with diabetes suffered complications and an early death ("diabetic coma") a short time after the onset of the disorder. This drug discovery extended the lives of millions of people worldwide who could not be treated and had a very poor prognosis. In fact, estimates show that today there are more than 15 million diabetic patients living near-normal lives while taking one or more types of insulin.

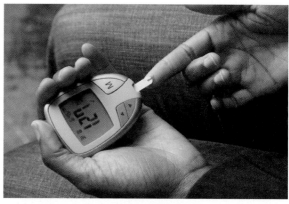

The dose of insulin needed by a diabetic patient is often determined by results of frequent finger-stick testing of blood glucose at home.

Safety Note

Many individuals are allergic to penicillin. In light of that, always check a patient's drug allergy history when receiving a prescription for penicillin or one of its derivatives. It is also considered good practice to update the patient's drug allergy history and to clean counting trays after contact with penicillin or its derivatives.

Penicillin—The First Antibiotic

An **antibiotic** is a chemical substance that kills or inhibits the growth of bacteria. Penicillin, the first antibiotic, was discovered by accident in 1928 by research scientist Dr. Alexander Fleming. After returning to his lab from a long vacation, Fleming noticed that many of his bacterial culture petri dishes were contaminated with a fungus. He also observed that, in some of the dishes, a bacteria-free zone surrounded the fungus. Fleming proceeded to isolate an extract from the bacteria-killing mold. He correctly identified it as being from the *Penicillium* genus and, therefore, named the agent *penicillin*. Penicillin saved many soldiers' lives during World War II, and, in 1945, this antibiotic was mass-produced and marketed. Penicillin and its derivatives are now the most widely used antibiotics in the world.

Today, there are hundreds of oral and injectable synthetic antibiotics, but continued research is needed to overcome increasing antibiotic resistance. Although a course of antibiotics might kill nearly all bacteria of a particular disease, the surviving bacteria reproduce, creating more resistant bacteria by natural selection and decreasing the effectiveness of the antibiotic. Consequently, stronger doses of the antibiotic are prescribed, which, in turn, creates a higher risk of side effects. An example of this chain-reaction effect can be seen with the antibiotic amoxicillin. Due to drug resistance, the required dose of amoxicillin to treat ear infections has doubled in the past 30 years.

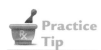
Practice Tip

For patients who have been prescribed antibiotics, pharmacy personnel should stress the importance of completing the entire course of therapy to reduce the incidence of antibiotic resistance and recurring infection.

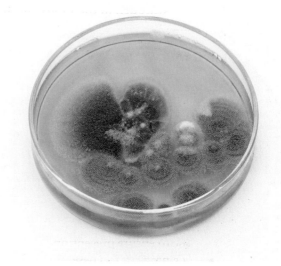

The clear areas around bacteria in the petri dish indicate the effective antimicrobial activity of penicillin.

The Scourge of Polio

Polio is considered one of the most destructive diseases of the twentieth century and reached pandemic proportions in North America, Europe, Australia, and New Zealand by the 1940s. Polio is characterized by muscle weakness and paralysis of the lower extremities. This disease typically affected children who, if they survived, often had residual paralysis that required braces and crutches for life. In 1952, more than 21,000 cases of the most serious form of polio—paralytic polio—were reported in the United States alone.

At the time, there was no cure for polio. The only way to treat severe symptoms was with the use of a noninvasive negative-pressure ventilator, more commonly called an *iron lung*. The iron lung would artificially maintain respiration during an acute polio infection until the patient could breathe independently. Typically, the treatment lasted about one to two weeks.

In 1953, American physician Jonas Salk created an injectable vaccine from animal cultures that contained the killed viruses of the three kinds of polio that were known at the time. (Earlier efforts were unsuccessful because the vaccines covered only one strain of the virus.) Salk developed a process using formalin, a chemical that inactivated or killed the whole virus. A "killed" or inactivated vaccine does not contain or transmit a live virus, preventing the risk of infection if administered correctly.

Mass immunization programs for American children were initiated in 1955, a year in which there were 28,000 reported cases of polio. One year later, there were only 15 cases of polio. In 1994, polio was declared eradicated in all of the Americas, and worldwide cases have dropped from hundreds of thousands to just under a thousand today, providing hope for the total eradication of a once-unstoppable disease.

The Pill

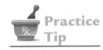
Practice Tip

Questions from a customer on the proper use of any birth control pill must be brought to the immediate attention of the pharmacist on duty. Pharmacy technicians may also be involved in the sale of the OTC "morning after" pill, which has legal age restrictions.

"The pill" is a colloquial name for the birth control pill. Before the birth control pill was developed, there were few contraceptive methods outside of abstinence, the rhythm method, and the use of condoms. Up until the mid-twentieth century, some state laws even prohibited teaching about contraceptive methods in medical schools. Despite this resistance, research on reproductive biology progressed and led to a major breakthrough in the 1930s: the identification of the female sex hormones estrogen and progesterone and the understanding of their functions. Though funding was scarce, and the hormones difficult and expensive to synthesize, research continued in the hands of a few passionate scientists and activists.

The early, approved birth control pills contained high doses of both estrogen and progesterone to ensure prevention of a pregnancy. These high doses contributed to a relatively high incidence of side effects, including

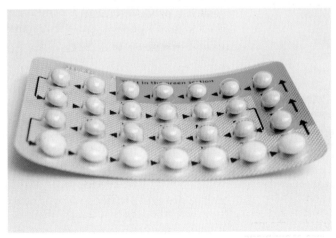

The birth control pill has had a major impact on reproductive rights and helped initiate the women's liberation movement in the 1960s.

nausea, headache, and blood clots. With time and additional research, the dosages of the sex hormones in the pill have steadily decreased, thus reducing the risk of adverse effects. Each prescription of birth control pills dispensed must contain written patient information on the risks of the pill.

Today, with an estimated 100 million women worldwide on the pill, there are many different combinations and names of brand and generic birth control pills. Some pills have different amounts of estrogen and progesterone during each week of the menstrual cycle. Some pills even decrease the number of menstrual periods. When taken appropriately, the pill is 99%+ effective in preventing pregnancy and is also useful in treating women with irregular or painful menstrual cycles.

HIV/AIDS

The emergence of a formidable virus—the human immunodeficiency virus (HIV)—occurred in the early 1980s when epidemiologists noted an outbreak of rare pneumonias and cancers in New York City. In 1983, HIV was independently isolated and verified by the Pasteur Institute in France and the National Cancer Institute in the United States. This virus progressively attacked the immune system and caused the development of acquired immunodeficiency syndrome, or AIDS. Transmitted through the exchange of bodily fluids during sexual contact or intravenous drug use, or through tainted blood transfusions, HIV quickly grew to epidemic proportions worldwide.

The cost for the lifetime treatment of HIV has been estimated at more than $400,000 per person. The first antiviral drug to treat HIV was FDA-approved in 1987. Further studies demonstrated limited efficacy of one drug alone due to the rapid development of resistance. Since 1987, many additional oral and injectable HIV drugs that attack the virus at different stages of its replication have been developed. Currently, combination therapy involving three or four drugs is commonly prescribed to control the virus. Medications given to a pregnant, HIV-infected patient have been shown to be effective in reducing the transmission of the virus to the newborn at delivery, although vaccines have so far been ineffective.

HIV drugs can cause many adverse side effects, are prohibitively expensive, and can interact with many medications. However, the fight against HIV is growing stronger. In the early days of the disease, a diagnosis of HIV or AIDS was virtually considered a death sentence. Today, approximately 50,000 new cases of HIV/AIDS are reported each year, with more than 1.2 million people living with the disease in the United States alone. For these patients, regimented medication therapy allows many of them to lead near-normal lives.

Sources of Drugs

Drugs are derived from various sources and can be classified as natural, synthetic (created artificially), synthesized (created artificially but in imitation of naturally occurring substances), and semisynthetic (containing both natural and synthetic components). The development of lifesaving and life-altering biogenetically engineered drugs is a major source of new drug development in the twenty-first century.

Natural Sources of Drugs

Some drugs are naturally occurring biological products and can be made or taken from single-celled organisms, plants, animals, minerals, and humans. Many herbal products come from natural sources. In addition to penicillin and insulin, other examples of modern-day drugs from natural sources are listed below:

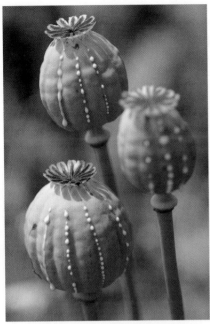

Morphine, codeine, and paregoric trace their ancestry to the opium poppy plant.

- The antibiotic streptomycin is produced from cultures of the bacterium *Streptomyces griseus*.
- Digitalis, a drug used to strengthen the heart and regulate its heartbeat, is formulated from the foxglove plant.
- The narcotic opium and its derivatives (morphine and codeine) come from the opium poppy plant.
- Quinine, used to treat malaria, and colchicine, used to treat acute gout, both come from the bark of the cinchona tree.
- Acetylsalicylic acid, more commonly known as aspirin, is derived from the bark of the white willow tree (which contains salicylic acid).
- USP thyroid extract is derived from the desiccated (dried) thyroid glands of pigs.
- The salts of minerals such as iron and potassium, which are commonly found in nature, are used for the treatment of iron deficiency and electrolyte replacement therapy.
- Milk of magnesia is an aqueous suspension of magnesium hydroxide and is used as an antacid or a laxative. Magnesium hydroxide is produced from sea water or the mineral brucite.
- Human growth hormone, or somatotropin, comes from the human brain.

Laboratory Sources of Drugs

In the modern era, many naturally occurring substances have been combined with other ingredients in a laboratory setting to produce synthetic, synthesized, and semi-synthetic drugs.

Synthetic Drugs A **synthetic drug** is a drug that has been created from a series of chemical reactions to produce a specific pharmacological effect. Phenobarbital—a barbiturate prescribed for seizure, nerve, or headache disorders—is an example of a synthetic drug. Another example is a sulfa antibiotic. Both phenobarbital and sulfa are considered synthetic drugs because these substances do not exist in nature.

Synthesized Drugs A **synthesized drug** is a drug created artificially in the laboratory but in imitation of a naturally occurring drug. Epinephrine hydrochloride is an example of a synthesized drug. A single dose of this lifesaving drug is contained in an auto-injector device called an EpiPen and is used by hypersensitive patients to treat severe allergic reactions to insect stings or other triggers. Epinephrine hydrochloride mimics the pharmacological action of the naturally occurring hormone adrenaline. Digoxin, aspirin, and quinine are all considered synthesized drugs that mimic the pharmacological action of their naturally occurring sources—foxglove, white willow (weeping willow) tree, and the cinchona tree, respectively. In addition, many antibiotics are produced by or derived from certain fungi, bacteria, and other organisms in the laboratory.

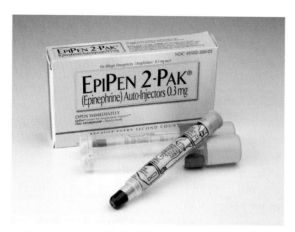

EpiPen is an example of a lifesaving injectable drug for severe allergies; it is often dispensed in a 2-Pak—one for home and one for school use.

Synthesized drugs have also found their way into the illegal drug market. Called designer drugs, these illegal drugs are produced in home chemistry laboratories by individuals who skirt drug control laws by modifying the chemical structure of existing drugs. The new drugs they create offer similar pharmacological effects to their drug counterparts. For example, a synthesized version of marijuana exerts a similar effect to the natural product but also produces more hallucinations. Methamphetamine, also known as "meth" or "speed," is another example of a synthesized drug. Because meth is produced from the common decongestant pseudoephedrine hydrochloride, community pharmacies are required by law to place restrictions on the sale of products containing this key ingredient.

Semisynthetic Drugs A **semisynthetic drug** is a natural drug that has been chemically modified in the laboratory to do one or more of the following actions: (1) improve the efficacy of the natural product; (2) reduce its side effects; (3) overcome developing bacterial resistance; or (4) broaden the spectrum of bacteria that can be treated. Many current antibiotics such as amoxicillin/clavulanate, azithromycin, and levofloxacin are modifications of the existing natural drugs. These antibiotics are more effective against different strains of bacteria or bacteria that have developed resistance to the natural product.

Biogenetically Engineered Drugs

Biotechnology combines the sciences of biology, chemistry, and immunology to produce synthetic, unique drugs with specific therapeutic effects. These drugs can be created by means of the recombinant deoxyribonucleic acid (recombinant DNA) techniques of genetic engineering. **Deoxyribonucleic acid (DNA)** is the complex, helically shaped molecule that carries the genetic code (see Figure 3.1). DNA is made up of four chemical base pairs. These pairs, which are abbreviated as A, T, C, and G, are repeated millions or billions of times throughout a genome. A **genome** is the entire DNA in an organism, including its genes. The DNA contains the instructions, or recipe, for creating messenger **ribonucleic acid (RNA)**, which in turn contains arranged sequences for making amino acids into proteins for living organisms. These proteins determine how an organism looks, how well its body metabolizes drugs or fights infection, and sometimes how it behaves. A defect in the DNA may increase the risk for developing certain diseases. If you can "unravel" the DNA code, you can more effectively prevent or treat diseases.

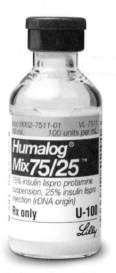

Biogenetically engineered drugs can treat many serious illnesses. Humalog is used primarily to treat Type I diabetes.

Genetic engineering is the process of utilizing DNA biotechnology to create a wide variety of drugs, such as insulin for diabetes; clotting factors for hemophilia; potent anti-inflammatory drugs for rheumatoid arthritis; and drugs for combating viral and bacterial infections, anemia, and some cancers. The development of biotechnology drugs has led to a new field of study that blends two scientific areas: pharmacology and genomics. Known as **pharmacogenomics**, this field of study examines the relationship between an individual's genes and his or her body's response to drugs. The vision of pharma-

FIGURE 3.1
Modeling DNA

(a) A single nucleotide. (b) A short section of a DNA molecule consisting of two rows of nucleotides connected by weak bonds between the bases adenine (A) and thymine (T) and between the bases guanine (G) and cytosine (C). (c) Long strands of DNA twisted to form a double helix.

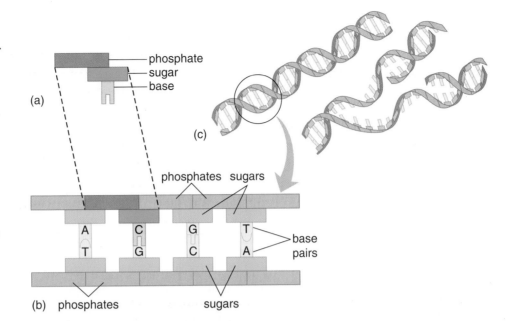

cogenomics is to be able to design and produce drugs that cater to an individual's genetic makeup. For example, blood thinners are metabolized by patients at different rates, thus altering its pharmacological and toxic effects. Genetic engineering would specify a blood thinner formula that would produce the intended pharmacological effect in a particular patient without the additional risk of adverse reactions.

Both biotechnology and genetic engineering promise to bring many new drugs to the market. Currently, more than 900 biogenetically engineered drugs are under development to treat more than 100 diseases.

Drug Classifications

Drugs are classified by the FDA as prescription, over-the-counter (OTC), or homeopathic. As discussed in Chapter 2, vitamins, minerals, and herbs are technically considered dietary supplements (not drugs) and are not directly regulated by the FDA. Because these drug classifications have unique characteristics, all pharmacy personnel must have a solid understanding of the different federal and state laws and regulations regarding the dispensing, marketing, and sale of the drugs that fall under these classifications.

Prescription Drugs

A **prescription drug**, formerly known as a *legend drug*, can be dispensed only upon receipt of a prescription from a healthcare professional licensed to practice in that state. Consequently, all prescription drugs are labeled with the legend "Rx only" (see Figure 3.2). A prescription drug may be available as a generic product (for example, clopidogrel), or it may be available as a brand name product (for example, Plavix). Therefore, it is important for the pharmacy technician to have a working knowledge of the top 200 generic and brand names of common drugs and their indications. (For a list of the top generic and brand name drugs, see Appendix A.)

Knowing the generic and brand names of drugs is also important in the discussion of insurance coverage with patients. In most cases, insurance will only cover the cost of

FIGURE 3.2
**Prescription
Drug Label**

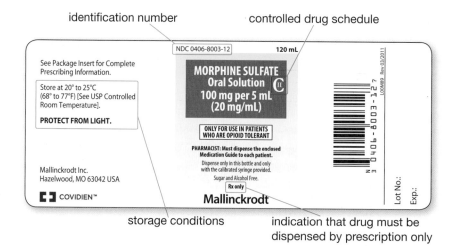

identification number   controlled drug schedule

See Package Insert for Complete
Prescribing Information.

Store at 20° to 25°C
(68° to 77°F) [See USP Controlled
Room Temperature].

PROTECT FROM LIGHT.

Mallinckrodt Inc.
Hazelwood, MO 63042 USA

C•3 COVIDIEN™

MORPHINE SULFATE
Oral Solution **CII**
100 mg per 5 mL
(20 mg/mL)

ONLY FOR USE IN PATIENTS
WHO ARE OPIOID TOLERANT

**PHARMACIST: Must dispense the enclosed
Medication Guide to each patient.**
Dispense only in this bottle and only
with the calibrated syringe provided.
Sugar and Alcohol Free.
Rx only

Mallinckrodt

NDC 0406-8003-12   120 mL

storage conditions   indication that drug must be
dispensed by prescription only

a generic product if it is available. If a patient does not have drug insurance, he or she
will often ask the pharmacy technician if a lower-cost generic product is available. If the
prescribed drug is not covered by insurance, the pharmacist or pharmacy technician
may need to call the physician's office to request a lower-cost alternative for the patient.

Controlled Substances Some prescription drugs are classified as controlled
substances by the Controlled Substances Act of 1970. These drugs are organized into
five schedules or classes according to their potential for abuse and addiction. (See
Table 2.1 on page 39.) Schedule II controlled substances, such as narcotics and
amphetamines, have the highest potential for abuse, drug tolerance, and psychological
or physical dependence.

Drug tolerance is a condition in which the body adapts to a drug so that higher
doses are needed to produce the same therapeutic effect achieved earlier with smaller
doses. For example, a patient who is taking a Schedule II or III narcotic on a continuous basis for pain relief may build up a drug tolerance, resulting in less pain relief at
the prescribed dosage. Consequently, that patient may take higher doses or more
frequent doses to achieve the pain relief he or she once had. Drug tolerance can lead to
psychological or physical dependence, or even to drug addiction.

Psychological dependence is defined as a condition in which a patient takes a
drug on a regular basis because it produces a sense of well-being. If the patient stops
taking the drug, he or she may experience anxiety or withdrawal symptoms due to a
psychological dependence on the medication. For example, a patient who takes a
sleeping pill every night may experience disruptive sleep patterns, yet the patient feels
that he or she must take the medication to get a good night's sleep.

Physical dependence is defined as taking a drug continuously so that when the
medication is stopped, physical withdrawal symptoms such as restlessness, anxiety,
insomnia, diarrhea, vomiting, and goose bumps occur. Withdrawal symptoms commonly occur with high doses of Schedule II and III drugs and, for some patients, may
occur after four weeks of continuous use.

Addiction is defined as compulsive and uncontrollable use of controlled substances,
especially narcotics. Addicted patients will do anything to support their drug habit.

If the major role of the profession of pharmacy is to protect the public, it is apparent that closely monitoring prescriptions for controlled drugs (including refills) is a
very important responsibility of the pharmacy technician. The technician must carefully review prescriptions for scheduled drugs for potential forgeries, prescribing by
multiple doctors, and requests from patients for early refills on their medications.

OTC Drugs

An **over-the-counter (OTC) drug** is a drug that can be purchased without a prescription. Before an OTC drug is approved for sale, the FDA must first recognize it as safe and effective when the labeled directions on the container, with regard to dose, frequency, precautions and contraindications, and duration of therapy, are followed. Most OTC drugs are indicated for self-limited conditions requiring accurate self-diagnosis and short-term therapy (usually less than seven days). Other OTC drugs such as baby aspirin or allergy medicine may be used on a long-term basis with physician permission.

The FDA has approved many OTC drugs after the expiration of the manufacturer's patent on the prescription drug. Such examples include Advil (ibuprofen), Aleve (naproxen), Claritin (loratadine), Zyrtec (cetirizine), and hydrocortisone. These drugs have been proven relatively safe over the years when appropriately used and sold as OTC medications. If used inappropriately, these drugs can cause side effects, adverse reactions, and interactions with prescription drugs.

It is very important that OTC drugs have adequate product labeling, written in easily understood terms, to assist the consumer in properly using the product, as there may be no contact with a pharmacist, nor any typed instructions from the physician. The FDA requires that labels contain a prominent "Drug Facts" box that lists the active ingredients, purposes, and use of the product, with any warnings and directions including age-appropriate dosing. This "Drug Facts" box allows the consumer to compare active ingredients and assess the benefits and risks of various OTC products. For example, if a customer is considering the purchase of multiple cold medications, a comparison of active ingredients can identify any overlap or duplication of drugs that may cause adverse effects. This information may be critically important if the medication is being purchased for a child or an elderly adult. In fact, many OTC medications have age restrictions on their package label such as "do not use < age 4 years" or "use under physician's care if under age 2 years." In addition to this information, drug labels are also required to have an expiration date as well as a list of inactive ingredients for those patients with allergies. Labeling requirements also assist the pharmacy technician in identifying a lower-cost generic or store brand OTC medication for the consumer.

Some OTC drugs and supplies are only sold in pharmacies "behind the counter." This restriction may be due to:

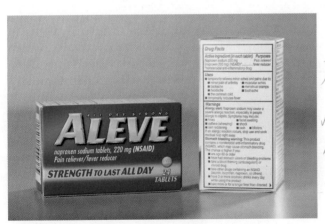

All OTC drugs must include "Drug Facts" labeling for the consumer to safely self-medicate with the product.

- federal or state laws and regulations (to control the dispensing of pseudoephedrine or codeine cough syrups)
- age requirements (to oversee the dispensing of Plan B and Next Choice)
- possible abuse/diversion (to monitor the use of insulin syringes)
- the need for additional pharmacist counseling (to discuss the use of certain asthma medications).

The role of the pharmacy technician in providing customer service on OTC drugs will be further discussed in Chapter 7.

Drug Facts

Active Ingredients .... Purpose

Conium maculatum 6X ....redness
Graphites 12X...dryness
Sulphur 12X .... tearing, burning

Uses:

According to homeopathic principles, the active ingredients in this medication temporarily relieve minor symptoms associated with styes, such as:
• redness • burning • dryness • tearing

Homeopathic medications contain one or more ingredients in a diluted form to stimulate the immune system. As with OTC medications, "Drug Facts" labeling is required.

 Safety Note

Most homeopathic medications are available without a prescription.

Homeopathic Medications

Another class of drugs under FDA control is called **homeopathic medications**. The term *homeopathy* is derived from the Greek root words *homos*, meaning "similar," and *pathos*, meaning "suffering or disease." Homeopathic practice uses subclinical doses of natural extracts or alcohol tinctures in which the active ingredient is diluted from one part per ten (1:10) to more than one part per thousand (1:1000), or even higher. The concept is that these small doses are sufficient to stimulate the body's own immune system to overcome the specifically targeted symptom.

Most homeopathic medications are OTC, but some are considered prescription only. An OTC homeopathic medication is labeled for a self-limiting condition, or a condition that does not require medical diagnosis or monitoring, and is nontoxic. The use of homeopathic medications was popular in the United States in the early nineteenth century and remains popular in many areas of Europe today. These medications are sometimes considered "natural treatments," and the risk of side effects is minimal.

Dietary Supplements

Most community pharmacies have a large inventory of vitamins, minerals, herbs, and dietary supplements. A **dietary supplement**, especially an herb, exerts weak pharmacological effects on the body similar to drugs. Consequently, dietary supplements may cause side effects, adverse reactions, and drug interactions. Glucosamine is an example of a dietary supplement that is used in humans and pets to provide nutrients for bone cartilage to treat mild arthritis symptoms. As with OTC drugs, consumers can purchase dietary supplements without a prescription and should read the labels carefully. Because dietary supplements are considered "food supplements" that maintain health, consumers should not exceed the recommended daily dose or "serving size."

As discussed in Chapter 2, these supplements do not have the same stringent controls as prescription and OTC medications and are loosely regulated by the Dietary Supplement Health and Education Act (DSHEA) of 1994. The FDA can only regulate

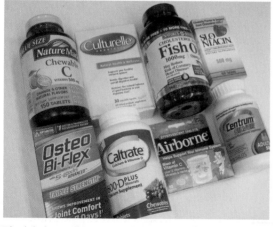

The labels on dietary supplements may not contain as much information for the consumer as labels on other OTC drugs.

dietary supplements when patient safety concerns exist, as in the case of weight-loss drugs. Consumers should be aware that the quality of many of these products is suspect when tested by independent consumer laboratories.

The use of herbs by patients poses a particular challenge to pharmacy personnel. Quite often, patients take herbal supplements and fail to disclose that information to their physician or pharmacist. As a result, some patients, particularly the elderly, may have an adverse reaction between their herbal supplement and their prescription medication. Therefore, a pharmacy technician can assist the pharmacist by gathering information about the patient's use of herbs or other dietary supplements and entering this data into the patient's computerized profile. (For more information about dietary supplements, refer to Chapter 7.)

USP and Dietary Supplements The USP Verified Mark is awarded by USP—a nonprofit, scientific organization with nearly 200 years of experience setting public standards for medicines and, more recently, dietary supplements and foods. As an independent entity, this organization is able to work with governments, manufacturers, and practitioners worldwide to set public health standards.

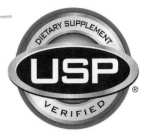

The USP verified mark for dietary supplements

The USP Verified Mark on a dietary supplement label tells consumers that the quality of the product has been verified under the U.S. Pharmacopeia's (USP's) rigorous USP Dietary Supplement Verification Program. This means that the dietary supplement:

- contains the ingredients listed on its label, in the declared potency and amounts
- does not contain harmful levels of specified contaminants
- will break down and release ingredients into the body within a specified period
- has been made according to current U.S. Food and Drug Administration (FDA) **good manufacturing practices (GMPs)**.

Process of USP Verification USP works with manufacturers who voluntarily participate in the USP Dietary Supplement Verification Program. The organization verifies the manufacturers' supplements through a comprehensive testing and evaluation process. USP's staff scientists:

- conduct an initial screening to help ensure that products or ingredients with known safety concerns are not admitted to the USP Dietary Supplement Verification Program.
- perform thorough audits of manufacturing facilities, practices, records, and quality control measures to determine whether the manufacturer follows good manufacturing practices
- test product samples in USP laboratories and other qualified laboratories
- allow use of the USP Verified Mark only on products that meet all of USP's stringent criteria
- conduct testing on products carrying the USP Verified Mark, sampled from the marketplace, to determine whether they continue to meet USP's standards.

Whereas others may provide testing and quality seals, USP is the only standard-setting organization recognized in U.S. federal law that offers third-party verification services. The USP's drug standards are FDA-enforceable per the Federal Food, Drug, and Cosmetic Act, and the organization's dietary supplement standards are recognized in the 1994 Dietary Supplement Health and Education Act.

Uses of Drugs

Today's medications are used not only to treat and cure illnesses but also to aid in their diagnosis and even prevent their onset. Because drugs serve a variety of purposes in a patient's healthcare regimen, pharmacy technicians in both community and hospital practice must be knowledgeable of the therapeutic uses of commonly prescribed drugs. Knowing this information is as important as learning the brand names and generic names of these medications. (To help you with learning this essential drug information, refer to Appendix A.)

Several classifications for uses of drugs exist, and most of these categories are not mutually exclusive. These classifications include therapeutic agents, pharmacodynamic agents, diagnostic agents, prophylactic agents, and destructive agents.

Therapeutic Agents

A **therapeutic agent** is a drug that targets a specific need in the body. Therapeutic agents are categorized according to the following functions:

- *Maintaining health*—Drugs with this purpose include vitamins and minerals to regulate metabolism and otherwise contribute to the maintenance of normal growth and functioning of the body. A specific example is the use of baby aspirin for patients identified as being at risk for a heart attack.
- *Relieving symptoms*—Drugs with this purpose include anti-inflammatory drugs such as ibuprofen used to treat fever, pain, or inflammation; narcotics to treat and prevent severe pain in terminally ill patients with cancer; or a diuretic or water pill to control excess fluid or high blood pressure.
- *Combating illness*—Drugs with this purpose include antibiotics to treat pneumonia, strep throat, or a bladder infection. Although antiviral medications do not cure HIV or AIDS, they may allow the immune system to remain sufficiently intact so as to delay disease progression. Drugs for Alzheimer's disease will not cure the patient but may delay both disease progression and loss of independence of the patient.
- *Reversing disease processes*—Drugs with this purpose include medications that control depression, blood pressure, or cholesterol levels.

Pharmacodynamic Agents

A **pharmacodynamic agent** is a medication that alters body functioning in a desired way. Pharmacodynamic agents can be used, for example, to stimulate or relax

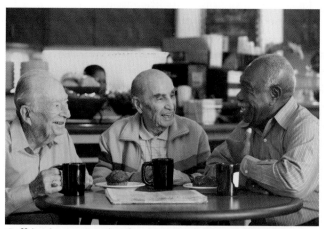

Caffeine is an example of a pharmacodynamic agent that can increase alertness.

muscles, to dilate or constrict pupils, or to increase or decrease blood glucose levels. Caffeine found in coffee, tea, or a soft drink is considered a pharmacodynamic agent because it stimulates the nervous system, allowing the consumer to remain alert. Other examples of these medications include decongestants for nasal stuffiness, oral contraceptives that depress hormones to prevent pregnancy, expectorants to thin fluid or loosen mucus in the respiratory tract, anesthetics to cause numbness or loss of consciousness, glucagon to increase blood glucose levels in diabetics, and digoxin to increase heart muscle contraction or slow heart conduction in patients with heart disease.

Diagnostic Agents

A **diagnostic agent** is a chemical containing radioactive isotopes that is used to diagnose or treat disease. Isotopes are forms of an element that contain the same number of protons but differing numbers of neutrons. Unstable, radioactive isotopes give off energy in the form of radiation. These isotopes act as radioactive tracers, helping healthcare practitioners pinpoint, diagnose, and treat certain disorders. Nuclear medicine uses radioactive isotopes such as technetium (^{99m}Tc) and iodine (^{131}I) for imaging regional function and biochemistry in the body. Technetium is also commonly used for imaging and functional studies of the brain, thyroid, lungs, liver, gallbladder, kidneys, and blood. The radiation exposure from the use of these isotopes is minimal and, therefore, has no harmful effects on a patient.

Working with these radioactive isotopes, called **radiopharmaceuticals**, is considered a specialization area of pharmacy practice. Pharmacists and pharmacy technicians who are involved in the procuring, storage, compounding, dispensing, and provision of information about these diagnostic agents work in a nuclear pharmacy and must have specialized training and certification in the handling of these agents.

Prophylactic Agents

A **prophylactic agent** prevents illness or disease from occurring. Examples of prophylactic agents include the antiseptic and germicidal liquid chemicals used for preoperative hand-washing procedures in order to prevent the spread of infection. Vaccines are also considered prophylactic agents, preventing the onset of diseases such as influenza, pneumonia, shingles, tetanus, measles, mumps, rubella, chicken pox, smallpox, poliomyelitis, and hepatitis. In fact, pharmacists are increasingly becoming involved in the administration of the influenza, pneumonia, and shingles vaccines to older adults and other high-risk individuals.

In certain situations, antibiotics are prophylactic agents as well. For example, a patient who has a history of rheumatic fever may be given a large, single dose of an antibiotic prior to a dental procedure. This preventive action decreases the patient's risk for acquiring a serious bacterial infection from the dental work.

Destructive Agents

A **destructive agent** has a *-cidal* action; that is, it kills bacteria, fungi, viruses—even normal cells or abnormal cancer cells. Many antibiotics, especially those given in high doses and/or as intravenous (IV) infusions, are **bactericidal**, meaning that these agents kill rather than inhibit bacteria that are sensitive to these drugs. Penicillin is an example of a bactericidal drug, though resistance by some bacterial organisms has developed over the years. Another example of a destructive agent is radioactive iodine, which is used to destroy some of the excess hormone secreted by the thyroid.

Another common example of a destructive agent is an **antineoplastic drug**, or a drug used in cancer chemotherapy to destroy malignant tumors. Cancer is often caused by an unregulated growth of abnormal dysfunctional cells. Different antineoplastic drugs are used in combination to slow the growth of cancer cells at different phases of their cell growth cycles. Unfortunately, most of these drugs cannot effectively distinguish cancer cells from normal cells, so side effects such as hair loss, immunosuppression, and ulcerations of the mouth or gastrointestinal (GI) tract commonly occur.

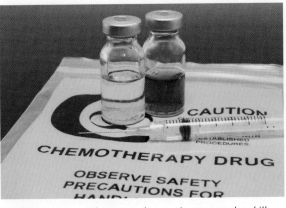

Traditional cancer drugs are destructive agents that kill both cancer and normal cells. Newer therapies in the future will be more selective.

Agents used in cancer chemotherapy are considered hazardous drugs. Consequently, these drugs require special storage, preparation, and monitoring in both the community and hospital pharmacy practice settings. Pharmacy personnel who handle these destructive agents must be specially trained, and women who are of childbearing age must limit their exposure to these medications. Women who are pregnant are generally reassigned in the pharmacy or excused from the sterile compounding of chemotherapeutic agents. (For more information on the preparation and handling of hazardous drugs, see Chapter 11.)

United States Pharmacopeia

As discussed in Chapter 2, the United States Pharmacopeia (USP) was charged by Congress in 1938 with the task of developing official compendia and public standards for all prescription and OTC drugs marketed in the United States. Today, this organization continues to develop authoritative, unbiased information on drug quality and disseminates this information to healthcare professionals. This drug reference is called the **United States Pharmacopeia–National Formulary (USP–NF)** and contains standards for medicines, dosage forms, drug substances, excipients or inactive substances, medical devices, and dietary supplements. These standards include drug name identification, strength, quality, and purity as well as guidelines for packaging, labeling, and storage of drug product. A manufactured drug product must conform to these standards to avoid possible charges of adulteration and misbranding and to be approved by the FDA.

Food and Drug Administration

The Food and Drug Administration (FDA) has the very important responsibility to assure the American public that the drugs that are approved are both safe *and* effective. New drugs must meet strict USP standards and undergo a fairly lengthy (and expensive) research process before they come to market. These stringent regulations were developed in response to a medication tragedy in the early 1960s. During that time period, a sedative called thalidomide was a popular sleep aid and marketed in 46 countries, particularly in Europe. When an Australian doctor discovered that the medication could also alleviate morning sickness in pregnant women, the drug was marketed as an antiemetic as well. In the United States, one FDA drug inspector was not convinced that thalidomide was adequately tested for this new therapeutic use and refused to approve this medication. Thalidomide was later proven to cause severe birth defects in fetuses, a discovery that spurred the FDA to tighten their drug approval process by requiring that all medications must pass trials for both safety and efficacy.

To gain a clear understanding of the FDA's impact on pharmacy practice, pharmacy technicians must be aware of the drug approval process. This process includes development of brand name drugs and their bioequivalent generics, the packaging and labeling of the products, and the continuing oversight by the FDA of all marketed medications.

Drug Approval Process

The FDA has regulations for manufacturers to follow while researching new chemical entities and developing those chemicals into brand or trade name drug products for the market. Before an **investigational new drug application (INDA)** is reviewed by the FDA or clinical studies are initiated, the pharmaceutical company must do extensive preclinical animal laboratory research; once an investigational new drug (IND) is approved by the FDA and the study has received approval by its institutional review board (IRB), human studies may begin.

The IRB, also known as the Human Use Committee, is comprised of scientists and practitioners from various disciplines as well as consumers from an institutional setting such as a university or hospital. The committee is charged with the responsibility to review, approve, and monitor all medical research involving humans. The proposed research must meet both scientific and ethical standards to be approved. Each research subject must sign an **informed consent**, a document that states, in easily understandable terms, the purpose and risks of the research.

Clinical Studies Scientists conduct three phases of clinical studies as part of the drug approval process. Phase 1 is the initial study or trial of new drugs in humans, usually completed on a small number of healthy volunteers. The main purpose of this phase is to gather sufficient data concerning the drug's actions and potential side effects. The information obtained is then used to design future clinical trials. A Phase 2 study is primarily meant to evaluate the effectiveness as well as the safety of a drug for a given indication or disease state. Phase 2 studies also involve a small number of patients and are well controlled and closely monitored by the FDA. If the results of Phase 1 and Phase 2 studies are promising, Phase 3 studies are conducted in larger clinical trials to better assess the benefits and risks of the investigational drug on patients.

New Drug Application for Brand Name Drugs If the investigational drug shows promise after Phase 3 studies are completed, the pharmaceutical manufacturer can apply for a new drug application (NDA) to the FDA. In the NDA, the applicant must prove the case for both the safety and the effectiveness of the drug before marketing. The results of the scientific studies are evaluated by an advisory panel of experts and recommendations are forwarded to the FDA. If the benefit of the drug outweighs the risk, generally the drug is approved (see Figure 3.3). The FDA may also request that additional studies be completed. The drug approval process may take a year or longer in most cases. Occasionally, when a medication appears to be very promising early on in the testing, the FDA may opt to fast-track the drug and grant early approval. A recent example of this accelerated process can be seen with the quick approval of drugs to control HIV.

Drug development is risky as well as costly. Out of 5,000 to 10,000 screened compounds, only 250 enter preclinical research testing, 5 enter human clinical trials, and 1 new compound is approved by the FDA. The cost of developing a new drug today is

FIGURE 3.3
The Three Phases of the Drug Approval Process

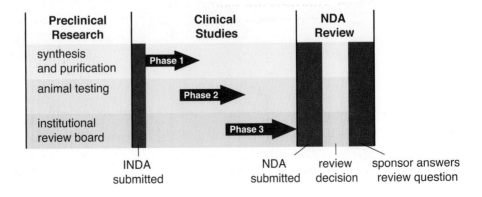

more than $1 billion, and it can take 15 years of research and development to bring a new medication from the laboratory to the pharmacy shelf.

Although the exorbitant costs and lengthy approval process can be daunting for pharmaceutical manufacturers, the financial incentive of patent protection on new drugs allows manufacturers to continue with their research and development of breakthrough drugs. The patent for a brand name drug is granted for an extended period, which allows the manufacturer sufficient time to recover the costs of clinical research. For this reason, brand name prescription drugs are costly for consumers—which may be a point of contention at the pharmacy counter during prescription pickup. Pharmacy personnel may want to address the issue of high-priced brand name drugs with their patients by explaining the relationship between the drug approval process and the high cost of brand name drugs.

Abbreviated New Drug Application for Generic Drugs   As discussed in Chapter 2, a **generic drug** contains the same active ingredients as the brand name product and delivers the same amount of medication to the body in the same way and in the same amount of time. Generic drugs are big business in any pharmacy. More than one billion generic prescriptions are dispensed every year, which accounts for nearly 80% of all prescription drugs. This number is expected to increase to 85% by 2016 as more brand name drugs become "off patent" (see Table 3.1).

Once the patent is due to expire on a brand name drug, a generic pharmaceutical company may submit an **abbreviated new drug application (aNDA)** to the FDA for drug approval. Generic drug applications are termed "abbreviated" because they are generally not required to include preclinical (animal) and clinical (human) data to establish safety and effectiveness. Instead, generic applicants must scientifically demonstrate that their product is **bioequivalent**, or performs in the same manner as an already approved brand name drug. Lipitor, for example, is a brand name drug that went "off patent" in 2012; atorvastatin is the generic name and is now available from several generic manufacturers who have formulated bioequivalent products.

One way scientists demonstrate bioequivalence between brand name and generic drugs is to measure the generic drug's **bioavailability**, or the time it takes the generic drug to reach the bloodstream in healthy volunteers and exert a pharmacological

TABLE 3.1 Blockbuster Drugs with Patent Expiration Years

Brand Name Drug	Generic Drug	Therapeutic Use	Patent Expiration Year
Nexium	esomeprazole	Heartburn, ulcers	2014
Celebrex	celecoxib	Arthritis	2014
Epogen	epoetin alfa	Anemia	2015
Crestor	rosuvastatin	High cholesterol	2016
Zetia	ezetimibe	High cholesterol	2016
Humira	adalimumab	Rheumatoid arthritis, etc.	2016
Cialis	tadalafil	Erectile dysfunction	2017
Remicade	infliximab	Rheumatoid arthritis, etc.	2018
Lyrica	pregabalin	Nerve pain, etc.	2019

effect. Bioavailability includes how a drug is absorbed, metabolized, distributed, or eliminated from the body. This study gives scientists the objective data necessary to compare the generic with that of the innovator (or brand name) drug. The generic version must deliver approximately the same amount of active ingredient into a patient's bloodstream in the same amount of time as the innovator drug.

The FDA is in the process of developing regulations for the approval of biogeneric or biosimilar versions of very expensive brand name biotechnology drugs. Unlike other generic drugs, "biosimilars" may require clinical trials for FDA approval.

Cost Savings of Generic Drugs

Most insurance plans, including the government-sponsored Medicare Part D plans, strongly encourage the widespread use of lower-cost generic drugs unless a physician states "brand name drug necessary" on the prescription. The pharmacy technician, under the supervision of the pharmacist, may encourage the use of available generic drugs to lower patients' out-of-pocket costs.

The dispensing of generic drugs is a major factor in containing the high cost of pharmaceuticals, with a cost savings of 30% to 80% over their brand name counterparts. In 2010, the average co-pay (not total retail cost) of a generic prescription drug was just over six dollars, whereas the co-pay of preferred and nonpreferred brand name prescription drugs was four to five times higher. Generic drugs have considerably slowed the rate of cost increases on pharmaceuticals.

The cost savings to patients and pharmacies occurs because, unlike the development of brand name drugs, generic manufacturers do not have to "front-end" the $1 billion in research costs that accompany each brand name drug discovery. With the possible exception of biogeneric drugs, generic manufacturers do not have to complete the Phase 1–3 studies to prove safety and efficacy of their products. These manufacturers only need to have evidence of their generic drugs' bioavailability. An added incentive for generic manufacturers is the FDA regulation that grants a 180-day exclusivity period for one or more manufacturers of aNDAs after the expiration of a patent. After this period, multiple generic companies—including many located outside the United States—may then manufacture the product, thus fostering competitive pricing.

National Drug Code Number

Under the Drug Listing Act of 1972, discussed in Chapter 2, once a brand name or generic drug receives FDA approval, each one is assigned a unique **National Drug Code (NDC) number** that appears on all drug stock labels as well as on copies of duplicate prescription labels filed in the pharmacy. The 10- to 11-character NDC number is made up of the following parts:

- a four- or five-digit *labeler code*, identifying the manufacturer or distributor of the drug
- a three- or four-digit *product code*, identifying the drug (active ingredient and its dosage form)
- a one- or two-digit *package code*, identifying the packaging size and type

The NDC number plays a crucial role for the pharmacy technician in the checks and balances of preventing avoidable medication errors during the dispensing process, a topic which is further discussed in Chapters 6 and 12. The pharmacy technician should focus on the three- or four-digit product code, or the middle number of the

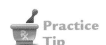
Practice Tip

When filling a prescription, pharmacy technicians should focus on the three- or four-digit product code, or the middle number of the NDC.

FIGURE 3.4
NDC Number and Bar Code

For both of these labels for Vistaril, the first four digits of the NDC number (0069) indicate Pfizer Labs. The second four digits indicate the product code. The last two digits of the NDC number define the packaging size and type. (a) The product code (5420) identifies the drug as hydroxyzine pamoate, 50 mg oral capsules. (b) The product code (5410) identifies the drug as hydroxyzine pamoate, 25 mg oral capsules.

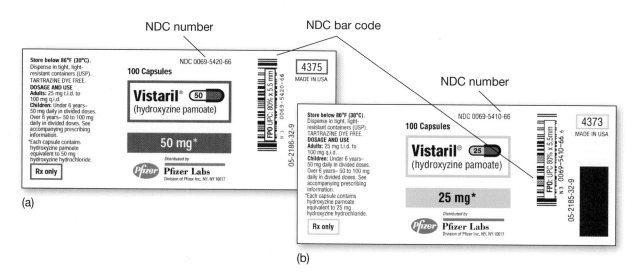

NDC, when filling a prescription. The NDC number bar code is commonly used by pharmacy personnel to verify that the correct drug is dispensed at time of filling.

Figure 3.4 shows NDC numbers and corresponding bar codes on labels for two different dosages of hydroxyzine pamoate.

Drug Information for Health Professionals

The FDA requires that manufacturers provide scientific information to the pharmacist with all prescription drug products. This information is contained in a **product package insert (PPI)** when the stock medication is sent to the pharmacy from the wholesaler. The information on the PPI is provided in a specific order as shown in Table 3.2. Of particular interest to the pharmacy technician is the information on storage and handling requirements.

The PPI is an information resource for the pharmacist and pharmacy technician, not for the patient. This insert provides pharmacy personnel with basic information on drug names, doses, indications, side effects, and adverse reactions. Pharmacy technicians should expand their knowledge of new drugs by reading these helpful documents when an opportunity arises in their workday.

Product package inserts are attached to or placed inside stock bottles. These inserts provide detailed information about the drug for the pharmacist and pharmacy technician.

TABLE 3.2   Organization of the Information in a Product Package Insert

- Description
- Clinical pharmacology
- Indications and usage
- Contraindications
- Warnings
- Precautions
- Adverse reactions
- Overdosage
- Dosage and administration
- Clinical studies
- How supplied/storage and handling
- Date of the most recent revision of the labeling

Side effects and adverse reactions noted on a PPI may also be highlighted within a black box. A **black box warning** (or boxed warning) is a warning statement on the PPI and patient medication guide indicating the possibility of a serious or even life-threatening adverse reaction from a drug. A thick black border surrounds the statement, hence the name. This box is required by the FDA and is based on the agency's postsurveillance studies of the adverse effects of approved drugs. To gather this data, physicians and pharmacists are encouraged to submit reports to the drugs' pharmaceutical manufacturers on potential and unexpected side effects. The manufacturers, in turn, are required to submit all reports to the FDA for further review and investigation. The FDA has two such reporting systems for adverse drug reactions (ADRs): MedWatch and Vaccine Adverse Event Reporting System (VAERS), which are discussed below. If the side effect or adverse reaction is being reported from different sources and is deemed a threat to patient safety, the FDA may then require the drug's manufacturer to insert a black box warning for healthcare professionals. Aside from its inclusion in the PPI, a black box warning is also published in the *Physician's Desk Reference*, or *PDR*. OTC drugs may also carry black box warnings on their labels.

The FDA recently mandated black box warning statements for several injectable biotechnology drugs including Enbrel, Remicade, and Humira. These drugs work by suppressing the immune system, thus increasing patient susceptibility to two rare but serious bacterial infections. Another black box warning was issued for Darvocet, a drug that had been on the market for 50 years. Further studies demonstrated that the pain medication had an adverse effect on the heart. One year later, Darvocet was withdrawn from the market.

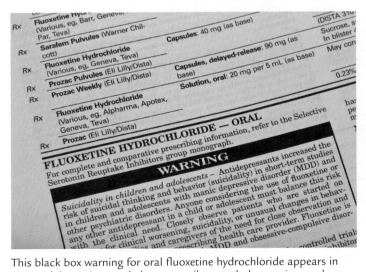

This black box warning for oral fluoxetine hydrochloride appears in *Facts and Comparisons* and alerts prescribers and pharmacists to the possibility of severe adverse reactions.

Drug Information for Consumers

For consumers, the FDA communicates side effects, adverse reactions, and black box warnings through either a patient package insert—such as the type accompanying birth control pills—or a supplemental printed medication guide called a **MedGuide**. The FDA develops the list of drugs requiring these information sheets and approves the information presented on the sheets. Common drugs that require an FDA-mandated MedGuide are listed in Table 3.3.

Based on the FDA mandate, the manufacturer of the drug is then responsible for providing the approved information in an easily understandable format to the pharmacy for sharing with patients. The information provided in the MedGuide is designed to further assist the patient in the proper use of the prescribed medication and to minimize the risk of serious adverse drug reactions. Therefore, each MedGuide is designed to:

- inform the patient about the drug product
- promote the safe and effective use of prescription drug products by the patient
- ensure that the patient has the opportunity to be informed of the benefits and risks involved in the use of that prescription drug product.

TABLE 3.3 Examples of Drugs Requiring a MedGuide

Drug	Risk Factor
Accutane	Causes birth defects in women of childbearing age; women must be on some form of birth control or be advised not to get pregnant while on this medication
Adderall	May cause insomnia, loss of appetite, and changes in pulse and blood pressure; monitor symptoms and vital signs
antidepressants	May be associated with an increase in suicide risk, especially in adolescent patients; watch for changes in behavior
birth control pills	Cause an increased risk of heart attack or stroke among smokers; the patient taking this type of drug should not smoke
Ciprofloxacin	May cause tendon rupture
Concerta	Is similar to Adderall
Coumadin	Reduces blood clotting, so the patient must be careful when working with sharp objects, shaving, and participating in contact sports while taking this drug; interacts with many drugs
NSAIDs	May cause an increase in the risk of stomach ulcers; take with food and no longer than necessary
Ritalin	Is similar to Adderall
Sildenafil	May cause dangerous lowering of blood pressure if taken with nitrates
Strattera	May interfere with growth and weight in children
Transmucosal Immediate-Release Fentanyl (TIRF)	Indicated only for breakthrough pain in cancer patients tolerant and maintained on around-the-clock opioid therapy; inappropriate conversions, dose, or misuse/abuse can lead to respiratory depression and even death

In pharmacy practice, the MedGuide is printed with supplemental medication information sheets for final verification of the prescription, medication, and label by the pharmacist. The medication information sheets and MedGuides are usually attached to the bag containing the medication(s) when the medications are given to the patient.

Legally, these medication guides are extensions of the labeling on the drug product, and the laws and regulations involving misbranding or mislabeling apply to them. If the required MedGuides are not distributed, the pharmacy is subject to heavy fines during an audit. The pharmacy technician should encourage the consumer to read this information, especially on all new drugs, and call the pharmacist with any questions or concerns.

Postmarketing Surveillance

Although every medication goes through a rigorous approval process, consumers should keep in mind that all drugs have a risk of toxicity. In recognition of this fact, the FDA continues to gather information about approved medications—in particular, about any serious adverse reactions that were not identified from research studies in the NDA. An **adverse drug reaction (ADR)** is defined as a negative consequence to a patient from taking a particular drug. Indeed, despite many years of research and clinical studies, some medications will enter the marketplace and place the patient at risk for a serious adverse reaction—an event that may not always be preventable or predictable. Once millions of prescriptions are written (or vaccine doses administered) for patients of all ages, rare adverse effects may suddenly appear in the general population.

Due to these potential risks, the FDA recognized the need to establish a nationwide postmarketing surveillance system to serve as a conduit for reporting serious adverse effects of certain medications. This adverse event reporting system (AERS) is a centralized database that stores information from two separate programs: MedWatch and VAERS. The AERS database publishes a quarterly newsletter that can be accessed online at www.paradigmcollege.net/pharmpractice5e/AERSdatabase.

MedWatch The FDA, in collaboration with the Institute of Safe Medication Practices (ISMP), provides a medication safety system called **MedWatch**, a voluntary program that allows any healthcare professional or consumer to report a serious adverse event associated with the use of any drug, biological device, or dietary supplement. Reports can be filed for all drugs online and are protected by privacy laws. Manufacturer labeling for all OTC drugs and dietary supplements must also include a toll-free number to report adverse effects. The FDA uses this information to track problems or issues that were not apparent when the medication was initially approved. In fact, the occurrence of some side effects may be so rare that it can only be detected in a large population after the drug comes to market. The recognition of a potential problem does not always mean the product will be removed from the market. Many times, other initiatives are implemented to reduce or eliminate a safety risk, such as improving prescribing information, increasing awareness by educating healthcare professionals or the public, or perhaps simply changing the name or labeling.

After gathering and assessing this reported information, the FDA may respond in two ways: (1) issuing safety alerts for drugs (including drug recalls), biologics, dietary supplements, and counterfeit drugs; and (2) requesting medication-labeling changes to the PPI, including contraindications, warnings, boxed warnings, precautions, and adverse reactions. For example, some research studies indicated that the diabetes drug

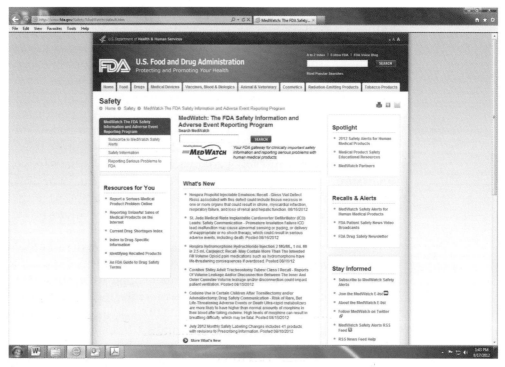

The FDA MedWatch website has the latest safety information for prescription drugs. The FDA also provides the MedWatch Online Voluntary Reporting Form (3500) for pharmacists to document an adverse drug reaction.

Avandia may increase the risk of a heart attack. Rather than recommend withdrawal of Avandia from the market, the FDA initially recommended labeling changes (black box warnings) in both the PPI for the pharmacist and the required MedGuide for the consumer. Further reports and scientific studies led the FDA to recommend that a risk evaluation and mitigation strategy (REMS) be developed by the pharmaceutical manufacturer further limiting the use of this drug. (For more information on REMS, refer to the section below.)

Safety alerts and labeling changes are published in a monthly newsletter. To review all medication safety alerts, go to www.paradigmcollege.net/pharmpractice5e/MedWatch and search "MedWatch," or sign up for the newsletter and alerts by e-mail.

Vaccine Adverse Event Reporting System (VAERS) A separate reporting system, called **Vaccine Adverse Event Reporting System (VAERS)**, is a postmarketing national safety surveillance system operated by the FDA and the Centers for Disease Control and Prevention (CDC) to collect and analyze information on adverse events that occur after an immunization. Since 1990, VAERS has received over 123,000 reports, most of which describe mild side effects such as fever. As with medications, hundreds of thousands of vaccine administrations may be required to detect a potential problem. In fact, it may take more than a million doses of a vaccine for a few adverse effects to occur and be investigated.

The FDA and the CDC use VAERS information to ensure the safest strategies of vaccine use and to further reduce the rare risks associated with vaccines. Although the benefits of immunization far outweigh the risks, some parents believe that administration of vaccines can result in autism, a developmental disorder, and have opted not to vaccinate their children. However, there is no scientific proof of this relationship. Pharmacists should continue to educate hesitant parents about the importance of childhood vaccinations.

Healthcare personnel are mandated by the National Childhood Vaccine Injury Act of 1986 to report serious adverse reactions from vaccines. Patients can report any problems with a vaccine as well. A VAERS report can be made online (www.paradigmcollege.net/ pharmpractice5e/VAERSonline), via an 800 number (1-800-822-7967), or by mail or fax on a downloaded form. With pharmacists and their technicians becoming more involved in vaccine administration, it is important to report any adverse effects.

Risk Evaluation and Mitigation Strategies

The FDA Amendments Act of 2007 gave the FDA the authority to require that a **risk evaluation and mitigation strategy (REMS)** be developed by drug manufacturers to ensure that the benefits of their drug outweigh the risks. One of the strategies authorized by this amendment was the development of MedGuides (discussed earlier) for consumer education on high-risk drugs.

Some drugs require more communications or an even more focused strategy—for example, isotretinoin for severe acne, fentanyl (Actiq) immediate-release narcotic for severe pain, Subutex and Suboxone for opioid dependence, and dofetilide (Tikosyn) for irregular heart rates. Drug manufacturers maintain a centralized database to more closely monitor patients on these high-risk drugs and must make periodic assessment reports to the FDA on the status of the REMS for each drug.

iPLEDGE Program This REMS program was designed for two reasons: (1) to prevent fetal exposure to the drug isotretinoin (Accutane, Claravis, Sotret); and (2) to inform and educate all healthcare providers and patients, male and female, on drug risks and how to use this medication safely. Isotretinoin is a drug with a very high incidence of teratogenicity or harm to the fetus. All prescribers, pharmacies, and drug wholesalers must be annually enrolled and certified to participate in this program; all patients must be registered and agree to meet all conditions required during treatment.

Prescribers must agree to provide contraception counseling to patients prior to and during treatment with this drug. If patients are sexually active, prescribers must document the forms of contraception the patients are currently using. For female patients with childbearing potential, a monthly pregnancy test is required and must have a negative result prior to prescribers issuing a prescription for this medication. Consequently, the quantity of medication written is limited to a 30-day supply with no refills. All pregnancies while on this drug must be reported.

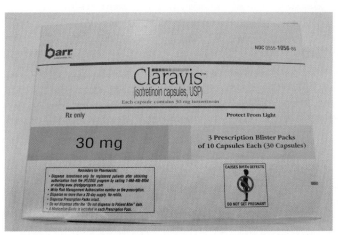

Claravis is a brand of isotretinoin that requires a REMS due to a high risk of birth defects.

In addition, pharmacies may only receive the drug from a certified wholesaler and can only dispense to patients registered in the iPLEDGE program with written prescriptions authorized by a certified prescriber. An assigned Risk Management Authorization (RMA) number must be placed on each prescription, and a MedGuide must be dispensed with each prescription. There are specified allowable time limits (usually seven days) to pick up the medication at the pharmacy.

Patients also share responsibilities while on this drug. Aside from registration and education, patients must agree not to share their medication with anyone or donate blood while on the medication and for one month after discontinuing the drug. Women of childbearing potential must agree to monthly pregnancy tests and, if sexually active, two forms of contraception while on the drug and for one month after discontinuation of the drug. In addition, they must agree to pick up the prescription within a specified period or the prescription is voided.

Transmucosal Immediate-Release Fentanyl (TIRF) Similar to the iPLEDGE program, this REMS program is designed to mitigate the risk of misuse, abuse, addiction, overdose, or severe complications due to various medication errors by the following actions: (1) prescribing only to appropriate opioid-dependent cancer patients; (2) preventing inappropriate dosage conversion from similar narcotics; (3) promoting safe storage to prevent accidental exposure to children; and (4) educating prescribers, pharmacists, and patients on the safe and appropriate use of fentanyl.

For participation in this program, prescribers, pharmacies (both hospital and retail), and wholesalers must enroll and be certified after completing an educational program; renewal is every two years. Prescribers must be aware that the drug is indicated only for the treatment of breakthrough pain in cancer patients who are tolerant to around-the-clock opioid therapy. Drug dose conversions are specified, as are definitions for opioid tolerance and dependence. The dose for brand and generic TIRF is interchangeable. Prescribers must agree to initiate therapy with the lowest dose, follow up on efficacy of dose titration, and document any signs of misuse or abuse. Pharmacies are responsible for training all staff including pharmacy technicians; hospital pharmacies can dispense TIRF to inpatients only.

Patients are also required to follow certain guidelines. They must sign an agreement with the prescriber, review and study the MedGuide, and follow prescribed instructions exactly. There can be no transfer of medication to others, and if, for any reason, the opioid therapy is discontinued, then the TIRF therapy must also be stopped. Patients must also agree to safely store and discard the medication to prevent harm to children and pets.

Subutex and Suboxone These sublingual (under the tongue) medications are prescribed by doctors certified to treat opioid dependence by the Drug Addiction and Treatment Act of 2000. The DEA number of certified physicians starts with an "x." Subutex is commonly prescribed for induction treatment, and Suboxone (sublingual tablets and dissolving film) for maintenance therapy. The goals of this REMS program are to mitigate the risks of accidental overdose, misuse, and abuse and to inform patients of serious risks. Prescribers must use low doses, conduct frequent follow-up visits for monitoring to assess efficacy, and provide counseling and psychosocial supports for the patient.

Pharmacies that dispense Subutex and Suboxone agree to provide a MedGuide on each prescription and to counsel the patient on the safe use of the medication, including potential drug interactions with alcohol, nerve/sleep pills (benzodiazepines), and antidepressants. The pharmacist should also counsel patients on securely and safely storing their medication to deter theft or access by children.

Tikosyn Many potent antiarrhythmic drugs used to treat an irregular heart rate, such as Tikosyn, can cause serious and sometimes fatal arrhythmias. To minimize this risk, a REMS program was developed by the drug manufacturer to establish dispensing and administration protocol for Tikosyn. This protocol dictates that the drug can only be prescribed and dispensed by those physicians and pharmacies that have been enrolled, educated, and certified in the program. In addition, physicians who are providing prescriptions for this medication must agree to follow manufacturer and FDA-approved guidelines for drug dosing and to inform their patients on the risks of the medication.

Initial therapy can only be conducted in healthcare facilities in which the drug can be carefully monitored for adverse effects; laboratory tests for kidney function, electrocardiograms, and cardiopulmonary resuscitation (CPR) equipment should be readily available. All pharmacy personnel must be trained in the protocol for Tikosyn, and each prescription dispensed must receive a special stamp provided by the drug manufacturer. Physicians and pharmacies achieve recertification one time based on their compliance with the REMS guidelines.

Drug Recall Process

Once a drug is approved, FDA oversight continues. A manufacturer is required to report any serious side effects and adverse reactions to the FDA. The FDA has the authority to obtain an injunction from the court and force the manufacturer to recall the drug product if it is contaminated or of poor quality or if it causes serious adverse reactions. In some cases in which the risk is greater than the perceived benefit, the FDA may issue a **drug recall** and withdraw the drug from the market; in other cases, the manufacturer may voluntarily withdraw the prescription or OTC drug due to future liability concerns. Such a case occurred in 2012: The pharmaceutical manufacturer Novartis withdrew Excedrin and Bufferin from the market due to suspected defects in some batches of product.

Three classes of recalls exist, and the FDA staff determines which class of recall is issued based on reports from the particular manufacturer and from healthcare providers. Table 3.4 describes the three types of recalls. A pharmacy wholesaler will commonly send a list of drugs with NDC and lot numbers that have been recalled so that the pharmacist or pharmacy technician can remove any such drugs from their pharmacy's inventory "to protect the patient." A Class I recall is serious and requires immediate action by pharmacy personnel. The role of the pharmacy technician in drug recalls is further explained in Chapter 7.

A resource web link to identify drug recalls is www.paradigmcollege.net/pharmpractice5e/drugrecalls. Consumers can return a recalled drug for refund or credit per store policy. The FDA's role under the guidelines is to monitor company recalls and assess the adequacy of the company's action. After a recall is completed, the FDA makes sure that the product is destroyed or suitably reconditioned and investigates why the product was defective.

TABLE 3.4 Recall Classes for Drugs

Class	Risk
I	A reasonable probability exists that use of the product will cause or lead to serious adverse health events or death. An example of a product that could fall into this category is a label mix-up on a lifesaving drug.
II	The probability exists that use of the product will cause adverse health events that are temporary or medically reversible. One example is a drug that is understrength but that is not used to treat life-threatening situations.
III	The use of the product will probably not cause an adverse health event. Examples might be a container defect, odd flavor, or wrong color in a liquid.

Pharmaceutical Equivalence and Pharmaceutical Alternatives

In addition to the manufacturer's PPI, printed medication information printouts, and MedGuides, other computerized and hard copy references may serve as a reference for pharmacy technicians. In all states, pharmacists or pharmacy technicians are permitted (or in some cases required) to substitute a lower-cost generic drug in place of a higher-cost brand name drug, as long as the generic drug is considered "equivalent." To help pharmacy personnel determine this, they can refer to the **FDA Online Orange Book** (also known as the *Approved Drug Products with Therapeutic Equivalence Evaluations*). This publication is available online and provides information on generic substitution of drugs that may have many different brand name or generic manufacturer sources. This online reference lists the drug products that the FDA considers to be (or not to be) therapeutically equivalent to other pharmaceutically equivalent products.

Pharmaceutically equivalent drug products are formulated to contain the same amount of active ingredient in the same dosage form in order to meet the same compendial or *USP–NF* standards (for strength, quality, purity, and identity) as an FDA-approved drug. However, pharmaceutically equivalent drug products may differ in characteristics such as shape, scoring configuration, release mechanisms, packaging, excipients (including colorings, flavors, and preservatives), expiration time, and—within certain limits—labeling. A vast majority of all FDA-approved drugs have a pharmaceutically equivalent generic product. A common example is the drug lisinopril 20 mg: The dosage unit may look different (i.e., have different markings), but the drug is absorbed in the same manner and exerts the same pharmacological effect (a decrease in blood pressure).

Pharmaceutical alternative drug products contain the same active therapeutic ingredient but contain different salts (for example, hydroxyzine hydrochloride rather than hydroxyzine pamoate) or are available in different dosage forms (a tablet rather than a capsule or an immediate-release tablet rather than an extended-release tablet). Different salts and dosage forms generally *cannot be substituted* without approval from the physician. Thus, for a prescription written for 100 mg of metoprolol succinate (an extended-release formulation), a pharmacy technician cannot substitute 100 mg of metoprolol tartrate (an immediate-release formulation). Although the active ingredients and dose are identical, the salts differ (succinate versus tartrate) and the release characteristics of the drug formulations differ. Dosage formulations will be discussed further in Chapter 4.

Some drug insurance companies may not allow coverage for a brand name pharmaceutical alternative drug with a unique salt or dosage formulation. If a pharmacy technician notes that insurance will not cover a prescribed drug, or the co-pay is too high for the patient, this observation should be brought to the immediate attention of the pharmacist. Often, once the prescriber is contacted, the prescription may be changed to a generic drug.

Drug products are considered to be therapeutic equivalents only if they are pharmaceutical equivalents and if they can be expected to have the same clinical effect and safety profile when administered to a patient under the conditions specified in the labeling. Under most circumstances, if a generic drug is both bioequivalent and therapeutically equivalent, it is "substitutable" for the brand name product by the pharmacist without prior approval of the physician. The laws and procedures governing generic substitution in the community pharmacy will be further discussed in Chapter 6.

Therapeutic equivalence evaluation codes are provided for all dosage forms—oral products, aerosols, topicals, and injectables. In general, if the specific generic product is listed as an "A" category, the drug is considered to be therapeutically equivalent and can safely be substituted; if the product is listed as a "B" category, then some discrepancy exists in its therapeutic effect and that product cannot be substituted.

The *FDA Online Orange Book* lists drugs and doses from generic manufacturers that may be safely substituted. For example, two brand name antihypertensive drugs such as Adalat CC and Procardia XL cannot be substituted for one another due to different drug release characteristics. There are, however, generic manufactured drugs that are compatible with either or both of the brand name drugs that can be substituted (see Table 3.5). The Actavis and Watson brands of nifedipine in doses of 30 mg and 60 mg can be substituted for Adalat CC; likewise, the Matrix Labs brand can be substituted for Procardia XL. Note that the Mylan brand can be substituted for either brand name drug. (Mylan had submitted sufficient evidence of therapeutic equivalence to the FDA to gain substitution approval for both Adalat CC and Procardia XL.) In most cases, the software your pharmacy utilizes will cross-reference the FDA-approved generic equivalents of a given brand name drug.

Each state may vary in procedures for dispensing generic or therapeutic equivalents. In most cases, a generic drug is freely substituted. Some physicians (and patients) do not like to substitute brands on their medications even if the medications are considered pharmaceutically and therapeutically equivalent; this is often the case with thyroid prescriptions written by an endocrinologist. The prescriber is permitted by law to write "brand medically necessary" on the prescription. For new prescriptions, pharmacy technicians should look for the words "brand medically necessary" on the prescription.

The patient may also request that a brand name product be dispensed even if the prescriber did not write "brand medically necessary" on the prescription; this often results in a higher co-pay from insurance. At times, a patient may request a lower-cost generic even though the physician wrote "brand necessary" on the prescription; a call to the physician's office is necessary to approve the generic over the brand name drug.

In general, it is not good practice for the patient to keep switching between brand name or generic products even if they are bioequivalent and therapeutically equivalent. Laboratory results may differ, though the brand name and generic product are prescribed at the same dose. For refills, it is important for the pharmacy technician to review the patient profile and see if a brand name or generic product was previously dispensed.

Just as with brand name drugs, not all patients will respond similarly to generic drugs. The pharmacy technician can, however, reassure the patient that the generic product in stock has received FDA approval. If in doubt, go online to the FDA website or ask the pharmacist before entering information into the computer or filling the prescription.

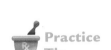

Practice Tip

When processing a prescription, pharmacy technicians may see either "brand medically necessary" or "dispense as written" expressed by the prescriber. These phrases are interchangeable and typically indicate that no substitution of medication can be made without the approval of the prescriber.

TABLE 3.5 Generic Drugs Therapeutically Equivalent to Adalat CC (AB1) and Procardia XL (AB2)

Therapeutic Equivalents Code	Generic Name	Manufacturer
AB1	Nifedipine 30 mg, 60 mg	Actavis
AB1	Nifedipine 30 mg, 60 mg	Watson
AB1, AB2	Nifedipine 30 mg, 60 mg, 90 mg	Mylan
AB2	Nifedipine 30 mg, 60 mg, 90 mg	Matrix Labs

Other Pharmacy Drug References

In addition to the *FDA Online Orange Book*, two reference works published by the USP establish the official legal standards for drugs in the United States: the *USP* (which describes drug substances and dosage forms) and the *National Formulary* (which describes pharmaceutical ingredients). Both are revised every five years, and supplements are published in between revisions. These two reference works are also printed in a combined edition known as the *United States Pharmacopeia–National Formulary (USP–NF)*. These detailed compendia drug standards are utilized by all pharmaceutical companies when submitting a new drug application to the FDA.

Several other reference books may also be helpful in various practice settings. Below is a summary of these important pharmacy drug references.

- *Physician's Desk Reference (PDR)* is published annually with reprints of PPIs from the pharmaceutical manufacturers of most drugs. This book is also useful for identifying unknown drugs by color, shape, and coding and for containing black box warnings for the pharmacist and pharmacy technician. Pharmacy technicians can learn more about the drugs that they are dispensing by studying the *PDR* and reading PPIs during any free or slow times in the pharmacy. This reference book is also available for consumer purchase in most bookstores.
- *Drug Facts and Comparisons* includes factual information on product availability, indications, administration and dose, pharmacological actions, contraindications, warnings, precautions, adverse reactions, overdose, and patient instructions. It is available as a hardbound copy, as a loose-leaf binder with monthly updates, and as a CD-ROM.
- *American Drug Index* is a commonly used reference in most pharmacies. This reference lists brand and generic drug names for all FDA-approved medications.
- Thomson Reuters Micromedex, an online computerized database, features monographs on more than 1,400 FDA-approved drugs including dosing, adverse reactions, and drug-drug interactions. This reference also includes an expanded, unbiased, evidence-based medicine ratings of drug indications.
- *Handbook of Nonprescription Drugs* is published by the American Pharmacists Association and provides a good background text reference for OTC drugs.
- *Remington: The Science and Practice of Pharmacy* is an excellent extensive text, especially for use in a compounding pharmacy where determinations of drug stability and compatibility are important. This reference covers the integration of scientific principles into clinical practice.
- *Homeopathic Pharmacopeia of the United States (HPUS)*, now called the *Homœopathic Pharmacopœia of the United States Revision Service (HPRS)*, is a compilation of standards for the source, composition, and preparation of homeopathic medications that may be sold in the community pharmacy.
- *American Hospital Formulary Service (AHFS)* is an excellent source of information, especially on parenteral drugs commonly used in hospital, long-term care, or home healthcare settings.
- Trissel's *Stability of Compounded Formulations* is an excellent reference for the pharmacy technician checking IV drug incompatibilities in the hospital or specialty compounding pharmacy. The book provides important stability and storage information in monographs on many compounded drug formulations (injectable, oral, enteral, topical, ophthalmic) in accordance with documented standards.
- *The Lawrence Review of Natural Products* provides up-to-date, objective, scientific monographs on more than 350 herbal medications.

Chapter Summary

- Within the past 300 years, several drug discoveries by various scientists have positively impacted the quality and quantity of life.
- Drugs are natural, synthetic, synthesized, or semisynthetic substances taken into or applied to the body to alter biochemical functions and achieve a desired pharmacological effect.
- Drugs can be classified as OTC, homeopathic, or prescription as regulated by the FDA.
- Overuse and abuse of controlled substances can lead to tolerance, psychological dependence, physical dependence, and addiction.
- The FDA requires manufacturers of OTC drugs to have extensive and easily understood labeling for consumers' self-use.
- Dietary supplements, which include vitamins, minerals, and herbs, are regulated under the DSHEA amendments.
- Uses of a drug may include one or more of the following: therapeutic, pharmacodynamic, diagnostic, prophylactic, or destructive agents.
- Congress charged the USP with developing adequate standards to protect the consumer.
- The approval process consists of many different phases of preclinical animal and clinical human studies leading to submission of a new drug application to the FDA.
- For approximately every 10,000 chemicals studied, only one product will be approved by the FDA at a research cost of more than $1 billion.
- For FDA approval, generic drugs need only show bioequivalence to an innovator or brand name product.
- Generic drugs provide a significant cost savings to consumers due to lower research expenditures and more competition in the marketplace.
- In order to substitute for a brand name prescription, a generic drug must show pharmaceutical and therapeutic equivalence.
- The NDC number is specific for each manufacturer, drug product, dose, and package size and is very important in preventing medication errors and in executing drug recalls.
- The FDA is charged with communicating various levels of drug recalls from time to time.
- The FDA monitors adverse effects of drugs and vaccines through its MedWatch and VAERS postmarketing surveillance programs.
- The FDA communicates serious or life-threatening effects of drugs through black box warnings to healthcare professionals in the PPI and to consumers in MedGuides.
- Drug manufacturers, with the encouragement of the FDA, develop REMS for select high-risk drugs to minimize serious adverse side effects.
- Pharmaceutically equivalent and alternative drug products from various manufacturers are listed in the *FDA Online Orange Book*.
- A multitude of good reference texts and websites exist that the practicing pharmacist and pharmacy technician can use to study various pharmaceutical products.

Key Terms

abbreviated new drug application (aNDA) the process by which applicants must scientifically demonstrate to the FDA that their generic product is bioequivalent to or performs in the same way as the innovator drug

active ingredient the biochemically active component of the drug that exerts a desired therapeutic effect

addiction compulsive and uncontrollable use of controlled substances, especially narcotics

adverse drug reaction (ADR) a negative consequence to a patient from taking a particular drug

antibiotic a chemical substance that is used in the treatment of bacterial infectious diseases and has the ability to either kill or inhibit the growth of certain harmful microorganisms

antibody the part of the immune system that neutralizes antigens or foreign substances in the body

antineoplastic drug a cancer-fighting drug

bactericidal having the ability to destroy bacteria

bioavailability the time it takes for a generic drug to reach the bloodstream in healthy volunteers

bioequivalent a generic drug that delivers approximately the same amount of active ingredient into a healthy volunteer's bloodstream in the same amount of time as the innovator or brand name drug

biotechnology the field of study that combines the sciences of biology, chemistry, and immunology to produce synthetic, unique drugs with specific therapeutic effects

black box warning a warning statement required by the FDA indicating a serious or even life-threatening adverse reaction from a drug; the warning statement is on the product package insert (PPI) for the pharmacy staff and in the MedGuide for consumers

deoxyribonucleic acid (DNA) the helix-shaped molecule that carries the genetic code

destructive agent a drug that kills bacteria, fungi, viruses, or even normal or cancer cells

diagnostic agent a chemical containing radioactive isotopes used to diagnose and treat disease

dietary supplement a category of nonprescription drugs that includes vitamins, minerals, and herbs that is not regulated by the FDA

drug any substance taken into or applied to the body for the purpose of altering the body's biochemical functions and thus its physiological processes

drug recall the process of withdrawing a drug from the market by the FDA or the drug manufacturer for serious adverse effects or other defects in the product

drug tolerance a situation that occurs when the body requires higher doses of a drug to produce the same therapeutic effect

FDA Online Orange Book an online reference that provides information on the generic and therapeutic equivalence of drugs that may have many different brand names or generic manufacturer sources

generic drug a drug that contains the same active ingredients as the brand name product and delivers the same amount of medication to the body in the same way and in the same duration of time; a drug that is not protected by a patent

genetic engineering process of using DNA biotechnology to create a variety of drugs

genome the entire DNA in an organism, including its genes

good manufacturing practices (GMPs) general principles and guidelines used during the manufacturing process to ensure a quality product

homeopathic medications a class of drugs in which very small dilutions of natural drugs are taken to stimulate the body's immune system

inert ingredient an inactive chemical—such as a filler, preservative, coloring, or flavoring—that is added to one or more active ingredients to improve drug formulations while causing little or no physiological effect; also called an *inactive ingredient*

informed consent a document that states, in easily understandable terms, the purpose and risks of the drug research

investigational new drug application (INDA) process by which a manufacturer submits research results from animal studies to the FDA to gain approval to gather data and investigate a new drug in humans

MedGuide written patient information mandated by the FDA for select high-risk drugs; also known as a *patient medication guide*

MedWatch a voluntary program run by the FDA for reporting serious adverse events, product problems, or medication errors; serves as a clearinghouse to provide information on safety alerts for drugs, biologics, dietary supplements, and medical devices as well as drug recalls

National Drug Code (NDC) number a unique number assigned to a brand name, generic, or OTC product to identify the manufacturer, drug, and packaging size

over-the-counter (OTC) drug a drug sold without a prescription

pharmaceutical alternative drug product a drug product that has the same active therapeutic ingredient but contains different salts or different dosage forms; cannot be substituted without prescriber authorization

pharmaceutically equivalent drug product a drug product that contains the same amount of active ingredient in the same dosage form and meets the same *USP–NF* compendial standards (i.e., strength, quality, purity, and identity); can be substituted without contacting the prescriber

pharmacodynamic agent a drug that alters body functions in a desired way

pharmacogenomics a field of study that examines the relationship between an individual's genes and his or her body's response to drugs

pharmacology the study of how drugs work inside the body for their intended purposes

physical dependence a state in which abruptly terminating a drug produces physical withdrawal symptoms such as restlessness, anxiety, insomnia, diarrhea, vomiting, and goose bumps

prescription drug a drug that requires a prescription from a licensed provider for a valid medical purpose; also known as a *legend drug*

product package insert (PPI) scientific information supplied to the pharmacist and technician by the manufacturer with all prescription drug products; the information must be approved by the FDA

prophylactic agent a drug used to prevent disease

psychological dependence a state in which taking a drug produces a sense of well-being and, consequently, the abrupt termination of the drug may create anxiety withdrawal symptoms

radiopharmaceutical a drug containing radioactive ingredients, often used for diagnostic or therapeutic purposes

ribonucleic acid (RNA) an important component of the genetic code that arranges amino acids into proteins

risk evaluation and mitigation strategy (REMS) a requirement by the FDA that procedures be developed by drug manufacturers to ensure that the benefits of selected high-risk drugs on the market outweigh their risks

semisynthetic drug a drug that contains both natural and synthetic components

synthesized drug a drug created artificially in the laboratory but in imitation of a naturally occurring drug

synthetic drug a drug that has been created from a series of chemical reactions to produce a specific pharmacological effect

therapeutic agent a drug that prevents, cures, diagnoses, or relieves symptoms of a disease

therapeutic effect the desired pharmacological action of a drug on the body

United States Pharmacopeia–National Formulary (USP–NF) a drug reference that contains standards for medicines, dosage forms, drug substances, excipients or inactive substances, medical devices, and dietary supplements

vaccine a substance introduced into the body to produce immunity to disease

Vaccine Adverse Event Reporting System (VAERS) a postmarketing surveillance system operated by the FDA and CDC that collects information on adverse events that occur after immunization

Chapter Review

Checking Your Understanding

To check your comprehension of this chapter's key concepts, read the following multiple-choice questions and then record your answers on a separate sheet of paper. Write your answers as modeled in these examples: 1d; 2c; 3b; etc.

1. Which type of FDA drug recall requires a pharmacy technician to immediately remove the product from the shelf?
   a. Class I
   b. Class II
   c. Class III
   d. Class IV

2. Jonas Salk is best known for his discovery of
   a. insulin.
   b. the HIV vaccine.
   c. the polio vaccine.
   d. the birth control pill.

3. Which of the following classifications of drugs is *not* directly under FDA control?
   a. homeopathic medications
   b. prescription drugs
   c. dietary supplements
   d. OTC drugs

4. What term can be defined as a condition in which a patient takes a drug on a regular basis because it produces a sense of well-being?
   a. addiction
   b. tolerance
   c. psychological dependence
   d. physical dependence

5. When a generic manufacturer files an aNDA with the FDA, it must prove
   a. bioequivalence.
   b. safety.
   c. efficacy.
   d. cost savings.

6. A radiopharmaceutical used for imaging is an example of a
   a. therapeutic agent.
   b. pharmacodynamic agent.
   c. diagnostic agent.
   d. prophylactic agent.

7. By which of the following means does the FDA communicate black box warnings to consumers on high-risk drugs?
   a. product package insert
   b. prescription label
   c. media (TV, radio, newspapers)
   d. MedGuide

8. What should you do if you receive a prescription with the words "brand medically necessary"?
   a. Substitute a lower-cost generic drug when filling the prescription.
   b. Check the *FDA Online Orange Book* for acceptable product substitutions.
   c. Realize that the prescription is written for a Schedule II drug that cannot be refilled.
   d. Fill the prescription as is with the brand name product.

9. The middle three- or four-digit code in a National Drug Code (NDC) number represents the
   a. product manufacturer.
   b. drug and dose.
   c. packaging size and type.
   d. schedule of the drug.

10. To determine generic equivalency of a brand name product, which reference source would you use?
    a. *Drug Facts and Comparisons*
    b. *FDA Online Orange Book*
    c. *Physician's Desk Reference*
    d. *Homeopathic Pharmacopeia Revision Service (HPRS)*

11. Which of the following drugs *is not* an FDA-required REMS?
    a. Avandia
    b. Accutane
    c. Actiq
    d. Adderall

12. The FDA monitors the incidence and risk of adverse drug reactions on the market with
    a. MedGuide.
    b. MedWatch.
    c. VAERS.
    d. DEA.

13. Which drug classification is comprised of antineoplastic drugs?
    a. therapeutic agents
    b. diagnostic agents
    c. prophylactic agents
    d. destructive agents

14. A written document that explains the risks and benefits of new drug research to a patient is called
    a. good research practice (GRP).
    b. therapeutic equivalence.
    c. informed consent.
    d. good manufacturing practice (GMP).

15. The text that describes USP standards for drug ingredients is called the
    a. *Physician's Desk Reference (PDR)*.
    b. *National Formulary*
    c. *Remington: The Science and Practice of Pharmacy*
    d. *Drug Facts and Comparisons*

Reinforcing Your Learning

To build on your understanding of the topics in this chapter, complete the following enrichment activities.

1. List all the various drug strengths of hydrocodone by drawing on your experience in the pharmacy where you work or by researching this topic on the Internet (www.paradigmcollege.net/pharmpractice5e/druginfo). What risks are associated with this drug? Find out how prevalent hydrocodone overuse and abuse is in your locality by asking a pharmacist. In light of your fact-finding, what recommendation would you make as to whether hydrocodone should be reclassified as a Schedule II drug by the federal government or your state board of pharmacy?

2. Determine the brand name, primary indications, precautions, storage conditions, and drug cost for the following gene therapy or biotechnology-based medications:
    a. etanercept
    b. adalimumab
    c. infliximab

3. Go to a community or chain pharmacy and make a list of five different package sizes of store-brand OTC products that contain dextromethorphan as the active ingredient. For each product on your list, write down the NDC number. Then compare the NDC numbers: Are some numbers the same? Are some numbers different? Based on what you learned, explain why the NDC number is critical for filling a prescription and for reducing medication errors in the pharmacy setting.

4. Visit a pharmacy and compare the boxed labeled directions and dose for the OTC product Aleve and the dietary supplement glucosamine. Which product label offers more safety information for the consumer? Why?

Thinking on Your Feet

To gain practice in handling challenging situations in the workplace, consider the following real-world scenarios and then use the guiding questions to help you formulate your responses.

1. A 51-year-old female patient requests information on the shingles (herpes zoster) vaccine that is administered at your pharmacy. You notice on the patient profile that she is taking Remicade. What rare but serious adverse reactions can occur with this medication? Is she a candidate for the vaccine? Knowing this information, how should you handle this patient's request?

2. A 75-year-old patient at your pharmacy counter is upset that he has to pay a higher amount for Spiriva because no generic equivalent exists. How would you explain to a patient in understandable terms the difference between a brand name product and a generic product? Are both approved by the FDA? Why does the generic drug cost so much less? Why is there not a generic equivalent for Spiriva on the market?

3. A mother brings in a prescription for Pulmozyme for her son. Which nebulizers are approved by the FDA for this drug? She has insurance, but the co-payment for Pulmozyme is still very expensive. Is there a coupon or discount program to help pay for the co-payment? How can you help the parent get some financial assistance? Go to www.paradigmcollege.net/pharmpractice5e/pulmozyme if you need help answering these questions in order to make a recommendation to the parent on how to lower the cost.

4. A 21-year-old female brings in a prescription for Claravis for the first time. She has no drug insurance and cannot afford the drug until her next paycheck. She returns to the pharmacy 10 days later to pick up the prescription, but it cannot be dispensed. Check www.paradigmcollege.net/pharmpractice5e/iPLEDGE and provide an explanation for the patient as to why the drug cannot be dispensed.

5. A patient brings in a prescription from her cardiologist for Coreg 6.25 mg 1 po bid #60 2 refills "brand necessary." She tells you that her drug insurance has expired since she lost her job and requests that you fill the prescription with a generic drug to save on cost. What do you do?

Acquiring Field Knowledge

To expand your knowledge of pharmacy practice, explore the following online activities that focus on research and information retrieval.

Reminder: *As you navigate the Internet, remember to exercise caution and good judgment when evaluating information. A thoughtful review of online text should take into consideration the following factors: the creator and sponsors of the website, the intended audience, the credentials of the authors and contributors, the reliability and validity of the posted information, the frequency of updates to the site, and the ease of navigation for a range of user skill levels.*

1. You are concerned for your own health because there is a high risk of breast cancer in your family. Is there a genetic test available to determine your risk? If you are at high risk, what are your choices for intervention? To find information on genetic screening for breast cancer, go to www.paradigmcollege.net/pharmpractice5e/breastcancer or conduct an online search using the phrase "breast cancer genetic testing." Record your findings to determine your course of action.

2. Go to the website of the Association of Natural Medicine Pharmacists (www.paradigmcollege.net/pharmpractice5e/ANMPginkgo) and locate the ginkgo biloba monograph; write up a summary of the primary indications, dosage, clinical efficacy, and safety of this herbal product.

3. Dietary supplements are not regulated by the FDA, yet the FDA recalled a dietary supplement in 2012: X-ROCK. Go to www.paradigmcollege.net/pharmpractice5e/X-ROCK and find a recall notice for X-ROCK. Why was this drug recalled? Upon what authority can the FDA recall this drug? With a partner, find other dietary supplements over the past 12 months that have required FDA intervention.

4. Compare the out-of-pocket cost of a 3-month or 90-day supply (quantity = #90) for the following generics or therapeutically equivalent drugs: Synthroid 100 mcg vs. levothyroxine 100 mcg, Nexium 40 mg vs. omeprazole 40 mg, and Crestor 10 mg vs. lovastatin 80 mg. Calculate the cost savings of the generic or therapeutic equivalent. Are the cost savings sufficient to justify the dispensing of the lower-cost product to save the consumer money?

Sampling the Certification Exam

To provide you with practice for the Certification Exam Review, read the following questions that have been patterned after the test format and then record your answers on a separate sheet of paper. Write your answers as modeled in these examples: 1d; 2c; 3b; *etc.*

1. Identify the generic drug name for the brand name drug Plavix.
   a. clopidogrel
   b. acetaminophen
   c. warfarin
   d. diphenhydramine

2. Which of the following is *not* an OTC drug?
   a. valcyclovir tablets
   b. hydrocortisone 1%
   c. cetirizine syrup
   d. Mucinex-D 12-hour tablets

3. Which of the following drug schedules has the highest potential for abuse?
   a. Schedule II
   b. Schedule III
   c. Schedule IV
   d. Schedule V

4. For a generic drug to be considered bioequivalent, it must contain the same active ingredient as the innovator drug, as well as be identical in strength, route of administration, and
   a. color.
   b. inactive ingredients.
   c. price.
   d. dosage form.

5. Which of the following OTC drugs must be sold "behind the counter"?
   a. Abreva
   b. Plan B
   c. Motrin IB
   d. Claritin

6. Standards for good manufacturing practices (GMPs) are developed by the
   a. FDA.
   b. USP.
   c. DEA.
   d. state boards of pharmacy.

7. Which drug is the correct brand name for the generic drug atorvastatin?
   a. Mevacor
   b. Pravachol
   c. Lipitor
   d. Zocor

8. If a prescription is written for Synthroid 100 mcg 1 po q am "brand necessary," the drug should be entered into the profile and filled by the pharmacy technician with
   a. Synthroid 100 mcg.
   b. Levoxyl brand 100 mcg.
   c. USP thyroid 1 gr.
   d. levothyroxine 100 mcg.

9. Hydromet 473 mL and ibuprofen 120 mL suspensions are made by the same drug manufacturer. What part of the NDC number will be identical?
   a. security code
   b. product code
   c. package code
   d. labeler code

10. Metroprolol is available in various doses as both a tartrate and a succinate salt. This type of drug cannot be interchanged and is considered a
    a. pharmaceutical equivalent drug product.
    b. pharmaceutical alternative drug product.
    c. brand name extension.
    d. bioequivalent drug.

Routes of Drug Administration and Dosage Formulations

4

Learning Objectives

- Differentiate between the terms *route of administration*, *dosage form*, and *drug delivery system*.
- Explain the properties of oral, topical, and parenteral dosage forms.
- Identify inactive ingredients and the various coatings of tablets and their functions.
- Differentiate between a suspension and an emulsion liquid dosage form.
- Identify dosage formulations utilizing the transmucosal route of administration.
- Define the emulsion characteristics of topical products such as ointments, creams, lotions, and gels.
- Explain the advantages and disadvantages of oral, topical, and parenteral dosage formulations.

- Discuss the importance of syringe selection for a diabetic patient.
- Contrast the advantages and disadvantages of insulin in multi-dose vials and prefilled insulin syringes.
- Understand the stability and expiration dates of insulin at room and refrigerated temperatures.
- Demonstrate correct techniques for administration of eyedrops, eardrops, metered-dose inhalers, and various parenteral injections.
- Differentiate among enteric-coated, sustained-release, and extended-release dosage formulations.

Preview chapter terms and definitions.

Healthcare providers have numerous pharmacological agents at their disposal and a wide variety of dosage forms with which to customize patient treatment. Before selecting the appropriate medications for their patients, however, providers must have a good understanding of two scientific areas in addition to pharmacology: pharmaceutics and pharmacokinetics. **Pharmaceutics** is the study of the release characteristics of various dosage forms or drug formulations. As you know, medications can be taken orally, inhaled, injected, inserted, or spread on the skin, and each of these routes affects the drugs' onset and duration of action. The characteristics of the drug formulation itself also impact the pharmacological action of any given drug. For example, a tablet or capsule may be formulated to release the drug immediately or slowly over a period of 8–12 hours, or even more slowly over a 24-hour period. **Pharmacokinetics** is the study of how drugs are absorbed into the bloodstream (absorption), circulated to tissues throughout the body (distribution), inactivated (metabolized), and eliminated from the body (excretion). Pharmacokinetic processes affect the medications' effectiveness, dosing schedule, and use.

A study of these scientific areas is well beyond the scope of this text, but the pharmacy technician student must gain an appreciation of the advantages and disadvantages of various routes of administration and drug formulations that are utilized in everyday pharmacy practice. A favorable patient outcome may well depend on selecting not only the most appropriate medication, but also the most appropriate drug formulation and route of administration to meet the patient's needs and reduce the risk of preventable medication errors.

Routes of Administration

Medications can be administered by several routes. A **route of administration** is a way to get a drug into or onto the body. The major routes of drug administration are oral, transmucosal, topical, inhalation, and parenteral. A **dosage form** is the physical manifestation of a drug—such as a tablet, capsule, suspension, ointment, cream, patch, or injection—that is designed to deliver the medication by one or more routes of administration. Many drugs, such as nitroglycerin, can be delivered to the body via different routes of administration: orally, as a tablet or capsule; transmucosally, as a transdermal patch; sublingually, as a tablet; topically, as an ointment; via inhalation, as an aerosol spray; or intravenously, as an infusion.

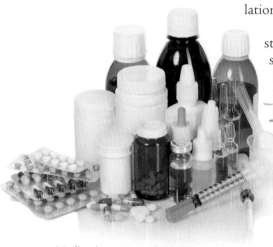

Oral dosage forms must proceed through a series of discrete steps: dissolution in the stomach; absorption in the stomach or small intestine; biotransformation in the liver; and, finally, distribution to the tissue or target organ. This series of steps to get a drug into the bloodstream to exert its therapeutic effect is called a **systemic effect**. Tablets, capsules, and oral liquids all have a delayed systemic effect. Parenteral injections, especially intravenous (IV) bolus and infusions, have an *immediate* systemic effect since they bypass the stomach and are rapidly absorbed and distributed into the bloodstream.

Most drugs administered by the transmucosal, topical, and inhalation routes of administration have a rapid onset of action and a more localized effect. A **localized effect** is when a drug exerts its pharmacologic action at or near the site of administration (for example, an eardrop in the ear).

Medications are available in many dosage forms that can be given by several routes of administration.

Oral Route of Administration

Medication administration for absorption along the gastrointestinal (GI) tract into the systemic circulation is referred to as the **oral route of administration**. However, the term *oral* can also refer to applying medication topically to the mouth (as in the local treatment of a cold sore). The abbreviation *PO* (from the Latin term *per os*, meaning "by mouth") is used to indicate the oral route of medication administration on a prescription.

Oral Dosage Forms

Tablets, capsules, solutions, suspensions, syrups, and elixirs are all common dosage forms for the oral administration of drugs. Tablets and capsules are the two most

Safety Note

The oral route is not appropriate for patients who are experiencing nausea or vomiting.

Safety Note

Although tablets and capsules may have distinctive markings and colors, the pharmacy technician should rely on the drug label and the National Drug Code (NDC) number—not the appearance of the medication—to identify the medication.

common types and are inexpensive to manufacture. The active ingredients in many tablets, capsules, and suspensions are often powders or **granules** that may contain a salt. Drugs are also available in salt form to add shelf life to the product and/or to affect the release characteristics of the drug into the bloodstream. For example, diclofenac potassium and diclofenac sodium both exist in tablet form; at equivalent doses, their therapeutic effect would be similar, but the pharmacy technician could not substitute one for the other without physician approval.

Tablets The **tablet** is a solid dosage form produced by compression. Tablets contain one or more active ingredients along with inert or inactive ingredients, or **excipients**. The common inert ingredients and their uses are listed in Table 4.1. All inert ingredients must be listed in the manufacturer product insert that accompanies the product. For over-the-counter (OTC) products, the inert ingredients must be listed for the consumer on the product labeling.

Tablets are available in a wide variety of shapes, sizes, surface markings, and coatings. Most tablets are imprinted with a distinctive letter and/or numerical code as well as coloring from their manufacturers for drug identification purposes. A variety of tablet dosage forms and their salts are available. Not all dosage forms and their salts are generically or therapeutically equivalent and thus cannot be substituted without the approval of the pharmacist and/or prescriber. Drugs designed to protect the stomach or to release their active ingredients more slowly will be discussed later in this chapter.

TABLE 4.1 Common Inert Tablet Ingredients and Their Uses

Ingredient	Use	Example
binder	Promotes adhesion of the materials in the tablet	methylcellulose
coating	Assists the patient's swallowing of the tablet; improves the flavor of the tablet; protects the stomach lining from the drug's side effects; delays the release of the medication once it has been consumed	saccharine
coloring	Provides tablet identification and elegance	FDA-approved coloring agents and dyes
diluent	Allows for the appropriate concentration of the medication in the tablet; provides bulk and cohesion	lactose
disintegrant	Helps break up the ingredients once the tablet has been consumed	starch
lubricating agent	Gives the tablet a sheen; aids in the manufacturing process	talc
solubilizer	Maintains the ingredients in solution; helps the ingredients pass into solution in the body	cyclodextrin

Types of Tablets Tablets can be designed to be easily swallowed, to mask taste, or to exert an immediate pharmacological response. Large pharmaceutical manufacturers use heavy tool and die machinery to make tablets by several methods. In the direct compression process, the powder or granular ingredients are compressed to produce a tablet end product. **Compression tablets** are the most inexpensive and common dosage form used today. Acetaminophen (Tylenol) is an example of a common compression tablet.

FIGURE 4.1
**Multiple
Compression
Tablets**

(a) Two layers or
compressions
(b) Three layers or
compressions

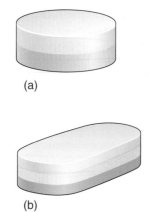

(a)

(b)

A **multiple compression tablet (MCT)** is produced by multiple compression cycles and is, in effect, either a tablet on top of a tablet or a tablet within a tablet. An MCT may contain a core and one or two outer shells (or two or three different layers, as shown in Figure 4.1), each containing a separate medication and colored differently. MCTs are created for appearance alone or to combine incompatible substances into a single medication. The Ambien CR brand is a common example of an MCT.

Some pharmaceutical companies manufacture an oblong tablet, a hybrid of the capsule and tablet, called a *caplet*. The **caplet** is simply a tablet shaped like a capsule and sometimes coated to look like a capsule. The inside of the caplet is solid rather than filled with powder or granular material like the inside of a capsule. Caplets have many beneficial properties: They are easier to swallow than large tablets, have a longer shelf life, and—unlike capsules—are tamper-proof. Caplet formulations on the market include the OTC drug Aleve and the prescription drug oxaprozin (Daypro).

Tablet Coatings Most compression tablets are uncoated, but some tablet dosage forms contain a special outside layer that dissolves or ruptures in the stomach or small intestine. Coatings on tablets can be used to improve appearance, flavor, or ease of swallowing. Common tablet coatings include sugar or film.

- A **sugar-coated tablet (SCT)** contains an outside layer of sugar that protects the medication and improves both appearance and flavor. Sugar coating masks the bitter taste of some drugs (quinine, ibuprofen) and increases the stability of the drug. The major disadvantage of a sugar coating is that it makes the tablets much larger and heavier and thus more difficult to swallow. An SCT could be crushed, but the bitterness of the drug would no longer be masked. Most multivitamins contain a sugar coating to mask the bitter smell and taste of the vitamins.

- A **film-coated tablet (FCT)** contains a thin outer layer of a polymer (a substance containing very large molecules) that can be either soluble or insoluble in water. Film coatings are thinner, lighter in weight, and more efficient and less expensive to manufacture than sugar coatings. These coatings are colored to provide an attractive appearance. The antibiotics erythromycin (Erythrocin) and metronidazole (Flagyl) have film coatings to prevent serious GI side effects that commonly occur with these drugs. An FCT can be crushed but may lose its taste-masking benefit.

Special Dosage Forms Most tablets are meant to be swallowed whole and to dissolve in the GI tract, but some tablets are designed to be chewed or dissolved on the tongue or in the mouth.

- A **chewable tablet** contains a base that is flavored and/or colored. The dosage form is designed to be masticated (or chewed) and absorbed quickly for a slightly faster onset of action. Chewing is preferred for antacids, antiflatulents, commercial vitamins, and tablets designed for children. Single chewable tablets, for example, can be prescribed for small children in lieu of other dosage forms. For example, the drug montelukast (Singulair), used to control asthma symptoms, and the drug amoxicillin, used to treat infections, are both available in chewable tablet form.

- An **oral disintegrating tablet (ODT)** is designed to melt in your mouth. ODTs are useful for pediatric and geriatric patients who have difficulty swallowing or for patients with nausea. Examples include ondansetron (Zofran), for the treatment of nausea and vomiting; Maxalt, for the treatment of migraine headaches; and donepezil (Aricept) for the treatment of Alzheimer's disease.

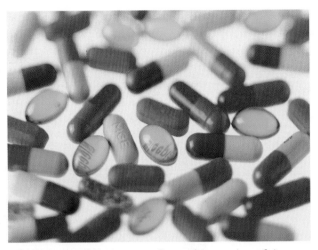

Capsules and tablets are manufactured in a variety of sizes and colors. Distinctive markings help patients identify the drugs.

Capsules The active ingredient(s) of a **capsule** is commonly in the form of a granular powder (sometimes a liquid gel) that is enclosed by a gelatin shell. Gelatin is a protein substance obtained from vegetable matter and from the skin, white connective tissue, and bones of animals. The gelatin shell of a capsule, which can be hard or soft, may be transparent, semitransparent, or opaque and may be colored or marked with a code to facilitate identification. In commercial manufacturing, the body and the cap may be sealed to protect the integrity of the drug within. This sealing practice has increased since the 1980s, when highly publicized incidents of capsule tampering occurred.

Like tablets, the active ingredients in capsules also contain a pharmacologically inert filler substance, or **diluent**. Capsules may also contain disintegrants, solubilizers, preservatives (which maintain the integrity of the ingredients), colorings, and other materials. Because a capsule encloses the components, flavorings are not common for this dosage form. Like tablets, capsules can also be formulated with delayed-release characteristics to allow less frequent dosing and/or side effects.

The active ingredients of capsules can also be manipulated by the crystalline size of the salt in the drug product. Macrodantin 100 mg contains 75 mg of the mononitrate salt and 25 mg of a controlled-release macrocrystalline mononitrate salt. This formulation has better absorption when taken with food, less nausea or GI upset, and a longer duration of action when compared with a generic drug that only contains 100 mg of the mononitrate salt.

Some drugs have salts for different dosage forms. For example, hydroxyzine 50 mg is available as the hydrochloride salt in the tablet formulation and a pamoate salt in the capsule formulation. In this case, the drugs *are considered therapeutically equivalent*. Therefore, if you are out of stock of one dosage form, the other dosage form could be safely substituted—but only with the approval of the pharmacist and/or prescriber. However, this substitution process is not always possible. For example, Zanaflex capsules 4 mg and Zanaflex tablets 4 mg are *not considered therapeutically equivalent*, and, consequently, cannot be substituted. In many cases, prescribers may not be familiar with which dosage forms are available, or the subtle differences in bioavailability or release characteristics among drug products. Pharmacist review of the medication substitution, therefore, is critical.

Powders and Effervescent Salts Other oral dosage forms, such as powders and effervescent salts, are used less frequently by patients. Still, these dosage forms offer some advantages over tablets and capsules. **Powders** are preparations in the form of fine particles. Commonly requested OTC powders include Goody's and BC headache powders, brewer's yeast, and fiber laxatives (Metamucil). The headache powders take less time to dissolve than tablets and are thought to work quicker than tablets in relieving a headache. In large-scale commercial manufacturing, as well as in compounding pharmacies, powders are milled and pulverized by machines and placed into gelatin capsules.

Effervescent salts are granules or coarse powders containing one or more medicinal agents (such as an analgesic), as well as some combination of sodium bicarbonate with citric acid, tartaric acid, or sodium biphosphate. When dissolved in water, effervescent salts release carbon dioxide gas, causing a distinctive bubbly or fizzy appearance and sound. Most people are familiar with effervescent tablets such as the Alka-Seltzer line of OTC products that are used to relieve headaches, hangovers, or indigestion.

Liquids **Liquids** consist of one or more active ingredients in a liquid vehicle such as a solution or suspension. Most liquids are commercially available as solutions (such as elixirs and syrups), suspensions, or emulsions for oral administration.

Common Solutions A **solution** is a liquid in which the active ingredients are completely dissolved in a liquid vehicle. Solutions may be classified by their vehicle as aqueous (water-based), alcoholic (alcohol-based), or hydroalcoholic (water-based and alcohol-based). The vehicle that makes up the greater part of a solution is known as a **solvent**. An ingredient dissolved in a solution is known as a **solute**. Promethazine hydrochloride is an example of a prescription drug for nausea that is available as a solution (also as a tablet and suppository).

 Safety Note

Because of their high sugar content, syrups should be used cautiously in diabetic patients.

Solutions are often classified by their ingredients. The most common dosage forms of solutions are elixirs and syrups. An **elixir** is a clear, sweetened, flavored solution containing water and ethanol (hydroalcoholic). An example of a drug in this dosage form is phenobarbital elixir, which contains phenobarbital, orange oil, propylene glycol, alcohol, sorbitol solution, color, and purified water. This elixir is used to treat anxiety and seizures.

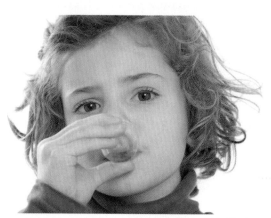

Many Rx and OTC medications are available for children in a flavored syrup formulation.

A **syrup** is an aqueous solution thickened with a large amount of sugar—generally sucrose—or a sugar substitute such as sorbitol or propylene glycol. Syrups may contain additional flavorings, colorings, or aromatic agents and are classified as medicated and nonmedicated. Medicated syrups include lithium citrate (for bipolar depression), ranitidine hydrochloride (for heartburn), or cetirizine hydrochloride (for allergies); nonmedicated syrups include cherry syrup or cocoa syrup. Cheratussin AC is a medicated prescription cough medicine that contains more than 10 inactive ingredients including several flavoring agents.

Most pediatric formulations are syrups or elixirs to mask the taste and ease the swallowing of the medication. Syrups are often the preferred vehicle of pediatric medications, such as cough medicines, because they do not contain alcohol.

Less Common Solutions Other available solutions include aromatic water, extracts, fluidextracts, tinctures, and spirits.

- An **aromatic water** is a solution of water containing oils or other substances that have a pungent, and usually pleasing, smell and that are volatile (i.e., easily released into the air). Rose water is an example.
- An **extract** is a potent dosage form derived from animal or plant sources from which most or all the solvent has been evaporated to produce a powder, an ointment-like form, or a solid. Extracts are produced from fluidextracts and are used in the formulation of medications.
- A **fluidextract** is a liquid dosage form prepared by extraction from plant sources and commonly used in the formulation of syrups. Vanilla extract is an example of a fluidextract.
- A **tincture** is an alcoholic or hydroalcoholic solution of extractions from plants. Examples include iodine and belladonna tincture and some herbal dietary supplements.
- A **spirit** is an alcoholic or hydroalcoholic solution containing volatile, aromatic ingredients. Examples include camphor and peppermint spirit, both of which can be used as medicines or flavorings.

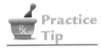

Practice Tip

Pharmacy technicians should always "shake well" a stock bottle of an oral suspension before transferring the medication to a smaller, labeled prescription bottle.

Suspensions Unlike a solution, a **suspension** is the state of a substance when its solid particles are mixed with but *undissolved* in a liquid. A suspension is considered a **dispersion** because the medication is simply dispersed or distributed throughout the vehicle, creating an incomplete mixture of the solid and liquid.

Suspensions contain many inactive ingredients such as colorings, flavorings, and coatings. Some suspensions are commercially available, such as Maalox, Mylanta, ibuprofen, sulfamethoxazole and trimethoprim, and Nystatin. Others come in the form of dry powders or granules that are mixed or reconstituted by the pharmacist or pharmacy technician with purified distilled water prior to dispensing to the patient.

Emulsions Another type of dispersion is known as an emulsion. An **emulsion** is a mixture of two immiscible or unblendable substances such as an oil-and-vinegar salad dressing; it must be shaken well to mix it evenly before use. One substance (the dispersed phase) is dispersed into the other (the continuous phase). Emulsions contain an emulsifying agent that renders the emulsion stable and less prone to separation. Emulsions are commercially available in some OTC oral dosage formulations, such as Creomulsion cough and cold products.

Colloids A **colloid** is a mixture having physical properties between those of a solution and a fine suspension. A **magma**, or milklike liquid, is an example of a dispersion containing ultrafine colloidal particles that remain distinct in a two-phase system. An example of a magma is milk of magnesia, which contains magnesium hydroxide and is used to neutralize gastric acid. Another type of colloidal

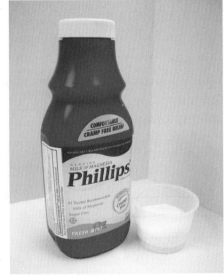

Milk of magnesia is an example of a colloid mixture.

dispersion is the **microemulsion**, or a liquid that is dispersed in another. Unlike other emulsions, however, it is clear because of the extremely fine size of the droplets of the dispersed phase. An example of a microemulsion is Haley's M-O.

Advantages and Disadvantages of Certain Oral Dosage Forms

In general, oral dosage forms offer convenience, safety, and ease of use for patients. However, these medications also have some disadvantages associated with their passing through the GI tract, including delayed onset and absorption and destruction of the drug by GI fluids. Furthermore, each dosage form has a unique set of benefits and drawbacks that pharmacy technicians must know to provide safe and effective care for the patients they serve.

Tablets Tablets provide several advantages for both manufacturers and patients: For manufacturers, tablets are easier and less costly to produce in bulk; offer high physical, chemical, and antimicrobial stability; and have a long shelf life. For patients, tablets offer low cost, more precise dosing, and increased palatability due to specialized coatings.

The major disadvantages of tablets include:

- delayed onset of action because the dosage form must disintegrate in the stomach and small intestine before being absorbed
- destruction of the drug by GI fluids
- local GI side effects in the stomach such as nausea, heartburn, or ulcers
- delayed absorption of medication because food is present in the stomach
- ineffectiveness for patients who are experiencing nausea or vomiting or who are comatose, sedated, or otherwise unable to swallow

Delayed-release (DR) tablets have their own specific advantages and disadvantages. This dosage form provides a longer duration of action and/or fewer side effects and has a reduced dosing schedule. Consequently, this tablet form improves patient compliance and, therefore, patient outcomes. DR tablets also have several disadvantages: They cannot be split or crushed, have a slower onset of action, have prolonged side effects, and are more expensive (higher co-pays) due to patent protection (see Table 4.2).

A patient can take one tablet, several tablets, or a portion of a tablet, as the prescribed dose requires. Many tablets are *scored* once or twice to facilitate breakage of the

TABLE 4.2 Common Delayed-Release Tablets and Capsules That Cannot Be Split

Adderall XR	Ditropan XL	oxycodone XR
Allegra-D 12/24	Effexor XR	potassium chloride
Alprazolam XR	GlipiZIDE XL	propranolol LA
Ambien CR	Glucotrol XL	SEROquel XR
Augmentin XR	indomethacin SR	Taztia XT
Avinza	Lamictal XR	theophylline XR
Budeprion XL/SR	metformin ER	verapamil XR
carbidopa/levodopa ER	methylphenidate LA	Voltaren XR
Concerta ER	Metoprolol ER	Wellbutrin XL
Depakote ER	MS Contin	
Diltia XT/diltiazem XL/ER	Niacin SR	
Divalproex ER/DR	nifedipine XL/CC	

tablet into portions for half (or even quarter) doses. The scoring of a tablet is designed to (almost) equally divide the dose in each section or quadrant. If a tablet is not scored, then it is generally recommended that it should not be split because the dose may not be equal in each piece. The Food and Drug Administration (FDA) has approved a limited number of prescription drugs for tablet splitting based on results of scientific studies.

Safety Note

Careful tablet splitting may reduce medication costs, but it is not recommended for all drugs.

Due to rising drug costs, it is not uncommon for patients to use a tablet splitter for breaking both scored and unscored tablets when treating conditions such as high blood pressure and high cholesterol. Scoring medications can save up to 50% for patients, with limited studies suggesting that this practice with select medications does not appreciably affect the control of the disease state. Patients should keep in mind that not all tablets can be split in equal doses, even with the use of a tablet splitter. For example, odd-shaped tablets such as Diovan or Cialis are particularly difficult to cut.

A tablet splitter can save money for patients taking high-cost medications.

Capsules Compared with tablets, capsules are typically easier to swallow, have a more rapid dissolution, and have a faster onset of action of the active ingredients. In addition to sharing the same disadvantages as tablets, capsules do not allow dosage manipulation like tablets or liquid formulations. The contents of most immediate-release capsules can be sprinkled over food such as applesauce or mixed with water and administered to a child or to a patient with an enteral or a nasogastric feeding tube.

Liquids Liquids have several advantages as a dosage form, including a faster onset of action than oral tablets or capsules, easy administration, and individualized dosing according to a patient's body weight. Liquid medications are also ideal for certain age-groups. For young children, liquids have easier dosage adjustments. For example, a flavored antibiotic liquid or suspension can be accurately dosed based on a patient's body weight and may be preferable over a tablet or capsule. For geriatric patients, liquid medications are easier to swallow, especially for those patients with swallowing difficulties due to Parkinson's disease or cancer. For patients who have to swallow large tablets, such as potassium chloride, prescribers can order a liquid formulation that offers the same dose and has the added benefit of less GI upset.

Liquids also have a few disadvantages. Liquid dosage forms are often less stable than their solid dosage tablet and capsule counterparts. Consequently, pharmacy personnel should monitor proper storage conditions of liquid medications, rotating and checking stock for expiration dates.

The higher sugar content of syrups can pose problems for diabetic patients; therefore, sugar-free OTC products should be recommended for this patient population. An unpleasant taste can be a disadvantage of some suspensions such as amoxicillin/clavulanate (Augmentin) and clindamycin (Cleocin). Although the medications' taste can be masked by various flavorings to promote compliance, certain flavorings may be physically incompatible with components of the suspension. With that in mind, pharmacy technicians must follow proven "recipes" in selecting the proper flavoring agent. (The role of the pharmacy technician in flavoring suspensions is further discussed in Chapter 6.)

Antibiotic suspensions are often mixed from irregular-shaped granules, which are not as likely as powders to float on the surface of a liquid. These suspensions have excellent flow characteristics and are more stable than those mixed from powders. A well-prepared suspension pours easily and settles slowly but can be redispersed quickly by gentle shaking.

Dispensing and Administration of Oral Dosage Forms

When dispensing oral medication, the pharmacist should discuss with the patient what drinks and foods to take with the medications, as well as which consumables to avoid.

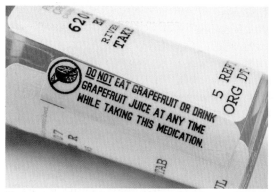

The pharmacist or the pharmacy technician under the pharmacist's direction often adds auxiliary labels to the prescription vial or container to further explain proper use to patients and to inform them of certain precautions.

For most medications, water is preferred to coffee, tea, juices, or carbonated drinks as an aid in swallowing. In fact, some beverages—such as milk, coffee, and tea—may inactivate certain antibiotics and osteoporosis medications. Pharmacists should also counsel patients as to behaviors to avoid while taking medications. Some of these curtailed behaviors include alcohol consumption, sun exposure, and driving. To remind patients of these medication restrictions, pharmacy personnel should affix colorful auxiliary labels to the drug containers to ensure that the medications are taken in the correct manner. (For more information on the use of auxiliary labels in pharmacy practice, see Chapter 6.)

Pharmacy technicians should also remind patients of proper storage conditions for liquid oral medications. Most antibiotics have a limited shelf life. In fact, the expiration date for most pediatric antibiotic suspensions reconstituted or mixed with water is 7–10 days at room temperature and 14 days if stored in the refrigerator. Pharmacy technicians should also be aware that some antibiotics, such as cefdinir and azithromycin, are best stored at room temperature after reconstitution and should not be placed in the refrigerator. Consequently, pharmacy personnel should be sure to address medication storage requirements with patients during pickup.

In addition to these general criteria, specific oral dosage forms have their unique dispensing and administration guidelines, as discussed below.

 Safety Note

Pharmacy technicians should always check the manufacturers' recommendations for storage and expiration dating of reconstituted products.

Tablets When swallowing tablets, patients who have difficulty swallowing solids should be instructed to place the medication on the back of the tongue and tilt the head forward. Tilting the head forward stimulates swallowing. Patients should also be reminded not to crush (or split) tablets that are intended to be swallowed whole, such as any delayed-release and enteric-coated drug. Both delayed-release and enteric-coated formulations have a special coating designed to resist destruction by gastric fluids. (For more discussion on enteric coatings, see the section titled "Drug Delivery Systems" later in this chapter.)

Capsules Like tablets, patients who have difficulty swallowing solids should place the capsule on the back of the tongue and tilt the head forward to ease the process. Some formulations, such as Theo-Dur and Divalproex capsules, are suitable to be opened up and sprinkled on food when swallowing proves difficult for a child or adult with asthma or seizures. Again, patients should be reminded not to open capsules that are intended to be swallowed whole, such as any delayed-release and enteric-coated drug.

Safety Note

To reduce medication measurement errors, it is recommended to use specific numerical volumes (for example, 5 mL) instead of the more traditional unit (1 teaspoonful).

Liquids Pharmacy personnel should remind patients (or parents or caregivers, if patients are minors) that bottles containing suspensions should be shaken before dosage administration. Another important reminder to communicate to patients is that liquid medication doses should be accurately measured in a medication cup or measuring spoon. Common household utensils are often inaccurate measurements of a "teaspoonful" (5 mL) or "tablespoonful" (15 mL). Oral and tuberculin syringes, measuring spoons, medication cups, and droppers are commonly dispensed in the hospital and community pharmacy settings to administer doses ranging from 0.1 mL to 30 mL. Specific information on these pharmacy measurement devices is discussed below.

Oral Syringes An **oral syringe** is used to measure and deliver oral liquid medications to pediatric patients. This type of syringe is a calibrated device consisting of a plunger and a cannula, or barrel, and is used *without a needle* to administer precise amounts of medication by mouth. Oral syringes may be used to slowly administer liquid medications to not only pediatric patients but patients who cannot open their mouths. For very small doses (less than 1 mL) for an infant, a 1 mL tuberculin syringe (again, without the needle) may be provided.

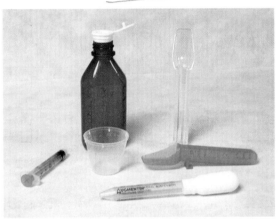
Infants or young children may have less difficulty taking liquid medication when it is administered with one of these devices, which also promote more accurate dosing.

Medication Cups Most manufacturers provide a medication cup for OTC liquids used to treat fever, cough, cold, and the like. These plastic cups contain specific dose demarcations in different units of measurement such as 1 teaspoonful (5 mL), 2 teaspoonsful (10 mL), and 1 tablespoonful (15 mL). Parents or caregivers should be directed to check the OTC package label for the specific dose appropriate for their child's age and weight or to ask the pharmacist.

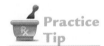
Practice Tip

Pharmacy technicians should be aware that the abbreviation *gtts* is used as a measurement for droppers as well as for IV infusions.

Droppers Droppers are critically important for delivering the correct dosage of smaller volumes of medication to infants and children. A **dropper** contains a small, squeezable bulb at one end and a hollow glass or plastic tube with a tapering point. Squeezing the bulb creates a vacuum for drawing up a liquid. A dropper is commonly calibrated to deliver 1.25 mL (one-fourth teaspoon) to 2.5 mL (one-half teaspoon). Because of the differing **viscosities** (the thicknesses and flow characteristics) of fluids, the size of a drop varies considerably among different suspensions and solutions. In light of that, droppers that are packaged with medications can only be used to measure those specific medications.

Transmucosal Route of Administration

The bioavailability of oral drugs may be adversely affected by rapid or premature degradation in the stomach or biotransformation in the liver. The **transmuscosal route of administration** circumvents these disadvantages by allowing a drug to be absorbed through or across the "sieve-like" or permeable mucous membranes of the mouth, eyes, ears, nose, rectum, vagina, and urethra. A more rapid and reliable onset of action and efficacy coupled with a lower incidence of unpleasant side effects make the transmucosal route a favored one in future drug development.

Transmucosal Dosage Forms

The transmucosal dosage forms include tablets, gum, and lozenges that are administered via the sublingual route or the buccal route of administration. These drugs are formulated to be administered in the oral cavity but not necessarily swallowed like most tablets. These unique dosage forms are able to bypass absorption delays in the stomach and proceed directly to the bloodstream to exert their beneficial therapeutic effect.

In addition to these formulations, ointments, solutions, suspensions, and sprays are dosage forms designed for absorption into the mucous membranes of the eyes, ears, and nose. Suppositories and solutions deliver medication through the mucous membrane linings of the rectum, urethra, and vagina.

Sublingual Medications In the **sublingual route of administration** (from *sub*, meaning "under," and *lingua*, meaning "tongue"), the tablet is placed under the tongue, where it is rapidly absorbed by blood vessels. One common medication that is administered via the sublingual route is the lifesaving drug nitroglycerin. Patients who are experiencing chest pain are instructed to place one nitroglycerin tablet under the tongue every five minutes until the pain is relieved or until three tablets have been administered. For these patients, the sublingual route provides a rapid onset of action, which is critical in this health crisis.

Buccal Medications In the **buccal route of administration**, a drug is absorbed by the blood vessels in the lining of the mouth. Common examples of drugs that are administered via this route are OTC nicotine gum (for nicotine addiction) or a lollipop-like lozenge such as oral transmucosal fentanyl citrate (OTFC), a narcotic. A **lozenge**, also known as a *troche*, is a solid dosage form containing active ingredients and flavorings, such as sweeteners, that are dissolved in the mouth. Lozenges generally have local therapeutic effects. Using proper technique when chewing nicotine gum or sucking on a lozenge is very important for appropriate drug release.

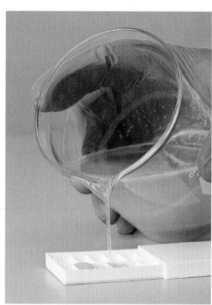

A pharmacy technician working in a compounding pharmacy may prepare lozenge formulations by pouring compounded solution into a lozenge mold.

Commercial OTC lozenges for relief of sore throats are quite common, although many other drugs, including such prescription drugs as nystatin or clotrimazole, are also available in a lozenge form. Compounding pharmacies may prepare lozenge formulations for specific indications in special needs pediatric or geriatric patients.

Ophthalmics, Otics, and Nasal Sprays/Solutions Ophthalmics, otics, and nasal products can all be delivered to a specific site with a minimum of systemic side effects. An **irrigating solution**, or a solution for cleansing or bathing an area of the body, can be used both topically in the ear (for example, acetic acid) as well as instilled in the eye (for example, normal saline).

Ophthalmics The **ocular route of administration** is the application of a drug into the eye. Ophthalmics are manufactured as sterile solutions, suspensions, or ointment formulations and administered via the ocular route. Betoptic and Betoptic S are examples of an ophthalmic solution and a suspension, respectively; the suspension should be shaken gently prior to use. The **conjunctival route of administration** is the application of a drug into the conjunctival mucosa, the lining of the inside of the eyelid. Placing the drug (commonly a sterile ointment) in the lining of the lower eye is usually an easier route of self-administration for the patient, which means he or she will achieve a higher concentration of drug at the site.

Safety Note

Eardrops can never be used in the eye, but eyedrops can be used in the ear.

The eye is more prone to infection than most areas of the body, so only sterile ophthalmic solutions, suspensions, or ointments should be used. A nonsterile otic medication for the ear *cannot be dispensed* as an ophthalmic medication even if it contains the same dose, drugs, and concentration. Ophthalmics are available as both OTC medications (for example, Visine for red eye irritation) and prescription drugs (for example, Sulamyd or sodium sulfacetamide for conjunctivitis [pink eye]).

Ophthalmic medications that are used repeatedly must contain a preservative to maintain antimicrobial sterility; examples of preservatives include methylparaben, propylparaben, thiomersal, and benzalkonium chloride. Some OTC and prescription sterile eye medications are dispensed in single unit-of-use packages for one-time use only. This type of packaging does not require a preservative but is typically more costly. After each use, the product is discarded. Restasis, a medication for the treatment of chronic dry eye syndrome, is an example of a single unit-of-use eye product.

Safety Note

Exercise caution when selecting ophthalmic and otic medications. Some products such as Neosporin are available as both an ophthalmic and an otic, and the otic product must *not* be used in the treatment of an eye disorder.

Otics Otics are nonsterile solutions or suspension drug formulations that are administered into one or both ears. The **otic route of administration** is the application of a drug into the ear canal. Otic medications can *never* be administered into the eye, although ophthalmic drugs may be administered into the ear. The analgesic otic antipyrine/benzocaine contains anhydrous glycerin and oxyquinolone sulfate as inactive ingredients; occasionally, these inactive ingredients can cause an allergic reaction.

Nasal Sprays/Solutions The **intranasal route of administration** is the application of a drug into the passages of the nasal cavity. Sprays are often used for OTC nasal decongestants. A **spray** is a dosage form that consists of a container having a valve assembly unit that, when activated, emits a fine dispersion of liquid. Examples of nasal sprays include Afrin for nasal congestion, intranasal steroids (Flonase, Nasonex) for the prevention of allergy symptoms, nitroglycerin for the relief of chest pain, and Imitrex for the treatment of migraine headaches.

Nasal sprays and solutions are commonly prescribed for administration in both nostrils. Some medications, however, are to be administered in one nostril daily, alternating nostrils to reduce irritation. The osteoporosis drug Miacalcin, for example, is administered using this alternating pattern. The administration dosage for nasal spray may differ as well. For example, the pediatric dose of steroid intranasal sprays is one spray; the adult dose is two sprays. Pharmacy technicians need to be aware of this dosage distinction when entering the dosage and patient instructions into the computer. Entering incorrect information could result in a twofold overdose for a pediatric patient.

Suppositories and Solutions A **suppository** is an example of a semisolid dosage form that is created from an inactive base ingredient (such as cocoa butter or glycerin) and formulated to melt at body temperature and release an active drug. Suppositories are designed for insertion into body orifices such as the rectum,

Safety Note

Some suppository ingredients, such as phenylephrine (used to shrink hemorrhoids), must be used with caution in patients with hypertension and other diseases. Refer patients to the pharmacist to assist in product selection.

vagina, or, less commonly, the urethra. These medications vary in size and shape according to their site of administration and the patient's age and gender. Some suppositories are meant for localized action, as in the treatment of external hemorrhoids; others are used for their systemic action, as in the treatment of internal hemorrhoids and ulcerative colitis. This dosage form is often formulated in a compounding pharmacy, especially if products are not commercially available.

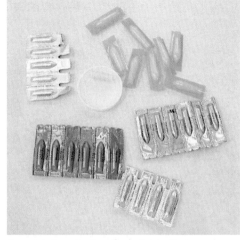

A suppository's site of administration determines the suppository's size and shape.

Rectal Suppositories/Solutions The **rectal route of administration** is used to deliver drugs into the rectum and includes dosage forms such as suppositories, solutions, ointments, creams, and foams. Rectal suppositories, solutions, or enemas are used for cleansing the bowel, for laxative or cathartic action, for hemorrhoids, or for drug administration in colon disease. Rectal suppositories, however, may also be used as vehicles for systemic drugs because the rich supply of blood and lymphatic vessels in the rectum provides for enhanced absorption.

Suppositories are often used in children or adults unable to take oral medication for the purpose of controlling fever, nausea, or vomiting, or for relieving constipation. OTC glycerin suppositories and promethazine (Phenergan) suppositories are two examples of suppositories that are administered to treat constipation and nausea respectively. The patient or caregiver should be instructed to be sure that the suppository is unwrapped and removed from its package. The suppository should then be inserted, small tapered end first, into the rectum with the index finger for the full length of the finger. It may be desirable, especially in infants and children, to ease suppository insertion by applying a lubricant such as petroleum jelly.

An **enema** is an example of a water-based solution administered rectally for cleansing or evacuating the bowel before a GI procedure, as a treatment for constipation, or for delivering an active drug. An evacuation enema, such as Fleet, is often administered to cleanse the bowels in preparation for a colonoscopy. A retention enema, such as Cortenema, is administered to deliver medication locally or systemically in the case of acute inflammatory bowel disease.

Vaginal Suppositories/Solutions The **vaginal route of administration** is the application of any drug within the vagina. Common dosage forms include vaginal tablets (or suppositories) and creams but may also include emulsion foams, inserts, ointments, solutions, and sponges. Typically, this route of administration is utilized for its local therapeutic effects such as cleansing (for example, douches), contraception, hormone replacement therapy, or treatment of common bacterial or yeast infections.

Urethral Suppositories/Solutions The **urethral route of administration** is the application of a drug within the urethra; common dosage forms include implants and urethral tablets (or suppositories). Drugs delivered by this route may be effective in treating cancer, incontinence, or impotence in men.

Advantages and Disadvantages of Certain Transmucosal Dosage Forms

Transmucosal dosage forms generally have a faster onset of action but a shorter duration of action and are prescribed for patients who need immediate relief of symptoms. A disadvantage of these dosage forms is the difficulty in reversing the effects of a drug that is rapidly absorbed in the bloodstream. For example, if a patient experiences an adverse drug reaction, it would be difficult to reverse the medication's effects.

Sublingual Medications The sublingual administration of medications has the advantage of a very rapid onset (less than 5 minutes) and is thus appropriate for immediate relief, as in the case of nitroglycerin sublingual tablets for treatment of chest pain. The rapid onset is the result of the medication entering the bloodstream directly without passage through the stomach or breakdown in the liver. A disadvantage of sublingual tablets is their short duration of action (less than 30 to 60 minutes), making this route of administration inappropriate for the routine delivery of medication.

Buccal Medications Advantages of buccal medications include a faster onset of action and, perhaps, fewer side effects than other formulations. General disadvantages of the buccal route are an unpleasant taste and local mouth irritation, as in the case of nicotine gum. Another disadvantage of this route is "dose dumping," a term used to describe a situation in which a patient does not follow the buccal medication's directions and, as a result, absorbs an excessive amount of drug in a short period.

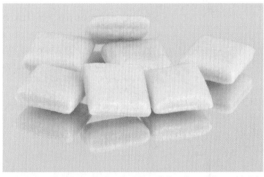

OTC nicotine gum must be carefully chewed to avoid unpleasant side effects (see Table 4.3).

Ophthalmics, Otics, and Nasal Sprays/Solutions Ophthalmics, otics, and nasal dosage formulations are almost always prescribed for their fast onset of action and localized therapeutic effects to treat conditions of the eye, ear, nose, or sinuses.

Ophthalmics Ophthalmic medications are available as both solutions and suspensions. Solutions have a more rapid onset of action, but suspensions have a longer duration of action. Pharmacy technicians should be aware that these two dosage forms should *not* be interchanged without the permission of the pharmacist and/or prescriber. An example of an ophthalmic solution is timolol maleate, a glaucoma medication that is available as both a solution and as a longer-acting gel-forming solution (GFS). These two products as well cannot be substituted without the permission of the prescriber. Pharmacy technicians must be extremely careful in selecting the right products from the shelf and comparing NDC numbers. Another example of an ophthalmic solution is Acular LS, a nonsteroidal anti-inflammatory drug for relieving pain and discomfort after eye surgery. This medication provides localized relief of symptoms without adverse effects on the GI tract. However, some medications prescribed for the eye have a systemic effect and can adversely affect blood pressure (in patients with hypertension) and breathing (in patients with lung disease). Pharmacy personnel should recommend that patients carefully read the labeled instructions and precautions on OTC ophthalmics and, if questions arise, seek out proper counseling from their pharmacist.

Otics Otics are available as solutions and suspensions. Like ophthalmics, these products should not be interchanged without the permission of the pharmacist and/or prescriber. Analgesic otic solutions can provide almost immediate pain relief to pediatric patients suffering from ear infections.

Nasal Sprays/Solutions Sprays for inhalation through the nose may be prescribed for either their local or systemic pharmacological effects. Proper dosing administration and frequency are crucial to therapeutic success, especially if patients are self-medicating with OTC medications. Overuse of common OTC nasal sprays and solutions for more than three days can lead to an adverse side effect known as chronic rebound congestion.

Antihistamine nasal sprays, such as Astelin and Astepro, offer relief of allergy symptoms without the disabling drowsiness that accompanies most potent oral antihistamines such as diphenhydramine or Benadryl. However, some nasal medications have systemic side effects, and precautions are advised for patients with certain medical conditions. Pharmacy personnel should recommend that patients carefully read the labeled instructions on OTC antihistamine nasal sprays and, if questions arise, seek out proper counseling from their pharmacist.

Suppositories and Solutions Rectal, vaginal, and urethral suppositories and solutions have unique benefits and drawbacks to their administration.

Rectal Suppositories/Solutions Rectal dosage forms, including suppositories and solutions, are used primarily to deliver systemic drugs if:

- an oral drug might be destroyed or diluted by acidic fluids in the stomach
- an oral drug might be too readily metabolized by the liver and eliminated from the body
- a patient is unconscious and needs medication
- a patient may be unable to take oral drugs because of nausea and vomiting or because of severe acute disorders of the GI tract

Because rectal doses do not transverse the digestive system for absorption, rectal dosage forms can be used in both young children and adults. For infants and young children, OTC glycerin suppositories are available for the safe treatment of mild constipation. Acetaminophen suppositories are also administered to young children who have a high fever but who will not or cannot take oral formulations of the medication. For adults, promethazine suppositories are prescribed for patients who are suffering from severe nausea and vomiting from a bad case of the flu or from the side effects of chemotherapy.

Disadvantages of rectal formulations include patient inconvenience and discomfort, premature expulsion of the suppository or solution, and erratic and irregular drug absorption.

Vaginal Suppositories/Solutions A variety of OTC vaginal suppositories are available for self-treatment of yeast infections that often occur as a side effect of oral antibiotic treatment. The pharmacist can assist with proper product selection.

Dispensing and Administration of Transmucosal Dosage Forms

Due to their unique design characteristics, transmucosal medications have certain dispensing and administration guidelines.

Safety Note

Sublingual nitroglycerin tablets are sensitive to air and light and, consequently, will lose potency over a certain period. These tablets should be kept in their original container and replaced every six months.

Safety Note

If nicotine gum is chewed vigorously, too much nicotine can be released, causing unpleasant side effects. Therefore, pharmacy personnel should instruct patients on the proper chewing technique for nicotine gum.

Sublingual Medications Nitroglycerin, a common sublingual medication, has specific storage requirements to safeguard the potency of the tablets. Because this medication is a relatively unstable drug, pharmacy technicians must instruct patients to store the nitroglycerin tablets in their original brown bottle (and not in a pillbox) to shield the medication from sunlight, which degrades its potency. Technicians should also remind patients to tightly secure the lid of the nitroglycerin container to avoid the introduction of air—another factor that lessens the medication's potency. Physicians usually advise patients to refill their nitroglycerin with a fresh bottle every three to six months.

Buccal Medications For buccally administered medications, it is important that the patient understand the difference between the technique for chewing regular gum and the technique for chewing nicotine gum. If the nicotine gum is chewed vigorously like chewing gum, then too much nicotine will be released, causing unpleasant side effects such as nausea and vomiting. Proper administration allows the gum to release the nicotine slowly, decreasing cravings. Counseling on the proper technique for administration of the nicotine gum is provided in Table 4.3.

Technique is also critical for oral transmucosal fentanyl citrate (OTFC), a narcotic analgesic lozenge. OTFC is available in multiple dosage strengths and is used in adults for relief of severe breakthrough pain. The lollipop is placed between the gums and the inner lining of the cheek, in the so-called buccal pouch; it is then sucked to slowly dissolve in the mouth (over approximately 15 minutes) to provide pain relief.

TABLE 4.3 Proper Technique for Administration of Nicotine Gum

1. Chew the gum slowly and stop chewing when you notice a tingling sensation in the mouth.
2. Park the gum between the cheek and gum and leave it there until the taste or tingling sensation is almost gone.
3. Resume slowly chewing a few more times until the taste or sensation returns.
4. Park the gum again in a different place in the mouth.
5. Continue this chewing and parking process until the taste or tingle no longer returns when the gum is chewed (usually after 30 minutes).
6. Do not eat or drink for 15 minutes before or while using the gum.

Ophthalmics, Otics, and Nasal Sprays/Solutions Ophthalmic, otic, and nasal medications have specific storage, handling, and administration guidelines that patients must be aware of for optimal treatment of their conditions.

Ophthalmic Medications Ophthalmics must be administered at or near room temperature before application into the eye. All medications should be stored according to the package insert to reduce bacterial growth and to ensure drug stability. Some ophthalmics—such as Travatan, Trifluridine, AzaSite, and Xalatan—require refrigeration and should be stored appropriately in the pharmacy before the prescription is picked up by the patient. During pickup, the pharmacy technician should remind the patient about proper storage at home.

Before application, patients should be advised to wash their hands to prevent contamination at the application site or of the medication. When applying the ophthalmic, patients should be careful not to touch the tube or dropper to the infected site. Any inadvertent contact between the container and the application site could contaminate the medication. To instill eyedrops or apply ophthalmic ointment, the patient's head should be tilted back and the medication should be administered to the

FIGURE 4.2
Administering Ophthalmic Medication

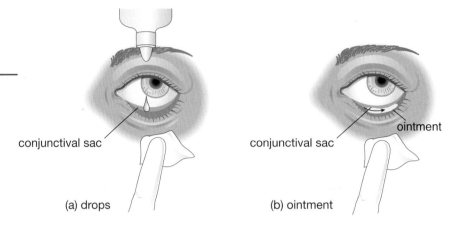

conjunctival sac

conjunctival sac

ointment

(a) drops

(b) ointment

outer surface of the eye or to the conjunctival sac, respectively (see Figure 4.2). Once the medication is administered, it is important for the patient to place a finger in the corner of the affected eye, next to the nose, to gently close the duct, thus preventing loss of medication through the tear duct. The patient should also keep the eye closed for one or two minutes after application.

When multiple drops of more than one medication are to be administered, the patient should be advised to wait five minutes between different medications lest the first medication be washed away. If an ointment and a drop are to be used together, then the patient should instill the drops first and then wait 10 minutes before applying the ointment. Previously applied medications should be cleaned away, as should any drainage from the eye. Cotton balls work well for this purpose.

Ophthalmic ointments are generally applied at night and are the formulation of choice when extended contact with the medication is desired because tears wash them out less easily. The patient should be reminded that he or she might experience some temporary blurring of vision after application.

Safety Note

Unused ophthalmic medication should be discarded 30 days after the container is opened. Manufacturer expirations do not apply once a patient has opened the medication.

Otic Medications Otics must be stored at room temperature. Heated drops may cause a rupturing of the tympanic membrane (eardrum), whereas cold drops can cause vertigo and discomfort. Certain ear conditions dictate the type of otic medication prescribed. For example, a patient with a ruptured eardrum would be treated with a solution or suspension containing no alcohol—a substance that would create more pain and a burning sensation in the ear. A patient who has suspected eardrum damage would most likely be prescribed a low-alcohol content otic solution or suspension.

Patients should be instructed in the proper technique for administering otic medications. This technique varies between children and adults (see Figure 4.3). To administer an otic medication to children under age three, parents or caregivers should tilt the child's head to the side with the ear facing up, pull the earlobe *down and back*, and instill the solution in the ear. Using this technique takes into account the child's inner ear anatomy and therefore allows the medication to reach the desired site. For patients over age three, the same procedure should be followed with the exception that the earlobe for this patient population should be pulled *up and back* to accommodate the inner ear anatomy.

After administration of the otic medication, the patient's head should remain tilted for two to five minutes. Cotton plugs placed in the ear after administration of eardrops will prevent excess medication from dripping out of the ear. The plugs will not reduce the amount of drug that is absorbed.

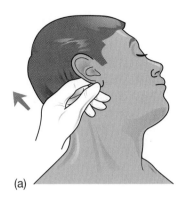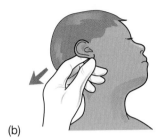

FIGURE 4.3
Administering Otic Medications

(a) Children over age three and adults should have the earlobe pulled up and back when otic medications are administered.
(b) Children under age three should have the earlobe pulled down and back.

(a)   (b)

Nasal Medications Nasal medications are applied by drops (instillation), sprays, or aerosols. Application may be for relief of nasal congestion or prevention of allergy symptoms. The patient should be instructed to tilt the head back; insert the dropper, spray, or aerosol tip into the nostril; point it toward the eyes; and apply the prescribed number of drops or sprays (repeating the process in the other nostril if indicated). Patients may experience a postnasal drip and taste the nasally administered medication. Breathing should be through the mouth to avoid sniffing the medication into the sinuses. Patients should be warned to not overuse OTC nasal decongestants (not more than three days) and to carefully follow the manufacturer's labeled instructions.

Suppositories and Solutions The insertion of rectal and vaginal suppositories and solutions may require certain preparatory steps and administrative techniques to ensure effective treatment, as outlined below.

Rectal Medications Prior to administration, rectal suppositories should be stored in the refrigerator to avoid melting in direct sunlight or high temperatures. Just prior to insertion, the suppository should be kept at room temperature for a few minutes, unwrapped, and lubricated with a small amount of petroleum jelly.

Rectal enemas should be used after a bowel movement. The patient should be instructed to lie on his or her left side with the left knee bent toward the chest. Next, the patient should shake the enema container, unwrap it, and gently insert the nozzle of the container into the rectum. Then the patient should firmly squeeze the bottle to release the entire drug into the rectum (unless otherwise directed). After administration of the medication, the patient should continue to lie on the left side, retaining the medicine in the rectum for as long as possible before evacuating the bowels.

Vaginal Medications Patients whose treatment includes a vaginal medication should be instructed to use the medication for the prescribed period to ensure effective treatment. Many vaginal creams are delivered to the site with the use of an applicator tube; the medication is dissolved and absorbed through the vaginal mucosa. Miconazole (Monistat) is an example of an OTC vaginal cream used to treat yeast infections. If the medication is to be applied with an applicator, then the application should follow the steps outlined in Table 4.4. Vaginal tablets may be less messy than equivalent cream formulations, although absorption of the active drug is less predictable.

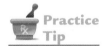

Practice Tip

Refrigeration is necessary to store most rectal suppository medications.

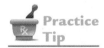

Practice Tip

Pharmacy personnel should remind patients who are using suppositories to remove the foil packaging prior to insertion.

TABLE 4.4 Proper Technique for Administration of Vaginal Medications

1. Empty the bladder and wash the hands.
2. Open the container and place the dose in the applicator.
3. Lubricate the applicator with a water-soluble lubricant if it is not prelubricated.
4. Lie down, spread the legs, and open the labia with one hand. With the other hand, insert the applicator about two inches into the vagina. (An alternative application is to insert the applicator and medication by standing with one foot on the edge of a bathtub.)
5. Release the labia; use the free hand to push the applicator plunger, releasing the medication.
6. Withdraw the applicator and wash the hands. Wash the applicator and dry it if reusing.

Topical Route of Administration

The **topical route of administration** is typically used to apply a drug directly to the surface of the skin. Most topically administered drugs do not have to be dissolved and absorbed in the stomach to exert their pharmacological effect; some may not even need to be absorbed into the bloodstream to work. These medications exert local pharmacological effects. By localizing the therapeutic effect, side effects of drugs administered to the intact skin are minimal. Caution is advised if certain topical medications are administered to broken skin due to an increase in systemic absorption and risk of hypersensitivity or side effects.

Topical Dosage Forms

Topical medications may include emulsions such as creams, ointments, lotions, and gels, which vary in viscosity. Other topical medications include sprays and aerosols, such as OTC local anesthetics to treat sunburn, antiseptics to clean wounds, and antifungals (for example, Lotrimin) to treat athlete's foot. In fact, topical medications can be found in many drug categories, including anesthetics, analgesics, anti-inflammatories, antibiotics, antifungals, antiseptics, astringents, moisturizers, pediculicides (for killing lice), protectants (for sun protection), and scabicides (for killing mites).

Ointments, Pastes, and Plasters Topical dosage forms such as ointments, pastes, and plasters have varying appearances and consistencies due to their base ingredients.

Ointments An **ointment** is a dosage form that is a water-in-oil (W/O) emulsion. A **water-in-oil (W/O) emulsion** is a formulation that contains a small amount of water dispersed in oil. Many cortisone-like medications and topical antibiotics such as Neosporin are available in both an ointment and a cream formulation. Ointments may be more therapeutically effective due to their skin adherence, but they are not as cosmetically acceptable as creams.

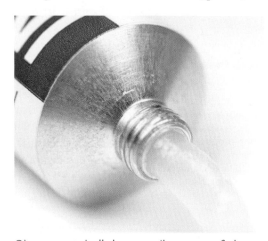

Ointments typically have an oily or greasy feel.

Ointments usually have an oily or greasy feel and may be medicated or nonmedicated. They may contain various kinds of bases, including:

- oleaginous or greasy bases made from hydrocarbons such as mineral oil or petroleum jelly (used in **liniments** for rubbing on the skin—for example, BENGAY)
- W/O emulsions such as lanolin or cold cream
- water-soluble or greaseless bases such as polyethylene glycol ointment (used in the topical antibiotic mupirocin)

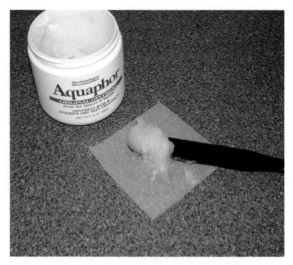

An ointment is referred to as a water-in-oil (W/O) preparation because it contains a small amount of water dispersed in oil. Often yelllowish or opaque in appearance, an ointment is easily applied to the skin but typically makes the skin feel oily or greasy.

Pastes A **paste** is like an ointment but contains more solid materials, creating a dense consistency. This consistency makes the application of a paste thicker than that of an ointment. Examples include zinc oxide paste, which is used as an astringent and a sunscreen, and triamcinolone acetonide dental paste (an anti-inflammatory preparation).

Plasters A **plaster** is a solid or semisolid that adheres to the body and contains a backing material such as paper, cotton, linen, silk, moleskin, or plastic. Plasters can be either medicated or nonmedicated preparations. An example is the OTC salicylic acid plaster used to remove corns. A corn is a painful thickening of the skin that typically occurs in areas of excessive pressure such as the toes.

Creams, Lotions, and Gels Topical dosage forms including creams, lotions, and gels have different formulations and are used to treat a variety of medical conditions.

Creams A **cream** is considered an **oil-in-water (O/W) emulsion** because it contains a small amount of oil dispersed in water. An example of an O/W emulsion base is the hydrophilic ointment containing petrolatum. Most creams are considered "vanishing," which means they are invisible once applied and rubbed into the skin. This quality makes creams more cosmetically acceptable to most patients. If not commercially available, many topical formulations such as hormonal creams are commonly prepared in a compounding pharmacy (see Chapter 8).

Lotions A **lotion** is another O/W emulsion for topical application. Containing insoluble dispersed solids or immiscible liquids, lotions are easily absorbed and can cover large areas of the skin. This topical treatment is especially effective for hairy areas of the body such as the scalp. Examples of lotions include calamine lotion, used for relief of itching, and benzoyl peroxide lotion, used to control acne.

Gels Much like a suspension, a **gel** contains solid particles in a liquid, but the particles are fine or ultrafine. Topically, gels apply evenly and leave a dry coat of the medication in contact with the area. One example of a gel is the prescription drug Voltaren, a topical medication used to treat arthritis. This anti-inflammatory drug can provide relief to an aching knee without the risk of GI effects associated with the oral formulation. Another marketed gel is MetroGel, which is available in two different strengths: for vaginal use (0.75%) and for adult acne or rosacea (1%). Still another prescribed gel is AndroGel, a pump spray used for the treatment of a male hormone deficiency.

Ultrafine gel dispersion dosage forms include jellies and glycerogelatins:

- A **jelly** is a gel that contains a higher proportion of water in combination with a drug substance and a thickening agent. Jellies are present in many antiseptics, antifungals, contraceptives, and lubricants. Lubricants are commonly used in pelvic and rectal examinations of body orifices. Lubricants are also used as an aid in sexual intercourse in postmenopausal women having vaginal dryness from an age-related hormone deficiency. Because of their high water content, jellies are subject to contamination and thus usually contain preservatives.
- A **glycerogelatin** is a topical preparation made with gelatin, glycerin, water, and medicinal substances. The hard substance is melted and brushed onto the skin, where it hardens again and is generally covered with a bandage. An example is zinc gelatin (Unna's Boot), used as a pressure bandage to treat varicose ulcers.

Colloids As mentioned earlier in this chapter, a colloid is a mixture with physical properties that fall between those of a solution and a fine suspension. A colloidal dispersion is a heterogeneous mixture in which ultrafine particles of one substance are evenly distributed throughout another substance. Aveeno is made with natural colloidal oatmeal milled into an ultrafine powder. When dispersed in water, this powder forms a soothing milky bath. It moisturizes and relieves dry, itchy, irritated skin caused by rashes, eczema, poison ivy, oak, sumac, and insect bites.

Collodion is an example of a topical microemulsion in which the vehicle is a liquid dissolved in a mixture of alcohol and ether. Upon application, the highly volatile alcohol and ether solvent vaporizes, leaving a film coating containing the active medication on the skin. The OTC product Compound W One-Step Wart Remover consists of acetic acid and salicylic acid in an acetone collodion base and is used to remove corns or warts.

Irrigating Solutions An irrigating solution, known as a *douche*, is often reconstituted from a powder and introduced into the vaginal cavity for local cleansing. Irrigating solutions are also used in the hospital postoperative setting to bathe the abdominal cavity after surgery. Irrigating powders, such as Neosporin-Polymyxin B sulfate and bacitracin zinc, are used topically to prevent bacterial infections. Domeboro effervescent tablets is an OTC product that contains aluminum acetate and is used topically on the skin as a soak or compress for minor "weeping" skin irritations, such as poison ivy.

Advantages and Disadvantages of Certain Topical Dosage Forms

The major advantage of topical formulations is that they have a fast onset of action with relatively few systemic side effects due to their localized therapeutic action. For example, most mild cases of poison ivy may be treated locally by applying an OTC topical formulation such as hydrocortisone cream. However, if the equivalent dose of Prednisone tablets were administered to treat this skin rash, the risk of GI side effects would be greater, especially if used on a long-term basis. Pharmacy technicians must keep in mind, however, that some topical products have the disadvantage of being absorbed systemically, resulting in potential side effects. For example, OTC hydrocortisone and similar cortisone-like products—if used over large areas of the body for extended periods—can cause systemic side effects. Topical dosage forms can also cause a hypersensitivity reaction in some patients.

Ointments Ointments are especially good for extremely dry areas of the skin where moisture needs to be retained, as well as for areas prone to friction from clothing or other body parts. Because they generally have a longer contact time with the skin, ointments have a longer duration of action than creams, lotions, and gels. However, the disadvantages of ointments are their appearance and their greasy residue on the skin.

Creams, Lotions, and Gels Creams, lotions, and gels apply more smoothly to the skin and leave a very thin film. They are also more readily absorbed and are more cosmetically acceptable for most patients. Topical vaginal medications are often prescribed because they treat an infection locally and therefore are less likely to be absorbed systemically and cause side effects. For example, a variety of OTC creams are available for the self-treatment of vaginal yeast infections that often occur as a side effect of oral antibiotic treatment. The major disadvantage of vaginally administered medications is the messiness of the creams (which is also true for ointments).

Like topical vaginal medications, topical hormone creams provide localized treatment and are less likely to cause systemic side effects. This dosage form also has seen increased use in light of recent studies that have shown a connection between long-term use of oral hormone medications and hormonal cancers. Compounding pharmacies can prepare individualized bioidentical hormone cream formulations based on saliva and blood tests; bioidentical hormones in a topical cream formulation provide individualized dosing, thus minimizing systemic absorption and risk of side effects.

Dispensing and Administration of Topical Dosage Forms

Depending on the dosage form, certain topical medications have specific application and handling guidelines that pharmacy personnel must relay to patients.

Ointments Certain products, such as nitroglycerin ointment, require the patient or caregiver to wear gloves during application to avoid absorbing excessive amounts of drug, which could cause headaches. A risk of increased absorption is also an issue in the application of topical potent corticosteroid ointments. Many of these ointments should be applied sparingly to affected areas of the body for short periods and—unless directed by a physician—should not be covered with bandages or other occlusive dressings (including diapers). Doing so can increase the absorption of the medication and the risk of side effects. Increased absorption of the product can also occur when select topical corticosteroids are applied to the face, underarms, or groin area. Pharmacy personnel should instruct patients to read medication instructions carefully when applying these topical medications.

Pharmacy personnel should also be aware that topical corticosteroid products are not all the same. For example, the topical corticosteroid betamethasone is commercially available as a valerate and dipropionate salt, and in a regular and "augmented" ointment (and cream) formulation. The potency of each of these products differs. The pharmacy technician must be careful to select the correct product during preparation and filling of the prescription. The overuse, or inappropriate use, of potent topical corticosteroids, such as the augmented formulations, can lead to serious local and systemic side effects.

Creams, Lotions, and Gels Like ointments, certain cream, lotion, and gel formulations also have specific precautions that patients should follow during application. For example, an OTC cream containing capsaicin (active ingredient in hot chili peppers) must be applied with gloves because severe irritation can occur if the cream is

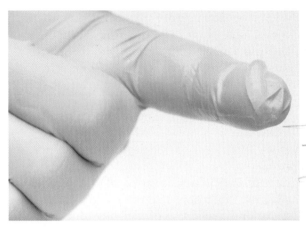

OTC Capsaicin (consisting of ground-up chili peppers) is used to treat patients with arthritis and must be applied with gloves.

inadvertently rubbed into the eyes. Capsaicin is available in both regular-potency and high-potency formulas and is used for treating arthritis symptoms. OTC hydrocortisone creams and lotions should be applied sparingly and cautiously, as previously discussed.

AndroGel, a product mentioned earlier that is used to treat adult males with low testosterone, is available as individual packets as well as a pump. The pump must be carefully primed three times prior to initial use; each pump thereafter delivers a specified amount of medication. The gel is applied by hand to the shoulders, upper arms, or stomach area. Once applied, the patient should not shower or swim for five hours.

Inhalation Route of Administration

The **inhalation route of administration** is defined as the application of a drug through inhalation into the lungs, typically through the mouth. The lungs are designed for the exchange of gases from the tissues into the bloodstream and serve as an excellent site for the absorption of medications. This route is primarily used to deliver bronchodilators and anti-inflammatory agents to asthma sufferers or those with chronic lung disease.

Inhalation Dosage Forms

Inhalation dosage forms are primarily aerosols and sprays intended to be inhaled via the oral respiratory route. However, sterile solutions, volatile medications, and micronized powders are inhalation medications that can be delivered through a variety of devices.

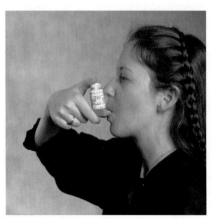

A metered-dose inhaler (MDI) is a common device used to administer a drug through inhalation into the lungs.

Aerosols and MDIs An **aerosol** is a spray in a pressurized metered-dose container that contains a propellant—an inert liquid or gas under pressure—designed to carry the active ingredient to its location of application. A **metered-dose inhaler (MDI)** is a handheld, propellant-driven device commonly used by patients who have been diagnosed with asthma or chronic lung disease. When activated, an MDI provides a specific measured amount of medication with compressed gas.

Aerosols such as Ventolin, Proventil, and ProAir HFA are MDIs that are commonly prescribed to relieve the symptom of shortness of breath in acute asthma. Symbicort and Advair HFA contain two active drugs in an aerosol form to reduce exacerbations of asthma. Depending on the formulation of the product and on the design of the valve, an aerosol may commonly emit a fine mist or a coarse liquid spray. Aerosols that contain chlorofluorocarbons or CFCs, such as Combivent and Maxair, will be phased out by December 2013 due to environmental concerns.

Sterile Solutions and Nebulizers Sterile solutions are sometimes used to deliver a drug into the lungs as well. These solutions are delivered as a mist through an atomizing machine called a **nebulizer**. This machine requires specialized tubing and a plastic mask (available in different sizes), which can be obtained from many community pharmacies. Common vehicles to deliver inhalation solutions into the lungs include sterile water for injection (SWI) and normal saline (NS). The solution is placed in the nebulizer, and the device will aerosolize both the medication and the vehicle. An example of a nebulizing solution is the "rescue" medication albuterol, which is available in different concentrations. Albuterol is often prescribed for the relief of bronchial spasms and wheezing in infants and children. This inhalant is also available as an aerosol.

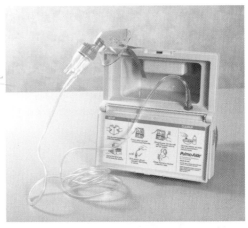

A nebulizer, also called an atomizing machine, is effective for delivering a mist or micronized powder to the lungs.

Volatile Medications and Vaporizers Vaporizers and humidifiers are other mechanical devices commonly used to deliver moisture to the air for relief of cold symptoms. Volatile medications, such as Vicks VapoSteam, can be used with some vaporizers.

Micronized Powders and Nonaerosolized Inhalers Some manufacturers use a nonaerosolized, breath-activated powder for inhalation to avoid propellants. This newer dosage uses a discus to administer a higher concentration of drug as a micronized powder into the lungs. The result may be a controlled release of active ingredients for prevention of recurring symptoms, with potentially fewer side effects. Advair Diskus and Spiriva HandiHaler are examples of inhalants in the prevention and long-term treatment of asthma or chronic lung disease symptoms. Patient counseling by the pharmacist is critical for proper use of these nonaerosolized inhalers.

A dry powder inhaler looks like a discus and is actuated by breathing in deeply at the opening of the device.

Advantages and Disadvantages of Certain Inhalation Dosage Forms

The main advantage of inhalation dosage forms is the rapid onset of action, which is second only to the IV route of administration. For example, a patient with asthma will obtain faster relief with an inhaled metered-dose medication rather than a tablet or capsule. However, a major disadvantage of all MDIs is poor inhalation technique by the patient, thus decreasing the amount of drug that reaches the pulmonary circulation. (Proper technique and use of spacer devices are addressed later in the chapter.)

Even more effective than an aerosol medication is a "nebulized" mist of medication, which delivers medication deeper into the lungs. The nebulizer delivers a higher dose of medication (commonly albuterol) to the lungs and has a faster onset of action, especially in infants and pediatric patients with acute shortness of breath or asthma. The larger amount of medication, however, may lead to a higher risk of side effects such as a rapid heart rate.

Dispensing and Administration of Inhalation Dosage Forms

Patients who are taking more than one MDI should administer the more immediate-acting drug first, followed by the second drug 5–10 minutes later. The pharmacist can review the drugs prescribed and assist the patient in suggesting a prioritized order of drug administration.

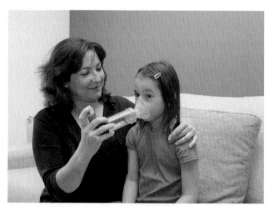

A spacer device improves the delivery of inhaled medications, especially in children and older adults.

Patients must also be instructed in the proper administration of aerosolized medications to control or relieve their respiratory symptoms. Following the correct inhalation technique ensures that the medication reaches the lungs. Table 4.5 lists steps patients should follow when administering MDIs. Hand-eye coordination and timing of inhalation are critical for optimum drug delivery with an MDI. Spacer devices are often recommended for use with pediatric and elderly patients. With a **spacer device**, the medication is released into a "storage chamber" where it can be more easily inhaled by the patient. Use of this device allows the patient to inhale a higher concentration of medication, thus providing better relief of symptoms. Spacer devices may be packaged with the medication or dispensed separately and are available in small, medium, and large sizes for infants, children, and adults, respectively.

After MDI administration of a cortisone-like drug, a patient should rinse the mouth thoroughly to prevent an oral fungal infection. The mouthpiece of the MDI device itself should also be washed with soap and water at least once weekly.

TABLE 4.5   Proper Technique for Administration of an MDI

1. Shake the canister well (or else only the propellant may be administered).
2. Prime the canister by pressing down and activating a practice dose. (Check priming instructions for each product as they vary depending on the manufacturer and active ingredient.)
3. Prepare the MDI by inserting the canister into a mouthpiece or spacer to reduce the amount of drug deposited on the back of the throat. (This is especially helpful for young children or older adults who may have difficulty with hand-eye coordination.)
4. Breathe out and hold the spacer between the lips, making a seal.
5. Activate the MDI and take a deep, slow inhalation at the same time.
6. Hold the breath briefly and slowly exhale through the nose.

Parenteral Route of Administration

A **parenteral solution** is a sterile or microbial-free solution (with or without medication) that is administered by means of a hollow needle or catheter inserted through one or more layers of the skin. The term *parenteral* comes from the Greek roots *para*, meaning "beside," and *enteron*, meaning "intestine." The derivation of the word indicates that this route of administration bypasses—or goes "beside" rather than through—the alimentary canal or GI tract. With that in mind, the **parenteral route of administration** includes the injection of any drug or fluid into the bloodstream, muscle, or skin.

Parenteral Dosage Forms

Safety Note

Although the abbreviations *SQ* or *SC* continue to be used by prescribers to indicate the subcutaneous route, this practice should be discouraged due to an enhanced risk of a medication error.

Parenteral dosage forms are administered through intravenous (IV), intramuscular (IM), subcutaneous, or intradermal (ID) routes. IV administration is defined as directly into the vein; IM, into the muscle; subcutaneous, under the skin; and ID, into the dermal layer of the skin.

IV Route One of the more common parenteral routes of drug and fluid administration is the IV route. An **intravenous (IV) infusion** is a method for delivering a large amount of fluid and/or a high concentration of medication directly into the bloodstream over a prolonged period and at a slow, steady rate.

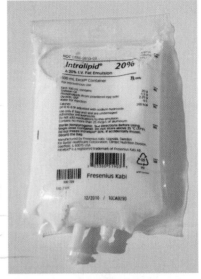

Liposyn is an example of an IV total parenteral nutrition solution for patients who are NPO (nothing by mouth).

Patients whose medical conditions preclude nothing by mouth (NPO, from the Latin term *nil per os*) may be maintained on IV solutions such as dextrose or normal saline (with or without added medication), as well as nutrient-containing products known as total parenteral nutrition (or TPN). In the hospital and in many home healthcare pharmacies, antibiotics, chemotherapy, nutrition, and critical care medications are administered via this route. Liposyn III is an example of a nutritional fat emulsion administered by the IV route of administration. (For more information on parenteral IV solutions and injections, see Chapter 11.)

IM Route The IM route is used to administer antibiotics, narcotics, medications for migraine headaches, vitamins, iron, male and female hormones, antipsychotic medications, and several vaccines including the influenza or flu vaccine administered in many community pharmacies. These medications are commonly administered by **injection**. For example, vitamin B_{12} and testosterone medications are commercially available as a single-dose vial and a multiple-dose vial in the community pharmacy. Testosterone injections are available as a cypionate salt (suspended in cottonseed oil) or as an enanthate salt (suspended in sesame oil). Though not interchangeable without prescriber permission, both of these salts deliver a similar amount of medication over a 10- to 14-day period.

The IM route is also used to deliver lifesaving medication, such as epinephrine, in an emergency. An EpiPen, an autoinjector device used for administering epinephrine, is available in both pediatric and adult dosages and can be administered IM (including through clothing) as well as subcutaneously. The medication device is commonly dispensed for children in a two-pack. It can be used for repeated injections, or one can be used at home and the other at school. Several states allow school personnel to legally administer epinephrine in emergency situations such as a hypersensitivity to insect stings or a severe allergic reaction to peanut butter.

Practice Tip

The shingles vaccine must be stored in a freezer; once reconstituted with sterile water, the vaccine must be administered subcutaneously within 30 minutes.

Subcutaneous Route Subcutaneous injections administer medications below the skin into the subcutaneous tissue. Common medications that are administered subcutaneously include epinephrine (or adrenaline) for emergency asthmatic attacks or allergic reactions, heparin to prevent blood clots, sumatriptan (Imitrex) for migraines, and the pneumonia and shingles vaccines. Besides these medications, almost all insulins and insulin-like products for diabetes are administered by the subcutaneous route. Insulins vary in their onset and duration of action; most of these medications work within 30–60 minutes, and some of these products may lower blood glucose levels for up to 24 hours. Insulins are also available as mixtures of rapid-acting and long-acting products, typically in a 75/25, 70/30, or 50/50 concentration. In the hospital or in the emergency room, regular or fast-acting insulin can also be administered via the IV route.

ID Route The ID route of administration is typically used for diagnostic and allergy skin testing, local anesthesia, and various diagnostic tests and immunizations. For allergy skin testing, small amounts of various allergens are administered (usually on the surface of the back) to detect allergies before beginning desensitization allergy shots. For diagnostic testing, such as for tuberculosis (TB), injections are given in the upper forearm, below where IV injections are given. If a patient is allergic or has been exposed to an allergen similar to TB, then the patient may experience a severe local reaction.

Advantages and Disadvantages of Certain Parenteral Dosage Forms

The parenteral route is often used for medications whose molecules are too unstable or large to be absorbed or for medications that are broken down so quickly in the stomach or liver that they cannot be taken orally. Parenteral administration in the hospital, skilled care facility, and home healthcare facility deserves special attention because of its complexity, widespread use, and potential for both therapeutic benefit and danger.

IV Route The IV route is the preferred route of administration to deliver medications in an emergency situation. IV medications act rapidly to control and treat symptoms and can be administered via any vein in the body. These medications are administered using two different methods: IV bolus (also referred to as IV push) and IV infusion.

With an **IV bolus injection**, the drug is administered all at once, such as the use of epinephrine or Adrenalin in the case of a cardiac arrest, or the use of glucagon when the blood glucose level of a patient with diabetes is dangerously low. These drugs can also be administered by the IM and subcutaneous routes.

An **IV infusion** provides a continuous amount of needed medication over a given period. The medication may be slowly infused over time (8 hours) in the IV solution, or it may be administered over 20–30 minutes in a smaller "minibag" connected to the IV solution. The advantage of an infusion is that there is less fluctuation in drug blood levels than is experienced with other routes of administration. The infusion rate can be adjusted to provide more or less medication as the situation dictates: a higher infusion rate for pain relief or a slower infusion rate if the patient experiences side effects such as shortness of breath.

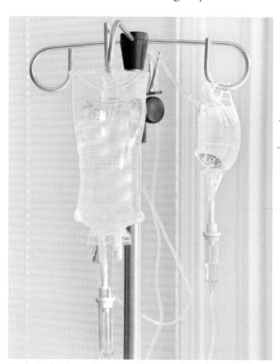

Both IV fluids and medications can be administered via infusions in the hospital.

The IV route does have associated inherent dangers, including the inability to retrieve the medication if an adverse or allergic reaction occurs. Another major disadvantage of administering a drug via the IV route is the potential for introducing toxic agents, microbes, or **pyrogens** (fever-producing by-products of microbial metabolism). Consequently, to minimize infection, IV products are prepared by pharmacy technicians in an isolated clean room environment using special techniques and equipment to ensure sterility. After preparation of each IV product, the technician as well as a pharmacist must inspect the solution for contaminants as well as salt precipitates, which is evidence of incompatibility. Particulate matter that is present in an IV solution may cause an **embolism** (blockage of a vessel) or **phlebitis** (a severe painful reaction at the injection site).

Before administration of the IV solution, the nurse must also inspect the solution for precipitates, swab the IV site with an alcohol wipe, and select the correct syringe and needle for the procedure. During administration of the IV product, the nurse must ensure that the solution is free of particulate matter and air bubbles—both of which may lead to embolism or phlebitis.

Failure to follow protocol for IV products may result in serious adverse effects for the patient recipient. (To learn more about germ theory and the importance of aseptic technique, see Chapter 10.)

IM Route The IM route of administration offers a more convenient way to deliver injectable medications. Although the onset of response to the medication is slower than with the IV route, the duration of action for an IM injection is much longer, making it more practical for use outside the hospital setting. In fact, some IM injections may exert a therapeutic effect for a period ranging from two weeks to three months. Still, a drawback of the IM route is its unpredictable absorption rate. For this reason, the IM route is not recommended for use on patients who are unconscious or in a shocklike state.

Dispensing and Administration of Parenteral Dosage Forms

Parenteral preparations are solutions in which ingredients are dissolved or reconstituted with solutions, including sterile solutions such as dextrose in water or normal saline. Because the body is primarily an aqueous, or water-containing, vehicle, most parenteral preparations introduced into the body are made up of ingredients placed in a sterile water medium. Some parenteral medications are available in single-use vials or ampules that contain no preservative; others may be available in a multi-dose vial of lyophilized powder with preservatives. All parenteral injections—whether administered via the IV, IM, subcutaneous, or ID route—must be sterile because they introduce medication directly into the body.

 Safety Note

Injections (including vaccines) should be given by trained healthcare professionals, not by pharmacy technicians.

Only trained professionals and healthcare providers are legally allowed to give parenteral injections. In recent years, however, patients (and their spouses or caregivers) have been taught by the home health nurse or pharmacist to administer injections or start infusions at home. In the pharmacy setting, many pharmacists are becoming increasingly involved in vaccine administration programs after completion of training and certification including cardiopulmonary resuscitation (CPR). Pharmacy technicians, however, must check their state regulations to determine if they are allowed to draw up or prepare injections for a final check by the pharmacist. Therefore, to better assist pharmacy and hospital personnel, pharmacy technicians must have a basic understanding of various syringe and needle sizes.

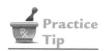

Practice & Tip

The word *hypodermic* comes from the Greek root words *hypo*, meaning "under or beneath," and *derma*, meaning "skin."

Safety Note

The syringes in Figure 4.4b are marked with the abbreviation *cc* (cubic centimeters). Because *cc* is considered a dangerous abbreviation, healthcare professionals, including the pharmacy technician, are encouraged to use the abbreviation for milliliters (mL) instead.

All parenteral injections are administered into the body (or IV bottle or minibag) with the use of a syringe and/or needle. A **syringe** is a calibrated device used to accurately draw up, measure, and deliver medication to a patient through a needle. Two types of syringes are commonly used for injections: glass and plastic. Glass syringes are fairly expensive and must be carefully sterilized between uses. Some drugs may require a glass syringe due to an incompatibility with plastic material. Plastic syringes are easier to store, handle, and dispose of after use; these syringes come from their manufacturers in sterile packaging. Plastic is clearly preferred and used both in and out of the hospital setting for most medications. For example, the blood thinner Lovenox is available in a prefilled plastic syringe in doses ranging from 30 mg per 0.3 mL to 100 mg per 1 mL. The proper disposal of plastic syringes and needles (and medications) is both a health and environmental concern; the use and sale of "sharps containers" is recommended for home and pharmacy use to safely dispose of used syringes and needles.

Common types of syringes include:

- the insulin syringe, which measures from 30 units to 100 units (equivalent to 0.3 mL to 1 mL)
- the tuberculin syringe, with a **cannula** (bore area inside the syringe) ranging from 0.1 mL to 1 mL
- the larger hypodermic syringe, with a cannula ranging from 3 mL to 60 mL

Insulin syringes are used by diabetic patients to administer insulin; tuberculin syringes are used for skin tests and for drawing up very small volumes of solution. Hypodermic syringes are used with hypodermic needles to inject parenteral drugs into the body or to remove blood from the body (see Figure 4.4). These syringes may be glass or—more commonly—disposable plastic with clear demarcations for accurate dosing. Hypodermic syringes (without a needle) are often used to more easily administer oral liquids to infants, children, and pets.

FIGURE 4.4
Common Types of Syringes

(a) Insulin syringes in 30 unit, 50 unit, and 100 unit sizes
(b) Tuberculin syringes marked with metric measures
(c) Hypodermic syringes in 6 mL and 3 mL sizes

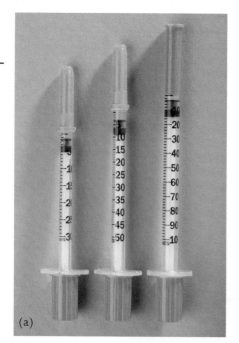

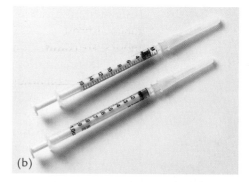

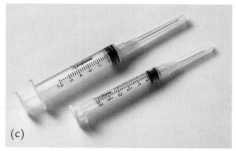

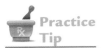
Remember that the larger the gauge number of a needle, the smaller the lumen and, consequently, the smaller the hole that the needle makes. Conversely, the smaller the gauge number of a needle, the larger the lumen, and, consequently, the larger the hole that the needle makes.

A **needle** is attached to the tip of a syringe and is used to either draw fluid into the syringe or push fluid out of the syringe. Needles come in various lengths and sizes. Needle length and size depend on the route of administration, patient factors such as body size, and drug formulation characteristics. Needles commonly range from 18 gauge to 32 gauge. The size of the gauge corresponds conversely to the size of the lumen (inner core) of the needle: the larger

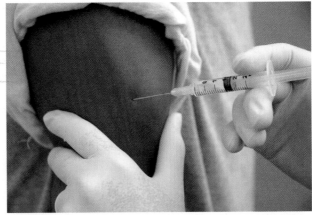

Disposable syringes and needles are used to administer drugs by injection. Different sizes are available depending on the type of medication and injection needed.

the gauge number, the smaller the lumen of the needle. (To learn more about needle gauges for parenteral injections, see the specific routes of administration below.)

Different states have different regulations on the sale of syringes and needles without a prescription because of their potential diversion for the injection of illegal drugs. Some states (or pharmacies) may require a prescription or the placement of syringes behind the prescription counter to control access to their sale. Many pharmacies will not sell syringes directly to the public unless they can provide proof of their diabetic status; the final decision may be at the discretion of the pharmacist.

IV Route As mentioned earlier, IV medications can be administered using two methods: IV bolus and IV infusions. IV bolus injections are needed when a rapid-onset pharmacological effect is desired, such as to deliver antiseizure drugs or clot-busting medications. IV infusions are administered when a steady level of medication is needed over a given period (usually eight hours). Blood, water, electrolytes, nutrients (such as proteins, amino acids, lipids, and sugars), and various drugs, including antibiotics, are commonly administered by IV infusion. Injections and infusions are usually administered into the superficial veins of the arm on the side opposite the elbow, although other sites are used as well. These injections are given at a 15- to 20-degree angle (see Figure 4.5).

FIGURE 4.5
Intravenous Injection

Intravenous (IV) injections are administered at a 15- to 20-degree angle.

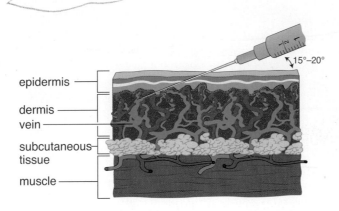

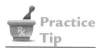

Practice Tip

Pharmacy personnel should be aware that PCA pumps are patient-controlled: Patients push a handheld controller to self-administer a dose of pain medication intravenously.

Infusion pumps are often used in the inpatient hospital setting to deliver IV infusions. These pumps continuously deliver medication 24/7 to regulate the amount, rate, and/or timing of infused fluid or medication. They are used primarily in the inpatient hospital setting. Examples of infusion pumps include:

- a **patient-controlled analgesia (PCA) infusion device**, which is a programmable machine that delivers small doses of painkillers upon patient demand
- a jet injector, such as epinephrine, which uses pressure rather than a needle to deliver the medication in an emergency
- an ambulatory injection device, such as an insulin pump, that the patient can wear while moving about and maintaining a normal lifestyle.

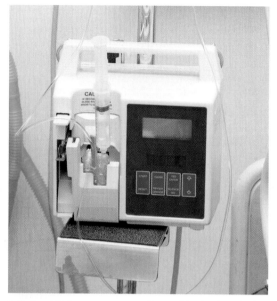

Infusion pumps are commonly used in the hospital to more accurately regulate the rate of IV drug infusions.

IM Route An IM injection does not work as fast as an IV injection (or infusion), but the pharmacological effect will last longer. Many narcotic pain medications are administered by IM injection in the hospital and nursing home. Certain drugs must be given via the IM route because they are known to irritate veins and cause phlebitis if given by the IV route. Some emergency medications, such as epinephrine, are also administered intramuscularly. The Twinject autoinjector is a device designed to administer a first dose of epinephrine in an emergency into the thigh muscle through clothing. The autoinjector must be held against the skin for 10 seconds for the medication to be released. A second dose may be administered into the muscle if needed.

IM injections typically are administered using a 22- to 25-gauge, 5/8 to 1½ inch needle. The needle must be sufficiently long to inject the drug through the dermal or skin layers into the muscle. The needle length for an IM injection may also be dependent on the adipose or fat content vs. lean muscle at the injection site of the patient. In light of that, a smaller-size needle can be used for an IM injection in a lean patient with average or smaller arm size or skin thickness. Though a large-gauge (smaller needle) is always preferable for patient comfort, some medications due to their viscosity (such as hormone injections) may require a small-gauge (larger needle) to withdraw the medication from the vial and inject the drug into the muscle.

The volume of injection is usually limited to less than 2 mL. Care must be taken during deep IM injections to avoid hitting a vein, artery, or nerve. In adults, IM injections are generally given into the upper, outer portion of the gluteus maximus, the

In an emergency such as a bee sting, an EpiPen can be administered IM through clothing.

FIGURE 4.6
Intramuscular Injection

Intramuscular (IM) injections are administered at a 90-degree angle.

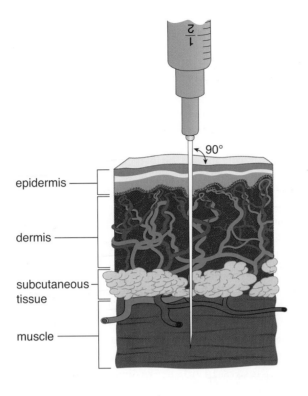

large muscle on either side of the buttocks. Another common site, especially for children, is the deltoid muscles beneath the shoulders. Figure 4.6 shows the needle angle and injection depth for an IM injection.

Subcutaneous Route Subcutaneous injections are typically administered on the outside of the upper arm, the top of the thigh, or the lower portion of each side of the abdomen. These injections should not be made into grossly adipose, hardened, inflamed, or swollen tissue. For the subcutaneous administration of insulin, the patient should be instructed by the pharmacist to carefully administer the medication while following a routine plan for site rotation. The site of insulin administration must be rotated from the abdomen, to each leg (upper thigh), and then to the arm to avoid or minimize local skin reactions and scarring.

FIGURE 4.7
Subcutaneous Injection

Subcutaneous injections usually are administered just below the skin at a 45-degree angle.

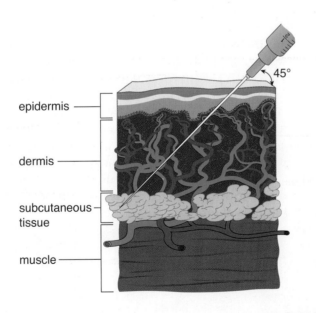

The needle used for subcutaneous injections is typically 3/8 to 5/8 of an inch in length, with a needle gauge in the range of 25 to 32. The gauge used by diabetic patients may vary from 28 to 32 with short, fine, or ultrafine needles. The correct length of the needle is determined by a skin pinch in the injection area. The proper needle length will be one-half the thickness of the pinch.

Subcutaneous injections are usually given just beneath the pinched skin with the syringe held at a 45-degree angle (see Figure 4.7). In lean older patients with less tissue, and in obese patients with more tissue, the syringe should be held nearer to a 90-degree angle. To avoid pressure on sensory nerves causing pain and discomfort, a volume of 1 mL or less is injected.

Administration of Insulin The most commonly used medication that is administered subcutaneously is insulin. Insulin is typically given several times a day with the administration time varying around mealtime or bedtime, depending on the type of insulin prescribed. Several types of insulin are available, including immediate, short-acting, intermediate-acting, and long-acting. These medications differ in onset and duration of action. The absorption of insulin may vary depending on the site of administration and the activity level of the patient. The patient should be cautioned about planning meals, exercise, and insulin administration to gain the best advantage of the medication and avoid the chances of creating hypoglycemia or low blood glucose levels.

Insulin Product Selection Syringe size, needle length, and needle gauge are critical factors in insulin product selection. For subcutaneous insulin injections, a higher gauge, smaller needle is used due to multiple daily injections.

Insulin dosage is prescribed in units rather than in milliliters. The concentration is 100 units per mL. Various insulins are available in both 10 mL vials (containing 1,000 units of insulin) and as a 3 mL prefilled insulin pen. A prefilled insulin pen would require replacement needles, which are available in a variety of sizes. The selection of pen needles is further discussed in Chapter 7.

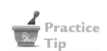

Practice Tip

Pharmacy personnel should inform patients taking insulin to roll the medication vials between their hands to agitate and warm the insulin. Insulin vials should never be shaken.

Insulin Vials The dose of insulin in a multi-dose vial is administered using a special syringe with the needle attached. The insulin syringe is available in several volume sizes such as 0.3 mL, 0.5 mL, and 1 mL; the proper size is determined by the dose of insulin needed. When preparing a vial of insulin for administration, the vial should be agitated and warmed by rolling the vial between the hands. Insulin vials should never be shaken. Then the rubber stopper of the vial should be cleaned with an alcohol wipe. An amount of air—equal to the amount of insulin to be withdrawn—should be injected into the vial by the needle-syringe unit. To remove air bubbles from the syringe containing the insulin, the patient should hold the syringe needle, tap it lightly, and then gently push the plunger to expel the air.

Insulin Pens An **insulin pen** is a portable device in which the prescribed dose of medication is "dialed up" to administer insulin. A prefilled insulin pen can deliver anywhere from 1 unit to 60 units of a prescribed insulin (see Figure 4.8). After priming, the patient simply "dials up" the correct units on the syringe and injects the medication.

Common insulin pens include Humalog KwikPens, NovoLog, Levemir FlexPens, Apidra, and Lantus SoloSTAR. BYETTA and Victoza are insulin-like products that are also available in a prefilled pen. Pharmacy personnel should be aware that prefilled pens cannot be mixed with other insulins, although Humalog KwikPen now is commercially available in a 75/25 and a 50/50 mixture of immediate and long-acting insulin. The insulin devices are packaged as five 3 mL prefilled insulin pens, with each pen containing 300 units of insulin.

FIGURE 4.8
Components of an Insulin Pen

The insulin pen is easy to learn, simple to use, and convenient to carry, especially while traveling.

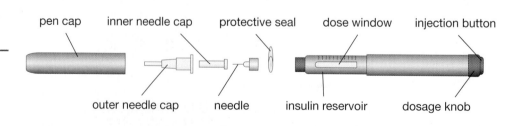

pen cap inner needle cap protective seal dose window injection button

outer needle cap needle insulin reservoir dosage knob

Insulin pens have many advantages for patients. The pens:

- are more convenient and easier to transport than traditional vials and syringes
- do not require the additional purchase of syringes and needles
- deliver more accurate dosages
- are easier to use for those with fine-motor skills impairment or visual impairments (such as a child or an elderly patient)
- cause less injection pain (as polished and coated needles are not dulled by insertion into a vial of insulin before a second insertion into the skin)
- retain a memory of past injections
- are disposable

The major disadvantage of the pens is their cost, with no or variable coverage from drug insurance plans.

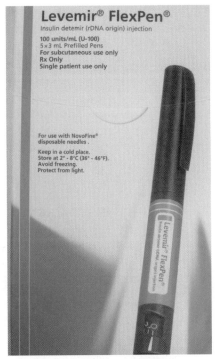

Insulin pens are a portable and convenient way for patients with diabetes to administer insulin.

Storage of Insulin All insulin must be protected from extremes in temperature. Patients should be instructed to keep insulin refrigerated and to check expiration dates frequently. Opened vials or insulin pens can be stored at room temperature and should generally be discarded after one month because the insulin can lose a portion of its potency even if stored under ideal conditions. Unopened vials or insulin pens should be refrigerated to maintain their potency until their time of expiration.

Insurance Coverage for Insulin Supplies Insurance companies, including Medicare, require a prescription for coverage of syringes, needles, and other diabetic supplies such as lancets, blood glucose monitors, and test strips. For patients over age 65, Medicare may cover some of the cost of diabetic supplies if proper paperwork is completed and on file. Assisting the diabetic patient is a very important role for the pharmacy technician and will be discussed further in Chapter 7.

ID Route ID injections are given into the capillary-rich skin layer just below the epidermis (see Figure 4.9). A small amount of medication is injected into the dermal layer of skin to form a wheal.

FIGURE 4.9
Intradermal Injection

Intradermal (ID) injections pierce the skin at a 10- to 15-degree angle. A small amount of medication (0.1 mL) is injected slowly into the dermal layer to form a wheal.

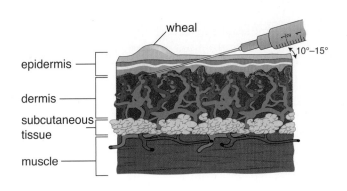

Drug Delivery Systems

A **drug delivery system** is most commonly a design feature of a dosage form that modifies the release of a drug by one or more pharmacokinetic parameters of the drug such as absorption, distribution, or elimination from the body. Formulating medications based on the pharmacokinetic process results in products with improved efficacy and safety, therefore optimizing disease control and patient outcomes. Tablets, capsules, and transdermal patches, in particular, have been redesigned for effectiveness as well as patient convenience and compliance to drug therapy. Dosage forms with specialized drug delivery systems include the oral disintegrating tablet, the sublingual tablet, and the buccal lozenge. These products have modified absorption and distribution phases of the pharmacokinetic process in order to enhance their therapeutic effects.

Other tablets and capsules have been formulated with an enteric coating to delay their release and protect the stomach or extend their release (SR, XR, XL) over a 12- to 24-hour period. These extended-release medications have a less frequent dosing schedule, which improves patient convenience and compliance and, ultimately, better disease control.

Transdermal patches are also formulated to release their medication slowly over 12 hours, 24 hours, 72 hours, or one week. For patients, this delayed release avoids or minimizes common side effects and provides convenience.

Lastly, vaginal rings and intrauterine devices are drug delivery systems that are inserted vaginally to prevent pregnancy. These contraceptive devices provide a slow release of hormones when placed in contact with the mucosa of the reproductive tract.

The pharmacy technician must be aware of the many drug products on the pharmacy shelf that may be available in various drug delivery systems—enteric coated, delayed release, sustained release, extended release, and so on. Many of these medications with special drug release characteristics do not have a generic equivalent.

Delayed-Release and Extended-Release Tablets and Capsules

Most tablet and capsule formulations are "immediate-release"; that is, the medication is designed to be activated or released shortly after the drug is taken. When treating an infection, immediate-release formulations are desirable to initiate a fast onset of action. However, when treating certain conditions, such as hypertension or hyperglycemia, immediate-release formulations would require a long-term, frequent dosage schedule, which may be an inconvenience to patients. For these patients, a medication designed to control blood pressure or blood glucose levels for 24 hours would be preferable.

Many tablets and capsules are available in a confusing alphabet of release formulations: DR, CR, CD, XR, SR, XT, and XL. Pharmaceutical manufacturers market these different release formulations to extend their existing product line, lengthen patent protection, and improve bottom-line profits. For example, Depakote—a medication commonly used for seizures—is available as both a DR enteric-coated drug and an ER or extended-release drug. However, these drugs are not interchangeable, and their inadvertent substitution could lead to toxicity, patient injury, or, possibly, patient death. Many other medications are also designated with release formulations. For example, the antihypertensive drug diltiazem and the antidepressant drug buproprion (Wellbutrin) have multiple immediate-release and extended-release products from several drug manufacturers on the market and, most likely, on your pharmacy shelf.

Safety Note

Pharmacy technicians should read drug labels carefully. A sustained-release (SR) dosage form is *not* the same as an extended-release (XL) dosage form of the same drug.

Safety Note

Pharmacy technicians should be aware that the protective or timed-release design characteristics of any delayed-release or extended-release oral formulations would be compromised if the medications were split or crushed.

In light of that, pharmacy personnel must exercise caution when filling prescription medication to avoid medication errors. (For more information on medication safety, refer to Chapter 12.) Technicians also need to be aware that many of these delayed-release and extended-release formulations come with a higher cost or co-payment for consumers.

A working definition of delayed-release and extended-release dosage formulations is as follows:

- Delayed-release (DR)—The United States Pharmacopeia (USP) defines the term *delayed-release tablet* as "enteric-coated to delay release of the medication until the tablet has passed through the stomach to prevent the drug from being destroyed or inactivated by gastric juices or where it may irritate the gastric mucosa."
- Extended-release (XL)—The USP defines *extended-release* as "formulated in such a manner to make the contained medicament available over an extended period of time following ingestion."

Delayed-Release Formulations Delayed-release (DR) formulations have a special coating designed to delay absorption of the medication and to resist breakdown by acidic gastric fluids. Consequently, the risk of side effects such as nausea or stomach upset is minimal. One delayed-release drug formulation is an **enteric-coated tablet (ECT)**. Examples of ECTs include aspirin, naproxen, and potassium chloride—all drugs that can be irritating to the stomach. Unlike an ECT, a tablet with a sugar or film coating makes the drug more palatable but does not impact or delay the release characteristics of the drug in the bloodstream. For example, an MCT can be formulated to provide controlled release in successive events or stages. Adalat CC for high blood pressure is an example of a delayed-release MCT.

Extended-Release Formulations Extended-release (XL) formulations allow a reduced frequency of dosing as compared with immediate-release medications. Both **sustained-release (SR) formulations** and **controlled-release (CR) formulations** belong to this category. For example, SR formulations, such as bupropion SR, allow a less-frequent dosing schedule (two doses 8–12 hours apart) than its immediate-release counterpart (three to four daily doses). CR formulations allow at least a twofold reduction in dosing frequency from that of immediate-release and most SR formulations. For example, Wellbutrin XL should be taken once a day in the morning; Wellbutrin SR should be taken every 8–12 hours.

Capsules and tablets can also be designed to extend drug release by altering the salt of the drug. The oral nitrate tablet isosorbide 30 mg is available as a mononitrate salt (with once daily dosing) and a dinitrate salt (twice daily dosing) to prevent chest pain. Another example is the antihypertensive drug metoprolol; it is available as an immediate-release tartrate salt and also as an extended-release succinate salt in doses of 25 mg, 50 mg, and 100 mg. Though the active ingredients are exactly the same, these drugs are not interchangeable—even at identical doses—and the correct stock bottle must be selected by the pharmacy technician.

Wax Matrix, Osmotic Pressure, and Targeted Release Systems

More recent drug delivery systems employ scientific and biotechnologic processes to design medications that produce long-term therapeutic effects. These innovative systems include matrix-controlled release formulations, osmotic pressure release formulations, and targeted drug delivery.

Matrix-Controlled Release Formulations Many unique and novel oral and trans-dermal drug delivery systems were developed by the ALZA Corporation, a company that was acquired by Johnson and Johnson in 2001. Many of these drug delivery systems are prepared using a wax matrix, a reservoir-controlled release utilizing an osmotic pressure principle or an ion exchange resin. In **wax matrix systems**, the drug is embedded in a polymer matrix, and the release takes place by the partitioning of the drug into the polymer matrix and surrounding medium. Drug release is controlled by diffusion of the drug through the coating membrane of the capsule. The narcotic drug Oxycontin is an example of a matrix-controlled release formulation in which the medication is released over a period of 12 hours.

Tussionex capsules, a narcotic cough medication, uses an ion exchange resin in its drug design to slowly release the active drug over 12 hours. In addition to an increase in the duration of action, the ion-exchange resin can mask taste, prevent tablet disintegration, and improve the chemical stability of the active ingredient.

Osmotic Pressure Release Formulations In the **osmotic pressure system**, the drug is delivered to the body by slowly being "pushed out" into the bloodstream. This drug delivery system has several therapeutic uses:

- to maintain a constant drug plasma concentration for behavioral control (Concerta, Adderall XR)
- to regulate blood glucose levels (Glucotrol XL)
- to manage depression (Effexor XR)
- to treat hypertension (Procardia XL) over a 24-hour period

Targeted Drug Delivery Systems In the near future, **targeted drug delivery systems** will become increasingly available. In this system, a drug is "carried" by a liposome, a biocompatible and biodegradable substance, and released at a targeted organ site (see Figure 4.10). Several chemotherapeutic agents are formulated for this drug delivery system, targeting only the cancerous organ. Employing this method avoids the adverse effects associated with chemotherapy, including decreased blood counts, alopecia (hair loss), and severe GI disturbances that occur when the toxic chemotherapeutic agent is distributed throughout other body systems.

FIGURE 4.10
Liposome

Liposomal drug delivery systems target specific cells for medication distribution, thus increasing the drug's effectiveness while decreasing its potential for toxicity.

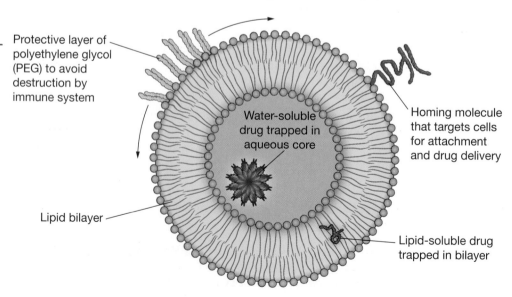

Protective layer of polyethylene glycol (PEG) to avoid destruction by immune system

Water-soluble drug trapped in aqueous core

Homing molecule that targets cells for attachment and drug delivery

Lipid bilayer

Lipid-soluble drug trapped in bilayer

Transdermal Patches

A **transdermal dosage form** is designed to deliver a drug contained within a patch or disk to the bloodstream via absorption through the skin. The patch consists of a backing, a drug core or reservoir, a rate-controlling membrane, an adhesive layer, and a protective strip. Once the strip is removed, the adhesive layer is attached to the skin. Chemicals in the patch or disk force the drug across the membranes of the skin and into the layer of skin where optimal absorption into the bloodstream will occur.

Transdermal patches provide a slow-release, steady level of drug in the system. In some patches, the membrane controls the rate of drug delivery, but in others the skin itself controls the rate. This mechanism of action is similar to controlled-release tablets or capsules but produces less side effects as less drug is released. Although the skin presents a barrier, absorption does occur slowly and is affected by patient-specific factors such as thickness of skin and blood flow, both of which vary with age. Transdermal patches administered to infants and young children may result in toxicity and are generally not recommended unless FDA approved for that age-group.

Therapeutic Uses Therapeutic effects may last from 24 hours to 1 week. Drugs such as nicotine, nitroglycerin, narcotic analgesics, clonidine, scopolamine, estrogen/progestin, estrogen, and testosterone are administered topically for their systemic effects on smoking cessation, chest pain, chronic pain, blood pressure, motion sickness, birth control, female hormone replacement levels, and male hormone replacement levels, respectively. For example, the nonsteroidal anti-inflammatory drug diclofenac (similar to ibuprofen) is available as a transdermal patch. This patch can deliver the medication directly to an injury site (strain, sprain, or contusion) for short-term treatment without the risk of severe adverse GI effects of its oral counterpart. Similarly, an estradiol transdermal patch (Vivelle-Dot) is administered twice a week and indicated for the topical treatment of postmenopausal symptoms with less risk of systemic side effects than an oral tablet formulation such as Premarin.

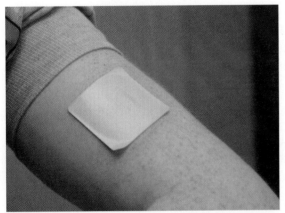

A transdermal patch offers a convenient delivery system for many medications. Transdermal patches should not be placed on skin that is overly hairy or on scar tissue or damaged skin.

Administration The site of administration for transdermal patches should be relatively hair-free (usually the upper arm); patches should not be placed over a large area of scar tissue or damaged skin, which may increase or decrease the release of the drug. Some patches are replaced every day, but others maintain their therapeutic effect for 3–7 days. The site of application should be rotated to minimize localized skin reactions.

One type of transdermal patch—a Lidoderm and nitroglycerin patch—provides 24 hours of relief from a 12-hour application. Most physicians advise their patients to remove the nitroglycerin and lidocaine patch at bedtime to prevent the development of drug tolerance. As defined in Chapter 3, drug tolerance occurs when the body requires higher doses of drug to produce the same therapeutic effect.

Another transdermal patch delivers fentanyl, a potent Schedule II opiate analgesic. This drug is slowly absorbed through the skin into the bloodstream and can relieve chronic pain for up to three days upon a single patch application. Sun exposure should be avoided, and heating pads, electric blankets, heat lamps, saunas, hot tubs, or heated water beds cannot be used with this drug. Localized heat speeds up the

Safety Note

Patients should be advised to carefully discard their used patches. The nicotine or narcotic patches, for example, could cause serious side effects if ingested by children or pets.

movement of fentanyl from the patch into the body. If the patch is damaged, then increased absorption of the active drug can occur. Both situations create a higher risk for a serious drug overdose.

Miscellaneous Delivery Systems

Other miscellaneous drug delivery systems include a vaginal ring delivery system and an intrauterine device, both of which continuously deliver hormones to a female's reproductive tract.

The NuvaRing is an example of a vaginal ring delivery system to prevent conception. The ring is 2 inches in diameter and is made of a flexible plastic that is inserted vaginally once a month. Once in contact with the vaginal mucosa, estrogen and progestin hormones are released and slowly absorbed and distributed into the bloodstream. This steady, consistent release of medication may result in fewer hormonal variations than when using other birth control methods. NuvaRing is as effective in preventing conception as birth control pills. In fact, a woman may be more compliant to therapy with a once monthly ring rather than the daily ingestion of a birth control pill. It is recommended that the contraceptive ring be refrigerated before being dispensed.

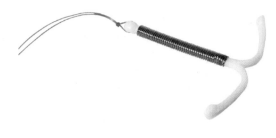

An IUD releases a progestin-only hormone within the uterus that prevents conception.

An **intrauterine device (IUD)** is another way to prevent conception via a drug delivery device. IUDs are available as hormonal drug and nondrug copper devices. For contraception, the IUD is inserted into the uterus via the vagina. The drug IUD contains a progestin-only hormone that is slowly released and localized in the uterus, thus decreasing the risk of long-term adverse effects. This device provides a higher degree of contraceptive protection with a lower failure rate than pills, patches, and contraceptive vaginal rings. As with the ring, the patient may experience side effects or discomfort or have difficulty with proper insertion.

Chapter Summary

- Drugs are administered in many dosage forms. Factors influencing the decision on route of administration include ease of administration; site, onset, and duration of action; quantity to be administered; drug metabolism by the liver or excretion by the kidney; and drug toxicity.
- Oral route of administration allows medication to travel through the digestive tract where it is absorbed for distribution.
- Oral dosage forms include tablets, capsules, powders, and liquids, with each dosage form offering convenience, safety, and ease of use for patients.
- Measuring spoons, oral syringes, medication cups, and droppers are critical for accurate dosing of liquid medication in infant and pediatric patients.
- Transmucosal route of administration allows medication to be absorbed through the mucous membranes of the mouth, eyes, ears, nose, rectum, vagina, and urethra.
- Transmucosal dosage forms include sublingual medications, buccal medications, ophthalmics, otics, nasal sprays/solutions, and suppositories; these dosage forms offer a fast onset of action when immediate relief is needed.
- Different routes of medication administration include the sublingual route (via the blood vessels under the tongue), the buccal route (through the mucosal lining of the cheek), the ocular and conjunctival routes (into the eye), the otic route (into the ear), the intranasal route (through the nose), and the rectal route (into the rectum).
- Topical route of administration allows medication to be absorbed through the skin.
- Topical dosage forms include ointments, pastes, plasters, creams, lotions, gels, and irrigating solutions; these dosage forms typically have a fast onset of action and minimal systemic side effects due to their localized therapeutic action.
- The inhalation or intrarespiratory route of administration allows medication to be inhaled through the oral respiratory route.
- Aerosols and sprays are common inhalation dosage forms and offer a rapid onset of action.
- MDIs, nebulizers, vaporizers, and discuses are devices used to deliver inhalation therapy.
- Parenteral route of administration includes the injection of any drug or fluid into the bloodstream, muscle, or skin.
- Parenteral administration commonly includes IV, IM, subcutaneous, and ID injections, as well as IV infusions.
- IV injections and infusions are injected directly into the bloodstream, and special precautions must be taken in their preparation and administration to maintain sterility and to prevent air embolisms.
- IV medications can be given by an IV bolus injection (when the entire drug is administered at once) or by IV infusion (when a drug is administered slowly over a designated period).
- IV infusions are given for a variety of purposes, including the delivery of fluids and electrolytes, nutrients, and drugs.
- Common types of syringes include the insulin syringe, the tuberculin syringe, and the hypodermic syringe.
- Needles come in various lengths and sizes; the size of the gauge corresponds conversely to the size of the lumen of the needle.
- Medications administered by IM injection include antibiotics, narcotics, vitamins, hormones, and vaccines.
- Insulin is a common medication administered via the subcutaneous route.
- ID route of administration is typically used for drug and allergy tests, local anesthesia, and various immunizations.
- Drug delivery systems are dosage forms whose design affects the delivery of the drug.

- Common drug delivery systems include delayed-release and extended-release tablets and capsules, matrix-controlled release formulations, osmotic pressure release formulations, and targeted drug delivery systems.

- Certain methods of contraception, such as the vaginal ring and the IUD, use drug delivery systems to release hormones and prevent pregnancy. The IUD is also used to deliver hormones to treat certain disorders of the reproductive tract.

Key Terms

aerosol a pressurized container with a propellant that is used to administer a drug through oral inhalation into the lungs

aromatic water a solution of water containing oils or other substances that has a pungent, and usually pleasing, smell and is easily released into the air

buccal route of administration a transmucosal route of administration in which a drug is placed between the gum and the inner lining of the cheek

cannula the barrel of a syringe or bore area inside the syringe that correlates with the volume of solution

caplet a hybrid solid dosage formulation sharing characteristics of both a tablet and a capsule

capsule the dosage form containing powder, liquid, or granules in a gelatin covering

chewable tablet a solid oral dosage form meant to be chewed that is readily absorbed; commonly prescribed for school-age children

colloid the dispersion of ultrafine particles in a liquid formulation

compression tablet a tablet consisting of an active ingredient and an inactive ingredient (diluent, binder, disintegrant, or lubricating agent) that is manufactured by means of great pressure

conjunctival route of administration the placement of sterile ophthalmic medications in the conjunctival sac of the eye(s)

controlled-release (CR) formulation a dosage form that is formulated to release medication over a long duration

cream a cosmetically acceptable oil-in-water (O/W) emulsion for topical use on the skin

delayed-release (DR) formulation a dosage form, such as an enteric-coated aspirin tablet, that contains a special coating designed to delay absorption of the medication and to resist breakdown by acidic gastric fluids

diluent an inactive ingredient that allows for the appropriate concentration of the medication in the tablet or capsule; also used to reconstitute parenteral products

discus a device that contains nonaerosolized powder used for inhalation

dispersion a liquid dosage form in which undissolved ingredients are mixed throughout a liquid vehicle

dosage form the physical manifestation of a drug (for example, a capsule or a tablet)

dropper a device used to accurately measure medication dosage for infants

drug delivery system a design feature of the dosage form that affects the delivery of the drug; such a system may protect the stomach or delay the release of the active drug

effervescent salts granular salts that release gas and dispense active ingredients into solution when placed in water

elixir a clear, sweetened, flavored solution containing water and ethanol

embolism a blockage of a blood vessel from a blood clot or inadvertent injection of an air bubble

emulsion the dispersion of a liquid in another liquid varying in viscosity

enema a solution, such as a Fleet enema, to be administered into the rectum to evacuate colon contents

enteric-coated tablet (ECT) a tablet coating designed to resist destruction by the acidic pH of the gastric fluids and to delay the release of the active ingredient

excipient an inert or inactive ingredient that forms a vehicle for a drug

extended-release (XL) formulation a tablet or capsule designed to reduce frequency of dosing compared with immediate-release and most sustained-release formulations

extract a potent dosage form derived from animal or plant sources from which most or all the solvent has been evaporated to produce a powder, an ointment-like form, or a solid

film-coated tablet (FCT) a tablet coated with a thin outer layer that prevents serious GI side effects

fluidextract a liquid dosage form prepared by extraction from plant sources and commonly used in the formulation of syrups

gel a dispersion containing fine particles for topical use on the skin

glycerogelatin a topical preparation made with gelatin, glycerin, water, and medicinal substances

granules a dosage form larger than powders that is formed by adding very small amounts of liquid to powders

inhalation route of administration the administration of a drug by inhalation into the lungs; also called *intrarespiratory route of administration*

injection the administration of a parenteral medication into the bloodstream, muscle, or skin

insulin pen a portable device in which the dose of insulin can be easily dialed up before administration

intranasal route of administration the placement of sprays or solutions into the nose

intrauterine device (IUD) a device that delivers medication to prevent conception

intravenous (IV) infusion the process of injecting fluid or medication into the veins, usually over a prolonged period

irrigating solution any solution used for cleansing or bathing an area of the body, such as the eyes or ears

IV bolus injection an injection in which a drug is administered intravenously all at once

IV infusion an infusion in which a drug is administered intravenously slowly over a given period

jelly a gel that contains a higher proportion of water in combination with a drug substance, as well as a thickening agent

liniment a medicated topical preparation, such as BENGAY, that is applied to the skin

liquid any free-flowing fluid that is commonly used to dissolve solids

localized effect the site-specific application of a drug

lotion a liquid for topical application that contains insoluble dispersed solids or immiscible liquids

lozenge a medication in a sweet-tasting formulation that is absorbed in the mouth; also known as a *troche*

magma a milklike liquid colloidal dispersion, such as milk of magnesia, in which particles remain distinct, in a two-phase system

metered-dose inhaler (MDI) a device used to administer a drug in the form of compressed gas through the mouth and into the lungs

microemulsion a clear formulation, such as Haley's M-O, that contains one liquid of tiny droplets dispersed in another liquid

multiple compression tablet (MCT) a tablet formulation on top of a tablet or a tablet within a tablet, produced by multiple compressions in manufacturing

nebulizer a device used to deliver medication in a fine-mist form to the lungs; often used in treating asthma

needle a thin, hollow transfer device used with a syringe to inject drugs into the body or withdraw fluids such as blood from the body

ocular route of administration the placement of sterile ophthalmic medications into the eye

oil-in-water (O/W) emulsion an emulsion containing a small amount of oil dispersed in water, as in a cream

ointment a semisolid emulsion for topical use on the skin

oral disintegrating tablet (ODT) a solid oral dosage form designed to dissolve quickly on the tongue for oral absorption and ease of administration without water

oral route of administration the administration of medication through swallowing for absorption along the GI tract into systemic circulation

oral syringe a needleless device used for administering medication to pediatric or older adult patients unable to swallow tablets or capsules

osmotic pressure system a drug delivery system in which the drug is slowly "pushed out" into the bloodstream

otic route of administration the placement of solutions or suspensions into the ear

parenteral route of administration the injection or infusion of fluids and/or medications into the body, bypassing the GI tract

parenteral solution a product that is prepared in a sterile environment for administration by injection

paste a water-in-oil (W/O) emulsion containing more solid material than an ointment

patient-controlled analgesia (PCA) infusion device a device controlled by a patient to deliver small doses of medication for chronic pain relief

pharmaceutics the study of the release characteristics of various dosage forms or drug formulations

pharmacokinetics the study of how drugs are absorbed into the bloodstream, circulated in tissues throughout the body, inactivated, and eliminated from the body

phlebitis an inflammation of the vein from the administration of drugs

plaster a solid or semisolid, medicated or non-medicated preparation that adheres to the skin

powders fine particles of medication used in tablets and capsules

pyrogen a fever-producing by-product of microbial metabolism

rectal route of administration the delivery of medication via the rectum

route of administration a way of getting a drug onto or into the body, such as orally, topically, or parenterally

solute an ingredient dissolved in a solution or dispersed in a suspension

solution a liquid dosage form in which the active ingredients are completely dissolved in a liquid vehicle

solvent the vehicle that makes up the greater part of a solution

spacer device a device commonly prescribed for children and older adults to assist in the administration of drugs from MDIs; medication can be inhaled at will rather than through timed, coordinated breathing movements

spirit an alcoholic or hydroalcoholic solution containing volatile, aromatic ingredients

spray the dosage form that consists of a container with a valve assembly that, when activated, emits a fine dispersion of liquid, solid, or gaseous material

sublingual route of administration oral administration in which a drug is placed under the tongue and is rapidly absorbed into the bloodstream

sugar-coated tablet (SCT) a tablet coated with an outside layer of sugar that protects the medication and improves both appearance and flavor

suppository a solid formulation containing a drug for rectal or vaginal administration

suspension the dispersion of a solid in a liquid

sustained-release (SR) formulation an extended-release dosage form that allows less frequent dosing than an immediate-release dosage form

syringe a device used to inject a parenteral solution into the bloodstream, muscle, or under the skin

syrup an aqueous solution thickened with a large amount of sugar (generally sucrose) or a sugar substitute such as sorbitol or propylene glycol

systemic effect the distribution of a drug throughout the body by absorption into the bloodstream

tablet the solid dosage form produced by compression and containing one or more active and inactive ingredients

targeted drug delivery system technology to deliver high concentrations of drugs to the diseased organ rather than expose the whole body to adverse side effects; commonly designed for cancer chemotherapy

tincture an alcoholic or hydroalcoholic solution of extractions from plants

topical route of administration the administration of a drug on the skin or any mucous membrane such as the eyes, nose, ears, lungs, vagina, urethra, or rectum; usually administered directly to the surface of the skin

transdermal dosage form a formulation designed to deliver a continuous supply of drug into the bloodstream by absorption through the skin via a patch or disk

transmucosal route of administration the absorption of drugs across any mucous membrane of the body including the mouth, eyes, ears, nose, rectum, vagina, and urethra

urethral route of administration the administration of a drug by insertion into the urethra

vaginal route of administration the administration of a drug by application of a cream or insertion of a tablet into the vagina

viscosity the thickness and flow characteristics of a fluid

water-in-oil (W/O) emulsion an emulsion containing a small amount of water dispersed in an oil, such as an ointment

wax matrix system a reservoir-controlled release drug delivery system using osmotic pressure or an ion exchange resin

Chapter Review

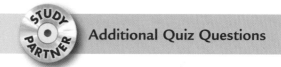

Additional Quiz Questions

Checking Your Understanding

To check your comprehension of this chapter's key concepts, read the following multiple-choice questions and then record your answers on a separate sheet of paper. Write your answers as modeled in these examples: 1d; 2c; 3b; *etc.*

1. The most common drug dosage form is a(n)
   a. compression tablet.
   b. extended-release capsule.
   c. enteric-coated tablet.
   d. inhalation aerosol.

2. Which of the following medications is available in a chewable tablet formulation?
   a. donepezil
   b. metronidazole
   c. ondansetron
   d. montelukast

3. The primary function of a film-coated tablet is to
   a. mask the smell and bitter taste.
   b. provide a faster onset of action.
   c. protect the stomach.
   d. rapidly dissolve in stomach acid.

4. Once reconstituted with water, antibiotic granules become a(n)
   a. suspension.
   b. tincture.
   c. syrup.
   d. elixir.

5. How much time will it take for most reconstituted antibiotics to expire, if stored in the refrigerator?
   a. 7 days
   b. 10 days
   c. 14 days
   d. 30 days

6. An opened bottle of nitroglycerin should be replaced
   a. every month.
   b. every 3–6 months.
   c. every year.
   d. when past expiration date on bottle.

7. An example of a water-in-oil emulsion is
   a. mupirocin ointment.
   b. hydrocortisone cream.
   c. clobetasol lotion.
   d. Aveeno oatmeal.

8. Which of the following topical medications must be applied with gloves?
   a. AndroGel pump
   b. metronidazole gel
   c. OTC capsaicin
   d. hydrocortisone lotion

9. Which of the following drugs is available as a nonaerosolized micronized powder?
   a. Advair
   b. Ventolin
   c. albuterol
   d. Combivent

10. The recommended route of administration of the shingles vaccine is
    a. intradermal.
    b. subcutaneous.
    c. intramuscular.
    d. intravenous.

11. If particulate matter gets into an IV solution during preparation, it may cause a painful inflammation of the veins, known as
    a. phlebitis.
    b. conjunctivitis.
    c. endocarditis.
    d. arthritis.

12. The word *parenteral* means, literally, "beside the _____."
    a. stomach
    b. intestine
    c. mouth
    d. liver

13. Which of the following is the major disadvantage of insulin pens?
    a. less accurate dosing
    b. inconvenience during travel
    c. cost
    d. increased injection pain

14. Opened vials of insulin kept at room temperature should be replaced every
    a. 7 days.
    b. 14 days.
    c. 30 days.
    d. 6 months.

15. Which of the following dosage formulations will have the longest duration of action?
    a. delayed-release formulations
    b. enteric-coated formulations
    c. controlled-release formulations
    d. sustained-release formulations

Reinforcing Your Learning

To build on your understanding of the topics in this chapter, complete the following enrichment activities.

1. Nitroglycerin is an example of a drug that comes in a wide variety of dosage forms appropriate for a wide variety of routes of administration. Research the different dosage forms, routes of administration, and advantages and disadvantages of nitroglycerin. To gather your information, refer to Internet sites or reference works, as well as ask healthcare professionals. Then fill in the following table with your findings.

2. Demonstrate in class the correct technique for the administration of:
    a. eyedrops
    b. eardrops
    c. a metered-dose inhaler (with and without a spacer device)
    d. an IM injection
    e. a subcutaneous injection

Dosage Form	Advantages	Disadvantages
a. sustained-release tablet		
b. sustained-release capsule		
c. sublingual tablet		
d. aerosol spray		
e. transdermal patch		
f. ointment		
g. IV		

3. Check the *Physician's Desk Reference (PDR)* for the following information on reconstituted antibiotic suspensions for these drugs: amoxicillin, amoxicillin/clavulanate, azithromycin, and cefdinir. How should each of these medications be stored? What expiration date is recommended after reconstitution at room temperature and under refrigeration? What auxiliary labels are needed for each?

4. Check the cash price of a 20 mg dose of Crestor, a brand name medication for cholesterol. If a patient asks you to get authorization from his prescriber for a new prescription for the 40 mg strength in order to split the tablets, would you be able to follow through on the patient's request? Does 40 mg Crestor meet FDA criteria for tablet splitting? What are the advantages and disadvantages of tablet splitting?

Thinking on Your Feet

To gain practice in handling challenging situations in the workplace, consider the following real-world scenarios and then use the guiding questions to help you formulate your responses.

1. A prescription has been brought in for a steroid cream (0.25%) to be applied to an infant's eczema on the cheeks. The mother states that she has a similar drug at home in an ointment formulation (1%) and wants to know whether she can use what she has at home because the drug is expensive. Creams and ointments are very different, and, in this case, the strength (and maybe the drug) is different as well. How should the pharmacy technician respond to this question? What should the pharmacist tell this mother about the differences between the two products?

2. A young man has come in to pick up some prescriptions for his asthma. His physician has just changed his prescription from oral prednisone to an inhaled steroid to control an exacerbation of his asthma. He is concerned about the inconvenience of the treatment and would rather take tablets than inhale a spray each day. The physician told the patient that the inhaled product would be safer for him in the long run. In addressing the patient's reservations about the inhalation therapy, what advantages could you provide as to the effectiveness of the inhaled product over the oral tablets?

3. An older man has just picked up two prescriptions for nitroglycerin: One prescription is for sublingual tablets, and the other prescription is for transdermal patches. When the patient asks why he has been prescribed two different formulations of the same drug, how would you respond?

4. A patient has come in to pick up some prescriptions for fertility drugs. Some of the medications are given subcutaneously and others are given IM. The pharmacist has selected the appropriate syringes for each of these routes.
   a. Which needle is appropriate for the IM injection, and which needle is appropriate for the subcutaneous injection?

   | 22G 1½ |
   | Needle |
   | Do not reshield used needles. Discard after single use. STERILE. |

   | 27G ½ |
   | Needle |
   | Do not reshield used needles. Discard after single use. STERILE. |

   b. Prepare a brief statement for the patient explaining which syringe is used for each type of injection.

5. An elderly patient with Type II diabetes has recently been placed on Humalog and Lantus insulin to control his blood glucose levels. The Humalog dose is 8 units before breakfast, 12 units before lunch, and 20 units before dinner. The Lantus dose is 40 units at bedtime. How soon before breakfast should the patient administer the Humalog insulin? What size insulin syringes are needed for the Humalog? the Lantus?

6. It is Saturday night and an out-of-town patient visits your pharmacy and requests a box of insulin syringes. What questions would you ask him or her? Can insulin syringes be legally dispensed without a prescription in your state? Check your response with a local pharmacist.

Acquiring Field Knowledge

To expand your knowledge of pharmacy practice, explore the following online activities that focus on research and information retrieval.

Reminder: *As you navigate the Internet, remember to exercise caution and good judgment when evaluating information. A thoughtful review of online text should take into consideration the following factors: the creator and sponsors of the website, the intended audience, the credentials of the authors and contributors, the reliability and validity of the posted information, the frequency of updates to the site, and the ease of navigation for a range of user skill levels.*

1. Visit a drug information site, such as www.paradigmcollege.net/ pharmpractice5e/drugs or www .paradigmcollege.net/pharmpractice5e/ rxlist, and research the drugs listed below. For each drug, write down the various dosage forms available and the route by which each dosage formulation is administered. (Each drug is available in at least two dosage forms.) Why are different routes of administration available?
   a. sumatriptan
   b. promethazine
   c. diazepam
   d. morphine
   e. triamcinolone
   f. albuterol

2. Visit www.paradigmcollege.net/ pharmpractice5e/duragesic, a website that provides information on the proper use of the Duragesic transdermal patch. Read the directions that discuss the appropriate sites for its use and the correct procedure for application. Create an informational patient brochure to share your findings.

3. Go to www.paradigmcollege.net/ pharmpractice5e/breastcancerprevention and research breast cancer prevention. Identify three factors that have been associated with a decrease in the risk of breast cancer.

4. TV media is actively promoting the Zostavax (or shingles) vaccine. Conduct an online search to find answers to the following questions: Who are candidates for this vaccine? What storage conditions are required for this vaccine? How stable is the drug once it is reconstituted? What is the recommended route of administration? What is the cash price of the vaccine?

5. Bupropion is available in three dosage formulations: immediate-release, SR, and XL. Currently, one of your customers is taking 100 mg tid of the immediate-release formulation. What dose and frequency are required if the patient switches to the SR formulation? the XL formulation? To help you find the answers, go to www .paradigmcollege.net/pharmpractice5e/ wellbutrin. Then click on the link that takes you to the Prescribing Information. Scroll through the text until you get to the subhead "Switching Patients from Wellbutrin tablets or from Wellbutrin SR Sustained-Release Tablets."

Sampling the Certification Exam

To provide you with practice for the Certification Exam, read the following questions that have been patterned after the test format and then record your answers on a separate sheet of paper. Write your answers as modeled in these examples: 1d; 2c; 3b; *etc.*

1. Which of the following dosage forms will deliver nitroglycerin (NTG) over a continuous 24-hour period?
   a. ointment
   b. sublingual tablets
   c. aerosol
   d. transdermal patch

2. The route of administration with the fastest onset of action is
   a. sublingual.
   b. subcutaneous.
   c. intramuscular.
   d. intravenous.

3. In a patient with severe nausea and vomiting, the most appropriate dosage form would be a
   a. liquid suspension.
   b. caplet.
   c. rectal suppository.
   d. magma.

4. A patient is administering 30 units of Novolin R insulin before each meal. Which of the following insulin syringes and needles would result in the most accurate reading and cause the least amount of pain at the injection site?
   a. 0.5 mL, 3/8 inch, 31 gauge
   b. 0.5 mL, ½ inch, 29 gauge
   c. 1 mL, 3/8 inch, 28 gauge
   d. 0.3 mL, 3/8 inch, 30 gauge

5. Which tablet dosage formulation is designed to melt in the mouth?
   a. sublingual tablet
   b. buccal tablet
   c. oral disintegrating tablet
   d. film-coated tablet

6. A liquid formulation thickened with sugar or a sugar substitute to mask taste is called a(n)
   a. elixir.
   b. syrup.
   c. emulsion.
   d. tincture.

7. You receive a prescription for an infant for Ranitidine in the dose of 0.8 mL po bid. To deliver the most accurate dosing, what measuring device should accompany the medication?
   a. 1 mL tuberculin syringe (without the needle)
   b. measuring cup
   c. dropper
   d. 5 mL oral syringe (without the needle)

8. A patient is prescribed an ophthalmic solution and ointment. How should they be administered?
   a. The solution and the ointment can be administered simultaneously.
   b. The ointment should be administered first; the solution should be administered 10 minutes later.
   c. The solution should be administered first; the ointment should be administered 10 minutes later.
   d. The ointment should be administered first; the solution should be administered 4 hours later.

9. The fastest onset of action to reverse shortness of breath is with a
   a. metered-dose inhaler.
   b. miconized powder.
   c. vaporized medication.
   d. nebulized medication.

10. A 10 mL vial of insulin will contain how many units of insulin?
    a. 10 units
    b. 100 units
    c. 500 units
    d. 1000 units

Pharmaceutical Measurements and Calculations

5

Learning Objectives

- Describe four systems of measurement commonly used in pharmacy and convert units from one system to another.
- Explain the meanings of the prefixes most commonly used in metric measurement.
- Convert from one metric unit to another (e.g., grams to milligrams, liters to milliliters).
- Convert Roman numerals to Arabic numerals.
- Convert standard time to military or 24-hour time.
- Convert temperatures to and from the Fahrenheit and Celsius scales.
- Round decimals up and down appropriately.
- Perform basic operations with proportions, including identifying equivalent ratios and finding an unknown quantity in a proportion.

- Convert percentages to and from fractions, ratios, and decimals.
- Perform fundamental dosage calculations and conversions.
- Solve problems involving powder solutions and dilutions.
- Use the alligation method to prepare solutions and topical products.
- Calculate the specific gravity of a liquid.

Preview chapter terms and definitions.

The daily activities of pharmacists and pharmacy technicians require making exact measurements. When pharmacy personnel measure liquids for reconstituted solutions (mixing water with a powder to make a solution), compound drugs, and prepare parenteral infusions, the amount, quantities, and calculations must always be precise. A mistake in a calculation can have severe consequences, such as drug toxicity or patient death. To give you a perspective on the importance of accuracy in pharmacy measurements and calculations, consider this comparison: While achieving 90% on your pharmacy calculations test would result in an exemplary grade of an A, achieving 90% of error-free medication preparation and dispensing in your daily pharmacy practice would result in a definite failing grade. Therefore, it is essential for pharmacy technicians to understand the basic measurement systems and mathematical calculations and formulas used in the healthcare field. A knowledge of the basic fundamentals of math, especially in the metric system, is critical to minimizing medication errors involving dosage, flow rates, and concentrations. This chapter lays the foundation for these mathematical skills. Additional math skills are covered in Chapter 7, "The Business of Community Pharmacy," as well as in Chapter 11, "Compounding Sterile Products and Hazardous Drugs."

Systems of Pharmaceutical Measurement

Systems of measurement are widely accepted standards used to determine such quantities as temperature, weight, distance (or length), area, volume, and time. Of these, temperature, weight, distance, and volume are the most important to the pharmacy profession.

- Quantities of temperature and weight are the simplest and most familiar measurements.
- Distance is a measurement of extension in space in one dimension.
- Volume, the least intuitive of these quantities, is a measurement of extension in space in three dimensions, or cubic volume.

Metric System

Developed in France in the 1700s, the **metric system** became the legal standard of measure in the United States in 1893 and is the system of measurement used in pharmacy practice.

The metric system has several distinct advantages over other measurement systems:

- The metric system is based on decimal notation, in which units are described as multiples of 10 (0.001, 0.01, 0.1, 1, 10, 100, 1000). This decimal notation makes calculation easier.
- The metric system contains clear correlations among the units of measurement of length, volume, and weight, which also helps to simplify calculation. For example, the standard metric unit for volume, the liter, is almost exactly equivalent to 1000 cubic centimeters.
- With slight variations in notation, the metric system is used worldwide, especially in scientific measurement, and therefore, like music, can be considered a "universal language."

The modern metric system makes use of the standardized units of the Système International (SI), adopted by agreement of governments worldwide in 1960. SI is a decimal system, with the prefixes denoting powers of 10 (see Table 5.1). In prescriptions using the metric system, numbers are also expressed as decimals rather than as fractions. To convert from one metric unit to another while performing calculations, healthcare personnel simply move the decimal point. Moving the decimal point to the left converts to larger units; moving the decimal point to the right converts to smaller units. For numbers less than one (1), a zero (0) is placed before the decimal point to prevent misreading, as

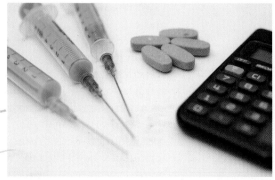

Injectable drugs in the hospital or oral dosage forms in the community pharmacy commonly use the metric system.

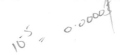

TABLE 5.1   Système International Prefixes

Prefix	Symbol	Meaning
micro-	mc	one-millionth (basic unit × 10^{-6}, or unit × 0.000001)
milli-	m	one-thousandth (basic unit × 10^{-3}, or unit × 0.001)
centi-	c	one-hundredth (basic unit × 10^{-2}, or unit × 0.01)
deci-	d	one-tenth (basic unit × 10^{-1}, or unit × 0.1)
hecto-	h	one hundred times (basic unit × 10^{2}, or unit × 100)
kilo-	k	one thousand times (basic unit × 10^{3}, or unit × 1000)

Safety Note

An error of a single decimal place is an error by a factor of 10.

in digoxin 0.25 mg. Note that an error of a single decimal place is an error by a factor of 10. Therefore, prescribers and pharmacy personnel must exercise due diligence when recording, interpreting, and measuring medication dosages containing decimals, for even minor errors can lead to serious medication errors.

Meter, Liter, and Gram Three basic units in the SI system are the meter, liter, and gram. The liter and the gram are the metric units most commonly used in pharmacy practice. Prefixes—syllables placed at the beginnings of words—can be added to these basic metric units to specify a particular measure. For example, the prefix *milli*– (meaning 1,000) can be added to the basic metric unit *liter* to form a new unit: *milliliter*, or one-thousandth of a liter. Each of these metric units has its own abbreviation, which is the same abbreviation for both single and plural measurements (for example, 1 mL, 3 mL; 1 g, 3 g). To understand these common metric units and their abbreviations, refer to Table 5.2.

TABLE 5.2   Common Metric Units

Measurement Unit	Equivalent
Length: Meter	
1 meter (m)	100 centimeters (cm)
1 centimeter (cm)	0.01 m; 10 millimeters (mm)
1 millimeter (mm)	0.001 m; 1000 micrometers, or microns (mcm)
Volume: Liter	
1 liter (L)	1000 milliliters (mL)
1 milliliter (mL)	0.001 L; 1000 microliters (mcL)
Weight: Gram	
1 gram (g)	1000 milligrams (mg)
1 milligram (mg)	1000 micrograms (mcg); one-thousandth of a gram (g)
1 kilogram (kg)	1000 grams (g)

FIGURE 5.1
Measurements in the Metric System

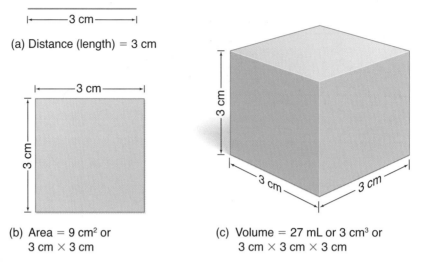

(a) Distance (length) = 3 cm

(b) Area = 9 cm² or
3 cm × 3 cm

(c) Volume = 27 mL or 3 cm³ or
3 cm × 3 cm × 3 cm

Meter The **meter** is the unit used for measuring distance, area, and volume and has limited application in pharmacy practice. Figure 5.1 shows the use of the meter in measuring distance, area, and volume.

Safety Note

Because the abbreviation *cc* has been associated with a higher risk of medication errors, the preferred unit of volume is milliliters (mL).

Liter The **liter** is the unit used for measuring the volume of liquid medications as well as liquids for oral and parenteral solutions. One liter is equivalent to 1000 cubic centimeters (abbreviated as *cc*), with each cubic centimeter equal to 1 mL or one-thousandth of a liter. An extremely small volume is measured in microliters, which is one-millionth of a liter. Directions for an antibiotic prescription may be to give 4 mL by mouth every 12 hours for 10 days. In the hospital or home healthcare setting, the antibiotic cefazolin at a dose of 1 g may be mixed in 50 mL of a sterile normal saline solution and administered over 30 minutes.

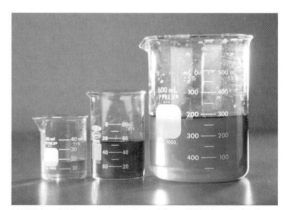

Liquid volumes are expressed in milliliters (which is the preferred unit) or in cubic centimeters. To measure the volumes of nonsterile liquids, volumetric flasks of varying sizes, such as the ones pictured here, are used.

Gram The **gram** is the unit used for 1) measuring the amount of medication in a solid dosage form, 2) indicating the amount of solid medication in a solution, and 3) expressing the weight of an object or a person. The gram is the weight of 1 cubic centimeter of water at 4 °C. The dose of many pharmaceuticals is commonly expressed in grams (g) or milligrams (mg). For example, community pharmacy personnel may see a prescription for the antiulcer medication sucralfate written as 1 g; hospital pharmacy personnel may see an order for an antibiotic suspension to be reconstituted or mixed with sterile water to result in a concentration of 600 mg per 5 mL.

The most common metric calculations in pharmacy involve conversions to and from grams, milligrams, and kilograms and to and from milliliters and liters. Table 5.3 shows how to easily perform these conversions.

TABLE 5.3 Common Metric Conversions

Conversion	Instruction	Example
kilograms (kg) to grams (g)	multiply by 1000 (move decimal point three places to the right)	6.25 kg = 6250 g
grams (g) to milligrams (mg)	multiply by 1000 (move decimal point three places to the right)	3.56 g = 3560 mg
milligrams (mg) to grams (g)	multiply by 0.001 (move decimal point three places to the left)	120 mg = 0.120 g
liters (L) to milliliters (mL)	multiply by 1000 (move decimal point three places to the right)	2.5 L = 2500 mL
milliliters (mL) to liters (L)	multiply by 0.001 (move decimal point three places to the left)	238 mL = 0.238 L

Other Systems of Pharmaceutical Measurement

Like languages, measurement systems tend to evolve by folk processes. For example, a foot was originally a length approximately equal to that of the average person's foot, and a cubit was equal to the length of a forearm from the elbow to the middle finger. To measure weight, stones, seeds, and grains were used as reference points; to measure volume, filled gourds and other containers were utilized. By nature, these common measures were *inconsistent* and *imprecise*—two terms that run counter to scientific disciplines such as chemistry, medicine, and pharmacy. The need for standardized measures among these various sciences resulted in the establishment of three different systems of pharmaceutical measurement over the centuries: the apothecary system, the avoirdupois system, and the household system.

Apothecary System The **apothecary system**, one of the oldest systems of measurement, is based on the weight system developed by the Romans. This system included such units of measurement as the dram (approximately equivalent to 4 mL) and the scruple (roughly equivalent to 1.3 g). These two units of measurement are rarely used today and could lead to medication errors if put into practice.

Another unit of measurement in the apothecary system is the **grain**, a dry weight measure that is the most commonly encountered nonmetric unit in pharmacy practice today. A common example of the use of the grain unit of measurement in modern-day pharmacy can be seen in aspirin and acetaminophen products, which are sometimes labeled as 5 grains (5 gr), an amount equivalent to approximately 325 mg. Prescriptions for phenobarbital and thyroid medications are also often written in grains. Phenobarbital is commercially available as ¼ grain (16.2 mg), ½ grain (32.4 mg), and 1 grain (64.8 mg). Another medication, USP thyroid, is often prescribed as ¼ grain (15 mg), ½ grain (30 mg), or 1 grain (60 mg). The use of the grain unit also occurs in extemporaneous nonsterile compounding, a practice in which pharmacists sometimes use a set of apothecary weights (designated from ½ grain to 5 grains) to measure powders.

Other units of measurement established by the apothecary system include the pint, quart, gallon, ounce, and pound—all of which have survived over the centuries (with changes to their equivalencies). The apothecary system was widely used until the

Safety Note

Pharmacy personnel should be aware that grain (gr) and gram (g) can be easily misinterpreted during the transcription and filling of medications and, therefore, may result in medication errors. With that in mind, pharmacy staff members should exercise care when handling prescriptions or medication orders that use these abbreviations.

TABLE 5.4 Apothecary Symbols

Volume		Weight	
Unit of Measure	**Symbol**	**Unit of Measure**	**Symbol**
minim	♏	grain	gr
fluidram	f3	scruple	Э
fluidounce	f3	dram	3
pint	pt	ounce	℥
quart	qt	pound	℔ or #
gallon	gal		

beginning of the twentieth century when most medications were still being compounded in the pharmacy setting. To familiarize yourself with the apothecary units of measure and their accompanying symbols, see Table 5.4.

Avoirdupois System The **avoirdupois system** of measurement originated in France and is considered the "everyday" system of measurement in the United States. This system includes such common units of measurement as feet and miles as well as grains, pounds, and ounces (units shared with the apothecary system).

Household System The **household system** of measurement is based on the apothecary system and was established to help patients take their medications at home. Like the apothecary and avoirdupois systems, this system includes such common units of measurement as the ounce and pound but also includes several liquid units that are still used in the food industry, some areas of pharmacy, and households today: the drop, teaspoon, tablespoon, and cup. Other household measurement units, such as the hogshead and the jigger, have become obsolete in pharmacy practice.

Conversion Equivalents Among Different Measurement Systems Prior to the nineteenth century, one challenge among pharmacy practitioners was the lack of standard equivalencies among these three measurement systems. Depending on which system they used, practitioners were dispensing widely differing doses. For example, a pound in the apothecary system is equivalent to 12 ounces, whereas a pound in the avoirdupois and household systems is equivalent to 16 ounces. An apothecary ounce is 31.1 g, but an avoirdupois ounce is 28.35 g. These discrepancies often resulted in medication errors. Consequently, a standardized system was needed to ensure accuracy in medication doses for patients, which led to the adoption of the metric system as the system of choice among U.S. pharmacies. In fact, many pharmacy computer systems are programmed to accept only amounts given in metric units. Occasionally, prescriptions or medication orders are written in the

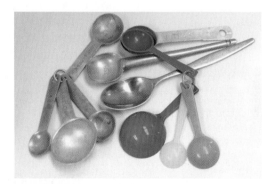

The volume held by a household teaspoon may vary, but a true teaspoon equals 5 mL.

other systems of measurement; therefore, pharmacy technicians should be familiar with all measurement systems to minimize dosing errors. To understand the variances among the apothecary, avoirdupois, and household units of measure and their metric equivalents, see Tables 5.5, 5.6, and 5.7, respectively.

 Safety Note

For safety reasons, the use of the apothecary system is discouraged. Use the metric system in your pharmacy calculations.

TABLE 5.5 Apothecary System

Measurement Unit	Equivalent within System	Metric Equivalent
Volume		
1 ♏ (minim)	–	0.06 mL
16.23 ♏	–	1 mL
1 f℈ (fluidram)	60 ♏	5 mL (3.75 mL)*
1 f℥ (fluid ounce)	6 f℈	30 mL (29.57 mL)†
1 pt (pint)	16 f℥	480 mL
1 qt (quart)	2 pt or 32 f℥	960 mL
1 gal (gallon)	4 qt or 8 pt	3840 mL
Weight		
1 gr (grain)	–	65 mg††
15.432 gr	–	1 g
1 ℈ (scruple)	20 gr	1.3 g
1 ʒ (dram)	3 ℈ or 60 gr	3.9 g
1 ℥ (ounce)	8 ʒ or 480 gr	30 g (31.1 g)
1 # (pound)	12 ℥ or 5760 gr	373.2 g

*In reality, 1 f℈ contains 3.75 mL; however, that number is usually rounded up to 5 mL or 1 tsp.
†In reality, 1 f℥ contains 29.57 mL; however, that number is usually rounded up to 30 mL.
††Many manufacturers use 60 mg instead of 65 mg as the equivalent for 1 gr (grain).

TABLE 5.6 Avoirdupois System

Measurement Unit	Equivalent within System	Metric Equivalent
1 gr (grain)	–	65 mg
1 oz (ounce)	437.5 gr	30 g (28.35 g)*
1 lb (pound)	16 oz or 7000 gr	454 g

*An avoirdupois ounce actually contains 28.34952 g; however, that number is usually rounded up to 30 g. It is common practice to use 454 g as the equivalent for a pound (28.35 g × 16 oz/lb = 453.6 g/lb, rounded to 454 g/lb).

TABLE 5.7 Household System

Measurement Unit	Equivalent within System	Metric Equivalent
Volume		
1 tsp (teaspoonful)	–	5 mL
1 tbsp (tablespoonful)	3 tsp	15 mL
1 fl oz (fluid ounce)	2 tbsp	30 mL (29.57 mL)*
1 cup	8 fl oz	240 mL
1 pt (pint)	2 cups	480 mL†
1 qt (quart)	2 pt	960 mL
1 gal (gallon)	4 qt	3840 mL
Weight		
1 oz (ounce)	–	30 g
1 lb (pound)	–	454 g
2.2 lb	–	1 kg

*In reality, 1 fl oz (household measure) contains less than 30 mL; however, 30 mL is usually used.
†When packaging a pint, companies will typically present 473 mL, rather than the full 480 mL, thus saving money over time.

Common Practice Issues with Conversions For each of the three measurement systems outlined in Tables 5.5, 5.6, and 5.7, you can observe that conversions of certain units of measurement to their metric equivalents resulted in decimals. To simplify and standardize these conversions, rounding up or down was universally adopted in pharmacy practice. These rounded decimals are designated on the three tables with an asterisk or a dagger. For example, on Table 5.5, when converting from fluid ounces to milliliters in pharmacy calculations, it is common practice to round 29.57 mL to 30 mL. When measuring this amount, it is often appropriate to make this estimation because the volume differs by such a small amount. However, the discrepancy becomes far more apparent when measuring multiple fluid ounces that have been rounded up to the 30 mL equivalent. For example, if asked to measure a household pint (16 fl oz), you would measure roughly 480 mL (16 oz multiplied by 30 mL). This calculation becomes problematic because 29.57 mL multiplied by 16 is equal to only 473.12 mL, not 480 mL. In fact, products in most one pint stock bottles are labeled 473 mL, yet pharmacies bill insurance according to the estimation of 480 mL and measure out fluid ounces in 30 mL increments. With that in mind, use the rounded 30 mL value for a fluid ounce and the rounded 480 mL for a pint when performing pharmacy calculations for this chapter.

Another calculation problem can occur with the ounce unit of measurement. The apothecary ounce is a weight measure and not a liquid measure. As you can see in Table 5.5 and Table 5.6, the ounce unit has been rounded down (from 31.1 g to 30 g) in the apothecary system and rounded up (from 28.35 g to 30 g) in the avoirdupois system. Today, many physicians are accustomed to writing prescription orders in ounces of medication for liquid dosage forms; however, the metric system is considered more accurate.

Safety Note

Always carefully check and double-check all calculations.

The grain unit also poses a conversion problem for pharmacy personnel. As noted in Table 5.5, most pharmacists consider 1 grain to be equal to 65 mg, but manufacturers often use a 60 mg conversion for 1 grain. In most cases, this difference in measurement is not clinically significant. However, for premature infants and neonates, precise calculations and uniform measurements must be used.

While slight differences in metric conversions do exist, the use of standardized metric equivalents among pharmacy personnel can aid accurate medication dosing and not adversely impact patient care. Pharmacy technicians should confer with the pharmacist if in doubt about any conversions to metric equivalents to ensure that the correct dose and product are selected.

Numeric Systems

Two types of numeric systems are used in pharmaceutical calculations: Arabic and Roman. The **Arabic system** uses numbers, fractions (such as ½), and decimals. In the **Roman system**, numerals are expressed in either capital letters or lowercase letters. (See Table 5.8 for a comparison of these two numeric systems.)

The most frequently used Roman numerals in pharmacy practice are the uppercase letters I, V, and X, which represent the Arabic numbers 1, 5, and 10, respectively. For example, tablet quantities of a narcotic prescription are often written in uppercase letters, such as XXX indicating 30 tablets.

The lowercase Roman numerals i, ii, and iii are also occasionally used in pharmacy practice. These numerals are commonly seen on prescriptions using apothecary measures and follow—rather than precede—the unit of measurement. For example, "aspirin gr vi" means "six grains of aspirin." Lowercase Roman numerals are also sometimes used to express other quantities such as volume (tbsp iii = 3 tablespoonsful). To prevent errors in interpretation, i, ii, and iii are often written with a line above the letters (ī, īi, īīi).

Safety Note

New safety guidelines discourage the use of Roman numerals in pharmacy practice.

Roman numerals are equal or smaller when reading left to right; the total value equals the sum of their individual values. Thus, iii = 3, and xi = 10 + 1 = 11. Otherwise, first subtract the value of each smaller numeral from the value of the larger numeral that it precedes, and then add the individual values. Thus, iv = 5 − 1 = 4, and xxiv = 10 + 10 + (5 − 1) = 10 + 10 + 4 = 24.

TABLE 5.8 Comparison of Roman and Arabic Numerals

Roman	Arabic	Roman	Arabic
s̄s̄	0.5 or ½	L or l	50
I or i or ī	1	C or c	100
V or v	5	D or d	500
X or x	10	M or m	1000

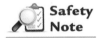

Time

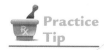
Practice Tip

Pharmacy technicians should be aware that midnight in the military time system may be referred to as 0000 or 2400, depending on hospital policy.

In the hospital setting, medication orders are commonly time-stamped with military or 24-hour time. Dosage administration schedules for unit dose and intravenous (IV) admixtures also use this method. **Military time** is based on a 24-hour clock, with midnight considered time 0000. The first two digits are the time in hours, and the second two digits are the time in minutes.

0000	Midnight
0600	6 AM
1200	Noon
1800	6 PM

Because no AM or PM designations are used, military time creates less confusion in the pharmacy workplace, resulting in fewer medication errors.

Example 1

At 0125, you receive an order for gentamicin 80 mg IV every 8 hours. The order is due to be administered at 0200, 1000, and 1800. When was the order received, and when should doses be prepared and sent to the patient care unit?

The order was received at 1:25 AM. The first dose is to be immediately prepared and sent to the patient care unit to be given at 2:00 AM. Follow-up doses are scheduled at 10:00 AM and 6:00 PM and will be delivered to the patient care unit later in the day.

Temperature

The United States is one of the few countries in the world that commonly uses Fahrenheit as its temperature scale. The **Fahrenheit temperature scale** uses 32 °F as the temperature when water freezes to ice and 212 °F as the temperature when water boils; the difference between these two extremes is 180 °F.

In the 1700s, a Swedish scientist with the last name of Celsius suggested a thermometer with a difference of 100 degrees between freezing and boiling. He used zero degrees (0 °C) as the freezing point and 100 °C as the boiling point. The **Celsius temperature scale** is commonly used in Europe and globally in science. Celsius is often the scale used in healthcare settings, including the pharmacy.

An understanding of the Fahrenheit and Celsius temperature scales is important to the proper storage of medication in the pharmacy. Storing unstable drugs at proper temperatures and maintaining refrigerator and freezer equipment at the appropriate temperatures are important responsibilities of the pharmacy technician. To ensure that these proper temperatures are maintained, technicians must monitor the refrigerator and document the temperatures

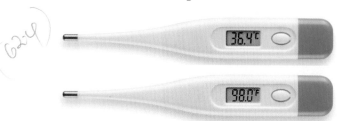

Pharmacy technicians may be asked to help patients convert between temperature readings in degrees Celsius and Fahrenheit. As with all conversions, this calculation must be done accurately.

TABLE 5.9   Temperature Equivalencies between Celsius and Fahrenheit

Celsius	Fahrenheit
0 °C	32 °F
5 °C	41 °F
10 °C	50 °F
15 °C	59 °F
20 °C	68 °F

once or twice daily, depending on their pharmacy's protocol. Most refrigerators in the pharmacy need to maintain a temperature of 2 °C to 8 °C. Technicians can find the storage temperature requirements, given in Celsius, on the manufacturers' drug package inserts or in their individual pharmacy's Policy and Procedure (P&P) manual. In addition, technicians may have the additional responsibility of monitoring and documenting the temperature conditions of medications in a freezer.

To help them fulfill these job responsibilities, pharmacy technicians must be able to perform conversions between the Celsius scale and the Fahrenheit scale. Table 5.9 shows the temperature equivalencies between these two scales. As you can see, every 5 °C change in temperature is equivalent to a 9 °F change.

In addition to using this chart, here are several mathematical methods of converting from Fahrenheit to Celsius and vice versa. One method uses the following equations:

$$°F = (1.8 \times °C) + 32°$$

$$°C = (°F - 32°) \div 1.8$$

An alternative method uses the following algebraic equation:

$$5 \times °F = 9 \times °C + 160$$

A temperature log documents the refrigerator and freezer temperature on a daily basis. Currently, most pharmacy temperature logs document to the tenth place for accuracy. If the log does not require a decimal, then the temperature should be rounded down if it is 0.1 to 0.4 and rounded up if it is 0.5 to 0.9.

Example 2

Convert 70 °F to degrees Celsius.

$$°C = (°F - 32°) \div 1.8$$
$$°C = (70° - 32°) \div 1.8$$
$$°C = 38° \div 1.8$$
$$°C = 21.1°, \text{ rounded down to } 21°$$

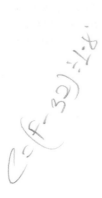

$(F - 32) \div 1.8$

$^{\circ}C$

$(1.8 \times ^{\circ}C + 32$

$^{\circ}F$

Example 3

Convert 30 °C to degrees Fahrenheit.

$$^{\circ}F = (1.8 \times {}^{\circ}C) + 32^{\circ}$$
$$^{\circ}F = (1.8 \times 30^{\circ}) + 32^{\circ}$$
$$^{\circ}F = 54^{\circ} + 32^{\circ}$$
$$^{\circ}F = 86^{\circ}$$

Example 4

According to the Enbrel package insert, the manufacturer requires that a syringe of this expensive biotechnology drug must be stored at a temperature from 2 to 8 °C. What should the range of the Fahrenheit temperature setting be on the thermostat in the refrigerator?

Step 1. Convert the degrees Celsius at the low end of the range.

$$^{\circ}F = (1.8 \times {}^{\circ}C) + 32^{\circ}$$
$$^{\circ}F = (1.8 \times 2^{\circ}) + 32^{\circ}$$
$$^{\circ}F = 3.6^{\circ} + 32^{\circ}$$
$$^{\circ}F = 35.6^{\circ}, \text{ rounded up to } 36^{\circ}$$

Step 2. Convert the degrees Celsius at the high end of the range.

$$^{\circ}F = (1.8 \times {}^{\circ}C) + 32^{\circ}$$
$$^{\circ}F = (1.8 \times 8^{\circ}) + 32^{\circ}$$
$$^{\circ}F = 14.4^{\circ} + 32^{\circ}$$
$$^{\circ}F = 46.4^{\circ}, \text{ rounded down to } 46^{\circ}$$

The pharmacy technician should be sure the thermostat setting in the refrigerator is between 36 and 46 °F, inclusively.

Example 5

Many community pharmacists today are trained and certified to administer vaccines. According to the Zostavax (shingles) vaccine package insert, the manufacturer requires that, due to instability, a vial of powder must be stored at a temperature in a range of -58 °F to 5 °F. The patient cost of each vial is more than $200, and you have a box of 20 vials that you just received from your local wholesaler. What should the Celsius temperature setting be at or below on the thermostat in the freezer?

Convert the degrees Fahrenheit to Celsius as follows:

$$^{\circ}C = ({}^{\circ}F - 32^{\circ}) \div 1.8$$
$$^{\circ}C = (5^{\circ} - 32^{\circ}) \div 1.8$$
$$^{\circ}C = (-27^{\circ}) \div 1.8$$
$$^{\circ}C = -15^{\circ}$$

The pharmacy technician must be sure that the thermostat setting in the freezer is less than –15 °C or 5 °F; otherwise, more than $4,000 worth of medication would have to be discarded!

Example 6

An anxious mother telephones the pharmacy on a Saturday night. Her six-month-old child has a fever. The only thermometer she has records a temperature of 38.5 °C. Her pediatrician told her to call if the child's temperature reached 101 °F. What is the child's temperature in degrees Fahrenheit? Should the mother call the pediatrician?

$$°F = (1.8 \times °C) + 32°$$
$$°F = (1.8 \times 38.5°) + 32°$$
$$°F = 69.3° + 32°$$
$$°F = 101.3°, \text{ rounded down to } 101°$$

The parent should call the child's pediatrician.

Basic Calculations Used in Pharmacy Practice

Many tasks in pharmacy—determining dosages, compounding medications, and preparing solutions—use calculations involving the units of measure given in the preceding section. Pharmacy work often requires performing fundamental operations involving fractions, decimals, ratios and proportions, and percents. A brief review of these basic mathematical skills is included in this section.

Fractions

When something is divided into parts, each part is considered a **fraction** of the whole. For example, a pie might be divided into eight slices, each one of which is a fraction, or $\frac{1}{8}$ of the whole pie. In this example, *1* is one slice of the pie, and *8* is the number of slices in the whole pie (see Figure 5.2). A simple fraction consists of two numbers: a **numerator** (the number on the top or the left) and a **denominator** (the number on the bottom or the right).

$$\frac{1}{8} \quad \begin{matrix} \leftarrow \text{ numerator} \\ \leftarrow \text{ denominator} \end{matrix}$$

A fraction is simply a convenient way of representing the division of the numerator by the denominator. For example, the fraction $\frac{6}{3}$ is 6 divided by 3, which equals 2. The fraction $\frac{7}{8}$ is 7 divided by 8, which equals the decimal value 0.875. Therefore, the number obtained upon dividing the numerator by the denominator is the value of the fraction.

FIGURE 5.2
Fractions of
the Whole Pie

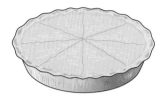
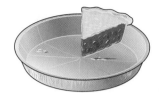

8 slices = 1 whole pie = $\frac{8}{8}$ of the whole pie   1 slice = $\frac{1}{8}$ of the whole pie

Decimals

An understanding of decimals is crucial to dosage calculations because most medication orders, such as the one shown below, are written using decimals.

> ℞   **Digoxin 0.125 mg #30**
> **Take 1 tablet every day to control heart rate.**

A **decimal** is any number that can be written in decimal notation using the integers 0, 1, 2, 3, 4, 5, 6, 7, 8, and 9 and a point (.) to divide the "ones" place from the "tenths" place. Figure 5.3 illustrates the relative value of each decimal unit and provides the names of the place values. Numbers to the left of the decimal point are whole numbers; numbers to the right of the decimal point are decimal fractions (parts of the whole). For example, in the decimal 2.09, the number to the left of the decimal point (in this case, *2*) is the whole number; the number to the right of the decimal point (in this case, *.09*) is the fraction.

If a decimal is less than one, a zero (0) is placed before the decimal point. This zero is called a **leading zero** and is used to prevent confusion and potential medication errors when reading decimals. For example, the decimal 0.131313 is less than one and therefore has a leading zero placed to the left of the decimal point.

A fraction can be expressed as a decimal by dividing the numerator by the denominator.

 Safety Note

For a decimal value less than one, use a leading zero to prevent errors.

$$\frac{1}{2} = 1 \div 2 = 0.5$$

$$\frac{1}{3} = 1 \div 3 = 0.33333\ldots$$

$$\frac{438}{64} = 438 \div 64 = 6.84375$$

Converting Decimals to Fractions The metric system generally uses numbers in decimal form. Any decimal number can be expressed as a decimal fraction that has a power of 10 as its denominator. The decimal-fraction equivalents shown in Table 5.10 correspond to the decimal place names presented in Figure 5.3.

FIGURE 5.3
Decimal Units
and Values

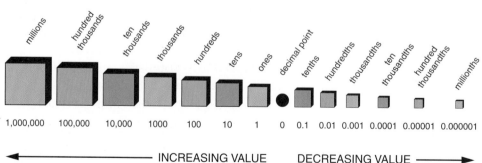

millions	hundred thousands	ten thousands	thousands	hundreds	tens	ones	decimal point	tenths	hundredths	thousandths	ten thousandths	hundred thousandths	millionths
1,000,000	100,000	10,000	1000	100	10	1	0	0.1	0.01	0.001	0.0001	0.00001	0.000001

◀——— INCREASING VALUE   DECREASING VALUE ———▶

TABLE 5.10   Decimals and Equivalent Decimal Fractions

$1 = \dfrac{1}{1}$	$0.01 = \dfrac{1}{100}$	$0.0001 = \dfrac{1}{10,000}$
$0.1 = \dfrac{1}{10}$	$0.001 = \dfrac{1}{1000}$	$0.00001 = \dfrac{1}{100,000}$

To express a decimal number as a fraction, remove the decimal point and use the resulting number as the numerator. To obtain the denominator, count the number of places to the right of the decimal point. Use Table 5.10 to find the corresponding power of 10 to put in the denominator.

$$2.33 = \frac{233}{100} \qquad 0.1234 = \frac{1234}{10,000} \qquad 0.00367 = \frac{367}{100,000}$$

Once a decimal number is expressed as a fraction, the fraction can be reduced or simplified by dividing it by a fraction equivalent to 1.

$$0.84 = \frac{84}{100} = \frac{84}{100} \div \frac{4}{4} = \frac{21}{25}$$

$$0.1234 = \frac{1234}{10,000} = \frac{1234}{10,000} \div \frac{2}{2} = \frac{617}{5,000}$$

Rounding Decimals   To round off an answer to the nearest tenth, carry the division out two places, to the hundredths place. If the number in the hundredths place is five or greater, add one to the tenths-place number. If the number in the hundredths place is less than five, round the number down by omitting the digit in the hundredths place.

5.65 becomes 5.7   4.24 becomes 4.2

The same procedure may be used when rounding to the nearest hundredths place or thousandths place.

3.8421 = 3.84 (hundredths)
41.2674 = 41.27 (hundredths)
0.3928 = 0.393 (thousandths)
4.1111 = 4.111 (thousandths)

Safety Note

When rounding calculations of IV fluid drops per minute (gtt/min), round partial drops down. So, if a calculation indicates 28.6 gtt/min, the answer is rounded down to 28 gtt/min, not rounded up to 29 gtt/min. Calculations involving drops are discussed in Chapter 11.

When rounding numbers used in pharmacy calculations, it is common to round off to the nearest tenth. However, sometimes a dose based on body weight is very small (as when prescribed for a child or an infant) and rounding to the nearest hundredth or thousandth may be more appropriate, as shown in the example below.

The exact dose calculated is 0.08752 g
Rounded to nearest tenth: 0.1 g
Rounded to nearest hundredth: 0.09 g
Rounded to nearest thousandth: 0.088 g

Check with the pharmacist to confirm proper rounding practices on a case-by-case basis.

Ratios and Proportions

A **ratio** is a comparison of two like quantities and can be expressed in a fraction or in ratio notation (using a colon). For example, if a beaker contains two parts water and three parts alcohol, then the ratio of water to alcohol in the beaker can be expressed as the fraction ²/₃ or as the ratio 2:3. The ratio is read not as a value (2 divided by 3) but as the expression "a ratio of 2 to 3."

As described in the previous example, one common use of ratios is to express the number of parts of one substance contained in a known number of parts of another substance. For example, suppose that 60 mL of sterile solution contains 3 mL of tetra-hydrozoline hydrochloride. This can be expressed as the ratio ³/₆₀ or ¹/₂₀. In other words, the ratio of the active ingredient to the sterile solution is 1 to 20, or 1 part in 20 parts.

Two ratios that have the same value, such as ½ and ⁴/₈, are said to be equivalent ratios. When ratios are equivalent, the product of the numerator of the first ratio and the denominator of the second ratio is equal to the product of the numerator of the second ratio and the denominator of the first ratio.

$$\text{Therefore if} \quad 2{:}3 = 6{:}9, \quad \text{then} \quad \frac{2}{3} = \frac{6}{9}; \quad \text{thus} \quad 2 \times 9 = 3 \times 6 = 18$$

The same thing is true of the reciprocals.

$$\text{Therefore if} \quad 3{:}2 = 9{:}6, \quad \text{then} \quad \frac{3}{2} = \frac{9}{6}; \quad \text{thus} \quad 3 \times 6 = 2 \times 9 = 18$$

Two equivalent ratios are said to be in the same proportion. Equivalent, or proportional, ratios can be expressed in three different ways.

$$\frac{a}{b} = \frac{c}{d} \qquad \text{example:} \quad \frac{1}{2} = \frac{4}{8}$$

$$a{:}b = c{:}d \qquad \text{example:} \quad 1{:}2 = 4{:}8$$

$$a{:}b :: c{:}d \qquad \text{example:} \quad 1{:}2 :: 4{:}8$$

Pairs of equivalent ratios are called a **proportion**. The first and fourth numbers, or outside numbers, are called the *extremes*, and the second and third numbers, or inside numbers, are called the *means*.

$$3{:}4 \quad = \quad 15{:}20$$

means

extremes

A very useful fact about proportions was illustrated in the previous examples: The product of the extremes equals the product of the means. If the proportion is expressed as a relationship between fractions, then the numerator of the first fraction times the denominator of the second is equal to the denominator of the first fraction times the numerator of the second. This can be stated as a rule:

$$\text{If} \quad \frac{a}{b} = \frac{c}{d} \quad \text{then} \quad a \times d = b \times c$$

This equation proves extremely valuable because it can be used to calculate an unknown quantity in a proportion when the other three variables are known. In

TABLE 5.11 Rules for Solving Proportions
■ Three of the four amounts must be known.
■ The numerators must have the same unit of measurement.
■ The denominators must have the same unit of measurement.

mathematics, it is common to express unknown quantities using letters from the lower end of the alphabet, especially x, y, and z.

When setting up ratios in the proportion, it is important that the numbers remain in the correct ratio and that the numbers have the correct units of measurement in both the numerator and denominator. Table 5.11 lists the rules for solving proportions. Example 7 will demonstrate the basic steps for solving for x using the ratio-proportion method.

Example 7

Solve for x.

$$\frac{x}{35} = \frac{2}{7}$$

By the proportion rule,

$$x \times 7 = 35 \times 2$$

$$7x = 70$$

Then, dividing both sides by 7,

$$\frac{7x}{7} = \frac{70}{7}$$

$$x = 10$$

The following example shows how the ratio-proportion method can be used to solve pharmacy calculation problems in both the community and hospital pharmacy settings. This method can be used to convert within or between different measurement systems, such as translating from household measure to the preferred metric system. The ratio-proportion method is also used to calculate specific dosages.

Example 8

A prescription for a sick child is received from the emergency room on Saturday night for amoxicillin/clavulanate 600 mg/5 mL for 4 mL po twice daily. No other pharmacies are open in town. The pharmacy technician discovers that the pharmacy is out-of-stock on the 600 mg/5 mL concentration of the prescribed drug, but the 400 mg/5 mL concentration is in stock. The prescribed concentration could be ordered, but the child would be without medication until Monday at noon. How could this common problem be solved by the pharmacy technician using the ratio-proportion method?

Step 1. Calculate the prescribed dose for the child:

$$\frac{x \text{ mg}}{4 \text{ mL}} = \frac{600 \text{ mg}}{5 \text{ mL}}$$

$$5x = 600 \text{ mg} \times 4 \text{ mL}$$

$$x = \frac{2400}{5}$$

$$x = 480 \text{ mg}$$

Step 2. Calculate the volume (mL) of the available concentration of 400 mg/5 mL:

$$\frac{480 \text{ mg}}{x \text{ mL}} = \frac{480 \text{ mg}}{5 \text{ mL}}$$

$$400x = 480 \text{ mg} \times 5 \text{ mL}$$

$$x = 2400 \div 400$$

$$x = 6 \text{ mL}$$

Safety Note

Pharmacy technicians should always have the pharmacist verify their calculations.

This value is the calculated volume of the 400 mg/5 mL concentration equal to the prescribed 480 mg dose. Therefore, 6 mL of the 400 mg/5 mL concentration given twice daily is equivalent to 4 mL of the 600 mg/5 mL concentration given twice daily. Consequently, the pharmacy fills the prescription, sends it the emergency room, and allows the sick child to begin treatment right away.

Converting Quantities between the Metric and Other Measurement Systems Many situations in pharmacy practice call for conversion of quantities within one measurement system or between different measurement systems. When possible, convert to the metric system because it is the preferred system. To convert between metric measurements and apothecary units, it is necessary to know the equivalent measures shown in Table 5.5. The following examples will demonstrate some common pharmacy conversions using the ratio-proportion method.

Example 9

How many milliliters are there in 1 gal, 12 fl oz?

According to the values in Table 5.7, 3840 mL are found in 1 gal. In addition, because 1 fl oz contains 30 mL, you can use the ratio-proportion method to calculate the amount of milliliters in 12 fl oz as follows:

$$\frac{x \text{ mL}}{12 \text{ fl oz}} = \frac{30 \text{ mL}}{1 \text{ fl oz}}$$

$$\frac{(12 \text{ fl oz}) \, x \text{ mL}}{12 \text{ fl oz}} = \frac{(12 \text{ fl oz}) \, 30 \text{ mL}}{1 \text{ fl oz}}$$

$$x \text{ mL} = 360 \text{ mL}$$

Add the two values:

$$3840 \text{ mL} + 360 \text{ mL} = 4200 \text{ mL}$$

Example 10

A solution is to be used to fill hypodermic syringes, each containing 60 mL. There are 3 L of the solution available. How many hypodermic syringes can be filled with the available solution?

According to Table 5.2, 1 L is equal to 1000 mL. The available supply of solution is therefore

$$3 \times 1000 \text{ mL} = 3000 \text{ mL}$$

Determine the number of syringes by using the ratio-proportion method:

$$\frac{x \text{ syringes}}{3000 \text{ mL}} = \frac{1 \text{ syringe}}{60 \text{ mL}}$$

$$\frac{(3000 \text{ mL}) \, x \text{ syringes}}{3000 \text{ mL}} = \frac{(3000 \text{ mL}) \, 1 \text{ syringe}}{60 \text{ mL}}$$

$$x \text{ syringes} = 50 \text{ syringes}$$

Therefore, 50 hypodermic syringes can be filled.

Example 11

You are to dispense 300 mL of a liquid preparation. If the medication amount (the dose) is 2 tsp, how many doses will there be in the final preparation?

Step 1. Begin solving this problem by converting to a common unit of measure using conversion values in Table 5.7.

$$1 \text{ dose} = 2 \text{ tsp} = 2 \times 5 \text{ mL} = 10 \text{ mL}$$

Step 2. Using these converted measurements, the solution can be determined using the ratio-proportion method.

$$\frac{x \text{ doses}}{300 \text{ mL}} = \frac{1 \text{ dose}}{10 \text{ mL}}$$

$$\frac{(300 \text{ mL}) \, x \text{ doses}}{300 \text{ mL}} = \frac{(300 \text{ mL}) \, 1 \text{ dose}}{10 \text{ mL}}$$

$$x \text{ doses} = 30 \text{ doses}$$

Example 12

A compounding prescription calls for acetaminophen 400 mg. How many grains of acetaminophen should be used in the prescription?

Solve this problem by using the ratio-proportion method. The unknown number of grains and the requested number of milligrams go on the left side, and the ratio of 1 gr = 65 mg goes on the right side, per Table 5.5.

$$\frac{x \text{ gr}}{400 \text{ mg}} = \frac{1 \text{ gr}}{65 \text{ mg}}$$

$$\frac{(\cancel{400 \text{ mg}}) \, x \text{ gr}}{\cancel{400 \text{ mg}}} = \frac{(400 \, \cancel{\text{mg}}) \, 1 \text{ gr}}{65 \, \cancel{\text{mg}}}$$

$$x \text{ gr} = 6.1538 \text{ gr, rounded to 6 gr}$$

Rounding to the nearest whole number, 6 gr should be measured and used in the prescription.

Example 13

A physician wants a patient to be given 0.8 mg of nitroglycerin. The available supply has tablets containing nitroglycerin 1/150 gr. How many tablets should be given to the patient?

Step 1. Begin solving this problem by determining the number of grains in a dose by setting up a proportion and solving for the unknown. The unknown number of grains and the requested number of milligrams go on the left side, and the ratio of 1 gr = 65 mg goes on the right side, per Table 5.5.

$$\frac{x \text{ gr}}{0.8 \text{ mg}} = \frac{1 \text{ gr}}{65 \text{ mg}}$$

$$\frac{(\cancel{0.8 \text{ mg}}) \, x \text{ gr}}{\cancel{0.8 \text{ mg}}} = \frac{(0.8 \, \cancel{\text{mg}}) \, 1 \text{ gr}}{65 \, \cancel{\text{mg}}}$$

$$x \text{ gr} = 0.0123076 \text{ gr, rounded to 0.012 gr}$$

Step 2. Determine the number of tablets that the patient should receive by first converting the fraction value to a decimal value:

$$1/150 \text{ gr} = 0.00666 \ldots \text{ gr, rounded to 0.0067 gr}$$

Step 3. Set up another proportion and solve for the unknown:

$$\frac{x \text{ tablets}}{0.012 \text{ gr}} = \frac{1 \text{ tablet}}{0.0067 \text{ gr}}$$

$$\frac{(\cancel{0.012 \text{ gr}}) \, x \text{ tablets}}{\cancel{0.012 \text{ gr}}} = \frac{(0.012 \text{ gr}) \, 1 \text{ tablet}}{0.0067 \cancel{\text{ gr}}}$$

$$x \text{ tablets} = 1.79 \text{ tablets, rounded to 2 tablets}$$

The dose of medications for pediatric patients is often based on body weight in kilograms, and sometimes the pharmacy technician will need to convert a patient's weight from pounds to kilograms. The following example will show this conversion using the ratio-proportion method.

Example 14

A patient weighs 44 lb. What is her weight in kilograms?

Because 1 kg equals 2.2 lb, using the ratio-proportion method,

$$\frac{x \text{ kg}}{44 \text{ lb}} = \frac{1 \text{ kg}}{2.2 \text{ lb}}$$

$$\frac{(\cancel{44 \text{ lb}}) \, x \text{ kg}}{\cancel{44 \text{ lb}}} = \frac{(\cancel{44 \text{ lb}}) \, 1 \text{ kg}}{2.2 \cancel{\text{ lb}}}$$

$$x \text{ kg} = 20 \text{ kg}$$

Practice Tip

Remember that 2.2 lb is equal to 1 kg.

Calculating Dosages One of the most common calculations in pharmacy practice is that of dosages. The available supply is usually labeled as a ratio of an active ingredient to a solution.

$$\frac{\text{active ingredient (available)}}{\text{solution (available)}}$$

The prescription received in the pharmacy gives the amount of the active ingredient to be administered. The unknown quantity to be calculated is the amount of solution needed to achieve the desired dose of the active ingredient. This yields another ratio.

$$\frac{\text{active ingredient (to be administered)}}{\text{solution (needed)}}$$

The amount of solution needed can be determined by setting the two ratios into a proportion.

$$\frac{\text{active ingredient (to be administered)}}{\text{solution (needed)}} = \frac{\text{active ingredient (available)}}{\text{solution (available)}}$$

 Safety Note

Pharmacy technicians should always double-check the units in a proportion and their calculations.

When solving medication-dosing problems, use ratios to describe the amount of drug in a dosage form (tablet, capsule, or volume of solution). It is important to remember that the numerators and denominators of both ratios must be in the same units. For example, in oral medications, the active ingredient is usually expressed in milligrams and the solution is expressed in milliliters. In both cases, the numerators are the same (mg), and the denominators are the same (mL). Similarly, the pharmacy stock will most likely be a milligram per milliliter solution. Because it is so easy to confuse units, setting up proportions with the units clearly shown is the safest way to solve these types of calculations.

Example 15

You have a stock solution that contains 10 mg of active ingredient per 5 mL of solution. The physician orders a dosage of 4 mg. How many milliliters of the stock solution will have to be administered?

Using the information provided, set up a proportion, but flip the ratios so that the unknown variable is in the upper left corner of the proportion.

$$\frac{\text{solution (needed)}}{\text{active ingredient (to be administered)}} = \frac{\text{solution (available)}}{\text{active ingredient (available)}}$$

$$\frac{x \text{ mL}}{4 \text{ mg}} = \frac{5 \text{ mL}}{10 \text{ mg}}$$

$$\frac{(4 \text{ mg}) \, x \text{ mL}}{4 \text{ mg}} = \frac{(4 \text{ mg}) \, 5 \text{ mL}}{10 \text{ mg}}$$

$$x \text{ mL} = 2 \text{ mL}$$

Thus, 2 mL of solution are needed to provide the 4 mg dose.

Example 16

An order calls for Demerol 75 mg IM q4 h prn pain. The supply available is in Demerol 100 mg/mL syringes. How many milliliters will the nurse give for one injection?

This order is calling for an intramuscular (IM) injection of 75 mg every 4 hours as needed for pain. Determine the number of milliliters in an injection by setting up a proportion:

$$\frac{\text{solution (needed)}}{\text{active ingredient (to be administered)}} = \frac{\text{solution (available)}}{\text{active ingredient (available)}}$$

$$\frac{x \text{ mL}}{75 \text{ mg}} = \frac{1 \text{ mL}}{100 \text{ mg}}$$

$$\frac{(\cancel{75 \text{ mg}})\, x \text{ mL}}{\cancel{75 \text{ mg}}} = \frac{(\cancel{75 \text{ mg}})\, 1 \text{ mL}}{100 \cancel{\text{ mg}}}$$

$$x \text{ mL} = 0.75 \text{ mL}$$

Notice that 0.75 mL is three quarters of a 1 mL syringe.

Proportions can be used to solve other types of dosage calculations, such as converting an adult dose, based on body surface area (BSA), to an appropriate child's dose. **Body surface area (BSA)** is an expression of a patient's weight and height, used to calculate patient-specific dosages. Many medications have a wide dosage range, and the patient's response and adverse reactions can vary widely, even in adults. For this reason, many physicians prefer to prescribe to children only those medications that have a known pediatric-suggested dose. As you will see in Example 17, the calculated pediatric dose is rounded down, rather than up, for safety reasons.

Example 17

Safety Note

Medication doses for premature infants, neonates, and pediatric patients may use two decimal places and are always rounded down.

An average adult has a BSA of 1.72 m² and requires a dose of 12 mg of a given medication. The same medication is to be given to a child in a pediatric dose. The child has a BSA of 0.60 m², and the proper dose for pediatric and adult patients is a linear function of the BSA (in other words, think of the child as a small adult). What is the proper pediatric dose? Round off the final answer.

The assumptions regarding the calculation of pediatric doses make it possible to use a proportion to answer this question.

$$\frac{\text{child's dose}}{\text{child's BSA}} = \frac{\text{adult dose}}{\text{adult BSA}}$$

$$\frac{x \text{ mg}}{0.6 \text{ m}^2} = \frac{12 \text{ mg}}{1.72 \text{ m}^2}$$

$$\frac{(\cancel{0.6 \text{ m}^2})\, x \text{ mg}}{\cancel{0.6 \text{ m}^2}} = \frac{(\cancel{0.6 \text{ m}^2})12 \text{ mg}}{1.72 \cancel{\text{ m}^2}}$$

$$x \text{ mg} = 4.186 \text{ mg, rounded to 4 mg}$$

Because this dose is for a child, it is appropriate for safety reasons to round the dosage down to 4 mg rather than up to 4.2 mg.

Percents

The word *percent* comes from the Latin phrase *per centum*, meaning "in one hundred." A **percent** is a given part or amount in a hundred. Percents can be expressed in many ways, and all of the following expressions are equivalent.

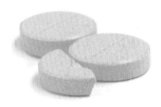

A pharmacy technician must be able to describe the piece of tablet as a ratio (1:2), a fraction (½), and a percentage (50%).

- a percent (e.g., 3%, or 3 percent)
- a fraction with 100 as the denominator (e.g., $^3/_{100}$)
- as a ratio (e.g., 3:100)
- as a decimal (e.g., 0.03)

Percent conversions from both ratios and decimals are often calculated by the pharmacy technician. Accuracy when calculating these conversions is critical to minimizing medication errors.

Converting Ratios and Percents To express a ratio as a percent, designate the first number of the ratio as the numerator and the second number as the denominator. Multiply the fraction by 100 and add a percent sign after the product.

$$5{:}1 = \frac{5}{1} \times 100 = 5 \times 100 = 500\%$$

$$1{:}5 = \frac{1}{5} \times 100 = \frac{100}{5} = 20\%$$

$$1{:}2 = \frac{1}{2} \times 100 = \frac{100}{2} = 50\%$$

To convert a percent to a ratio, first change it to a fraction by dividing it by 100 and then reduce the fraction to its lowest terms. Express this as a ratio by making the numerator the first number of the ratio and the denominator the second number.

$$2\% = 2 \div 100 = \frac{2}{100} = \frac{1}{50} = 1{:}50$$

$$10\% = 10 \div 100 = \frac{10}{100} = \frac{1}{10} = 1{:}10$$

$$75\% = 75 \div 100 = \frac{75}{100} = \frac{3}{4} = 3{:}4$$

$$\frac{1}{2}\% = \frac{1}{2} \div 100 = \frac{^1/_2}{100} = \frac{1}{2} \times \frac{1}{100} = \frac{1}{200} = 1{:}200$$

Converting Percents and Decimals To convert a percent to a decimal, drop the percent symbol and divide the number by 100. Dividing a number by 100 is equivalent to moving the decimal two places to the left and inserting zeros if necessary.

$$0.75\% = 0.75 \div 100 = 0.0075$$

$$4\% = 4 \div 100 = 0.04$$

$$200\% = 200 \div 100 = 2$$

To change a decimal to a percent, multiply by 100 or move the decimal point two places to the right and add a percent symbol.

$$0.25 = 0.25 \times 100 = 25\%$$

$$1.35 = 1.35 \times 100 = 135\%$$

$$0.015 = 0.015 \times 100 = 1.5\%$$

Dimensional Analysis

The dimensional analysis method, also known as "calculation by cancellation," is an approach that many medical, pharmacy, and nursing students utilize to solve pharmacy calculation problems. Drug calculations have units of measure or "dimensions" attached to them. The dimensional analysis method is based on the principle that any number can be multiplied by one without changing its value. This process helps to break down mathematical problems and assist in conversion to desired units of measurement. Below is a real-world example of solving a pharmacy calculation problem using this method.

Example 18

A mother visits your pharmacy on a Saturday night. She asks for the correct dose of Infants' Tylenol Oral Suspension Liquid for her child, who is 3 months old and weighs 15 lb. Infants' Tylenol Oral Suspension Liquid is 160 mg/5 mL, and the dose is 10 mg/kg. What is the correct dose in milligrams (mg) and volume in milliliters (mL) that the mother should administer to her child?

Step 1. To solve, break down this problem into smaller problems. Begin by recording what is known and include units of measurement or dimensions:

- Infant weighs 15 lb.
- Dose for Tylenol is 10 mg/kg.
- Concentration of the Infants' Tylenol Oral Suspension Liquid is 160 mg/5 mL.

Step 2. Because the dose for Tylenol is in kilograms, solve for *x* to determine the infant's weight in kilograms. As you can see from the example below, pounds (lb) cancel out, so the unit of measure for *x* is given in kilograms (kg).

$$\frac{1 \text{ kg}}{2.2 \text{ lb}} = \frac{x \text{ kg}}{15 \text{ lb}}$$

$$x = \frac{15}{2.2}$$

$$x = 6.8 \text{ kg (weight of the infant)}$$

Step 3. Next, solve for *y* to determine the dose of Tylenol to be administered to the infant. As you can see from the example below, kilograms (kg) cancel out, so the unit of measure for *y* is given in milligrams (mg).

$$\frac{10 \text{ mg}}{\text{kg}} = \frac{y \text{ mg}}{6.8 \text{ kg}}$$

$$y = 6.8 \times 10$$

$$y = 68 \text{ mg (the dose of Tylenol required for the infant)}$$

Step 4. You now know the weight of the infant in kilograms (kg) and the infant's dose in milligrams (mg). You can now use the ratio and proportion calculation to determine the amount of Tylenol suspension to be drawn up in the oral syringe. The milligrams (mg) cancel out, so the unit of measure for *x* is given in milliliters (mL).

$$\frac{160 \text{ mg}}{5 \text{ mL}} = \frac{68 \text{ mg}}{x \text{ mL}}$$

$$x = 68 \times \frac{5}{160}$$

$$x = 2.1 \text{ mL, rounded down to 2 mL (the amount of Infants' Tylenol Oral}$$
$$\text{Suspension Liquid to be administered to the infant)}$$

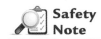

Safety Note

Pharmacy personnel should remind parents or caregivers to only use the oral syringe provided with their child's product to administer the medication.

Advanced Calculations Used in Pharmacy Practice

The pharmacy technician will need to calculate the amount of ingredients required to create prescribed solutions. For example, parenteral products are often reconstituted by adding a diluent to a lyophilized or freeze-dried powder to prepare a solution for IV administration. The product is commercially manufactured in powder form because of the instability of the drug in solution over a long period. In addition, the pharmacy technician may be asked to create solutions of a specific concentration by combining measured amounts of solutions of more and less concentrated ingredients. This section will present these types of calculations.

Preparing Solutions Using Powders

When preparing solutions using powders, pharmacy technicians should be aware that the active ingredient (the powder) is discussed by weight but that the substance also occupies a certain amount of space or volume. This space is referred to as **powder volume (pv)**. It is equal to the difference between the final volume (fv) and the volume of the diluting ingredient, or the diluent volume (dv), as expressed in the following equation:

$$\text{powder volume} = \text{final volume} - \text{diluent volume}$$

or

$$pv = fv - dv$$

Example 19

A dry powder antibiotic must be reconstituted for use. The label states that the dry powder occupies 0.5 mL. Using the formula for solving for powder volume, determine the diluent volume (the amount of solvent added). You are given the final volume for three different examples with the same powder volume.

Final Volume	Powder Volume
(1) 2 mL	0.5 mL
(2) 5 mL	0.5 mL
(3) 10 mL	0.5 mL

$$dv = fv - pv$$

(1) $dv = 2 \text{ mL} - 0.5 \text{ mL} = 1.5 \text{ mL}$

(2) $dv = 5 \text{ mL} - 0.5 \text{ mL} = 4.5 \text{ mL}$

(3) $dv = 10 \text{ mL} - 0.5 \text{ mL} = 9.5 \text{ mL}$

Example 20

You are to reconstitute 1 g of dry powder. The label states that you are to add 9.3 mL of diluent to make a final solution of 100 mg/mL. What is the powder volume?

Step 1. Calculate the final volume. The strength of the final solution will be 100 mg/mL. Since you start with 1 g = 1000 mg of powder, for a final volume x of the solution, it will have a strength 1000 mg/x mL. Using the ratio-proportion method,

$$\frac{x \text{ mL}}{1000 \text{ mg}} = \frac{1 \text{ mL}}{100 \text{ mg}}$$

$$x \text{ mL} = \frac{(1000 \text{ mg}) \times 1 \text{ mL}}{100 \text{ mg}} = 10 \text{ mL}$$

Step 2. Using the calculated final volume and the given diluent volume, calculate the powder volume.

$$pv = fv - dv$$

$$pv = 10 \text{ mL} - 9.3 \text{ mL} = 0.7 \text{ mL}$$

Working with Dilutions

Medications may be diluted for several reasons. They are sometimes diluted prior to administration to children, infants, and older adults to meet the dosage requirements of those patients. Medications may also be diluted so that they can be measured more accurately and easily. For example, volumes less than 0.1 mL are usually considered too small to measure accurately. Therefore, they must be diluted further. Many pharmacies have a policy as to how much an injection can be diluted. A rule of thumb is for the required dose to have a volume greater than 0.1 mL and less than 1 mL.

The following example will demonstrate the method for solving typical dilution problems. The first step is to use the ratio-proportion method to solve for the volume of the final product by using a ratio of diluted solution to desired concentration. The second step is to determine the amount of diluent simply by subtracting the concentrate from the total volume. Both of these volumes are approximate because they depend on the calibration and accuracy of the measuring devices used.

Although the second step is used to determine the amount of diluent added, the amount will actually be determined by adding "up to" the desired total quantity. The abbreviation QS for "sufficient quantity" is used to describe the process of adding enough of the last ingredient in a compound to reach the desired volume. It is helpful to calculate the necessary amount beforehand so that an adequate supply of medication is available.

Example 21

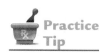
Practice Tip

An injected dose generally has a volume greater than 0.1 mL and less than 1 mL.

Dexamethasone sodium phosphate is available as a 4 mg/mL sterile preparation for injection. An infant is to receive 0.35 mg. The volume needed would be a miniscule 0.08 mL, which is very difficult to accurately measure. Prepare a dilution so that the final concentration is 1 mg/mL. How much diluent will you need if the original product is in a 1 mL vial and you dilute the entire vial? What is the volume of final dose to be measured?

Step 1. Determine the volume (in milliliters) of the final product. Because the strength of the dexamethasone is 4 mg/mL, a 1 mL vial will contain 4 mg of the active ingredient. Then, for a final volume x of solution, you will have a concentration of 4 mg/x mL.

Diluted solution	Desired concentration

$$\frac{x \text{ mL}}{4 \text{ mg}} = \frac{1 \text{ mL}}{1 \text{ mg}}$$

$$x \text{ mL} = \frac{(4 \text{ mg} \times 1 \text{ mL})}{1 \text{ mg}} = 4 \text{ mL final product}$$

Step 2. Subtract the volume of the concentrate from the total volume to determine the volume of diluent needed.

$$4 \text{ mL total volume} - 1 \text{ mL concentrate} = 3 \text{ mL diluent needed}$$

Therefore, an additional 3 mL of diluent are needed to dilute the original 1 mL of preparation to arrive at a final concentration of 1 mg/mL.

Step 3. Set up a ratio-proportion to determine the volume of medication to be prepared from the diluted medication.

$$\frac{x \text{ mL}}{0.35 \text{ mg}} = \frac{1 \text{ mL}}{1 \text{ mg}}$$

$$x \text{ mL} = 0.35 \text{ mL}$$

This volume is much more accurately measured in a tuberculin syringe.

Using Alligation to Prepare Compounded Products

Physicians often prescribe concentrations of medications that are not commercially available, and these prescriptions must be compounded (added together) at the pharmacy. When an ordered concentration is not commercially available, it may be necessary to combine two different products with the same active ingredient in differing strengths. The resulting concentration will be greater than the weaker strength, but less than the stronger strength. For example, 1% and 5% hydrocortisone ointments may be combined to provide a 3% ointment. This is called

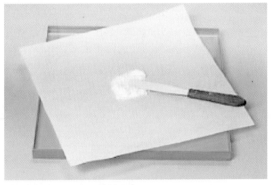

When the desired concentration of a cream is not available, the pharmacy technician must use an alligation to calculate how much cream of the lesser concentration, and how much of the greater concentration, should be mixed together.

alligation. An alligation is used when the two quantities needed to prepare the desired concentration are both relatively large. (To learn more about the techniques for mixing topical creams of different strengths to produce a pharmaceutically elegant final product, refer to Chapter 8.)

The amount of each stock product to be added together is calculated by using the alligation alternate method. In this method, pharmacy personnel change the percentages to parts of a proportion and then use the proportion to obtain the amounts of the two ingredients needed to prepare the desired concentration. The answer can then be checked using the following formula.

$$\text{milliliters} \times \text{percent (expressed as a decimal)} = \text{grams}$$

It is important to note that this formula works for any strength solution. The following examples will demonstrate the application of the alligation alternate method.

Example 22

Prepare 250 mL of dextrose 7.5% weight in volume (w/v) using dextrose 5% (D_5W) w/v and dextrose 50% ($D_{50}W$) w/v. How many milliliters of each will be needed?

Step 1. Set up a box arrangement and at the upper left corner write the percent of the highest concentration (50%) as a whole number. At the lower left corner, write the percent of the lowest concentration (5%) as a whole number, and in the center, write the desired concentration.

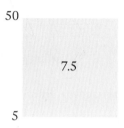

Step 2. Subtract the center number from the upper left number (i.e., the smaller from the larger) and put it at the lower-right corner. Now subtract the lower left number from the center number (i.e., the smaller from the larger), and put it at the upper right corner.

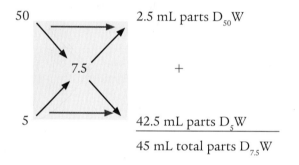

The number 2.5 mL represents the number of parts of the 50% solution that will be needed to make the final 7.5% solution, and the number 42.5 mL represents the number of parts of the 5% solution that will be needed. The sum of these two numbers, 2.5 mL + 42.5 mL = 45 mL, is the total number of parts of the 7.5% solution. In terms of ratios, the ratio of the 5% solution to the 7.5% solution is 42.5:45, and the ratio of the 50% solution to the 7.5% solution is 2.5:45. Much less of the more concentrated 50% solution (2.5 mL) is needed to make the final 7.5% solution.

Step 3. Calculate the volume needed of each dextrose solution.

50% Dextrose

$$\frac{x \text{ mL of } 50\%}{250 \text{ mL}} = \frac{2.5 \text{ mL parts D}_{50}\text{W}}{45 \text{ mL total parts D}_{7.5}\text{W}}$$

$$x \text{ mL} = \frac{(250 \text{ mL}) \times 2.5 \text{ mL parts}}{45 \text{ mL total parts}}$$

$$x \text{ mL} = 13.8888 \text{ mL D}_{50}\text{W, rounded to } 13.9 \text{ mL}$$

5% Dextrose

$$\frac{x \text{ mL of } 5\%}{250 \text{ mL}} = \frac{42.5 \text{ mL parts D}_5\text{W}}{45 \text{ mL total parts D}_{7.5}\text{W}}$$

$$x \text{ mL} = \frac{(250 \text{ mL}) \times 42.5 \text{ mL parts}}{45 \text{ mL total parts}}$$

$$x \text{ mL} = 236.11 \text{ mL D}_5\text{W, rounded to } 236.1 \text{ mL}$$

Step 4. Add the volumes of the two solutions together. The sum should equal the required volume of dextrose 7.5%.

$$236.1 \text{ mL}$$

$$+ \ 13.9 \text{ mL}$$

$$250.0 \text{ mL}$$

Step 5. Check your answer by calculating the amount of solute (dextrose) in all three solutions. The number of grams of solute should equal the sum of the grams of solutes from the 50% solution and the 5% solution, using the following formula.

$$\text{mL} \times \% \text{ (as a decimal)} = \text{g}$$

$$250 \text{ mL} \times 0.075 = 18.75 \text{ g}$$

$$13.9 \text{ mL D}_{50}\text{W} \times 0.5 = 6.95 \text{ g}$$

$$236.1 \text{ mL D}_5\text{W} \times 0.05 = 11.805 \text{ g, rounded to } 11.8 \text{ g}$$

$$11.805 \text{ g}$$

$$+ \ 6.945 \text{ g}$$

$$18.750 \text{ g}$$

The amounts measured to prepare this prescription will be rounded to the nearest milliliter: 14 mL D$_{50}$W and 236 mL D$_5$W.

Example 23

You are instructed to make 454 g of 3% zinc oxide cream. You have in stock 10% and 1% zinc oxide cream. How much of each percent will you use?

Step 1.

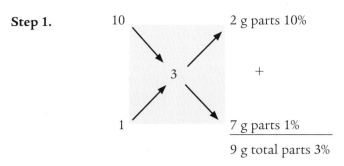

10   2 g parts 10%

3   +

1   7 g parts 1%

9 g total parts 3%

Step 2. 10% zinc oxide cream

$$\frac{x \text{ g of } 10\%}{454 \text{ g}} = \frac{2 \text{ g parts } 10\%}{9 \text{ g total parts } 3\%}$$

x g of 10% = 101 g of 10% zinc oxide cream

1% zinc oxide cream

$$\frac{x \text{ g of } 1\%}{454 \text{ g}} = \frac{7 \text{ g parts } 1\%}{9 \text{ g total parts } 3\%}$$

x g of 1% = 353 g of 1% zinc oxide cream

Step 3. Check your work.

$$353 \text{ g} + 101 \text{ g} = 454 \text{ g}$$

Calculating Specific Gravity

Calculating specific gravity is another example of a ratio-proportion application. **Specific gravity** is the ratio of the weight of a substance to the weight of an equal volume of water, the standard, when both are at the same temperature. Final weight can be measured in grams because 1 mL of water weighs 1 g.

1 mL, volume of water = 1 g, weight of water

specific gravity of water = 1

The specific gravity represents the weight of 1 mL of the substance and has no units of measure. The ratio called specific gravity is in essence a comparison of the weight of a liquid to the weight of water when exactly 1 mL of each is measured out. Water is the standard that is used, and the specific gravity assigned to it is one (1). The formula for determining specific gravity is as follows:

$$\text{specific gravity} = \frac{\text{weight of a substance}}{\text{weight of an equal volume of water}}$$

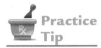

Practice Tip

Usually numbers are not written without units, but no units exist for specific gravity.

When the specific gravity is known, certain assumptions can be made regarding the physical properties of a liquid. Solutions that are thick (or viscous) or have particles floating in them often have specific gravities higher than one (1), or heavier than water. Solutions that contain volatile chemicals (or something prone to quick evaporation), such as alcohol, often have a specific gravity lower than one (1), or lighter than water.

Example 24

If the weight of 100 mL of dextrose solution is 117 g, what is the specific gravity of the dextrose solution?

$$\text{specific gravity} = \frac{\text{weight of a substance}}{\text{weight of an equal volume of water}}$$

$$= \frac{117 \text{ g}}{100 \text{ g}}$$

$$= 1.17$$

If the specific gravity is known, you can determine the weight of a volume of a liquid.

Example 25

If a liquid has a specific gravity of 0.85, how much does 125 mL of it weigh?

Because the specific gravity of the liquid is 0.85,

$$\text{specific gravity} = \frac{\text{weight of a substance}}{\text{weight of an equal volume of water}}$$

$$0.85 = \frac{85 \text{ g (weight of 100 mL of the liquid)}}{100 \text{ g (weight of 100 mL of water)}}$$

Now, use the ratio-proportion method to find the weight of 125 mL.

$$\frac{x \text{ g}}{125 \text{ mL}} = \frac{85 \text{ g}}{100 \text{ mL}}$$

$$\frac{(125 \text{ mL}) x \text{ g}}{125 \text{ mL}} = \frac{(125 \text{ mL}) 85 \text{ g}}{100 \text{ mL}}$$

$$x \text{ g} = \frac{10,625 \text{ g}}{100}$$

$$x \text{ g} = 106.25 \text{ g}$$

Chapter Summary

- The metric system is preferred worldwide for making accurate, standard measurements.
- The metric system of measurement makes use of decimal units, including the basic units of the gram (for weight) and the liter (for volume).
- Pharmacy professionals should be able to convert between different systems such as metric, avoirdupois, apothecary, and household measures.
- The most widely used units of measure in pharmacy include milligrams, grams, kilograms, milliliters, liters, and grains.
- Pharmacy technicians working in hospital pharmacies must be comfortable reading military time (also called 24-hour time or international time).
- In the pharmacy, technicians must be able to convert temperatures from Fahrenheit to Celsius.

- Pharmacists and pharmacy technicians should be familiar with the standard prefixes for abbreviating metric quantities and with the basic mathematical principles used to calculate and convert doses and prepare reconstituted solutions from powdered drug products.
- Pharmacy personnel should be able to find an unknown quantity in a proportion when three elements of the proportion are known; they should also be able to use the alligation method to compound a product from products having different concentrations.

Key Terms

alligation the compounding of two or more products to obtain a desired concentration

apothecary system a weight-based measurement system developed by the Romans

Arabic system a mathematical system using numbers, fractions, and decimals

avoirdupois system a system of measurement that originated in France and is used for common measurements in the United States; units of measure include the foot, mile, grain, pound, and ounce

body surface area (BSA) a measurement related to a patient's weight and height, expressed in meters squared (m^2), and used to calculate patient-specific dosages of medications

Celsius temperature scale the temperature scale that uses 0 °C as the temperature at which water freezes at sea level and 100 °C as the temperature at which it boils

decimal any number that can be written in decimal notation using the integers 0 through 9 and a point (.) to divide the "ones" place from the "tenths" place (e.g., 10.25 is equal to 10¼)

denominator the number on the bottom part of a fraction that represents the whole

Fahrenheit temperature scale the temperature scale that uses 32 °F as the temperature at which water freezes at sea level and 212 °F as the temperature at which it boils

fraction a portion of a whole that is represented as a ratio

grain a dry weight unit of measurement in the apothecary system (e.g., 5 grains [5 gr] of aspirin are equivalent to approximately 325 mg)

gram the metric system's base unit for measuring weight

household system a system of measurement based on the apothecary system; units of measure include the ounce, pound, drop, teaspoon, tablespoon, and cup

leading zero a zero that is placed in the ones place in a number less than zero that is being represented by a decimal value

liter the metric system's base unit for measuring volume

meter the metric system's base unit for measuring length

metric system a measurement system based on subdivisions and multiples of 10; made up of three basic units: meter, gram, and liter

military time a measure of time based on a 24-hour clock in which midnight is 0000, noon is 1200, and the minute before midnight is 2359; also referred to as *24-hour time* or *international time*

numerator the number on the upper part of a fraction that represents the part of the whole

percent the number or ratio per 100

powder volume (pv) the amount of space occupied by a freeze-dried medication in a sterile vial, used for reconstitution; equal to the difference between the final volume (fv) and the volume of the diluting ingredient, or the diluent volume (dv)

proportion a comparison of equal ratios; the product of the means equals the product of the extremes

ratio a comparison of numeric values

Roman system a mathematical system in which numerals are expressed in either capital letters or lowercase letters

specific gravity the ratio of the weight of a substance compared to an equal volume of water when both have the same temperature

Chapter Review

 Additional Quiz Questions

Checking Your Understanding

To check your comprehension of this chapter's key concepts, read the following multiple-choice questions and then record your answers on a separate sheet of paper. Write your answers as modeled in these examples: 1d; 2c; 3b; etc.

1. The modern metric system makes use of the standardized units of the
   a. avoirdupois system.
   b. Système International (SI).
   c. household system.
   d. apothecary system.

2. _____ is the metric prefix that indicates thousandth.
   a. *Nano-*
   b. *Micro-*
   c. *Milli-*
   d. *Deci-*

3. A kilogram is equal to
   a. 1000 micrograms.
   b. 1000 milligrams.
   c. 1000 centigrams.
   d. 1000 grams.

4. In the metric system, the liter is a standard measurement of
   a. distance.
   b. area.
   c. volume.
   d. weight.

5. The varicella (chicken pox/shingles) vaccine requires a storage temperature of –15 °C or colder. What is the equivalent temperature in degrees Fahrenheit?
   a. 0 °F
   b. 5 °F
   c. 10 °F
   d. 32 °F

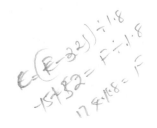

6. A decimal fraction has as its denominator a power of
   a. 2.
   b. 5.
   c. 10.
   d. 25.

7. Another way to look at 58% is 58 out of one
   a. hundred.
   b. thousand.
   c. million.
   d. billion.

8. Liposyn III has a specific gravity of 0.985. How much will 1 L of the IV solution weigh?
   a. 985 g
   b. 1000 g
   c. 1001.5 g
   d. 0

9. The only unit of measure that is the same in the apothecary system and avoirdupois system is the
   a. grain.
   b. gram.
   c. liter.
   d. ounce.

10. Which measurement is commonly used to convert an adult dose to an appropriate child's dose?
    a. height
    b. age
    c. body surface area (BSA)
    d. body mass index (BMI)

11. A prescription is written for Cephalexin 125 mg/5 mL with the directions for the patient to take 8 mL po bid. You are out-of-stock on the 125 mg/5 mL bottle but have a 250 mg/5 mL bottle on the shelf. What is the amount of suspension (in mL) for each dose of the higher concentration bottle in stock?
    a. 4 mL
    b. 5 mL
    c. 8 mL
    d. 16 mL

12. You are asked to prepare 1 g of Ancef for an IV. The label states that you are to use 2.5 mL of diluent to make a final concentration of 330 mg/mL. Calculate the powder volume.
    a. 0.5 mL
    b. 2.5 mL
    c. 3 mL
    d. 10 mL

13. In common pharmacy practice, how many grams of weight are in 1 oz?
    a. 28.35 g
    b. 30 g
    c. 31.1 g
    d. 454 g

14. An IV medication order is received in the hospital with the first dose to be started at 2200 hours. What time is that?
    a. 10:00 AM
    b. 10:00 PM
    c. 2:00 AM
    d. 2:00 PM

15. A prescription is received at your compounding pharmacy to make 100 g of 2% hydrocortisone cream. You have 2.5% hydrocortisone available in stock to mix with Aquaphor. Using the alligation method, how many grams of Aquaphor will be needed to mix with the 2.5% hydrocortisone to make a final concentration of 2%?
    a. 80 grams
    b. 50 grams
    c. 20 grams
    d. 2.5 grams

Reinforcing Your Learning

To build on your understanding of the topics in this chapter, complete the following enrichment activities.

1. Convert the following:
   a. 34.6 g = _____ mg
   b. 735 mg = _____ g
   c. 3400 mL = _____ L
   d. 1.2 L = _____ mL
   e. 7.48 kg = _____ g
   f. 473 mL = _____ L

2. Convert the following:
   a. 24 fl oz = _____ pt
   b. 40 gr (apothecary) = _____ Э (apothecary)
   c. 6 Ʒ (apothecary) = _____ # (apothecary)
   d. 6.25 tbsp = _____ tsp
   e. 8 qt = _____ gal
   f. viii = _____ (Arabic numeral)
   g. C = _____ (Arabic numeral)

3. Create a series of flash cards for Table 5.7: Household Measures. Record the measurement units for weight and volume on one side of a card and their metric equivalents on the other side. Choose a partner and help each other with the memorization of these conversions.

4. Obtain a 1 mL tuberculin syringe (without a needle) and a 5 mL oral syringe (without a needle) from a local pharmacy for an experiment. Measure 0.09 mL of water and 0.35 mL of water. Which syringe and volume is easier and more accurate?

Thinking on Your Feet

To gain practice in handling challenging situations in the workplace, consider the following real-world scenarios and then use the guiding questions to help you formulate your responses.

1. Solve the following conversion problems:
   a. You have 2 L of irrigating solution in stock. The solution is to be used to fill vials that hold 50 mL each. How many vials can you fill with the 2 L of solution?
   b. The patient has received a bottle containing 200 mL of a liquid medication. The patient is to take 5 tsp of the medication per day. How many days will the bottle last?
   c. A compound prescription calls for codeine sulfate 16.25 mg. How many grains of codeine sulfate should be used in the prescription? (Assume 65 mg = 1 gr)
   d. A patient takes two $1/150$ gr nitroglycerin tablets per day. How many milligrams of nitroglycerin does the patient receive each day?

2. Solve the following problems:
   a. In stock you have a solution that contains 8 mg of active ingredient per 10 mL of solution. A customer has a prescription calling for a quantity of 4 doses of 6 mg each of the active ingredient. How many milliliters of the solution should the customer be given?
   b. A medication order calls for phenobarbital 60 mg. The supply available is phenobarbital 100 mg/mL of solution. How many milliliters of the solution will the patient be given?
   c. If the adult dose of a medication is 30 mg and the average adult body surface area (BSA) is 1.72 m², what would be the appropriate pediatric dose for a child with a BSA of 0.50 m²?

3. Solve the following solution preparation problems:
   a. You have been asked to prepare a solution containing a powder with a volume of 0.7 mL. The total volume of the solution that you are to prepare should be 30 mL. How much diluent will you use in the solution, and what will be the percentage, by volume, of powder in the solution?
   b. You are instructed to make 240 mL of a 0.45% w/v solution. You have a 3% concentrate in stock. How much of the full-strength solution will you use, and how much diluent will be needed?
   c. You must prepare 300 mL of a solution containing 42.5% dextrose. In stock you have solutions containing 5% dextrose (solution 1) and 50% dextrose (solution 2). How many milliliters of each stock solution must you use in the solution that you prepare?

Acquiring Field Knowledge

To expand your knowledge of pharmacy practice, explore the following online activities that focus on research and information retrieval.

Reminder: As you navigate the Internet, remember to exercise caution and good judgment when evaluating information. A thoughtful review of online text should take into consideration the following factors: the creator and sponsors of the website, the intended audience, the credentials of the authors and contributors, the reliability and validity of the posted information, the frequency of updates to the site, and the ease of navigation for a range of user skill levels.

1. Go to www.paradigmcollege.net/pharmpractice5e/mederrorprevention and conduct a search for medication error prevention. What measures are recommended to minimize errors in the pharmacy workplace? Discuss your findings with the class.

2. Heparin is available in many concentrations in the hospital: 1 mg/mL, 10 mg/mL, 100 mg/mL, 1000 mg/mL, 5000 mg/mL, and 10,000 mg/mL. This wide variety of concentrations has led to many medication errors and even deaths in the neonatal and pediatric populations. Develop a written policy and procedure for your hospital to reduce the risk of heparin dosing errors. Use www.paradigmcollege.net/pharmpractice5e/heparinerrors as a resource.

3. Check www.paradigmcollege.net/pharmpractice5e/codeine and see how many milligrams of codeine are in Tylenol #2, #3, and #4. For extra credit, can you identify three other medications that are commonly dosed in grains?

Sampling the Certification Exam

To provide you with practice for the Certification Exam, read the following questions that have been patterned after the test format and then record your answers on a separate sheet of paper. Write your answers as modeled in these examples: 1d; 2c; 3b; *etc.*

1. The dose of diazepam for seizures lasting greater than 10 minutes is 0.2 mg/kg rectal (with a maximum dose of 10 mg). For a 5 kg child, what would be the appropriate dose (in mg) of diazepam?
   a. 0.2 mg
   b. 1 mg
   c. 2 mg
   d. 10 mg

2. You receive a stat order for Narcan 2.5 mg. The medication is available in a concentration of 0.4 mg/mL. How much drug do you need to prepare for the needed dose?
   a. 0.4 mL
   b. 1 mL
   c. 6.25 mL
   d. 10 mL

3. What is the temperature range allowed for an item requiring refrigeration?
   a. 35 °F to 45 °F
   b. 15 °C to 30 °C
   c. 25 °C to 2 °C
   d. 15 °F to 30 °F

4. What measurement is used to identify the size of an amber vial for liquids or syrups?
   a. ounces
   b. grains
   c. scruples
   d. drams

5. What is the proper way to write warfarin *five milligrams* to prevent a medication error?
   a. 5.0 mg
   b. 5 mg
   c. 0.5 mg
   d. 0.005 g

6. A prescription is written for phenobarbital 1 grain. How many milligrams is that equivalent to?
   a. 15 mg
   b. 30 mg
   c. 65 mg
   d. 100 mg

7. Which calculation method is used when pharmacy personnel need to mix two different strengths of the same active ingredient in order to create the desired strength?
   a. rounding up
   b. dimensional analysis
   c. ratio and proportion
   d. alligation

8. What is the specific gravity of 250 mL of water?
   a. 0.25
   b. 0.5
   c. 1.0
   d. 1.25

9. You receive a prescription for amoxicillin/clavulanate (Augmentin) 250 mg/mL, 3.5 mL po bid for 10 days. What volume must be dispensed?
   a. 35 mL
   b. 70 mL
   c. 100 mL
   d. 250 mL

10. How many milligrams are in 5 grains of ferrous sulfate?
    a. 5 mg
    b. 65 mg
    c. 162.5 mg
    d. 325 mg

Unit

2

Community Pharmacy

Dispensing Medications in the Community Pharmacy

6

Learning Objectives

- Discuss overall community pharmacy operations and general responsibilities of the pharmacy technician with regard to the dispensing of prescription drugs.

- Identify the parts of a prescription and recognize the most commonly used abbreviations for amounts, dosage forms, times of administration, and sites of administration.

- Discuss the various types of prescriptions that are processed in a community pharmacy.

- List the advantages of electronic prescribing in modern-day community pharmacy practice.

- Know the federal laws on the filling, refilling, and transferring of controlled substances.

- Describe controls necessary for reviewing prescriptions of scheduled drugs, including the identification of possible forgeries.

- Identify the parts of a patient profile, detail the steps required to select a patient from the database, and discuss the importance of including up-to-date insurance, allergy, and adverse drug reaction information.

- Identify the parts of a stock drug label and know the importance of comparing National Drug Code numbers in medication selection and filling.

- Describe the parts of a medication container label.

- Explain the step-by-step procedures for processing both new and refill prescription orders.

- Discuss how automation is utilized in community pharmacy to minimize medication errors.

- Discuss the importance of a final check and verification by the pharmacist prior to dispensing prescription drugs to the patient.

- Identify the OBRA-90 mandated regulation that must be executed by pharmacy technicians prior to dispensing medications to patients.

Preview chapter terms and definitions.

T he primary role of the pharmacist is to dispense medications safely, accurately, and in accordance with state and federal laws upon receipt of valid medication orders from licensed prescribers. Prescribers are most often physicians but may also include dentists, veterinarians, nurse practitioners, or physician's assistants. The pharmacy technician plays a critical role assisting in customer service, updating patient demographics and insurance information, entering prescriptions into a patient profile, and accurately filling prescription orders. By supporting the pharmacist, the technician frees the pharmacist to spend more time resolving medication-related problems and counseling patients about their medications.

A vast majority of all pharmacy technician positions are in chain or independent community pharmacy settings. This chapter discusses in detail the major responsibilities of both the pharmacist and the pharmacy technician in dispensing new and refill prescriptions in a typical community pharmacy. The exact procedures outlined in this chapter may vary within a specific community pharmacy, but the basic tasks are similar and must be learned by the aspiring pharmacy technician.

Because pharmacy practice laws vary among states, pharmacists and pharmacy technicians need to be aware of the legal regulations for the state in which they practice. Consequently, this chapter includes a clarification of the legal responsibilities of the pharmacist and pharmacy technician in the dispensing process, including the dual responsibility of the identification of potential medication errors.

Community Pharmacy Operations

More than four billion prescriptions are dispensed annually in all pharmacies in the United States, and the majority of prescriptions are filled in a community pharmacy. In addition to dispensing prescriptions, community pharmacies also offer specialized services, such as compounding noncommercially available medications and preparing and delivering prescriptions to nontraditional healthcare sites such as nursing homes, personal care homes, and prisons. Other patient services provided by community pharmacies include vaccine administration, blood pressure checks, and laboratory testing for blood glucose and cholesterol levels. These specialized services will only grow exponentially over the next few decades in response to an increasingly older patient population.

The pharmacy dispensing area is locked and restricted to pharmacists and pharmacy technicians. "Rx only" and select OTC drugs are stored in this secured area.

Community Pharmacy Facility

A community pharmacy, or retail pharmacy, is divided into two areas: a front area that houses over-the-counter (OTC) drugs, medical supplies, dietary supplements, and other merchandise, and a back area that is restricted to pharmacy personnel only. The pharmacy counter separates these two areas. To limit the access to prescription medications, the area of the pharmacy behind the counter where the prescription medications are stored and prepared for sale is usually secured by code or key and is off-limits to the public. The secured area where the prescription drugs are stored may be entered only by authorized employees, such as the pharmacist and the pharmacy technician. No family or friends are allowed in this secured work area. If there is no pharmacist on duty, this area of the pharmacy must be locked and closed to the public or secured as per state law. The remainder of the store may remain open to sell any other merchandise or products, including OTC drugs and dietary supplements.

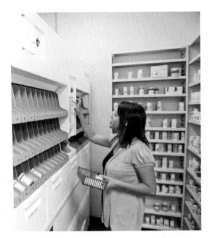

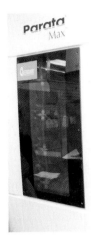

Parata Max® is a high-speed, high-accuracy automated dispensing system.

To meet customer needs, community pharmacies must focus on service and convenience. Many pharmacies use automation technology to dispense with greater speed and accuracy and to allow the pharmacist more time during operational hours to provide patient counseling. Parata Systems offers an automated system called Parata Max®, which labels, fills, caps, sorts, and stores up to 232 prescriptions, processing up to 60% of total prescription volume with 100% accuracy for drug and strength. Automation reduces the number of manual fills by pharmacy staff, helping to lower the cost per prescription.

Convenience is also an important factor when fulfilling the healthcare needs of patients. For that reason, several community pharmacies have hours of operation that vary from 40 to 168 hours a week, with many of these facilities offering home deliveries and after-hours availability for working families, shift workers, and patients recently discharged from emergency rooms and hospitals. As an added convenience, many community pharmacies offer a drive-thru area for prescription drop-off and pickup.

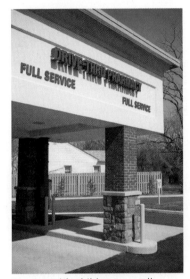

Parents with children, as well as older patients and patients with disabilities, often prefer the convenience of a drive-thru pharmacy.

Customer service and convenience provided by the community pharmacy are important because patients can also choose to send their prescription orders to large, less expensive, out-of-state, mail-order pharmacy warehouses. Mail-order pharmacies can fill prescriptions for less cost because they use automation and have round-the-clock filling operations. Many national chain pharmacies offer a mail-order option, and the Veterans Administration (VA) operates several regional centralized warehouses that use the mail-order drug distribution system. These operations differ from a local community pharmacy primarily by their sheer workload volume and lack of direct contact with patients.

Some prescription insurance programs encourage patients to use mail-order pharmacies by offering lower co-payments on a 90-day supply of a medication. The potential cost savings of mail-order pharmacies may be partially offset by delays in the receipt of a needed medication (to the potential detriment of health), drug wastage, and minimal counseling offered to the patient. For example, patient information on mail-order prescriptions is usually limited to preprinted typed sheets or toll-free numbers. On the other hand, patients receiving prescription medications from a community pharmacy always have direct access to the on-duty pharmacist during operational hours.

Community Pharmacy Personnel

Community pharmacies are staffed by pharmacists and pharmacy technicians who work in tandem to fulfill the healthcare needs of their customers.

Pharmacists As mentioned in Chapter 1, a community pharmacist has many responsibilities. Some of these tasks include gathering medical, medication, and allergy histories; checking computer warnings about drug interactions; verifying, preparing, and dispensing prescriptions; counseling patients about their prescribed medications as well as OTC drugs and healthcare devices; monitoring controlled substances; and administering vaccinations such as influenza, pneumonia, and shingles. Pharmacists—particularly in independent pharmacies—are also involved in the managerial tasks of running a business, including the hiring and firing of employees, evaluating insurance contracts, reconciling insurance claims, and ordering and maintaining inventory.

Pharmacy Technicians A pharmacy technician working in the community pharmacy is involved in selling medications and healthcare-related products to customers. The sale of prescription medications, called *legend drugs*, is regulated and carefully monitored. Customers cannot buy these drugs without an appropriate prescription from a licensed healthcare provider. Legend drugs are identified on their stock bottle with the label "Rx only" (see Figure 6.1); controlled drugs are labeled as C–II, C–III, C–IV, and C–V, depending on their Drug Enforcement Administration (DEA) classification.

FIGURE 6.1
The Rx Only Designation

The "Rx only" on this medication label designates that this medication can only be dispensed according to a prescription.

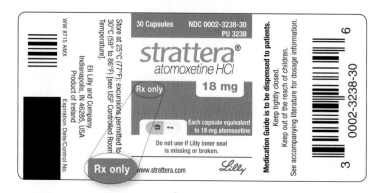

In the community pharmacy, a technician's role in the dispensing of prescription drugs often changes during the day. He or she is typically juggling several different tasks at once, with each task requiring due diligence to ensure accuracy. A list of these general tasks can be seen in Table 6.1, but these duties may fluctuate, depending on a facility's approved policies and procedures. A community pharmacy's regulations are typically explained during an on-the-job training program for new pharmacy technicians or—in some cases— in a written Policy and Procedure (P&P) manual. The training program or manual not only reflects the requirements of the relevant state laws and regulations (as discussed in Chapter 2) but also provides guidelines for the safe and effective operation of the pharmacy as defined by the facility itself. It is important for the pharmacy technician to understand these policies and procedures and to follow them carefully.

In addition to assisting in prescription processing, the pharmacy technician is expected to help maintain a clean work environment by vacuuming the pharmacy restricted area, cleaning counters and counting trays, bundling and removing trash, and securing the disposal of patient-specific information. Lastly, the pharmacy technician is involved in the business operations of the

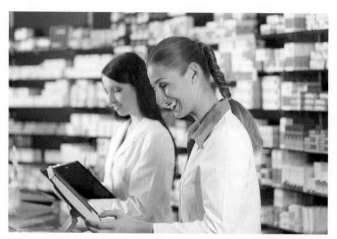

The pharmacist and technician work together as a team to provide customer service as well as efficient and safe dispensing of medications.

TABLE 6.1 Key Pharmacy Technician Duties in the Community Pharmacy

- Greeting customers at the pharmacy counter or drive-thru window and receiving written prescriptions
- Answering the telephone and referring call-in prescriptions or transfers to the pharmacist
- Initiating refills requested by patients in person or by telephone
- Clarifying and resolving questions about the prescription (name, directions, and so on) with the prescriber's office
- Updating patient profiles, including patient demographics, allergies, and health conditions
- Entering or updating billing information for third-party reimbursement
- Scanning and entering new prescriptions (or refill requests) into the patient profile
- Submitting prescription claims online to insurance providers
- Contacting insurance companies to resolve eligibility or prescription processing issues
- Counting, reconstituting, packaging, and repackaging products
- Preparing and affixing medication container labels for prescriptions
- Retrieving and counting drug products from storage in the restricted prescription area
- Returning stock bottles to their proper storage locations
- Distributing labeled medications to the patient after final verification by the pharmacist
- Storing completed prescriptions for future patient pickup
- Retrieving medications for patient pickup
- Offering a medication counseling opportunity for the patient
- Accepting payments and co-payments for prescription(s)

community pharmacy, including inventory control; the processing and resolution of prescription claims to insurance; and the sale of nonprescription products, dietary supplements, and supplies. These business responsibilities will be discussed in detail in Chapter 7.

Reviewing a Prescription

The reason many people go to a community pharmacy is to fill a prescription. A **prescription** is defined as an order of medication for a patient, issued by a physician or a qualified licensed practitioner for a valid medical condition and then filled by a pharmacist. The prescription is usually recorded on a preprinted form bearing the name, address, and telephone and fax numbers of the prescriber. Patients may hand you the hard copy of a prescription, or prescribers may deliver the prescription to the pharmacy via phone, fax, or electronic transmission. As new technologies develop, the use of hard copy prescriptions is diminishing, with more prescriptions being delivered by electronic transmission, called *e-prescribing*. No

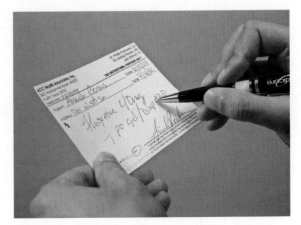

Reviewing a prescription for completeness and accuracy is an important responsibility of a pharmacy technician.

TABLE 6.2 Parts of a Prescription

Part	Description
Prescriber information	Name, address, telephone number, and other information identifying the prescriber; NPI and DEA numbers; and, sometimes, the state license number
Date	Date on which the prescription was written; this date may differ from the date on which the prescription was received
Patient information	Full name, address, telephone number, and date of birth of the patient
℞	Symbol ℞, from the Latin word *recipere* meaning "to take"
Inscription	Medication prescribed, including generic or brand name, strength, and amount
Subscription	Instructions to the pharmacist on dispensing the medication
Signa	Directions for the patient to follow (commonly called the sig)
Additional instructions	Any additional instructions that the prescriber deems necessary
Signature	Signature of the prescriber

matter what form a prescription takes, the pharmacy technician must be familiar with the basic components of a prescription in order to review the order for completeness (see Table 6.2).

Basic Components of a Prescription

Pharmacy technicians are responsible for checking each prescription for completeness and accuracy. (See Figure 6.2 for an example of a complete prescription.) The technician performs this review under the supervision of the pharmacist. In order to complete an accurate review, the technician must have an understanding of the components of a prescription and their individual purposes, as listed below:

- The **DEA number** is issued by the Drug Enforcement Administration (DEA) to a prescriber authorizing him or her to prescribe controlled substances. In most cases, for security reasons and to prevent forgeries, the DEA number of the prescribing physician may be handwritten rather than preprinted on the prescription form.
- The National Provider Identifier or **NPI number** is required to file a third-party insurance claim on all noncontrolled prescriptions as well as other reimbursable healthcare services. Any healthcare provider, including a pharmacist, may be assigned an NPI number.
- The patient's name should be given in full, including first and last names. Initials alone are not acceptable. If the writing is illegible, then the technician should rewrite the patient's name in full above the name on the prescription and verify the spelling of the patient's name at the time the prescription is received.
- The patient's address and telephone number are needed for patient records. Requesting the telephone number aids patient identification and minimizes dispensing errors. Asking for a secondary phone number (cell or business) is helpful if additional information is needed from the patient. If this information is missing, then the pharmacy technician should request it from the patient and add it to the prescription or patient profile.

FIGURE 6.2
A Complete Prescription

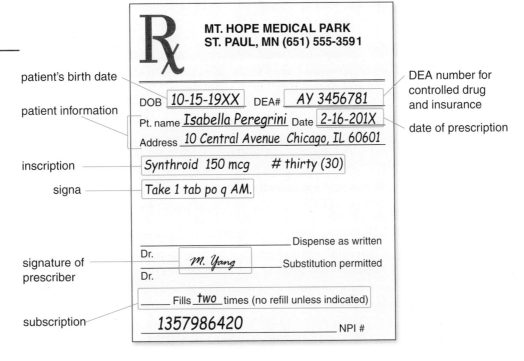

patient's birth date

DEA number for controlled drug and insurance

patient information

date of prescription

R℞ MT. HOPE MEDICAL PARK
ST. PAUL, MN (651) 555-3591

DOB _10-15-19XX_ DEA# _AY 3456781_

Pt. name _Isabella Peregrini_ Date _2-16-201X_

Address _10 Central Avenue Chicago, IL 60601_

inscription —— _Synthroid 150 mcg   # thirty (30)_

signa —— _Take 1 tab po q AM._

_____ Dispense as written

signature of prescriber

Dr. _M. Yang_ ____ Substitution permitted

Dr.

subscription

_____ Fills _two_ times (no refill unless indicated)

_1357986420_ _____ NPI #

- Preprinted prescriptions often contain a space for the patient's birth date. If this space is not filled in, then the technician should request this information. The patient's birth date is necessary for third-party billing and for correct identification among patients having the same name. Knowing the patient's age also helps the pharmacist evaluate the appropriateness of the drug, its quantity, and the dosage form prescribed, thus minimizing medication errors.

- The date the physician wrote the prescription should be provided. For pharmacy records, the date when the prescription is received should be typed into the computerized patient profile as well, if different from the current date. If no date is written on the prescription, then the date the prescription is brought into the pharmacy should be recorded and noted as such. If the undated prescription is for an antibiotic, then the pharmacist may wish to verify that the patient is under the current care of a physician. The need for an antibiotic may no longer be necessary and, in fact, could be harmful. The date on a prescription holds special importance for controlled substances (see the section titled "Controlled Substances" later in this chapter).

- The **inscription** is the part of the prescription that lists the medication prescribed, including the strength and amount. A medication may be listed on a prescription using a brand or generic name. As discussed in Chapter 3, a given drug (i.e., one with a particular generic name) may be marketed under various brand names. For example, Prinivil and Zestril are two brand names under which the generic drug lisinopril is marketed by pharmaceutical companies. Generic drugs are often less expensive than brand name drugs and are often automatically substituted for brand name drugs in the pharmacy software, under regulations now existing in every state. If the prescription for a brand name drug is filled with a generic equivalent, then the name, strength, and manufacturer of the generic substitution may be included on the dispensed medication container label.

- The **subscription** is the part of the prescription that lists the instructions to the pharmacist about dispensing the medication, including compounding instructions, labeling instructions, refill information, and information about the appropriateness of dispensing drug equivalents.

Safety Note

Amounts on prescriptions should be written out to prevent alterations.

- A **refill** is an approval by the prescriber to dispense the medication again without requiring a new order. If the refill section on the prescription is left blank, then the prescription cannot be refilled. The words *no refill* (sometime abbreviated NR) will appear on the medication container label, and *no refill* will be entered into the patient's record. Even if the refill blank on the prescription indicates *as needed*, or *prn*, unlimited duration is not allowed. Most pharmacies and state laws require at least yearly updates on *prn*, or as needed, prescriptions.

- Regulations in a given state may require two signature lines at the bottom of the prescription: one stating *dispense as written* and the other stating *substitution permitted*. If the **dispense as written (DAW)** line is signed, then substitution of a generic equivalent is not permitted. Other states may require only one signature line; **brand name medically necessary**, which is sometimes shortened to *brand necessary*, must be designated on the prescription if a prescriber wishes that only the brand name product be dispensed. At times, a patient may request a brand name to be dispensed in lieu of a generic drug. This request is abbreviated as *DAW2* and often results in an increased patient co-pay.

- The **signa** (or *sig* for short) is the part of the prescription that communicates the directions for use. This information is transferred from the prescription onto the label that is placed on the medication container for patient use.

- The signature of each local physician in black ink should be recognizable by both the pharmacy technician and pharmacist to detect possible forged prescriptions. An electronic signature may be utilized on a faxed prescription for all medications except for controlled substances.

Authenticity of a Prescription

Safety Note

Show all prescriptions with questionable authenticity or illegible handwriting to the pharmacist.

If there are any doubts about the authenticity or completeness of a prescription, the pharmacy technician should alert the pharmacist immediately. A telephone call from the pharmacy technician or the pharmacist to the prescriber's office might be necessary to clarify an order. The technician is allowed to clarify a prescription in some states, but all changes should be documented on the prescription (and/or in the patient profile), including the name of the nurse who clarified the prescription, and initialed by the technician or pharmacist.

Types of Prescriptions

A new prescription arrives in the pharmacy as a written hard copy from the patient, a verbal order reduced to writing by a pharmacist, an electronic prescription (or e-prescription), a telephone or fax order from a prescriber, a prescription not yet due, or a transfer prescription from another pharmacy. In addition to newly written prescriptions, the community pharmacy also receives refill requests from the patient, partial fills, emergency fills with prescriptions having no refills by the pharmacist, and transfer prescriptions to another pharmacy. These prescriptions—as well as handling new and refill prescriptions for controlled substances—deserve special attention.

Written Rx

A written prescription is a preprinted form that contains the name, address, and telephone number of the prescriber; information about the patient; the date; and the

FIGURE 6.3
**Humalog
Prescription**

The prescription
should contain all
necessary informa-
tion for the techni-
cian and pharmacist
to accurately fill the
prescription.

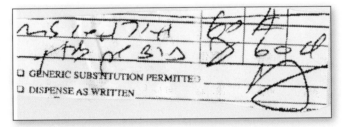

R

Simona Brushfield, MD
2222 IH-35 South
Austin, TX 78703
(512) 555-1212   fax: (512) 555-1313

DOB _Sept 12, 1953_ DEA# _____

Pt. name _Miguel Esparza_ Date _01/15/2015_

Address _7583 E 11Th St_

Austin, TX 78705

Humalog
100 units/mL vial
1 vial
12 units sub Q qAM;
18 units sub Q qPM pc

Refill _PRN_ times (no refill unless indicated)

Simona Brushfield, MD MD

_____ License #

FIGURE 6.4
**Hard-to-Read
Prescription**

This prescription
is for morphine
sulfate (MS)
60 mg, but it
is unclear if the
prescriber is
ordering MS ER
(extended release)
or MS IR (imme-
diate release). A
follow-up call to
the physician's
office is necessary.

❑ GENERIC SUBSTITUTION PERMITTED
❑ DISPENSE AS WRITTEN

medication(s) prescribed. This type of prescription is typically dropped off at the pharmacy counter or at the drive-thru window.

Upon review of a written prescription, the technician most likely will see abbreviations used by the prescriber in the subscription (see Figure 6.3). In order to read and interpret the medication order, the pharmacy technician should be familiar with common prescription abbreviations, as shown in Table 6.3 on the following page. (A more complete listing of abbreviations can be found in Appendix C.) This knowledge is critical in pharmacy practice, for any misinterpretation of pre-scription abbreviations could result in a serious medication error from the wrong drug, wrong dose, or wrong directions.

If the prescription is handwritten by the pre-scriber, then the combina-tion of the use of abbrevia-tions and the handwriting style might make the prescription difficult to read. Figure 6.4 shows an example of a hard-to-read prescrip-tion. If any part of the prescription is unclear or undecipherable, then the technician must check with the pharmacist prior to beginning the prescription-filling process. If the pharmacist is unclear on a component of the prescription, the technician should call the prescriber's office for clarification; the name of the nurse along with the clarification should be entered onto the hard copy of the prescription and into the computerized patient profile.

Medicaid Prescriptions and TRPPs Written prescriptions for Medicaid patients have distinct requirements. The Centers for Medicare and Medicaid Services (CMS), in cooperation with each state board of pharmacy, now require that all prescriptions for Medicaid patients be written on a tamper-resistant prescription pad. A **tamper-resistant prescription pad (TRPP)** is a paper pad that is specifically designed to prevent copying, erasure, or alteration. A prescription written on a TRPP will be noted on the back of the original prescription. If a prescription for a Medicaid patient is not written on a TRPP, then pharmacy personnel must contact the prescriber's office to authenticate the order. After verification of the prescription, the date, time, nurse's name, and initials of the pharmacist or technician must be documented on the back

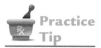**Practice Tip**

To access the ISMP's List of Error-Prone Abbreviations, Symbols, and Dose Designations, pharmacy technicians should visit www .paradigmcollege .net/pharmprac tice5e/ISMP.

TABLE 6.3   Common Prescription Abbreviations

Category	Abbreviation	Meaning
Amount	cc *	cubic centimeter (mL)
	g	gram
	gr	grain
	gtt	drop
	mg	milligram
	mL	milliliter
	qs	a sufficient quantity
	tbsp	tablespoonful
	tsp	teaspoonful
Dosage form	cap	capsule
	MDI	metered-dose inhaler
	sol	solution
	supp	suppository
	susp	suspension
	tab	tablet
	ung	ointment
Time of administration	ac	before meals
	am	morning, before noon
	bid	twice a day
	hs *	at bedtime
	pc	after meals
	pm	evening, after noon
	prn	as needed
	q6 h	every 6 hours
	qid	four times a day
	tid	three times a day
	tiw	three times a week
Site of administration	ad *	right ear
	as *	left ear
	au *	each ear
	od *	right eye
	os *	left eye
	ou *	each eye
	po	oral, by mouth
	pr	per rectum
	sl	sublingual (under the tongue)
	top	topical (skin)
	vag	vaginally

*These abbreviations, although commonly utilized by practitioners, are easily misread. Consequently, the abbreviations have been designated as dangerous by the Institute for Safe Medication Practices (ISMP).

of the prescription along with the word "verified." Awareness of this pharmacy practice is critical. If a pharmacy audit reveals prescriptions for Medicaid patients that are not written on TRPP or authenticated by pharmacy personnel, claims for reimbursement may be denied.

Computer Entry of Written Prescriptions When entering written prescriptions into the computerized patient profile, the pharmacy technician must exercise diligent care and effort during the transcription. It is critical that the correct patient be selected, for many patients have the same or similar names. To avoid any confusion, the technician should verify with all patients their date of birth and/or address. Many drugs also have similar names, and the incorrect drug or dose can be easily chosen from the drop-down menus in the computer database. Any subscription comments written on the prescription by the prescriber *must* be included on the medication label. For example, a narcotic prescription may include any of the following instructions: "may cause sedation," "do not fill until XX date," or "refill no sooner than every 30 days." Likewise, a prescription for an antibiotic may include the following directions: "take for 10 days" or "take with food." All of these instructions must appear on the medication container label.

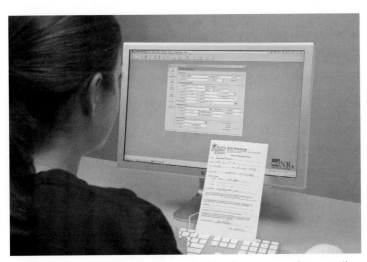

An important responsibility of the technician is to accurately transcribe the hard copy prescription into the computer database.

e-Prescriptions

Pharmacy personnel are seeing an increase in e-prescriptions as health information technology is being embraced by medical practitioners (see Figure 6.5 on the following page). **E-prescriptions**, or electronic prescriptions, are prescriptions that are transmitted electronically from prescribers to pharmacies, typically via examination room personal computers or by personal digital assistants (PDAs). This form of prescription, approved by all state boards, is gaining in popularity due to financial incentives offered by the federal government as well as the advantages this system provides in ensuring safe and effective patient care. This growth can be seen in the following statistic: In 2011, more than 570 million prescriptions were written; more than one-third of those prescriptions were e-prescriptions. This statistic reflects a 75% increase in e-prescribing from the previous year, a trend that will continue in the coming years. In fact, the projected cost savings of e-prescriptions over the next 10 years is estimated to be as high as $240 billion in improved health outcomes.

Many e-prescribing software systems are available to prescribers, including Surescripts—a system that connects prescribers with pharmacies and insurance providers. More than 60,000 community pharmacies (95%) can now receive e-prescriptions from medical offices that utilize Surescripts.

FIGURE 6.5
e-Prescription

An e-prescription greatly minimizes transcription errors, thus improving the safety and accuracy of processing prescriptions.

```
-------------------------------------------------------------------
!!! -- START SECURED ELECTRONIC PRESCRIPTION TRANSMISSION -- !!!
-------------------------------------------------------------------
FROM THE OFFICES OF PHIL JACKSON, MD; ETHEL JACOBSON, MD;
                     PETER JARKOWSKI, PA; EUGENE JOHNSON, DO

OFFICE ADDRESS:           67 EAST ELM
                          CEDAR RAPIDS, IA 52411
OFFICE TELEPHONE:         (319) 555-1212   TRANSMIT DATE: FEB 20, 2015
OFFICE FAX:               (319) 555-1313   WRITTEN DATE:  FEB 20, 2015
-------------------------------------------------------------------
TRANSMITTED TO            THE CORNER DRUG STORE
PHARMACY ADDRESS:         875 PARADIGM WAY
                          CEDAR RAPIDS, IA 52410
PHARMACY TELEPHONE:       (319) 555-1414
-------------------------------------------------------------------
PATIENT NAME:             JEFFREY KLEIN      D.O.B.: OCT 18, 1979
PATIENT ADDRESS:          1157 NORTH PLAZA AVE
                          CEDAR RAPIDS, IA 52411
-------------------------------------------------------------------
PRESCRIBED MEDICATION:    FLUOXETINE 20 MG
SIGNA:                    i PO QD
DISPENSE QUANTITY:        30
REFILL(S):                PRN
-------------------------------------------------------------------
PHYSICIAN SIGNATURE:      [[ ELECTRONIC SIGNATURE ON FILE ]]
                          [[ FOR DR. ETHEL JACOBSON ]]
-------------------------------------------------------------------
!!! -- END SECURED ELECTRONIC PRESCRIPTION TRANSMISSION -- !!!
-------------------------------------------------------------------
```

Advantages of e-Prescriptions For prescribers and pharmacy personnel, the advantages of e-prescribing are speed, accuracy, improved billing, and decreased potential for prescription forgeries and medication errors. In addition, e-prescribing minimizes the risk of potential medication errors due to a prescriber's handwriting, misinterpretation of abbreviations, and illegible faxes. E-prescribing also offers a variety of optional applications that benefit healthcare personnel, including: (1) e-refills automatically sent from the pharmacy to the prescriber; (2) prescriber access to patient pharmacy databases of community pharmacies and insurance providers; and (3) access to insurance eligibility and preferred drug lists of each insurance provider. These applications reduce the risk of drug interactions and adverse drug reactions as well as the time spent on getting approvals for prior authorizations on nonformulary drugs.

For patients, e-prescribing offers several advantages as well, including increased accuracy and decreased wait times. In fact, because e-prescriptions are forwarded from the prescriber's office directly to the pharmacy, the prescriptions are typically filled and ready to be dispensed to patients upon their arrival at the pharmacy. Another benefit of e-prescriptions is improved patient compliance. In 2011, Surescripts partnered with pharmacy benefits managers and retail pharmacies and reviewed more than 40 million prescription records to compare the effectiveness of e-prescriptions and paper prescriptions on first-fill medication adherence, or new prescriptions filled and picked up by the patient. Their findings revealed that first-fill medication adherence on e-prescriptions improved by 10% over traditional written, verbal, and faxed prescriptions.

e-Prescribing and Controlled Substances Although e-prescribing is gaining momentum, pharmacy technicians need to be aware that, at present, most states are requiring that prescriptions for Schedule II controlled substances must remain as hard copy or print documents with a signature from a prescriber licensed with the

DEA. Electronic prescribing of controlled substances (EPCS) must be approved by each state board of pharmacy before it can be implemented.

Telephone/Fax Orders

Other types of prescriptions that are commonly used by prescribers are telephone and fax orders. These prescriptions may be received by pharmacy technicians but must always be referred to a pharmacist for processing. Once the pharmacist transcribes the order into a written prescription and verifies its accuracy, the technician can enter the information into the computerized patient profile, as with a new prescription. The prescription is then verified a second time by the pharmacist after technician order entry.

Medical offices that are not yet equipped to send e-prescribed medication orders to the pharmacy may elect to fax new (or refill) medication orders to a dedicated fax line in the pharmacy. Some software in pharmacies automatically sends a request to the prescriber for a new prescription if the patient has no remaining refills on the requested medication. Fax orders contain all the necessary patient demographic, prescriber, and medication information to fill the prescription. Faxed orders are entered into the patient profile and verified by the pharmacist before being filled. At times, the medical office may deny the faxed refill request or require that the patient make an appointment before additional refills are authorized. Schedule II prescriptions cannot be faxed and require a hard copy and signature from an authorized prescriber registered with the DEA.

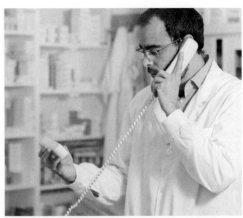

In most states, only the pharmacist may take verbal prescriptions over the telephone.

Prescriptions Not Yet Due

Often a patient may present a new written prescription, or the pharmacy may receive a verbal, faxed, or electronic prescription that does not have to be (or cannot be) filled until a future date. This type of prescription is referred to as a "prescription not yet due" and may be on hold for a variety of reasons. For example, the patient may have sufficient medication at home, especially if the dose was changed, and doesn't need to have the prescription filled just yet. Or the prescription is being held because the patient may not have the cash on hand to pay for all prescribed medications. A prescription may also not be filled due to lack of insurance coverage until a future date. In these situations, the prescription is typically held or stored in an alphabetized file box or in the computerized patient profile for easy retrieval at a later date.

Pharmacy technicians should follow their pharmacy's protocol regarding prescriptions not yet due. With the exception of controlled drugs, prescriptions are valid to be filled from one year of the original date written. Most state boards of pharmacy—as well as the policy and procedure manuals of individual pharmacies—do not permit the storage of Schedule II prescriptions for future use, and these medications must be returned to the patient.

Transfers In

At the patient's request, most prescriptions can be legally transferred between pharmacies. A "transfer" pharmacy may call the "originating" pharmacy that filled (or holds) an original prescription to copy or transfer all relevant information (including any remaining refills on the prescription) to the transfer pharmacy. This type of prescription is referred to as a "transfer in." This process is easier if the patient presents to the transfer pharmacy the medication vial containing the name of the medication, the dosage, the prescription number, and the pharmacy's name and telephone number. However, the transfer can also be made if the patient supplies the following information to the transfer pharmacy: his or her name and birth date, the name and phone number of the originating pharmacy, and the name of the medication to be transferred. Figure 6.6 shows an example of a form used to document information that must be received for each transfer prescription.

FIGURE 6.6
Information Needed for a Transfer Prescription

The Corner Drug Store   **Transferred Rx**   Copy from Competitor

Patient Name _____ Date _____

Address _____

Phone Number _____ Birth Date _____

Allergies/Health Conditions _____ Hold ☐ DAW ☐

Pharmacy Phone # _____ Pharmacy _____

RPh _____

Rx # _____

Last Fill _____

Original Date _____

Remaining Refills _____

Prescriber _____

Prescriber Phone # _____

MD DEA _____ Pharmacist initials _____

Pharmacy DEA (if controlled substance) _____

Processing of Transfers In Pharmacies provide prescription transfers as a service to patients, but careful documentation is required. Common reasons for a transfer may be cost, insurance coverage, and customer service issues, including the pharmacy's hours of operation or the convenience of the pharmacy's location. According to the law in most states, only a licensed pharmacist can transfer or copy a prescription from (or to) another pharmacy. In states that do not allow pharmacy technicians to receive these orders, the pharmacist must talk to a pharmacist at the originating pharmacy. The originating pharmacy must "close" the prescription to any remaining refills once it is transferred out to another pharmacy. Pharmacy personnel should be aware that there are limits on transfers of controlled drugs.

The processing of transfer prescriptions requires additional time to make a telephone call, initiate a hard copy prescription after talking to a pharmacist, and enter the prescription into the patient profile. If the prescription is for a new patient, then more time is needed to get necessary demographic, allergy, and health and insurance information to complete the patient profile. The technician should resolve any difficulty reading or interpreting the pharmacist's transcribing prior to entry into the patient profile to minimize medication errors. If a transfer prescription has no remaining refills (or the date is beyond one year or, in some cases, six months), then the physician's office must be called to request a new prescription before it can be filled by the transferring pharmacy.

Refill Requests

Pharmacy technicians often receive a telephone call or personal request from a patient at the pharmacy to refill a medication. These refill requests are relatively easy to process if the patient has the prescription container and can tell you the prescription number that is on the label. Most pharmacy software has the capability to record automatic refills when their time is due. Unlike new prescriptions, the prescription information for refills has already been previously entered (and verified by the pharmacist) into the computerized patient profile. Consequently, the process for filling a refill request requires less computer entry and verification, thus shortening the wait time for dispensing to the patient.

The role of the pharmacy technician in handling a refill request is to verify that a refill does indeed exist for the requested medication and, if so, to forward the request for pharmacist review and approval. Most pharmacies and insurance plans allow medications to be refilled approximately five days prior to the next refill date.

Early Refills If a refill request is made too early (or more than five days before the refill date), then the request will be rejected by third-party insurance. For example, suppose a patient requests a refill of Motrin 600 mg #90 with the sig: 1 tab tid prn; this prescription represents a 30-day supply of this drug. The patient's profile indicates the prescription was filled on April 1. Because this is a 30-day supply, the refill is due May 1, which means that the technician can initiate the refill request on or after April 25. Each pharmacy and insurance provider has its own policy defining the procedure for handling early refills, especially for controlled substances. Pharmacy technicians should explain the early refill policy of their facility to patients, if asked.

At times, a patient may ask pharmacy personnel for an early refill of a medication due to special circumstances, such as an upcoming vacation or a lost prescription. Insurance companies often will not pay for an early refill automatically. In response to that patient request, the pharmacy technician may offer to call the insurance provider and get approval for a "one time" early refill. If prior approval is not granted by the insurance provider, the patient may need to pay for the prescription and send in the receipt for possible reimbursement at a later date.

No Refills Under certain circumstances, no refills are permitted—despite what the medication label indicates. Prescriptions that fall under this restriction include:

- a prescription that is more than 12 months old
- a prescription for a controlled drug (Schedules III–IV) that was written more than six months ago or refilled five times
- a prescription for a controlled drug that has been previously transferred to another pharmacy

Pharmacy personnel should also understand that all prescriptions written in the emergency room (ER) for antibiotics or other medications are commonly prescribed for short-term use with no refills. In most cases, the ER prescriber will not authorize refills. Pharmacy technicians should communicate this protocol to patients and instruct them to contact their primary care physicians about their prescriptions.

Partial Fills

At times, the pharmacy may have insufficient drug inventory to fill or refill a prescription for the required quantity. In those instances, the pharmacy will dispense a **partial fill**, or a two- to five-day supply of medication to hold over the patient until new drug inventory is received. For example, a patient may give a prescription to the technician for Gabapentin 300 mg po tid #270, which is a three-month or 90-day supply, but the technician discovers that the pharmacy inventory only has stock bottles containing 150 capsules. Common practice is to issue a five-day supply of medication (in this case, 15 capsules) and order the remaining medication for the next business day. The five-day supply hopefully will not inconvenience the patient and cover weekends and holidays. The remaining 135 capsules in inventory can be used for other patients' prescriptions for Gabapentin received later that day. The patient is typically billed only for the amount of drug dispensed. The technician must alert the patient to the partial fill and let them know when the remainder of the prescription can be picked up.

Emergency Fills

An emergency fill is a short-term emergency supply of needed medication for chronic conditions such as high blood pressure, diabetes, high cholesterol, or epilepsy. Patients with these conditions typically have prescriptions with limited refills, which require them to schedule follow-up visits with their primary care physicians for monitoring and blood work. At times, the patient may ask for an emergency refill to bridge the gap when refill authorization is not feasible, such as at night or on weekends. Most states allow pharmacists to use their best professional judgment to provide a short-term emergency supply (usually two to three days) of medication.

Typically, there is no patient charge for a temporary emergency fill of needed medication for a chronic disease. When the prescription is renewed by the prescriber, the amount of medication "loaned" to the patient is commonly subtracted from the refill. For example, if three tablets of amlodipine 10 mg are loaned and a new prescription is received the next day for #90, then 87 tablets will be dispensed, but 90 tablets will be billed to insurance. Emergency fills of controlled drugs are seldom permitted except under extremely unusual circumstances, as discussed later in this chapter.

Transfers Out

A "transfer out" is a prescription refill in which pharmacy personnel, at the request of a patient, contact another pharmacy to transfer a prescription. Typically, this patient request may stem from convenience (such as the patient running errands near another pharmacy location) or from circumstances (such as the patient being out of town on business or vacation).

When the pharmacy technician receives such a request, he or she must notify the pharmacist so that the appropriate medication information and refills are communicated to the "transfer" pharmacy. The pharmacist must then verify that refills are indicated and that the prescription is eligible for transfer. Controlled prescription drugs cannot be refilled "early" and can only be transferred one time. The pharmacist must "close" the prescription once the transfer of information to another pharmacy is complete. If the medication was already filled at your pharmacy, but not yet dispensed to the patient, then it must be retrieved from the storage bins and returned to inventory. The medication charges must then be reversed with the insurance provider.

Many chain community pharmacies have a shared database of patient profiles. For example, a Walgreens pharmacy in Alabama can access the profile of the originating Walgreens pharmacy in Georgia and fill the prescription. The transfer can occur without the need of a telephone call and verification of patient and medication information. The pharmacy in Alabama would typically send an electronic message to the pharmacy in Georgia to notify personnel of the transfer.

Controlled Substances

As discussed earlier, a prescription for a controlled substance (Schedule II–V) requires additional care because of the potential for a patient to intentionally or unintentionally abuse the drug. Many of these drugs have a high likelihood of tolerance or physical or psychological dependence, as discussed in Chapter 3. Because the role of the pharmacy profession is to safeguard public health, the pharmacy technician and the pharmacist must carefully review, assess, and monitor the legitimate use of all new and refilled scheduled substances.

A controlled drug can only be dispensed upon receipt of a valid prescription written for a valid medical condition. The date of the original prescription on all controlled drugs should be entered into the profile, rather than the date the prescription was filled. Federal law requires a name and physical address (not a post office box) on all prescriptions for controlled substances.

Safety Note

Pharmacy technicians must be thoroughly familiar with regulations concerning scheduled substances for the state in which they practice.

Schedule II Prescription Requirements Prescriptions for Schedule II controlled substances should be handwritten or typed, and they cannot be e-prescribed, faxed, or phoned in to the pharmacy. Most states do allow a nurse, nurse practitioner, or physician's assistant to write a prescription for a Schedule II medication, but it must be signed by the physician. Signatures on all Schedule II prescriptions should be handwritten in black ink; a stamped or electronic signature is not acceptable. The drug, dose, and quantity of a prescription for a Schedule II drug cannot be altered in any way by the physician, nurse, pharmacist, or technician and can never be refilled. A new prescription is required each time it is dispensed. If in doubt, the pharmacy technician should call the prescriber to verify the authenticity of the prescription.

State laws or regulations may control the time period for initially filling a Schedule II prescription. In some states, a Schedule II prescription must be filled within seven days of issue; in other states, it must be filled within 72 hours. Other states may have no time frame, but a six-month maximum would be consistent with other regulations on C–III and C–IV drugs. There may also be limits on the quantity of a controlled drug that may be dispensed. In some states, the limit may be 120 units (tablets or capsules) or a 30-day supply, whichever is less. Many pharmacies have a policy of dispensing only a 30-day supply of a controlled substance. Insurance company policies may limit the supply as well.

Refills for Controlled Substances Pharmacy technicians must be aware that refills for controlled drugs depend on their schedules.

Safety Note

Schedule II drugs cannot be refilled but require a new prescription.

Schedule II Refills There are no refills on a Schedule II medication. At times, the patient may request a "partial fill" of such a prescription due to cost or insufficient inventory at the community pharmacy. If it is a legitimate prescription, a partial fill can be approved, but the remainder of the prescription is voided. In other words, if a prescription for Ritalin LA 20 mg #60 is presented to the pharmacy, but only 30 tablets are in stock, the prescription could be filled but the remaining 30 tablets could

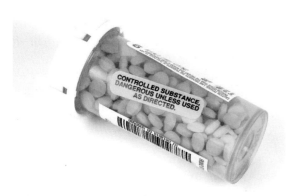

Pharmacy technicians must be aware that refills for controlled substances depend on their schedules.

not be filled at a later date. A new prescription would be required. In such situations, often the patient will take the hard copy prescription to another pharmacy that can completely fill the quantity of medication prescribed.

The safeguard of not allowing the refill of Schedule II drugs frequently causes an inconvenience to a parent whose child may be treated with a Schedule II drug for attention-deficit hyperactivity disorder, commonly known as ADHD. In many states, a prescriber is permitted to write two additional future-dated prescriptions for such medications for a patient, or the patient's representative, to hold until needed. It is illegal in most states for pharmacies to store or "hold" future prescriptions of Schedule II drugs, so it must be retained by the patient (or parent).

Schedule III and IV Refills A prescription for a Schedule III or IV drug (see Figure 6.7) may be refilled up to five times if allowed by the physician, but these refills must occur within a six-month period, after which time a new prescription is required. Pharmacy personnel should be aware that the six-month time frame starts with the date the prescription was written, not with the date it was filled. The five refills may include both completely and partially filled prescriptions. Pharmacy technicians who are unsure as to whether a prescription (or refill) is for a controlled drug should check the medication stock bottles on the shelf (or the medication container label) for a C–III or C–IV designation.

Early refill requests by patients for Schedule III or IV drugs must be carefully monitored by the pharmacy technician. If refills are indicated for a controlled drug, then prescriptions are typically refilled no sooner than one or two days before the customer's supply is scheduled to run out (although this is not a hard-and-fast rule). If the request for refill is too early for a controlled medication such as pain or nerve medications, then it may be rejected by the pharmacist and/or insurance. Each pharmacy has a policy defining the procedure for handling early refills of Schedule III and IV controlled substances.

Generally, by federal and state law, refills for prescriptions of controlled medications can only be transferred to another pharmacy one time. Careful attention must be given to the transfer and documentation of Schedule III and IV prescriptions. If a controlled substance is transferred between pharmacies, then the DEA numbers of both the

FIGURE 6.7
Controlled-Substance Prescription

Lorazepam is a C–IV drug that is prescribed with a maximum of five refills. A prescriber DEA number must be on the Rx or on file at the pharmacy.

R͟x

Sunjita Patel, MD
7612 N. HWY 27
Cedar Rapids, IA 52404
(319) 555-1212   fax: (319) 555-1313

DOB _Aug 24, 1949_ DEA# _AP4756687_

Pt. name_Amala Gupta_ Date _02/16/2015_

Address _5473 W 70th Street_
Cedar Rapids, IA 52401

Lorazepam
_0.5 mg_
120 (one hundred twenty)
i po q 4-6 h prn anxiety

Refill _5_ times (no refill unless indicated)

_Sunjita Patel, MD_____ MD
_____ License #

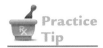

Practice Tip

By law, refills for Schedule III and IV drugs must occur within a six-month period. That period begins on the date that the prescription was *written*, not the date that the prescription was filled.

originating and receiving (or transfer) pharmacy must be exchanged and reduced to writing on the prescription form or in the computerized pharmacy database.

If a Schedule III or IV prescription was filled and in the storage bin at the originating pharmacy, then the technician may be directed by the pharmacist to reverse the charge (or credit to insurance, if covered) via online billing and to remove the medication from the storage bin and place the unused medication back into inventory. This prevents patients from transferring narcotics to one pharmacy but returning to the original pharmacy to pick up the original prescription before the drug is taken out of storage.

Schedule V Refills A prescription for a Schedule V controlled substance (required in some states) may be refilled only if authorized by a prescribing physician. Some states allow patients to purchase a limited supply of a Schedule V medication without a prescription (see Chapter 7 for further discussion). Most Schedule V medications contain codeine in a cough syrup formulation. Due to their abuse potential, some state boards of pharmacy have reclassified codeine-containing cough syrups to Schedule III.

Emergency Dispensing A Schedule II medication is rarely dispensed without an authorized prescription. Occasions may arise in which the usual and customary procedures for filling and dispensing a Schedule II drug will result in the delay of a medication urgently needed by a patient. Pursuant to a valid medical reason, an emergency supply of a drug—known as emergency dispensing—can be provided to a patient in most but not all states. The prescriber may provide an oral or a faxed prescription. Again, the stricter of state versus federal regulations apply. An emergency procedure is described as follows:

- A controlled substance administration is to be immediate if the patient is to receive proper treatment.
- The pharmacist immediately converts a verbal order into writing.
- The pharmacist documents the need for the emergency dispensing of the Schedule II prescription by writing something similar to "authorization for emergency dispensing" on the front of the temporary prescription.
- If the pharmacist does not know the prescriber, then good faith efforts are made by the pharmacy to verify that the prescriber is authentic.
- Within seven days (72 hours in some states), the prescriber must deliver a written version of the emergency verbal order to the pharmacy.

Most state boards of pharmacy have made a provision for the emergency dispensing of a limited supply of pain-relieving narcotic medications for terminally ill hospice patients. In this situation, the pharmacist takes a verbal order from a prescriber or his/her representative, reduces the order to writing, indicates "hospice" on the prescription, records the name and DEA number of the prescriber, and fills the prescription. A follow-up hard copy may or may not be required under these special circumstances, depending on the regulations of that state.

Authentication A controlled substance prescription must be carefully reviewed by both the pharmacy technician and the pharmacist for authenticity because this type of prescription is more likely to be forged or altered by individuals who abuse drugs. Forgeries may be written on stolen or preprinted facsimiles of prescriptions and are often difficult to recognize, especially during a busy pharmacy workday. However, there are some telltale signs of possible forgeries that pharmacy technicians should recognize.

TABLE 6.4 Indicators of a Potentially Forged Prescription or Drug-Seeking Behavior

- The prescription is altered (for example, a change in quantity).
- Prescription pads have been reported missing from local doctors' offices.
- The prescription is presented as a clever computerized fax on non–tamper-proof safety paper.
- There are misspellings on the prescription.
- A refill is indicated for a Schedule II drug.
- A prescription from the emergency department is written for more than a #30 count or seven-day supply.
- A prescription is cut and pasted from a preprinted, signed prescription.
- A second or third prescription is added to a legal prescription written by a physician.
- A patient presents a prescription containing several medications but only wants the pharmacy to fill the narcotic prescription.
- The prescription is signed with different handwriting or in different ink, or the prescription is not signed by the physician.
- The DEA number is missing, illegible, or incorrect.
- The prescription is written by an out-of-state physician or a physician practicing in an area far from the pharmacy. This event is particularly suspicious if the prescription is received at night or on the weekend, when it would be difficult to confirm.
- An individual other than the patient drops off the prescription. Pharmacy personnel should require a photo ID such as a driver's license and document this information.
- A new patient specifies a brand name narcotic.
- A new patient wants to pay for the prescription with cash, even though he or she has insurance. Doing so avoids a paper trail.

These indicators are listed in Table 6.4. In addition to forged prescriptions, pharmacy personnel must also be alert to drug-seeking behaviors of patients in the pharmacy workplace. To address these deceptive practices, both pharmacy employees and prescribers must exercise vigilance as well as implement safeguards in their practice settings.

Preventive Measures in the Pharmacy Workplace Pharmacy technicians should learn to recognize the legal signatures of the local prescribers who send prescriptions to the pharmacy. Some physicians have their DEA number preprinted on their prescriptions, but others write it on the prescription when writing out a prescription order for a controlled substance medication. Most pharmacies have a computerized physician database containing DEA, NPI, state license number, and contact information. In fact, all insurance plans require a pharmacy to have a physician's DEA number on file to be reimbursed for prescriptions for all controlled medications. Pharmacy personnel can also check for a falsified DEA number by following the procedure listed in Table 6.5.

Technicians should exercise caution when another person (other than the patient or a family member) attempts to call in a refill or to pick up a prescription for a controlled substance. When in doubt, the technician should call the patient to relay the situation and to verify approval for medication pickup. Some pharmacies request a photo ID such as a driver's license in order to confirm information written on a received prescription, or for documenting those picking up controlled medications for someone else. If another individual picks up the prescription, pharmacy personnel may ask him or her to confirm the patient's address and/or date of birth.

TABLE 6.5 Steps for Checking a DEA Number

1. Add the first, third, and fifth digits of the DEA number.
2. Add the second, fourth, and sixth digits of the number, and multiply the sum by two.
3. Add the results of steps 1 and 2. The last digit of this sum should be the same as the last digit of the DEA number.
4. The second letter of the DEA number should be the same as the first letter of the physician's last name.

Pharmacy personnel should be on the alert for **drug seekers**, or patients who may receive prescriptions for the same or similar controlled drugs from several physicians or who constantly request "early refills." A drug seeker may be tolerant, psychologically dependent, or physically addicted to the medication or may be illegally selling the drugs. Many drug-seeking patients pay with cash to minimize computerized insurance tracking and use more than one pharmacy, physician, or dentist. Drug seekers are very skilled and often try to become "best buddies" with pharmacy technicians and pharmacists to gain their friendship and allay any concerns about drug abuse or diversion. If these individuals have been dispensed a narcotic and an antibiotic from an ER, they will often request that only the pain medication be filled. If a pharmacy technician suspects that a patient may have illegal intentions, he or she should seek the professional judgment of the pharmacist.

Caution must also be exercised when accepting prescriptions from out-of-state patients, especially at night or on weekends when the authenticity of the prescription cannot be proven. Some pharmacies only fill controlled substances for patients residing in their immediate geographical area and for prescribers who practice in the community.

If a forgery or drug-seeking behavior is suspected, pharmacy technicians should always alert the pharmacist. Follow-up actions should include retention of the prescription, detainment of the individual, and police notification. One way to detain the individual is by saying, "I will need to confirm some information with the doctor. Please give me a few minutes to fill your prescription." Another way that a technician can stall the filling of the prescription is by saying, "This prescription may take some time to fill. Can you come back in one hour?" Pharmacy personnel should always keep the name and phone number of the local agent from the state drug and narcotic agency on hand in case suspicious activity is observed in the pharmacy workplace.

Preventive Measures in the Medical Office Prescribers are encouraged to carry their prescription pads on them or to lock their prescription pads in the drawers of the examination rooms. These measures prevent patients and other healthcare personnel from accessing blank prescriptions for illegal use. Prescribers are also encouraged to write out quantities so that 12 tablets of a narcotic cannot be altered by adding a zero, thus creating 120.

In addition, many medical offices utilize some type of TRPP to eliminate forgeries. In Georgia, for example, the prescription for a Medicaid patient must meet one or more of the following requirements approved by the State Board of Pharmacy:

- gray security background; the word "VOID" appears when script is photocopied
- identifier production batch number in the margin on the front of the sheet
- consecutive number in the upper left-hand corner of the sheet
- erasure protection; white mark appears when erased with ink eraser

FIGURE 6.8
Coin-Activated Security Mark on a Prescription

Many states now require that all controlled drugs be written on tamper-resistant prescriptions to eliminate forgeries.

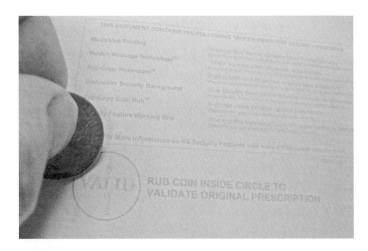

- security watermark on back of sheet; hold up to the light at a 45-degree angle to view (when duplicated, the artificial watermark is not visible on copy)
- coin-activated security on back of script; rub with coin to validate script (see Figure 6.8)

Preventive Measures Taken by State Boards of Pharmacy Many state boards of pharmacy have implemented a regional multi-state database to more effectively identify forgeries and drug seekers. Pharmacy personnel should also be aware that each state has its own requirements and definitions for a "tamper-resistant" prescription. Consequently, a prescription for a controlled substance that was written out of state will probably not meet in-state requirements and thus can only be filled in the state it was written.

Safety Note

A pharmacist has the right to refuse to fill a prescription for a controlled substance.

The Right of Refusal A pharmacist has the right to refuse to fill any controlled-substance prescription; this practice is known as *the right of refusal*. For example, it may not make sense to have a narcotic prescription for severe pain filled three months after the date it was written. If a legitimate concern exists that a prescription was not written in good faith, or not for a legitimate medical use, then the pharmacist's duty is to refuse to fill that prescription from the prescriber and return the prescription to the patient. Most pharmacists will make some sort of notation on the prescription to alert another pharmacist to a potential problem in filling the prescription. Many local pharmacies activate a "tree calling list" to alert other pharmacies of a potential problem prescription circulating in the community.

If there is concern that the patient is abusing a legal prescription or receiving controlled substances from more than one prescriber or more than one pharmacy, then the pharmacist should contact the prescriber. Even if the prescriber approves the order, the pharmacist can exercise the option to not fill the prescription. For example, if the prescriber orders an excessive amount of narcotic that could do harm to the patient, then the pharmacist may elect not to fill the prescription. However, if a diagnosis of cancer is known, or the patient is under care of a hospice team or oncologist (cancer physician), then use of high-dose narcotics for comfort and pain relief is medically necessary.

It is illegal for a physician to write a prescription for a Schedule II drug for a family member; it is considered unethical for a prescriber to write a Schedule III or IV prescription for a family member. Circumstances vary and it will be up to the professional judgment of the pharmacist to fill or refuse to fill such a prescription.

Processing a Prescription

The processing of prescriptions is a complex procedure with skills being gained only with experience in the community pharmacy. This process must be efficient but accurate and requires teamwork and communication from the pharmacy technician and pharmacist. In addition to correctly filling and dispensing the prescription, it is important that the patient understand how to appropriately take the medication from the labeled information and/or with additional counseling from the pharmacist.

No matter what type of prescription is ordered by a physician or qualified licensed practitioner, the prescription follows the same critical path once it crosses the threshold of a community pharmacy (see Table 6.6). A discussion of the details of each step

 Safety Note

Steps 6, 7, 10, 11, 13, and 14 in Table 6.6 should include verification that the proper product has been selected.

TABLE 6.6 The Critical Path of a New Prescription

1. After the patient drops off the prescription, the pharmacy technician checks the prescription to make certain it is legible, complete, and authentic.
2. The pharmacy technician verifies that the patient information is contained in the pharmacy database. If the patient is not in the pharmacy database, then the technician obtains necessary demographic, insurance, allergy, and health information from the patient and enters that information into the computer.
3. The pharmacy technician enters (types or scans) the prescription into the computer database from the written prescription, faxed prescription, or e-prescription, billing the insurance company or calculating the cost to the patient.
4. The pharmacist then verifies the accuracy of the technician's computerized entry against the original prescription (or a photocopied image) and generates the medication information sheet and then the medication container label.
5. The pharmacy technician asks the pharmacist to check the drug utilization review (DUR) or drug interaction warning screen when required.
6. The pharmacy technician selects the appropriate medication and verifies the National Drug Code (NDC) number on the stock drug bottle against the computer-generated medication information sheet. In some pharmacies, the bar codes on the stock bottle and medication container label are compared for accuracy.
7. The pharmacy technician prepares the medication (the prescribed number of tablets or capsules are counted or the prescribed amount of liquid measured). Controlled drugs are often double-counted and initialed.
8. The pharmacy technician packages the medication in the appropriate container.
9. The pharmacy technician (or the pharmacist, depending on state law) affixes the computer-generated medication label to the prescription container.
10. The pharmacy technician prepares the filled prescription (including original prescription, medication information sheet, stock drug bottle, medication container label, and medication container) for the pharmacist to make a final check.
11. The pharmacist checks the prescription and may initial the label and prescription.
12. The pharmacist "bags" the approved prescription(s) for patient sale and attaches the medication information sheet (and MedGuide, if required) about the prescription, including indications, interactions, and possible side effects.
13. The pharmacy technician returns the stock drug bottle to the shelf. If the bottle is opened, then the bottle is so marked or labeled for inventory ordering.
14. The pharmacist or pharmacy technician delivers the packaged prescription to the cash register area for patient pickup (or storage) and pharmacist counseling. The pharmacy technician verifies that the correct patient is receiving the prescription by asking for address or birth date verification. If someone other than the patient is picking up a controlled drug prescription, then a photo ID may be required.
15. If payment is due, then the patient pays by cash, credit card, or check. Some insurance providers require the patient to sign a form verifying that the prescription was picked up.

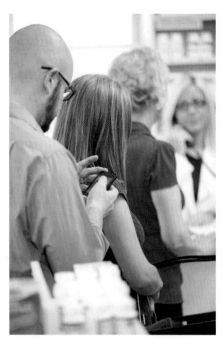

While no one likes to wait in line, the accurate and safe processing of a prescription is a priority.

in this critical pathway is important to the education of a pharmacy technician.

The prescription filling process, which begins with the receipt and review of the prescription and ends with the dispensing to the patient, takes about 5–10 minutes per prescription (without interruptions, such as phone calls, patients dropping off prescriptions, and so on). Most likely, there will be many interruptions during a pharmacy shift, so at times it may take 15–20 minutes to process a prescription. If there are insurance issues, a longer time delay can be expected. The pharmacy technician should ask the patient whether he or she prefers to wait for the prescription to be filled and, based on workload and staffing, should provide a good estimate for the waiting time should the patient elect to shop or run errands.

Some independent pharmacies have a computer dedicated for the pharmacist and one for the pharmacy technician. In chain pharmacies, both pharmacists and technicians may be working at one or more computers throughout the pharmacy during the shift. It is important that technicians "sign on" with their user names and passwords for each computer they will be working on; a pharmacist must do likewise. Technicians do not have the capability on their computers to provide a final check for any prescription or document a required consultation with the patient.

Most chain and mail-order pharmacies utilize a conveyor belt to improve the efficiency of processing a prescription. As each medication order is filled for each patient, the labeled medication, the original prescription (if available), and the medication information leaflet are placed in a plastic bin or tray and then onto a conveyor belt— like a mini-assembly line—for a final check by the pharmacist.

Pharmacy Laws and Protocol

Pharmacy technicians should check with their state board of pharmacy to review regulations for processing various types of prescriptions. Each state board of pharmacy defines what practices are allowable in their state. For example, in some states (South Carolina being one of them), certified pharmacy technicians may receive and take verbal prescriptions over the telephone as well as handle transfers in or out of the pharmacy. Other states may not allow technicians to perform these tasks.

State regulations also define dispensing policies. For example, a patient may request that a three-month supply of medication be filled in order to save on co-payments or to avoid the inconvenience of traveling to the pharmacy each month. If a prescriber writes a prescription for a three-month or 90-day supply and insurance approves the prescription, then the patient request can be granted. If, however, the prescriber writes a prescription for a 30-day supply with two refills, the pharmacy technician or pharmacist often must call the prescriber's office to get approval to fill a 90-day supply. If approval is not sought and documented, then some state boards of pharmacy consider this action the practice of medicine rather than pharmacy—and possible legal ramifications may ensue.

Technicians should also be aware of federal laws regarding patient counseling and confidentiality on prescriptions. The Health Insurance Portability and Accountability Act (HIPAA) of 1996 provides safeguards to protect patient privacy and medical records. (This act is discussed in greater detail in Chapter 13.) It is important that all pharmacy personnel understand the rules that govern patient privacy and the serious ramifications that can occur if patient confidentiality has been breached—including termination of employment.

Pharmacists are also mandated to follow all federal and state regulations when receiving prescriptions. However, under certain circumstances, pharmacists may elect not to fill a prescription based on religious or ethical convictions. For example, in some states, a pharmacist may refuse to fill (or sell) Plan B (the "morning after" pill), birth control pills, drugs used for abortion, or narcotics intended for assisted suicide. For legal reasons, any refusal to fill must be documented by the pharmacist. The pharmacist may also refuse to fill any narcotic prescription if he or she is not convinced of the legitimate medical use of the narcotic—even on a valid prescription. In those cases, the pharmacist expresses a concern to the patient or simply states that the pharmacy does not have the drug or quantity of drug in stock.

Special Processing of Certain Drugs Because of their potential for abuse or toxicity, certain drugs must be processed differently. These drugs include Accutane, Suboxone, and Tikosyn, among others. As mentioned in Chapter 3, these high-risk drugs require more communication and monitoring of patients. For example, Accutane is a prescription drug used for the treatment of severe acne, most likely in teenagers. It is also a Category X drug—that is, it is highly likely to cause birth defects. To dispense this medication, both the prescriber and the pharmacy must enroll in an iPLEDGE program. Female patients must undergo monthly pregnancy tests, and those who are sexually active must be on some form of birth control. Even males must be educated, as the risk of the drug passing to the female during sexual intercourse could cause birth defects. In addition, there are strict time limits on dispensing the drug to the patient due to careful monitoring and the need for frequent laboratory testing.

The Patient Profile

After initial review of the prescription, the processing of the order begins by accessing the patient profile. A **patient profile** is a confidential database that contains demographic information to track all prescriptions that have been dispensed at that pharmacy for that individual patient. Some chain pharmacies use a common database, allowing prescription information in the patient profile to be shared among all of their affiliated pharmacies nationwide. In many pharmacies, the hard copy prescription is scanned and recorded permanently into the patient profile. The original information from the written or scanned prescription may then be entered into a central database and be accessed at a pharmacy other than the one where the prescription was originally received. The patient may pick up the prescription at the receiving pharmacy rather than the originating pharmacy. This is extremely helpful for patients with medication needs who travel frequently or share residencies in two or more states.

Components of a Patient Profile Every patient who presents a prescription to the pharmacy must have a current updated profile (see Figure 6.9 on the following page). Components of the patient profile include patient demographics; insurance and billing information; medical, allergy, and prescription histories; and prescription preferences, such as no childproof caps, large-print medication sheets, foreign language specifications, and so on. (For an explanation of all of these components, see Table 6.7 on the following page.) The medication and prescription history section

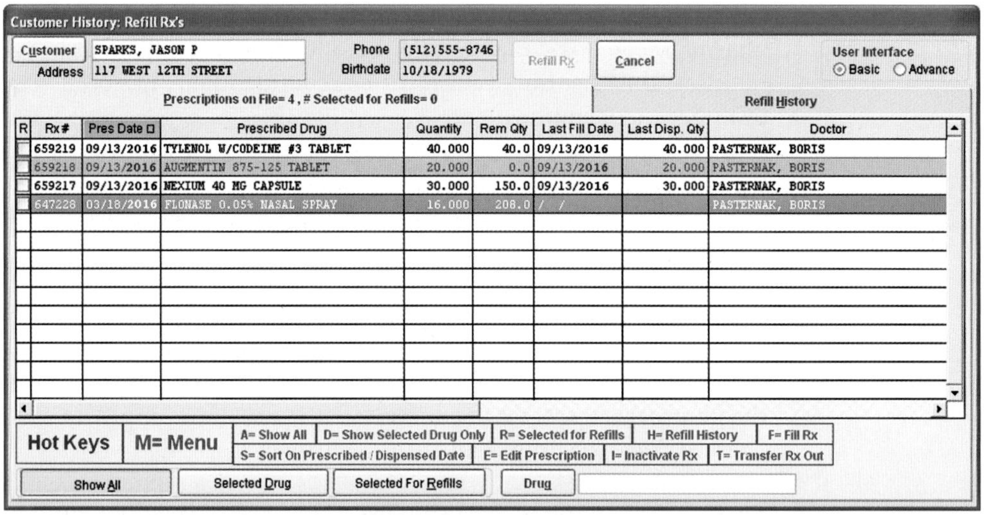

FIGURE 6.9
Computerized Patient Profile

A computerized profile is maintained for each patient receiving a prescription from the pharmacy. This profile is part of a confidential database that helps the pharmacist and pharmacy technician confirm that medications are dispensed safely.

Customer History: Refill Rx's

| Customer | SPARKS, JASON P | | Phone | (512) 555-8746 | | Refill Rx | Cancel | | | User Interface ⊙ Basic ○ Advance |
| Address | 117 WEST 12TH STREET | | Birthdate | 10/18/1979 | | | | | | |

Prescriptions on File= 4 , # Selected for Refills= 0   Refill History

R	Rx #	Pres Date □	Prescribed Drug	Quantity	Rem Qty	Last Fill Date	Last Disp. Qty	Doctor
☐	659219	09/13/2016	TYLENOL W/CODEINE #3 TABLET	40.000	40.0	09/13/2016	40.000	PASTERNAK, BORIS
☐	659218	09/13/2016	AUGMENTIN 875-125 TABLET	20.000	0.0	09/13/2016	20.000	PASTERNAK, BORIS
☐	659217	09/13/2016	NEXIUM 40 MG CAPSULE	30.000	150.0	09/13/2016	30.000	PASTERNAK, BORIS
☐	647228	03/18/2016	FLONASE 0.05% NASAL SPRAY	16.000	208.0	/ /		PASTERNAK, BORIS

Hot Keys **M= Menu**

| A= Show All | D= Show Selected Drug Only | R= Selected for Refills | H= Refill History | F= Fill Rx |
| S= Sort On Prescribed / Dispensed Date | E= Edit Prescription | I= Inactivate Rx | T= Transfer Rx Out |

| Show All | Selected Drug | Selected For Refills | Drug | |

TABLE 6.7 Components of the Patient Profile

Component	Content
Identifying information	Patient's full name (including middle initial in some cases), street address, telephone number, birth date, and gender. Increasingly, some programs are entering e-mail addresses so that refill notifications and other communications can be made.
Insurance and billing information	Information necessary for billing. More information on insurance billing is discussed in Chapter 7.
Medical and allergy history	Information concerning existing conditions (for example, diabetes or heart disease) and known allergies and adverse drug reactions the patient has experienced. (The pharmacy software reviews the medical history for the pharmacist to make sure that the prescription is safe to fill for a given patient.)
Medication and prescription history	Most databases allow the listing of any prescriptions filled at this pharmacy location; some software may allow listing of OTC medications. The new prescription will be compared with previously filled prescriptions in the database. (The pharmacy software reviews this information for the pharmacist to make sure that the prescription will not cause adverse drug interactions [i.e., negative consequences] because of the combined effects of drugs and/or drugs and foods.)
Prescription preferences	Patient preferences as they apply to prescriptions (for example, child-resistant or non–child-resistant containers, generic substitutions, large-print labels, foreign language preference, and so on).
HIPAA confidentiality	Each new patient is required by law to receive a statement on patient confidentiality of information on the patient profile, which must be documented. (This statement is for the protection of the pharmacy.)

contains the prescription number (automatically assigned), drug prescribed, dosage form, quantity, number of refills authorized (if any), prescriber name and identifiers, and patient cost or co-payment for the prescription. Drugs may be entered by brand or generic name, but the software will commonly default to the lower cost generic name. All information entered into the patient profile by the pharmacy technician must be verified by the pharmacist before the prescription can be filled.

A major part of the pharmacy technician's job is maintaining a profile for each patient receiving prescription medications from the pharmacy and updating this profile as necessary. The procedure for managing a patient profile varies, depending on whether the patient is a current customer or a new customer.

Patient Profile for Current Customer If a patient profile already exists, then it is important for the pharmacy technician to verify that the correct one is selected. The technician must match the patient name with the correct address. This step is critical, for more than one patient may have the same name (Bob Smith) or a similar name (Michael vs. Michelle Courier) or may have more than one address listed in the patient profile. Also, the technician needs to be careful when searching for hyphenated names in the database to ensure that the correct patient profile has been accessed. As a safeguard, a second patient identifier, in addition to the patient's name, is used for verification of the information. For new prescriptions, this identifier is commonly the date of birth. The birth date for each patient is typically written (or circled) on the hard copy prescription. Failure to verify an identifier may result in a serious medication error—a prescription entered and filled for the wrong patient.

In addition to matching the patient name and address, the pharmacy technician needs to verify that the name, address, and phone number of the prescriber on the prescription match the information in the patient profile. If an incorrect phone number is entered into the profile, refill requests will be faxed or telephoned to the wrong medical office.

Patient Profile for a New Customer If a patient is a new customer to the pharmacy, then a profile will need to be created, either at the time the prescription is submitted to the pharmacy or—in the case of phoned-in prescriptions, faxed prescriptions, or e-prescriptions—prior to dispensing the medication(s) to the patient. Figure 6.10 on the following page is an example of a written patient profile form that may be used to obtain information from the patient. Pharmacy technicians should ask new customers to fill in the form and should encourage them to ask questions if any difficulties arise during its completion. Additional information can be obtained through a conversation with the patient, patient representative, or parent and can be directly entered into the computerized database.

At the time of an initial visit, the patient will likely be given a copy of the store's confidentiality policy to comply with the Health Insurance Portability and Accountability Act (HIPAA) of 1996. Documentation of patient receipt and sign-off of this information is commonly saved in the patient profile. It is extremely important that confidentiality of patient medical information be maintained at all times. (For more information on patient confidentiality protocol, see Chapter 13.)

Documenting Medication Allergies and Adverse Drug Reactions Whether creating or maintaining a patient profile, it is extremely important for the pharmacy technician to ask the patient about allergies to medications, as well as about past history of adverse drug reactions. An **allergy** is a hypersensitivity to a specific substance that may be manifested as a rash, shortness of breath, runny nose, watery

Safety Note

All drug allergies and adverse drug reactions must be documented in the patient profile.

Safety Note

Patients with allergies to foods such as eggs, peanuts, gluten (wheat), dyes, and soy may experience a cross-reaction with medications.

FIGURE 6.10
Written
Patient Profile
Form

PATIENT PROFILE

Patient Name

| Last | First | Middle Initial |

Street or PO Box

| City | State | ZIP |

| Phone | Date of Birth | | Social Security No. |
| (___)___ ____ | Month Day Year | □ Male □ Female | ___ __ _____ |

□ Yes, I would like medication dispensed in a child-resistant container.
□ No, I do not want medication dispensed in a child-resistant container.

Medication Insurance   Card Holder Name _____
□ Yes   □ Card Holder   □ Child   □ Disabled Dependent
□ No   □ Spouse   □ Dependent Parent □ Full Time Student

MEDICAL HISTORY

HEALTH

		ALLERGIES AND DRUG REACTIONS
□ Angina	□ Epilepsy	□ No known drug allergies or reactions
□ Anemia	□ Glaucoma	□ Aspirin
□ Arthritis	□ Heart condition	□ Cephalosporins
□ Asthma	□ Kidney disease	□ Codeine
□ Blood clotting disorders	□ Liver disease	□ Erythromycin
□ High blood pressure	□ Lung disease	□ Penicillin
□ Breast feeding	□ Parkinson disease	□ Sulfa drugs
□ Cancer	□ Pregnancy	□ Tetracyclines
□ Diabetes	□ Ulcers	□ Xanthines
Other conditions _____		□ Other allergies/reactions _____

Prescription Medication(s) Being Taken   OTC Medication(s) Currently Being Taken

Would you like generic medication when possible? □ Yes □ No

Comments

Health information changes periodically. Please notify the pharmacy of any new medications, allergies, drug reactions, or health conditions.

_____ Signature _____ Date □ I do not wish to provide this information.

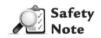

Safety Note

Patients can develop allergies to antibiotics, even if they have taken antibiotics without adverse reactions in the past.

eyes, or swelling. In extreme cases, allergic reactions can lead to shock, coma, or death. An **adverse drug reaction (ADR)** is any unexpected negative consequence from taking a particular drug.

If a new patient indicates that he or she does not have any allergies, then the notation NKA (meaning *no known allergies*) or NKMA (meaning *no known medication allergies*) should be recorded on the back of the prescription form and in the computerized patient profile. If the patient indicates that he or she does have an allergy, then that specific medication allergy must be documented and entered into the patient profile. This information may assist the pharmacist in reviewing the prescription for potential medication-related problems prior to filling the prescription.

FIGURE 6.11
**Drug Allergy
Screen of
Computerized
Patient Profile**

Many computer
profiles have
drop-down
menus to list drug
allergies.

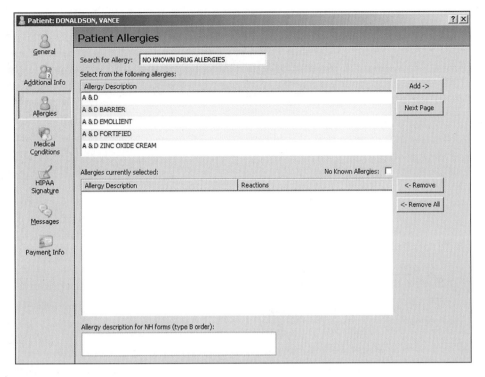

Many community pharmacies will require the pharmacy technician to ask patients at each visit about changes in allergies, medical conditions, or new medications, including OTC drugs and dietary supplements, in order to keep the patient profile current. Inquiring about allergies every time a patient comes to the pharmacy with a prescription for an antibiotic is a good practice. Antibiotics, especially penicillin and sulfa drugs, are the most common types of medication allergies, and allergies can begin at any age. A patient could have safely taken an antibiotic several times in the past and become allergic to it on a subsequent occasion.

Patients can be allergic to any medication or ingredient. Other common medications that can cause allergic reactions include aspirin, nonsteroidal anti-inflammatory drugs (NSAIDs) such as ibuprofen, codeine, and anesthetics. Some patients who report stomach upset or nausea may believe that they are experiencing an allergic reaction. However, this is more likely an expected side effect of the prescribed medication, not a true allergy or adverse drug reaction. Therefore, the technician should ask the patient to describe the symptoms before documenting the allergy into the patient profile; if unsure, ask the pharmacist for help in determining the allergy history (see Figure 6.11).

Once the patient profile contains allergy-related information, the computer software will always alert the pharmacist that a potential allergy or a hypersensitivity reaction may occur if a prescription is filled for that drug. For example, if hydrocodone, a codeine derivative, is being prescribed to a patient whose profile indicates that he or she may be allergic to codeine, then the pharmacist will receive a precautionary message on the computer screen. The pharmacist may ask the patient whether he or she remembers taking hydrocodone in the past without an allergic reaction. In addition to potentially causing patient harm, a missed drug allergy could trigger a major negligence lawsuit.

Documenting Insurance Information Once the demographic and prescription information is reviewed and entered into the correct patient profile, the pharmacy technician often submits an online claim to an insurance plan. Prescription insurance

**Safety
Note**

If a pharmacy
technician is
unsure whether a
patient's reported
allergy is truly an
allergy, he or she
should ask the
pharmacist before
including the
information in the
patient profile.

eligibility must be verified often; some insurance will change every year or with the start of new employment. Unlike most hospitals and medical and dental offices, a pharmacy processes a claim *prior to* the patient receiving the medication. This is done to more quickly recover the cost of the drug product. If there is a problem with insurance eligibility (incorrect ID number, group number, or date of birth) or drug coverage (drug not covered), then the pharmacy technician must try to call the insurance provider and resolve the issue. If the feedback from the online processing is "insurance expired," the pharmacy technician may need to ask if a new insurance card was issued to the patient.

As mentioned earlier in this chapter, a provider NPI number is required to bill insurance on noncontrolled medications. An NPI number is a unique National Provider Identifier for any healthcare provider involved in writing prescriptions or billing insurance for any healthcare-related service. As such, each physician, physician's assistant, nurse practitioner, and some pharmacists have been assigned an NPI number by the government (Center for Medicare and Medicaid Services). At times, the nurse practitioner or physician's assistant may not have an NPI number, or one that is on file with the insurance provider. In those situations, the NPI number of the supervising physician is utilized to process and bill the prescription. In the case of controlled medication, the prescriber must have a DEA number in order for the prescription to be processed and billed correctly.

It is not uncommon for insurance to only cover a 30-day supply of medication, even if the prescriber approved a higher quantity. For example, a prescriber may write a 90-day supply of Nexium for heartburn, but insurance may only cover a 30-day supply. Or, the pharmacy may receive a prescription for Ambien CR 12.5 mg #30 for sleep, but insurance may only cover 18 tablets per 30 days, giving the patient the option of purchasing the other 12 tablets out of his or her own pocket. The rationale is that insurance does not want to pay for expensive drugs or those that may be overused.

If the drug on the prescription is not covered by insurance (usually expensive drugs), or if it is not included on a preferred drug list (PDL), then a prior authorization may be required. A **prior authorization (PA)** requires the pharmacy technician or pharmacist to call or fax the prescriber's office so that the prescriber (or his or her representative) can explain the justification for the use of the drug with the patient's insurer. This often delays processing the prescription for 72 hours or longer. Another option for the prescriber is to order an alternative lower-cost drug that is covered by insurance. The patient always has the option to pay for the medication in full instead of waiting for the outcome of the PA, but many drugs are very expensive. If insurance approves the PA, then the technician can notify the patient and process the prescription claim online and fill the prescription. Chapter 7 provides more details about online billing and insurance claims.

Pharmacist Review and Verification

Once all information has been entered into the patient profile, the data must be verified by the pharmacist before it can be filled. The pharmacist will verify that the correct date, patient, drug, dose, directions, refills, and prescriber were selected. During this verification process, most pharmacy software applications will also provide for a drug utilization review if necessary.

Drug Utilization Review A **drug utilization review (DUR)** requires a closer review of the patient profile for potential medication problems with other drugs in the profile. Pharmacy software will compare a prescription with others the patient has received to determine whether a further review of the prescription by the pharmacist is necessary.

This software is specifically designed for pharmacies and insurance companies to provide an additional level of protection with which to detect a potentially serious medication error. This safeguard also addresses two real-world pharmacy practice issues: (1) It is nearly impossible for any pharmacist (or physician) to remember doses, adverse effects, and drug interactions for all medications, especially while juggling a typically busy pharmacy workload; and (2) a complete centralized medication profile may not exist because patients may go to more than one pharmacy or more than one physician.

The DUR is an extremely important responsibility for the pharmacist. It is at this step in the process that a potential allergy, hypersensitivity, adverse reaction, or drug interaction will be recognized. The necessity of a DUR by a pharmacist is triggered by a number of factors—for example, if the prescribed medication may:

- interact with existing or past medications on the patient's profile (for example, blood thinners such as warfarin)
- be contraindicated because of the patient's allergy or medical history (penicillin allergy, diabetes, or asthma)
- be a duplicate of a similar drug prescribed in the past (for example, two different migraine headache drugs or narcotics)
- have been prescribed in doses too low (subtherapeutic) or too high (toxic) for this patient
- not be indicated or may be used with caution in certain patient populations (for example, pregnant, pediatric, or geriatric patients)

Most DUR notifications will be categorized by their potential severity: mild, moderate, or severe. In most pharmacies, the action taken on "severe" DURs must be documented. The pharmacist must use his or her professional judgment to review the profile, assess the significance of the potential interaction or adverse reaction, and determine what type of action, if any, is necessary. These options include:

- reviewing the patient medication profile
- contacting the prescribing physician
- counseling the patient on potential issues prior to dispensing
- overriding the DUR and filling the prescription

Safety Note

Pharmacy technicians should understand that only a pharmacist can override a DUR.

The pharmacy technician will not be able to fill or dispense the prescription to the patient until the verification is complete and the DUR, if any, is resolved by the pharmacist. It is important for the technician to alert the pharmacist that a DUR exists and effectively communicate to the patient that a potential problem exists with the prescribed medication that must be resolved prior to dispensing. Often the pharmacist will write a reminder note to counsel the patient at the time of prescription pickup to increase awareness of a potential side effect or adverse reaction. Many times a computer program will require an action by the pharmacist before the drug is dispensed.

A DUR is a good example of medication therapy management (MTM) services in which the pharmacy is reimbursed an additional fee for identifying, resolving, and documenting a potentially severe—and costly—adverse drug effect.

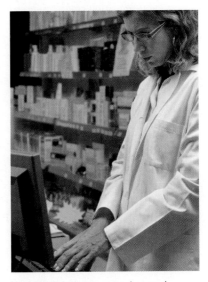

The pharmacist must review and document all potentially severe drug utilization reviews in the computer database.

Reimbursement is available from some insurance and all Medicare Part D providers. MTM services would not be possible without the assistance of pharmacy technicians in other steps of the processing of the prescription.

Pharmacist Verification Once verification from the pharmacist is complete, the prescription is safe to fill. A patient-specific medication information sheet is printed to initiate the filling process. This sheet includes a bar code for the prescription, patient demographics, insurance billing information and co-payments, detailed information on the drug being dispensed, the National Drug Code (NDC), drug identifier (picture or description of the tablet or capsule), and any remaining refills on the prescription. Used by the pharmacy technician to fill the order, the medication sheet accompanies the medication that is dispensed to the patient.

Medication Selection and Preparation

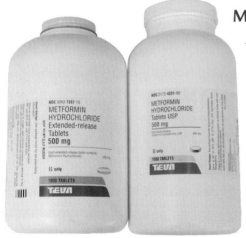

As mentioned above, the medication information sheet serves as the prescription order; it will contain patient demographics; the drug's name, strength, and quantity; and the NDC number. The pharmacy technician must retrieve the stock bottle, match the NDC numbers of the medication sheet and the stock bottle, and then fill the prescription from inventory. After filling the prescription, it is common practice to mark an "X" on the bottle or cap to indicate an opened bottle. Care should be taken not to cover up the drug name, expiration date, or NDC number when marking the bottle. The stock drug bottle should then be returned to the inventory shelf.

The pharmacy technician should carefully check the drug's name, strength, and formulation when selecting it from stock. In this case, both drugs are metformin 500 mg, but one bottle is immediate-release and the other is extended-release. Selecting the wrong formulation could result in a serious medication error.

Drug Inventory In order to efficiently and accurately select medications from the pharmacy stock to fill a prescription, the technician must become familiar with the drug inventory and its precise location. Figure 6.12 reviews the standard parts of a label on a pharmacy stock bottle. The drug name, strength, package size, and NDC number of the pharmacy stock bottle should always be checked immediately and compared with the medication sheet printout before the technician counts out and places the medication in a smaller container for dispensing to a patient. On the unit

FIGURE 6.12
Parts of a Stock Drug Label

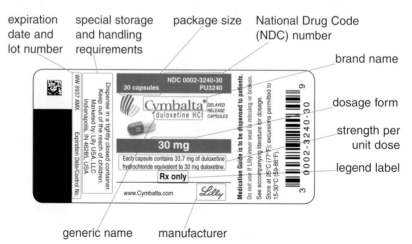

stock bottle, the brand name is often in bold print, and the generic name is in smaller print under or beside the brand name. The dosage form such as delayed-release, sustained-release, or extended-release is also indicated in this area. The dose or strength per unit is prominently displayed near the drug name. The package size is commonly a stock drug bottle of 30, 60, 90, 100, or 500 tablets or capsules. Although expiration dates are checked routinely, the dating should be reviewed prior to dispensing.

Safety Note

The expiration date of a product should always be checked by the pharmacy technician before filling, especially on an infrequently used medication.

Drugs are often arranged alphabetically, with those of similar spellings and strengths or similar generic manufacturers shelved near one another. Packaging and labeling of the same drug in various doses, dosage forms, strengths, or concentrations may be similar. To minimize dispensing errors, some drugs may be purposely stocked slightly out of order to get the attention of pharmacy personnel when retrieving a stock drug bottle from the shelf. Pharmacy technicians are often in a better position to identify potential sources of medication errors related to filling the prescription order.

Storage Locations Drugs are usually stocked by brand or generic drug name. High-volume pharmacies may have an additional section of the pharmacy dedicated to fast-moving Top 200 drugs, enhancing filling efficiency. (For detailed information on the most commonly dispensed generic drugs, see Appendix A.) Antibiotic powders for reconstitution are usually stocked in a separate area (as are all solutions, syrups, and suspensions). Some pharmacies may also have a separate shelving section for birth control pills, topical creams, ointments and gels, nasal and lung sprays and inhalers, and otic (ear) and ophthalmic (eye) medications.

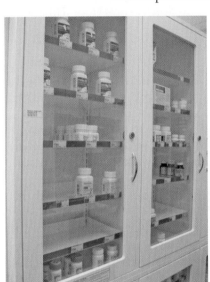

Schedule II drugs are most commonly stored in a locked cabinet. In most pharmacies, access to these medications is limited to the pharmacist. This requires the pharmacist to unlock the cabinet, select the appropriate stock bottle, compare the NDC number with the medication container label, and count out the medication. Other controlled Schedule III, IV, and V substances may be distributed throughout the stock drug inventory. Pharmacy technicians must be aware of the policy and procedure for filling controlled substance prescription orders in their pharmacy. For example, some pharmacies may have the technician "double count" all controlled drug prescriptions or initial the medication label.

All C–II drugs are stored in a locked and secured safe or cabinet with access generally restricted to the pharmacist.

Organization of Inventory Pharmacy personnel must maintain a highly organized drug inventory. They should also implement precautionary measures to prevent inadvertent drug mix-ups during the selection process. These measures may include:

- providing distant storage areas for look-alike, sound-alike drugs
- using alert labels, tall-man lettering (such as hydrOXYzine), or color-coded shelving bins for all high-risk drugs
- reshelving all stock bottles in their proper locations after filling prescription orders
- using bar-code scanning to compare the NDCs of stock drug bottles to medication information sheets
- noting computer reminders to double-check sound-alike drugs during the verification process
- using bar-code scanning to compare labeled medications with original prescriptions

Special Procedures In some cases, the drug dose or quantity prescribed may not be available in the drug inventory. For example, a pharmacy technician may read a prescription order for Nystatin Cream 30 g but discover that the package size is not on the inventory shelf. In that situation, the technician has two options: (1) He or she could "**out-of-stock**" the medication on the computer, and the product would be automatically ordered and received from the wholesaler the next business day; or (2) the technician could change the order with pharmacist approval and dispense two 15 g tubes of Nystatin Cream instead. Technicians may also encounter discrepancies between the ordered quantity of pills or capsules and the package size available in inventory. For example, a technician may read a prescription order for cephalexin 500 mg 1 cap po bid #20 but discover that only 250 mg capsules are in stock. With pharmacist approval, the prescription order may be changed to cephalexin 250 mg 2 caps po bid #40. Making this exchange allows the patient to receive a needed antibiotic without unnecessary delay.

Technicians will also encounter many drug products that have more than one generic manufacturer. If on computer entry the right drug but wrong NDC number were selected, then the NDC number on the medication information sheet will not match the NDC number of the stock drug bottle in inventory. Most likely, the tablets or capsules will have different colors, shapes, and markings. In this situation, "a change of manufacturer" request must be placed and the prescription order with the NDC of the drug in stock must be selected. The prescription must be re-verified by the pharmacist before a "new" medication information sheet with the corrected NDC number is printed.

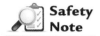
Safety Note

Pharmacy technicians should use a medication's NDC number to confirm that the correct medication has been pulled from inventory.

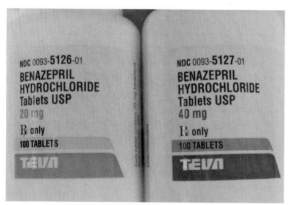

It is important that the pharmacy technician select the correct drug from stock. In this case, the drug is the same and so is the manufacturer and the package size. The NDC number ensures that the proper dose of drug is selected.

Filling a Prescription When filling a prescription, the NDC number is used by many pharmacists and technicians to aid in identifying the exact drug, dose, and package size. It is very important that the technician compare the NDC number of the stock bottle with the medication information sheet printout. Automation in some pharmacies allows the comparison of the bar code of the printout and the stock drug bottle, minimizing the chance of human error. After the technician confirms the NDC on the stock bottle with the printed medication sheet, a patient- and drug-specific medication container label will be printed. This label will be affixed to the appropriate plastic or glass container (or package) holding the medication. The medication container label's instructions must read exactly as indicated on the prescription's signa on the original prescription.

Occasionally, the NDC number of the prescription order will not match the stock drug bottle. The pharmacy (or wholesaler) may have changed the package size or generic manufacturer source of a drug product. Thus, a patient may receive tablets or capsules with a different color or shape upon refill because of this "change of manufacturer." A new printout of the medication sheet and/or medication container label will reflect this new NDC number. It is important that the technician notify the patient at the time of pickup that the appearance of the medication may have changed but that the drug and dose are identical to the medication that was prescribed and dispensed previously. Informing the patient of this change will alleviate the patient's concern about receiving the wrong medication.

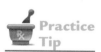
Practice Tip

To review a list of common look-alike and sound-alike medications created by the Institute for Safe Medication Practices, go to www.paradigmcollege.net/pharmpractice5e/lookandsoundalike drugs.

Safety Note

Pharmacy technicians should exercise caution when selecting insulin from the refrigerator. Insulin mix-ups are a common medication error.

 Safety Note

Technicians should implement three verification checks during the filling process to confirm that the correct drug was selected.

Safety Note

In pharmacy practice, 100% accuracy is expected with all prescriptions.

Accuracy Checks When filling a prescription, technicians need to pay careful attention to product selection. A common error is the selection of the wrong stock drug bottle or dose or package size because two products look alike (similar labeling), have different formulations available (SR, XL, XR, DR), or have names that sound alike. In fact, selecting the wrong insulin from the refrigerator is one of the most common medication errors. For example, the names of several types of insulin manufactured by Eli Lilly are quite similar: Humulin R, Humulin N, Humalog, Humalog mix 50/50, Humulin mix 70/30, and Humalog mix 75/25. Some types of insulin are available in 10 mL vials; other insulin is administered through the use of a KwikPen. It would be easy to inadvertently select the incorrect insulin from the refrigerator; however, barcode scanning of the NDC would detect the error.

To avoid medication errors, pharmacy technicians need to develop good work habits, including carefully reading and comparing the stock drug label with the medication information sheet, utilizing bar code technology if available, and avoiding product identification based on drug manufacturer label design. The technician should also implement three separate checks during the filling process to ensure that the correct drug was selected: (1) when the product is initially being pulled from the inventory shelf; (2) at the time of preparation; and (3) when the product is returned to the shelf.

Although speed is important, 100% accuracy is paramount. If prescriptions filled in a given day were 99% correct, then the average pharmacy filling 200 prescriptions daily would have filled two prescriptions incorrectly. This is unacceptable. In order to strive to eliminate errors, a cross-check system using pharmacy technicians, pharmacists, and automation is utilized in the filling process. Each prescription is checked several times for accuracy during the filling process. Automation using bar code technology to scan prescriptions and NDC codes further ensures that the right drug and dose were selected for the right patient. For more information on medication safety practices, see Chapter 12.

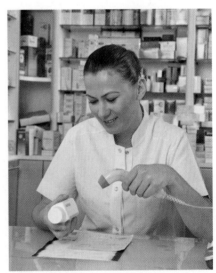

Before filling the prescription, the technician should scan the stock bottle to ensure that the correct drug was selected from inventory.

Preparing Oral Dosage Forms Oral drug products are available in many different dosage forms, each of which has its own dispensing requirements.

 Safety Note

Equipment should be cleaned after counting sulfa, penicillin, or aspirin products.

Tablets and Capsules The most commonly dispensed drug formulation is the tablet or capsule. Tablets and capsules must be counted out from a stock drug bottle (in most cases) and placed in the appropriately sized vial or medication container. Figure 6.13 on the following page shows the equipment and procedure for counting tablets and capsules. A special counting tray is used that has a trough on one side to hold counted tablets or capsules and a spout on the opposite side to pour unused medication back into the stock bottle.

When handling oral dosage forms such as tablets or capsules, pharmacy technicians should minimize any direct finger contact with the medications because germs and oils from the skin could contaminate the products. The tablets and capsules should always be counted with a clean spatula and picked up with forceps if they are

FIGURE 6.13   Counting Tablets

(a) Tablets should be counted by fives and moved to the trough with a spatula. (b) The unneeded tablets should be returned to the stock container by pouring them from the spout. (c) The counted tablets should then be poured into the appropriately sized medication vial.

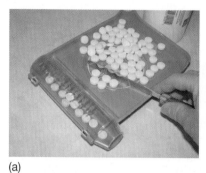

(a)

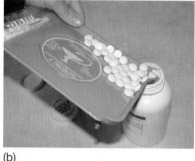

(b)

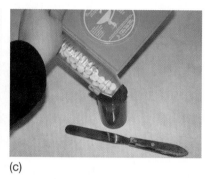

(c)

dropped on the counter. The spatula, tray, and forceps should be cleaned often throughout the workday with 70% isopropyl alcohol, and these items should always be cleaned after handling a product that leaves a powder residue. Because of the frequency of severe patient allergies, this equipment should also be cleaned immediately after counting sulfa, penicillin, or aspirin products.

Controlled Substances   Most pharmacies allow the pharmacy technician to fill Schedule III and IV drugs (those controlled substances typically not stored in a locked cabinet). As stated earlier, many pharmacies' procedures may require a manual count of all controlled substances (Schedules II, III, and IV) by both a pharmacist and pharmacy technician as well as the recording of their initials on the medication container label. This practice prevents potential abusing or drug-seeking patients from returning to the pharmacy to complain that the pharmacist or technician shorted the count on their prescription.

Safety Note

The pharmacist must check all drugs prepared by the pharmacy technician.

Liquid Formulations   Liquid products, such as pediatric cough and cold syrups and suspensions, are sometimes dispensed in their original packaging. They are also commonly poured from a stock bottle directly into an appropriately sized dispensing bottle (from 2 fl oz to 16 fl oz). The pharmacy technician should present the original stock bottle to the pharmacist for final check along with the original prescription, the patient information leaflet, and the medication on the labeled container.

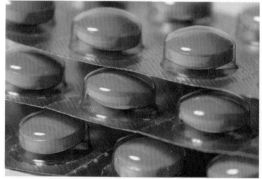

Several medications are available in unit dose blister packs. These packs are exempt from childproof packaging requirements.

Handling Prepackaged Drugs   Many medications are commercially available in unit-dose or unit-of-use packaging. These products simplify the filling process: The technician retrieves the drug from inventory by matching the correct name, manufacturer, quantity, and strength with the order. (Counting out the medication is often not necessary.) Even though these medications are prepackaged, the pharmacist must still verify the quality of the technician's work, ensuring that the proper drug, dosage form, and amount were chosen and placed in the proper container; a proper label was prepared; and, if appropriate, the correct amount of distilled water was added for reconstitution.

Unit-Dose Packaging As the name implies, unit-dose packaging means that each **unit dose** of a tablet or capsule is individually packaged in sealed foil and considered tamper-proof. Drugs may be available in unit-dose packaging for stability reasons or for cost savings and are more commonly seen in the hospital and nursing home setting. The packaging must be labeled with the manufacturer's name, lot number, and expiration date in addition to the drug's name and strength. For example, a prescription of Ondansetron 8 mg ODT #8 for nausea and vomiting requires that eight individually packaged unit doses be placed in a medication container or plastic, ziplock bag with a medication label. Other medications commonly available in unit doses include suppositories and migraine medications. Unopened unit doses may be legally returned to pharmacy stock. (For more information on the use of unit-dose packaging in hospital pharmacy practice, see Chapter 9.)

Unit-of-Use Packaging A drug may be commercially available in a prepackaged, unit-of-use form. A **unit of use** is a fixed number of dosage units in a stock drug container. Examples of such packaging include birth control pills, topical ointments and creams, eyedrops, and eardrops. Several of these drugs are prescribed once or twice daily, and many insurance companies reimburse for a one-month or three-month supply of medication. Unit-of-use packaging consists of a month's supply, which is often 30, 60, or 90 tablets or capsules. Filling a prescription with a medication in unit-of-use packaging amounts to little more than locating the correct drug in the correct strength, verifying the NDC number, and affixing the correct medication container label.

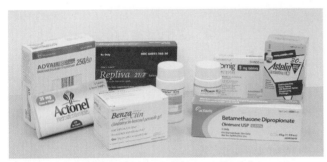

Unit-of-use packaging for commonly prescribed drugs saves time and reduces medication preparation errors.

An antibiotic powder is another common example of unit-of-use packaging. Prior to dispensing, the antibiotic must be reconstituted with a given amount of distilled water. Medications such as antibiotic powders are often available in multiple strengths and volumes, so checking the drug labels for dose, volume, and NDC number is critical to minimizing mistakes. These medications should always be dispensed with an appropriate measuring device and are commonly labeled "Shake well and give [child's name] 1 teaspoonful (or 5 mL) by mouth every eight hours." In most cases, due to a short expiration date, the antibiotic suspension is not prepared (adding the distilled water) until the patient (or parent) picks up the medication.

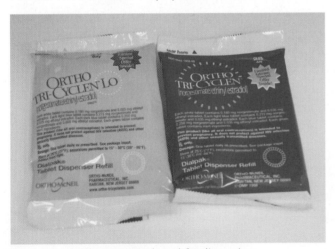

Birth control pills are prepackaged for dispensing.

Flavoring Drugs Children as well as pets may benefit from flavoring prescribed medication to improve compliance or adherence to drug therapy. Most pediatric suspensions are available with some flavor from the manufacturer once they are reconstituted with distilled water. However, in many cases, the taste may still be unacceptable to the child. Many pharmacies have the capability to flavor medications upon

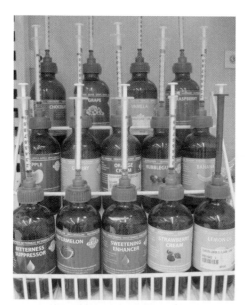

Formulas for adding various flavors to medications to improve taste are available to the pharmacy technician.

request from a patient or parent at a minimal additional charge. The flavoring formulas for each drug and dose are provided in the computer database. For several "unpleasant tasting" drugs, such as amoxicillin/clavulanate and clindamycin, pharmacy technicians often flavor the medications without an additional charge. Although some flavors may be incompatible with the prescribed medication, most flavors will not interfere with the drug's active ingredient(s). Flavors are free from dyes and sugar and are hypoallergenic, so they are safe to use in those with allergies, diabetes, or even those who are gluten or casein (milk) sensitive.

Flavoring agents have sweetening enhancers as well as bitterness suppressors and are available in many flavors: apple, banana, bubblegum, cherry, chocolate, grape, lemon oil, orange crème, raspberry, strawberry cream, vanilla, and watermelon. Formulas for flavoring agents often combine one or more agents to result in the desired flavor. Flavors are then drawn up in an oral syringe and added to the suspension. In most cases, the amount of distilled water to be added to the antibiotic powder may be slightly adjusted to account for the volume of the flavoring agents.

The flavoring of drugs is a patient service that can improve customer loyalty and, therefore, customer retention. More importantly, this service improves patient compliance with the prescribed medication regimen, resulting in a happy child, a happy parent, and a happy prescriber.

Choosing Medication Containers A wide variety of plastic vial sizes are available for tablets and capsules in various dram sizes (from 10 to 60 drams). Selecting the proper vial size is a skill that becomes easy with experience. The pharmacy software printout on the patient medication information sheet may even recommend a vial size based on the count and size of the specific drug product. Most containers in the pharmacy are amber-colored to prevent ultraviolet (UV) light exposure and subsequent degradation of the medication.

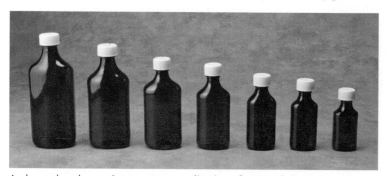

Amber-colored containers protect medications from UV light exposure.

Other containers common to the retail pharmacy include amber liquid containers (from 2 oz to 16 oz) and solid white ointment jars for creams or ointments. Various size boxes are available as well for products such as suppositories, unit-of-use packages, or injectable syringes. Many products, such as antibiotic suspensions, metered-dose inhalers (MDIs), and oral contraceptives, are available in a manufacturer-provided container; the prescription label is attached directly to the product or the box.

All medications should be dispensed in child-resistant containers that are designed to be difficult for children to open. The Poison Prevention Packaging Act of 1970 requires (with some exceptions, such as sublingual nitroglycerin tablets, unit-of-use, and unit dose) that all prescription drugs be packaged in child-resistant containers but states that a non–child-resistant container may be used if the patient receiving it makes a request for such a container. For example, many older patients, especially those with arthritis, may have difficulty opening child-resistant containers and may request an exemption from child-resistant containers. The regulations of a given state may require the patient to initiate a special request for dispensing a prescription in a non–child-resistant container. Some state laws allow pharmacy patients to complete a blanket request form for non–child-resistant containers. Other states require patients to sign such a request for each prescription. Often pharmacies make use of a stamp on the back of the prescription for this purpose. All patient requests for non–child-resistant containers must be added to the patients' profiles for future reference. Pharmacy personnel should also be aware that certain OTC drugs, such as aspirin and iron, must be marketed in child-resistant containers due to their potential toxic effects in children.

Medication Information for the Patient

It is important to provide each patient with sufficient information to correctly take the prescribed medication. Written information is delivered through the medication container label, auxiliary labels, patient medication information sheets, and—with some high-risk drugs—an FDA-mandated MedGuide. From a legal point of view, a medication should be accompanied by information to help a patient understand the appropriate use and common side effects of the dispensed medication.

Medication Container Label A **medication container label** is a label stating the dosage directions from the prescriber and is affixed to the container of the dispensed medication. In addition, the label customarily contains the date; the name, address, and phone number of the pharmacy; the Rx number; the patient's name; the number of refills; the prescriber's name; the drug name; and the name of the drug's manufacturer (see Table 6.8). However, this label information may vary somewhat, depending on the laws and regulations of a given state. Some states require veterinary labels to carry the name and address of the animal owner and the species of the animal.

The prescription label is usually generated by the computer after review and verification by the pharmacist. In some pharmacies, the label is generated only after the bar code of the medication information sheet is compared with the bar code of the stock

---

TABLE 6.8 Medication Container Label Information

- Date when prescription filled
- Prescription's serial number
- Pharmacy's name, address, and telephone number
- Patient's name
- Prescriber's name
- All directions for use given on the prescription
- All necessary auxiliary labels containing patient precautions
- Medication name, whether generic or brand
- Medication strength
- Drug manufacturer's name
- Drug quantity
- Drug expiration date or date after which drug should not be used because of possible loss of potency or efficacy
- Initials of the licensed pharmacist
- Number of refills allowed, or the phrase "No Refills"

FIGURE 6.14
Prescription and Label Comparison

(a) The original prescription contains the information that should be included on the label.
(b) The medication container label transcribes the instructions for the patient.

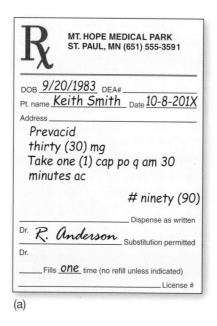

R̥ MT. HOPE MEDICAL PARK
ST. PAUL, MN (651) 555-3591

DOB 9/20/1983 DEA# _____
Pt. name Keith Smith Date 10-8-201X
Address _____

Prevacid
thirty (30) mg
Take one (1) cap po q am 30
minutes ac

ninety (90)

_____ Dispense as written
Dr. R. Anderson ___ Substitution permitted
Dr. _____
_____ Fills one time (no refill unless indicated)
_____ License #

(a)

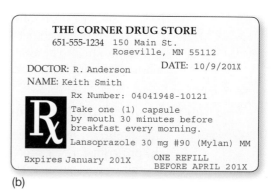

THE CORNER DRUG STORE
651-555-1234 150 Main St.
Roseville, MN 55112

DOCTOR: R. Anderson DATE: 10/9/201X
NAME: Keith Smith

R̥ Rx Number: 04041948-10121
Take one (1) capsule
by mouth 30 minutes before
breakfast every morning.
Lansoprazole 30 mg #90 (Mylan) MM

Expires January 201X ONE REFILL
BEFORE APRIL 201X

(b)

drug bottle. This practice provides additional protection from selecting the wrong drug or dose. Medication container labels typically reinforce the dosing instructions of the prescriber (see Figure 6.14). However, some prescription orders simply state "take as directed." If that is the case, the pharmacy technician must verify that the prescriber did indeed give the patient specific directions or make a request that the pharmacist counsel the patient on the appropriate use of the medication. To avoid insurance rejections during an audit, such prescriptions should be clarified with the prescriber's office and documented on the prescription and/or in the patient profile.

Medication container labels for Schedule II through Schedule V drugs must contain the transfer warning "Caution: Federal law prohibits the transfer of this drug to any person other than the patient for whom it was prescribed." It is common practice for this statement to be placed in small print on all medication container labels.

Once the prescribed medication is in the appropriate container, the medication container label is affixed directly to the container by the person generating the label or may be kept separate for review by the pharmacist before being affixed, depending on state laws and regulations. Some pharmacists prefer to affix prescription labels for unit-of-use drugs on the box in which the product is packaged. On any unit-of-use packaging, care should be exercised by the technician to not place the label over the drug name; otherwise, the final check by the pharmacist is made more difficult. A disadvantage of the latter method is that if the box is lost or discarded, then the physician's directions to the patient have been lost as well. Most small items such as unit doses, tubes of cream or ointment, or bottles of an ophthalmic or otic medication are often placed in an appropriately sized, child-resistant prescription vial and labeled.

Auxiliary Label In addition to medication container labels typed with prescriber directions, a medication may be labeled with an auxiliary label (see Figure 6.15). An **auxiliary label** is a small, colorful label that is added to a dispensed medication to supplement the directions on the medication container label. The application of these auxiliary labels requires a thorough knowledge and understanding of the drug and is thus usually restricted to the professional judgment of the pharmacist. Some pharmacy software may automatically print drug-specific auxiliary labels when the medication

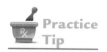

Practice Tip

In some states, the law requires the pharmacist to affix the medication container label to the container.

FIGURE 6.15
Auxiliary Labels

Auxiliary labels are affixed to the medication container by the pharmacist or the pharmacy technician under his or her direct supervision. These labels aid the patient in taking the medication in the safest and most appropriate manner.

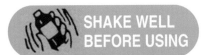
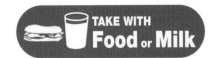
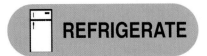
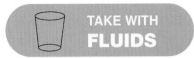
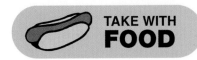
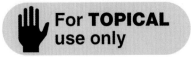

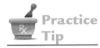
Practice Tip

Computer-generated medication information sheets provide package insert information in a format that can be understood by the patient.

container label is printed. Auxiliary labels may include warnings such as to avoid exposure to sunlight, take with food, take on an empty stomach, and avoid alcohol. With experience, the pharmacist may allow the technician to add auxiliary labels to medication containers. However, if the technician is in doubt about the appropriateness of any auxiliary labels, he or she should ask for confirmation from the pharmacist.

Medication Information Sheet Additional written drug information in easily understood terms is given to the patient to take home and review for each new and refill medication with a medication information sheet. A **medication information sheet** is a computerized printout that provides details on how to safely take the prescribed medication. This information always accompanies the medication and also includes patient demographics and prescription specific information such as directions, Rx number, and refills remaining.

This medication information sheet contains information in the following categories:

- Ingredient Name
- Common Uses
- Before Using this Medication
- How to Use this Medication
- Cautions
- Possible Side Effects
- Overuse
- Additional Information

The medication sheet may also contain a section called Product Identification, which includes the shape, color, and any markings of the tablet or capsule. This information allows patients to compare the product identifiers with the medication contained in the bottles, providing an added verification check that the correct drug was dispensed. In the event that the manufacturer was changed on a generic product, the pharmacy technician should inform patients seeking a refill so that they understand the reason for any altered appearance of their medication.

Although the medication information sheet does not replace the counseling provided by the pharmacist or prescriber, the patient may not remember the counseling details if only verbal instructions are given. The written information will provide more detailed information that the patient can review at home when actually taking the medication.

Medication Guide As discussed in Chapter 3, a patient medication guide, or MedGuide, must be provided to patients receiving a select number of high-risk drugs. The MedGuide is commonly printed after the final check of the prescription by the pharmacist. In the past, this information was called the patient package insert or PPI. The MedGuide is basically a "black box" warning advising consumers of a potential adverse reaction or of the proper use of a medication with a special dosage formulation, such as the inhaled pulmonary drugs Advair or Serevent. Some medications, notably all birth control pills, have their own MedGuide that is automatically dispensed with the product.

Final Check of the Prescription

It is extremely important—and required by law—that the pharmacist checks every prescription before it is dispensed to the patient to verify its accuracy. Typically, the pharmacy technician will present the original hard copy prescription (if available), the medication information sheet, and the labeled container with the prescribed medication for this final check. Often the unit stock bottles of tablets, capsules, or liquids will be provided to check the source (and NDC number) of the medication.

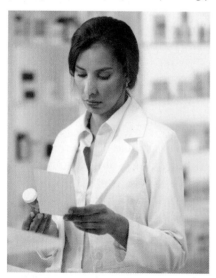

The pharmacy technician must have all prepared prescriptions checked by the supervising pharmacist.

The pharmacist reviews the original prescription order, compares it with the patient profile, confirms that the medication information sheet has been printed, verifies that the drug selected by the technician (from the stock bottle) is correct, and checks the accuracy of the medication container label. At the discretion of the pharmacist, a personal note may be added to the medication information sheet; comments such as "caution in sun" or "no alcohol" or "do not take with acetaminophen (Tylenol)" may emphasize counseling. Additionally, the price or insurance eligibility is often checked to see whether the prescribed drug is covered or billed to the correct insurance plan, especially if more than one plan is available.

Automation is often used to enhance human double checks and minimize the risk of medication errors. Some chain pharmacies may use a scanner to compare the labeled medication container via drug identification software. The bar code may suggest that the prescription for 250 mg of cephalexin should contain red and gray capsules with certain markings. A pharmacist will often do a visual scan (sometimes with the help of a light and magnifying glass) of the medication contained in the vial to verify the contents; some experienced pharmacists can identify the characteristic smells and scents of liquids. MedGuides and medication information sheets are attached to the paper bag containing the prescription by the pharmacist after the final check.

Before dispensing to a patient, the pharmacist will compare the original prescription with the labeled instructions and perform a visual check of the medication.

After this review, the pharmacist may initialize the medication container label and/or the original prescription. In doing so, the pharmacist assumes legal responsibility for the correctness of the prescription. However, the pharmacist does not necessarily assume sole responsibility. Technicians have been held legally responsible for dispensing and labeling mistakes, especially in situations in which the dispensing error was the result of negligence on their part or not following established policies and procedures.

A duplicate of the computer-generated copy of the medication container label is usually affixed to the back of the original new prescription by the pharmacist or pharmacy technician. This provides a paper trail of exactly which product (drug, dose and quantity, directions, and NDC number) was used in filling the prescription for each patient. It is not uncommon for the filling technician and the verifying pharmacist to initial this copy, especially in the case of a controlled substance. If the prescription is filled with a drug from a different manufacturer, then a duplicate label with the new NDC number is also filed for documentation.

Once the original prescription has completed the final check and the copy of the label has been affixed to the medication container, the original prescription is filed numerically. Prescription records must be stored and readily retrievable for potential review and audit. Before filing a prescription for a controlled Schedule II substance, the pharmacist must, by law, sign and date the back of the prescription. Some pharmacies require the pharmacist to maintain a perpetual inventory (exact unit count) of these Schedule II drugs. If the technician records this information, then it must be cosigned by the pharmacist. Even minor discrepancies must be reported immediately to state and federal authorities.

Dispensing to the Patient

After the final verification and filing of the original prescription, the medication is available for immediate or future distribution to the patient. Completed prescriptions are stored alphabetically or numerically for future pickup; patients generally have seven days to pick up the prescription before it is returned to stock. Patients may also elect to have the prescription status sent to an e-mail address or to a cell phone via a text message.

Some medications—in particular, insulins, injections, and suppositories—should be stored in the refrigerator once the final verification by the pharmacist is completed. Other medications, such as antibiotic suspensions, must be mixed just prior to dispensing. Suitable measuring devices should be provided on all pediatric suspensions and liquids.

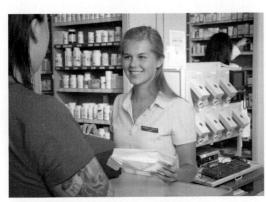

When a patient receives a prescription, the medication will be provided with written information as well as the opportunity to discuss any questions about the medication with the pharmacist.

Medications may be picked up at the pharmacy window (inside the store) or, in some cases, at a pharmacy drive-thru window. It is very important for the pharmacy technician to verify that the correct patient is receiving the dispensed medication, especially if someone else (such as a family member or a friend) picks up the prescription. To ring up the purchase, it is standard practice to verify patient address and/or birth date and to "sign or log on" to the computer in order to use bar-code scanning technology. In the case of controlled substances, a good practice is to require a photo ID to be presented and subsequently documented.

If the prescription is a "partial fill" or "change of manufacturer," then the pharmacy technician should be sure to relay this information to the patient; in case of a partial fill, the technician should provide the patient

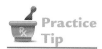

Practice Tip

By law, the pharmacy technician must offer the patient (or the patient's representative or parent) the opportunity for verbal counseling by the pharmacist.

with a promised time when the remainder of the prescription can be filled. In the case of a "change of manufacturer," the dosage unit may have a different color or shape. If "half-tablets" are prescribed, then the pharmacist or technician may recommend that the customer purchase a **tablet splitter** to more easily divide the tablets, especially if the tablets are scored.

Although the pharmacy technician is not allowed to counsel patients, the pharmacy technician is legally bound to offer the patient verbal counseling to be provided by the pharmacist. The pharmacy technician also assists the pharmacist in ensuring that educational resources and counseling are available to the patient. Most pharmacists try to make an effort to counsel every patient on a new prescription and to be available for counseling for any questions on refill medications. The pharmacist may initiate a request to counsel a patient if a questionable allergy, duplicate therapy, potential side effect, or drug–drug interaction warning appeared during the prescription filling process; a computer reminder for mandatory counseling may be prompted from a DUR. A private or semiprivate area should be available for medication counseling. The acceptance or decline of counseling by the patient is often documented by the pharmacy technician in the pharmacy software.

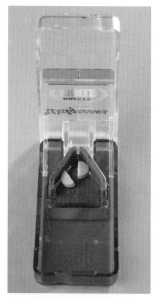

A tablet splitter may be needed if the prescription calls for half-tablet doses.

Chapter Summary

- In the community pharmacy, a pharmacy technician assumes a number of responsibilities related to prescription drugs; these depend on federal and state laws and regulations.
- The technician assists in the filling of prescriptions, which commonly involves retrieving stock bottles of drugs, counting the prescribed quantity of medications, filling the appropriate containers, and affixing medication container labels.
- The technician can legally take written prescriptions from walk-in customers but cannot, in most states, take new or transfer prescriptions by telephone and transcribe them.
- The parts of a prescription include prescriber information, the date, patient information, the symbol ℞, the inscription (the medication or medications prescribed and their amounts), the subscription (the instructions to the pharmacist), the signa (directions to the patient), additional instructions, and the prescriber's signature.
- The pharmacy technician is often responsible for entering the new prescription orders and creating or updating the computerized patient profile, including identifying information, medical history, medication/prescription history, drug allergy information, insurance/billing information, and prescription preferences.
- The pharmacy technician must become familiar with common abbreviations that are needed to interpret prescriptions and enter information into the patient profile database.
- Both technicians and pharmacists must be able to identify possible forged prescriptions or patients with drug-seeking behaviors when dispensing controlled drugs.
- Prescriptions for controlled substances require special record-keeping procedures. Pharmacy technicians should be sure to follow any labeling requirements given under state and federal laws.
- The patient receives medication information by way of drug and auxiliary labeling on the medication container, a medication information sheet for each drug dispensed, MedGuide, and counseling by the pharmacist.
- Medication container labels must contain a unique prescription number, the name of the patient, the date of the prescription, directions for use, the name and strength of the medication, the manufacturer of the medication, the quantity of the drug, the expiration date or beyond-use date, the initials of the pharmacist, and the number of refills. Auxiliary labels may also be affixed to the container at the discretion of the pharmacist. The name, address, and phone number of the pharmacy must also be on the label.
- The pharmacist is responsible for the final check of the original prescription and for reviewing the patient profile, the accuracy of the drug and quantity used, and the medication container label.

Key Terms

adverse drug reaction (ADR) an unexpected negative consequence from taking a particular drug

allergy a hypersensitivity to a specific substance, manifested in a physiological disorder

auxiliary label a supplementary label added to a medication container at the discretion of the pharmacist that provides additional directions

brand name medically necessary a designation on the prescription by the physician indicating that a generic substitution by the pharmacist is not allowed; commonly seen on prescriptions for thyroid medication; often abbreviated as "brand necessary"

DEA number an identification number assigned by the Drug Enforcement Administration (DEA) to identify someone authorized to handle or prescribe controlled substances within the United States

dispense as written (DAW) a notation identical to "brand name medically necessary"; indicates on a prescription that a brand name drug is necessary or that a generic substitution is not allowed; DAW2 is often used to indicate patient preference for a brand name drug

drug seeker one who requests early refills on medications or gets prescriptions from multiple physicians or multiple pharmacies for controlled substances to obtain more than the typically prescribed amount of medication

drug utilization review (DUR) a procedure built into pharmacy software designed to help pharmacists check for potential medication errors in dosage, drug interactions, allergies, and so on

e-prescriptions prescriptions that are transmitted via electronic means

inscription the part of the prescription listing the medication or medications prescribed, including the drug names, strengths, and amounts

medication container label a label containing the dosage directions from the prescriber, affixed to the container of the dispensed medication; the pharmacy technician may use this copy to select the correct stock drug bottle and to fill the prescription

medication information sheet a leaflet printed from the prescription software and provided to patients on each medication dispensed; the technician may use this copy to select the correct stock drug bottle and fill the prescription

NPI number a unique National Provider Identifier for any healthcare provider involved in writing prescriptions or billing insurance for any healthcare-related service

out of stock (OOS) a medication not in stock in the pharmacy; a drug that must be specially ordered from a drug wholesaler

partial fill a supply dispensed to hold the patient until a new supply is received from the wholesaler; this practice is due to an insufficient inventory in the pharmacy, which prevents completely filling the prescription

patient profile a record kept by the pharmacy that lists a patient's identifying information, insurance information, medical and prescription history, and prescription preferences

prescription an order written by a qualified, licensed practitioner for a medication to be filled by a pharmacist to treat a patient's medical condition

prior authorization (PA) approval for coverage of a high-cost medication or a medication not on the insurer's approved formulary, obtained after a prescriber calls the insurer to justify the use of the drug; must be obtained before the drug is dispensed by the pharmacy to be covered by insurance

refill an approval by the prescriber to dispense the prescribed medication again without the need for a new prescription order

signa ("sig") the part of the prescription that indicates the directions for the patient to follow when taking the medication

subscription the part of the prescription that lists instructions to the pharmacist about dispensing the medication, including information about compounding or packaging instructions, labeling instructions, refill information, and information about the appropriateness of dispensing drug equivalencies

tablet splitter a device used to manually split or score tablets

tamper-resistant prescription pad (TRPP) a paper pad that is specifically designed to prevent copying, erasure, or alteration

unit dose a dosage unit that is individually labeled and packaged by the manufacturer in sealed foil and considered tamper-proof

unit of use a fixed number of dose units in a stock drug container, usually consisting of a month's supply of tablets or capsules, or 30 tablets or capsules

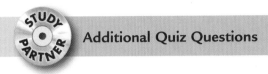
Checking Your Understanding

To check your comprehension of this chapter's key concepts, read the following multiple-choice questions and then record your answers on a separate sheet of paper. Write your answers as modeled in these examples: 1d; 2c; 3b; *etc.*

1. The pharmacy technician's duties with regard to Schedule II drugs include all of the following *except*
   a. receiving the prescription from the patient.
   b. entering the prescription information into the computerized patient profile.
   c. retrieving the drug from the secured storage area.
   d. dispensing the drug to the patient.

2. In a prescription, the signa is the
   a. signature of the prescriber.
   b. initials of the pharmacist.
   c. directions for the patient to follow.
   d. instructions to the pharmacist on dispensing the medication.

3. The symbol ℞ stands for the Latin word *recipere* and means
   a. "to give."
   b. "to take."
   c. "to prepare."
   d. "to mix."

4. A signature on a prescription for a Schedule II controlled substance
   a. may be stamped.
   b. must be handwritten in black ink.
   c. is not necessary if the prescription is faxed directly from the physician's office.
   d. may be that of the prescriber's agent, such as a nurse, physician assistant, or nurse practitioner.

5. A generic drug may be substituted for a brand name or proprietary drug provided the generic drug
   a. is the same color and shape as the brand name drug.
   b. has undergone clinical efficacy trials.
   c. is bioequivalent to the brand name or proprietary drug.
   d. is nontoxic.

6. Pharmacy personnel can check to see whether a DEA number has been falsified by
   a. looking up the number in the *FDA Online Orange Book*.
   b. performing a mathematical calculation.
   c. checking the number in *Drug Facts and Comparisons*.
   d. using a code to translate the number into an alphabetic form, which is the name of the prescriber.

7. Refills are commonly dispensed for a one-month supply of a Schedule III drug
   a. whenever the patient requests it.
   b. when approved by online claims processing to an insurer.
   c. no sooner than 21 days after the last refill.
   d. no sooner than 28 days after the last refill.

8. In all states, a pharmacy technician may
   a. receive a new prescription from a patient.
   b. take a new prescription over the phone and immediately transcribe it.
   c. counsel patients on medications when the pharmacist is busy.
   d. check another technician's work before dispensing the drug to the patient.

9. A Schedule III prescription may be refilled a maximum of
   a. once.
   b. twice.
   c. five times, or within six months.
   d. twelve times, or within one year.

10. For select high-risk drugs, the FDA requires
    a. auxiliary labels.
    b. a patient information sheet.
    c. a medication container label.
    d. a MedGuide.

11. For processing noncontrolled drugs to insurance, the technician will need the prescriber's
    a. NPI number.
    b. DEA number.
    c. state license number.
    d. medical office telephone number.

12. The term *DAW2* means
    a. a prescriber wants a medication to be dispensed as written.
    b. a patient requests a brand name to be dispensed.
    c. a patient requests a generic drug to be dispensed.
    d. a pharmacist is permitted to substitute a therapeutic equivalent drug.

13. Which of the following drugs requires special handling and processing?
    a. Accutane
    b. Bystolic
    c. Coreg
    d. doxycycline

14. A pharmacy technician may not
    a. place the medication label on the container.
    b. dispense Schedule III and Schedule IV medications.
    c. override a drug utilization review.
    d. discuss OTC label information with the patient.

15. The transfer warning "Caution: Federal law prohibits the transfer of this drug to any person other than the patient for whom it was prescribed" must, by law, appear on all
    a. C–II drugs only.
    b. controlled drugs.
    c. birth control pills.
    d. prescriptions.

Reinforcing Your Learning

To build on your understanding of the topics in this chapter, complete the following enrichment activities.

1. Determine which of the following is a valid DEA number for Dr. Barry Middleton:
   BM 6473218
   AM 1234563
   SM 1737622
   PM 5732459

2. Break into small groups and discuss how you would handle the receipt of a prescription for a controlled substance that you suspect is a forgery or belongs to a drug seeker. What indicators might point to suspicious behavior? What actions should be taken by pharmacy personnel? Share your group's observations and recommendations and compare your plans of action.

3. Find a partner to help you role-play several common community pharmacy scenarios. Begin by deciding who will assume the role of the pharmacy technician and who will be the patient. Then write a script for each of the following scenarios that reflects good communication and problem-solving skills.
   a. A prescribed medication that is not in stock in the pharmacy
   b. A prescribed medication that can only be a partial fill due to an insufficient amount in stock
   c. A prescribed medication that cannot be filled as written without a prior authorization
   d. A prescribed medication that cannot be filled due to the possibility of a serious interaction

4. Review the patient profile below and then answer the following questions.
   a. What essential information is missing from this patient profile?
   b. What allergies and drug reactions does the patient have?
   c. What known medical conditions does the patient have?
   d. What prescriptions and OTC medications is the patient currently taking?
   e. Should the customer's prescription be filled in a child-resistant container? Explain why or why not.
   f. Does the customer have prescription insurance? If so, then in whose name is this insurance held?

PATIENT PROFILE

Patient Name

Fisher   *Patrick*   *R.*
Last   First   Middle Initial

199 E. Church St.
Street or PO Box
Alpharetta   *GA*   *30005*
City   State   ZIP

Phone   Date of Birth
(__)__ ___   _____   □ Male
                    Month   Day   Year   □ Female

☒ Yes, I would like medication dispensed in a child-resistant container.
□ No, I do not want medication dispensed in a child-resistant container.

Medication Insurance	Card Holder Name	*Patrick Fisher*	
□ Yes	☒ Card Holder	□ Child	□ Disabled Dependent
☒ No	□ Spouse	□ Dependent Parent	□ Full Time Student

MEDICAL HISTORY

HEALTH
□ Angina
□ Anemia
☒ Arthritis
□ Asthma
□ Blood clotting disorders
□ High blood pressure
□ Breast feeding
□ Cancer
□ Diabetes
Other conditions _____

□ Epilepsy
□ Glaucoma
☒ Heart condition
□ Kidney disease
□ Liver disease
□ Lung disease
□ Parkinson disease
□ Pregnancy
□ Ulcers

ALLERGIES AND DRUG REACTIONS
□ No known drug allergies or reactions
□ Aspirin
□ Cephalosporins
□ Codeine
□ Erythromycin
□ Penicillin
□ Sulfa drugs
□ Tetracyclines
□ Xanthines
□ Other allergies/reactions _____

Prescription Medication(s) Being Taken
Ibuprofen 200 mg
Amlodipine 10 mg

OTC Medication(s) Currently Being Taken
Aleve

Would you like generic medication when possible? ☒ Yes □ No

Comments

Health information changes periodically. Please notify the pharmacy of any new medications, allergies, drug reactions, or health conditions.

Shania Tanguma _____ Signature *9-9-20IX* Date   □ I do not wish to provide this information.

Thinking on Your Feet

To gain practice in handling challenging situations in the workplace, consider the following real-world scenarios and then use the guiding questions to help you formulate your responses.

1. Abby Gee approaches you at the pharmacy counter and presents you with the following prescription:

```
MT. HOPE MEDICAL PARK
MY TOWN, USA  (305) 555-3591

                        DEA # _____
PT. NAME  Abby Gee          DATE  9-10-201X
ADDRESS _____     DOB _____
        _____

Rx    Nexium 40 mg
      Take 1 cap ac daily


REFILLS  Ø  TIMES
C. Janew
_____  M.D.  _____  M.D.
DISPENSE AS WRITTEN      SUBSTITUTE PERMITTED
```

   a. Are any essential items missing from the prescription? If so, what are these items?
   b. What medication has been prescribed? In what strength? In what amount?
   c. When should this drug be taken?
   d. Can generic pantoprazole be dispensed? Why or why not?

2. While you are servicing the drive-thru window customers, Tomas Riviera pulls up and hands you the following prescription to fill:

```
CANTERBURY GARDENS MEDICAL OFFICE
MARKHAM, IL  (606) 555-8310

                        DEA # _____
PT. NAME  Tomas Riviera      DATE _____
ADDRESS _____     DOB _____

Rx    Prednisone    QS
      Take AM       5 tabs day 1
                    3   "   2
                    2   "   3
                    1 tab "  4 and 5
REFILLS  Ø  TIMES
_____  M.D.  A Demomis  M.D.
DISPENSE AS WRITTEN      SUBSTITUTE PERMITTED
```

   a. Are any essential items missing from the prescription? If so, what are these items?
   b. What medication has been prescribed?

3. Mr. Rubbins, a regular customer, drops off the following prescription at the pharmacy counter while shopping in your store:

```
                    WELLSTAR MEDICAL OFFICE
                         ROSWELL, GA
                                   DEA # _____
    PT. NAME  H. R. Rubbins          DATE  11-24-201X
    ADDRESS _____        DOB _____
            _____

    Rx      Tylenol/Codeine No.4
            Take 1 prn pain q4-6 h
                            #30
    REFILLS  6  TIMES
    _____ M.D.  J. Jutten _____ M.D.
       DISPENSE AS WRITTEN        SUBSTITUTE PERMITTED
```

a. Are any essential items missing from the prescription? If so, what are these items?
b. What information is needed for this scheduled drug that is not needed for the prescriptions in exercises 1 and 2 of this section?
c. What information is incorrect on this Rx?

Acquiring Field Knowledge

To expand your knowledge of pharmacy practice, explore the following online activities that focus on research and information retrieval.

Reminder: As you navigate the Internet, remember to exercise caution and good judgment when evaluating information. A thoughtful review of online text should take into consideration the following factors: the creator and sponsors of the website, the intended audience, the credentials of the authors and contributors, the reliability and validity of the posted information, the frequency of updates to the site, and the ease of navigation for a range of user skill levels.

1. Information about potential drug interactions is available on many community pharmacy websites. To view an example, visit www.paradigmcollege .net/pharmpractice5e/walgreens. Hover over the Pharmacy and Health tab and then scroll down to Health Information and click on this link. Look under the Health Center heading and click on Check Drug Interactions. Follow the prompts to determine if there is a drug–drug interaction between the following medications:

   - Zocor and amiodarone
   - Protonix and Plavix
   - Bactrim DS and warfarin

2. Research the drug thalidomide and the controversy surrounding its use in the early 1960s. Then visit www.paradigmcollege .net/pharmpractice5e/STEPS to gain an understanding of the regulatory organization's role in this pivotal event. In light of this history, what boxed warning appears on Thalomid today? What is the S.T.E.P.S. program, and why was it initiated? What is the pharmacy's role in the S.T.E.P.S. program? Use your research findings to write a brief history of the thalidomide crisis and its impact on the marketing and dispensing of the drug today.

3. Electronic prescribing, commonly known as *e-prescribing*, is a major trend in community pharmacy practice. To obtain current information on the use of e-prescribing in the United States, visit www.paradigmcollege.net/pharmpractice5e/surescripts and click on the "E-Prescribing" tab in the top bar. Then click on the link "See your state's progress report" at the bottom of the screen. Next, hover over the state in which you practice to show capsule information on the status of e-prescribing in your state. Using this information, address the following questions: Where does your state rank in e-prescribing? How many physicians and pharmacies are enrolled in e-prescriptions? What percentage of patients have insurance beneficiary and history information available?

Sampling the Certification Exam

To provide you with practice for the Certification Exam, read the following questions that have been patterned after the test format and then record your answers on a separate sheet of paper. Write your answers as modeled in these examples: 1d; 2c; 3b; *etc.*

1. Which of the following pieces of information is *not* legally required on a prescription?
   a. prescriber's name
   b. date written
   c. responsible party for payment
   d. refill information

2. What is required on a controlled substance prescription for OxyContin that is *not* needed for a prescription written for tramadol?
   a. DEA number
   b. physician's signature
   c. address of physician
   d. date written

3. A pharmacy technician is filling a prescription for eyedrops that reads "2 gtt OU t.i.d." How many drops will the patient use a day?
   a. 12 gtt
   b. 8 gtt
   c. 6 gtt
   d. 3 gtt

4. How often should a patient's allergy information be updated?
   a. only at the patient's first visit
   b. once a year
   c. never
   d. at every visit with a new prescription

5. The following prescription is received at the pharmacy:

   Zithromax 200 mg tablets
   Disp: 5
   Sig. ii stat then i PO daily × 4D

   What is wrong with the prescription?
   a. The drug should be taken for 10 days total and needs to be written for 11 tablets.
   b. The drug is only available intravenously (IV) and given in a hospital.
   c. The drug is not available in this strength.
   d. The drug is only available as a capsule and must be ordered that way.

6. A prescription for Advair Diskus is received with the sig: 1 b.i.d. What is the appropriate direction to type on the label?
   a. Take one dose every 12 hours.
   b. Inhale one dose two times a day as needed.
   c. Inhale one puff by mouth two times a day.
   d. Take one capsule twice a day.

7. A prescription for Cortisporin reads "AU." What do you type on the label?
   a. both ears
   b. both eyes
   c. right eye
   d. right ear

8. Which of the following is exempt from the Poison Prevention Packaging Act of 1970?
   a. hormone replacement therapy
   b. OTC iron tablets
   c. sublingual nitroglycerin tablets
   d. potassium chloride tablets

9. A technician may be suspicious of a forged prescription for Vicodin if he or she notices
   a. no date on the written prescription.
   b. no DEA number on the written prescription.
   c. the quantity has been changed.
   d. the Rx is written by an oncology physician.

10. To minimize the risk of medication errors, the technician should add what information to the original prescription upon its receipt?
    a. the patient's primary insurance provider
    b. the patient's address
    c. the patient's cell phone number
    d. the patient's date of birth

The Business of Community Pharmacy

7

Learning Objectives

- Understand the roles, responsibilities, and limitations of the pharmacy technician in the sale of over-the-counter drugs, dietary supplements, and medical supplies, especially for patients with diabetes.

- Accurately process special over-the-counter sales, such as Schedule V cough syrups, decongestants containing pseudoephedrine, and emergency contraceptives.

- Understand the importance of necessary cash register management functions.

- Identify procedures for managing the purchasing, receiving, and posting of drug inventory, including controlled substances.

- Understand mathematical principles in calculating markup, discounts, and average wholesale price.

- Define and explain the terms *pharmacy benefits manager*, *deductible*, *co-payment*, *coinsurance*, *tiered co-pay*, and *prior authorization*.

- Discuss drug insurance coverage for private, Medicaid, Tricare, and Medicare plans.

- Know how to process a workers' compensation insurance claim.

- Define the term *coordination of benefits*.

- List options for lower prescription costs for uninsured patients.

- Identify the necessary insurance information needed to process online claims for prescription drugs.

- Calculate days' supply of medication for online billing.

- Resolve problems with online claims processing, audits, and charge-backs.

Preview chapter terms and definitions.

A side from assisting pharmacists in serving the healthcare needs of patients, pharmacy technicians are also responsible for performing several business tasks that are vital to the daily operation of a community pharmacy. This chapter provides an overview of these business functions, including the operation of a cash register, computer system (including a bar-code scanner), and automated dispensing and counting devices; the assistance of customers in the purchase of over-the-counter (OTC) drugs and various products; the online billing of third-party insurance; and the management of inventory. To effectively complete these tasks, technicians need to have an understanding of basic math principles as well as business math concepts such as markup, discount, and average wholesale price (AWP). Learning these skills not only gives technicians a view into the business operations of a community pharmacy but also gives them a vested interest in the profitability of their workplace.

Nonprescription Sales

Community pharmacies are typically organized into two distinct areas: a back area that contains prescription medications and other related items and a front area that houses over-the-counter (OTC) drugs, dietary supplements, medical supplies, and other merchandise. These OTC drugs, or nonprescription products, are commonly stocked by drug class or by indication, such as pain relievers, fever reducers, allergy medicine, contraceptive products (condoms, jellies), first-aid care, antacids, laxatives, foot care products, and so on. The concept of self-service for nonprescription products and other merchandise was popularized by Walgreens in 1960, with other retailers adopting this business model shortly thereafter. This concept required more shelf space for a wider variety of products. Today's community pharmacies offer many brand name and generic OTC drugs as well as vitamins, herbs, and dietary supplements in a variety of package sizes. Although self-service has become a popular business model for retailers, customer service remains paramount to the success of a community pharmacy. The pharmacy technician plays a major role in assisting customers in locating products in the front area of the pharmacy and in bringing any questions they may have on OTC drug selection, dose, and side effects or interactions to the attention of the pharmacist.

Over-the-Counter Drugs

An **over-the-counter (OTC) drug** is one that is approved for sale without a prescription. The Food and Drug Administration (FDA) approves and regulates OTC drugs only after the drug and dosage are generally recognized as *safe and effective* for the approved indication when taken according to labeled directions. A broad definition of nonprescription products includes not only OTC drugs but also vitamins, minerals, herbal medications, and other products that are sometimes classified as dietary supplements.

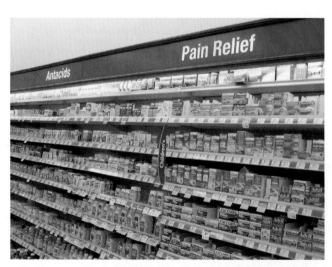

OTC medications are commonly stocked by indication, such as pain relief, antacids, and so on.

Common OTC drugs are listed in Table 7.1. Many of these popular OTC drugs, such as hydrocortisone and ibuprofen, once required a prescription. Although OTC medications may be purchased without a prescription, the active ingredients are often the same as those found in higher-strength prescription formulations. For example, ibuprofen is available in an OTC strength of 200 mg, whereas the prescription strengths are 400 mg, 600 mg, and 800 mg. Pharmacy technicians should also be aware that a few refrigerated drugs located in the back area—in particular, fast-acting regular insulins such as Novolin and Humulin—can also be sold to a patient with or without a prescription.

TABLE 7.1 Common OTC Drugs and Their Indications

Brand Name	Generic Name	Indication(s)
Advil/Motrin	Ibuprofen	Headache, pain
Afrin	Oxymetazoline	Nasal decongestant
Aleve	Naproxen	Headache, pain
Allegra	Fexofenadine	Allergy
Benadryl	Diphenhydramine	Allergy
Claritin	Loratadine	Allergy
Cortizone-10	Hydrocortisone	Itching, inflammation
Imodium	Loperamide	Diarrhea, irritable bowel syndrome
Lotrimin	Clotrimazole	Topical antifungal
Monistat	Miconazole	Vaginal antifungal
Mucinex	Guaifenesin	Expectorant
Neosporin	Triple antibiotic	Topical anti-infective
Prevacid	Lansoprazole	Heartburn
Prilosec	Omeprazole	Heartburn
Zantac	Ranitidine	Heartburn
Zyrtec	Cetirizine	Allergy

At times, the pharmacy technician may receive a prescription for an OTC medication; in most cases, the drug will not be covered by insurance. However, in some cases, such as with pediatric cough, cold, and allergy medicines, insurance may cover the prescribed OTC drug. Some pharmacies elect to fill such a prescription to increase the number of prescriptions dispensed and to provide an opportunity for the patient to receive counseling on the appropriate use of the product. If the OTC drug is on sale, the pharmacy technician should direct the patient to the lower-priced OTC purchase.

Benefits of OTC Drugs Because OTC drugs can be purchased in many retail outlets as well as in the pharmacy, customers are purchasing these products for self-administration at an ever-increasing rate. The increase in the use of OTC drugs is related to a number of factors, including the increased cost and inconvenience of physician visits, the rising cost of prescription medications, and the lack of health or drug insurance coverage. With OTC products, patients can obtain medications to treat symptoms of illness or to maintain health. This self-medication practice, however, places a high importance on product labeling.

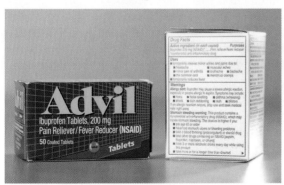

The FDA requires complete labeling for the safe and effective self-medication use of all OTC products.

Labeling of OTC Products Manufacturers of OTC products must include on their labels all information necessary for the safe and effective use of the products by consumers. Therefore, the language on each product label must be both understandable and readable. Such information should include active ingredients, inactive ingredients (in case of an allergic reaction), purpose or use of the product, dosage and frequency of administration for different age-groups, any precautions or warnings, any special storage requirements, and the product's expiration date. Manufacturers typically provide a toll-free number as well, in the event that consumers have a question or concern.

Safety Note

Most OTC drugs should be used for a limited time, which is typically defined as seven days or less.

Consumer Precautions Consumers using OTC drugs need to remember that these products should be used for a restricted period (usually less than seven days) for self-limiting indications such as a cold or cough, unless directed by a physician. For example, a physician may direct an adult patient to take a baby aspirin on a long-term daily basis in order to lower a patient's risk of heart disease. If the pharmacist cannot determine the source of a self-limited problem, or if the patient has self-medicated with an OTC drug for seven or more days, the patient should be referred to the appropriate healthcare professional.

The consumer must also remember that no drug, even an OTC product, is completely safe and without side effects or adverse reactions. OTC cough medicines, for example, can be misused if the dosage recommended by the manufacturer is exceeded. In fact, the use of OTC cough and cold products for children under age six is strongly discouraged by the FDA because the risk of adverse reactions is greater than the benefit. OTC products that contain the cough suppressant dextromethorphan (DM) may cause auditory and visual hallucinations in high doses. Because DM products have a history of abuse among adolescents, consumers must be age 18 or older to buy these products and must provide an ID to pharmacy personnel upon purchase.

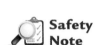

Safety Note

The FDA discourages the use of OTC cough and cold products for children under age six.

OTC Products and Pharmacy Personnel When selecting a product, customers often seek the advice of pharmacy personnel. With that in mind, pharmacists and pharmacy technicians should be aware of their responsibilities in the sale of these OTC products.

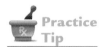

Practice Tip

Pharmacy technicians should not counsel patients about the use of OTC products without the approval of the pharmacist.

Role of the Pharmacist Customers often seek the counsel of the pharmacist to help them choose an appropriate product. For example, a pharmacist may need to identify and select a sugar-free cough syrup for a young patient who is diabetic, a laxative for a pregnant patient who is taking a prenatal vitamin and iron, or an appropriate nasal decongestant for a patient with high blood pressure. The pharmacy technician's support allows the pharmacist to take the necessary time away from prescription-filling duties to assess the problem, make an appropriate drug product selection, and counsel the patient. Only pharmacists can address questions about drug product selection, indications, dosage and administration, expected therapeutic effect, side effects, contraindications, and interactions.

Role of the Pharmacy Technician OTC drugs are becoming an increasingly important part of the technician's responsibilities. Technicians often carry out such functions as selling and stocking OTC products, ordering or rearranging inventory, and removing stock when the shelf life has expired or a product is recalled. Customers may also approach technicians with questions about OTC products, but technicians should direct them to the pharmacist for questions about any of the topics listed at the end of the Role of the Pharmacist section above.

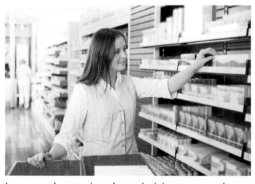

In many pharmacies, the technician may need to restock the OTC shelves or check for expiration dates.

Sale of Certain OTC Products Pharmacy personnel need to be aware that certain OTC products have specific restrictions and procedures that must be followed during consumer purchase. These products include Schedule V drugs, drugs that contain pseudoephedrine and ephedrine, and emergency contraceptives.

Schedule V Drugs A **Schedule V drug** is a medication with a low potential for abuse and a limited potential for creating physical or psychological dependence. A common example of a Schedule V medication is a cough medication containing codeine. Although federal law allows the dispensing of Schedule V medications without a prescription, there are restrictions and requirements for their sale, as listed below:

- The drugs must be stored behind the counter, in the prescription area.
- The amount of cough syrups sold to a single customer is generally limited to a specific volume (such as 120 fl oz or 4 fl oz) within a 48-hour period.
- Only a pharmacist (or the pharmacy technician under direct supervision) can make the sale.
- The purchaser must be 18 years of age and have proof of identity.

Safety Note

Some states require a signed prescription in order to dispense a Schedule V drug. The pharmacy technician must follow the appropriate state laws.

A state—and even an individual pharmacy—may have more stringent laws for Schedule V drugs than the federal government. For example, some states require a signed prescription from a licensed healthcare professional for Schedule V drugs. Other state boards of pharmacy (Minnesota, for example) have reclassified Schedule V codeine-containing cough syrups as Schedule III and follow Drug Enforcement Administration (DEA) limitations (five refills or six months from original date of prescription). In Texas, a Schedule V drug (including refills) is treated like a Schedule III or IV drug.

Individual pharmacies have also instituted more stringent protocols for the dispensing of Schedule V drugs. Some pharmacies, for example, require a signed prescription from a physician—even if state guidelines don't require one—to discourage potential drug abuse. Therefore, because of these varying regulations, pharmacy personnel must be sure to check the laws in their state of practice as well as the protocol outlined in their facility's policy for guidance on Schedule V drugs.

If the sale of an OTC drug that is also a Schedule V drug is allowed, then the pharmacy technician or the pharmacist must record all sales in a record book. This record must include the following information:

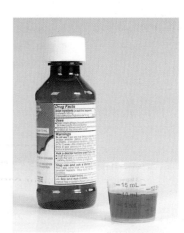

Most codeine-containing cough syrups are classified as Schedule V drugs and are stored behind the counter. State laws require written documentation before their sale without a prescription.

- name and address of the purchaser
- date of birth of the purchaser
- date of purchase
- name and quantity of the Schedule V drug sold
- name and initials of the pharmacist handling or approving the sale

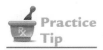

Practice Tip

Pharmacy technicians should be familiar with the Combat Methamphetamine Epidemic Act of 2005 and the protocol that must be followed when dispensing drugs containing pseudoephedrine and ephedrine. For a review of these regulations, see Chapter 2.

Drugs That Contain Pseudoephedrine and Ephedrine The federal government and many states have passed legislation restricting the access and sale of OTC products that contain pseudoephedrine and ephedrine. These products include cold and sinus medications, ephedrine-containing tablets, and metered-dose inhalers (MDIs) for the treatment of asthma. These restrictions have been put in place because the common ingredients in these medications have been used as raw products in the illegal manufacture of methamphetamine. Consequently, all products containing pseudoephedrine and ephedrine must be stocked behind the prescription counter. In addition, many states limit the purchase of these products to "prescription only," and several states require that the sale be conducted by pharmacists only. Mandated limits determine how many "units" of these drugs can be legally purchased at one time at one

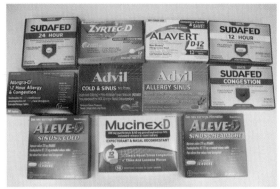

OTC products that contain pseudoephedrine must be stored in the prescription area, and certain conditions must be met before a sale is completed.

location. The limits for pseudoephedrine are 3.6 grams (maximum purchase in one day) and 9 grams (maximum purchase in 30 days).

The sale of pseudoephedrine or ephedrine requires written (or computerized) documentation such as a logbook similar to that for Schedule V drugs (see Figure 7.1). The documentation must be kept for a minimum of two years. The information required prior to the sale of these products includes:

- a validated and current photo ID, which is usually a driver's license; the number may be entered or the license scanned at the point of sale
- proof that the customer is age 18 or older
- date and time of purchase
- product being purchased
- the street address, state, and ZIP code of the customer
- the customer's signature in the logbook or electronically

Pharmacists and pharmacy technicians should also be aware of a practice called **smurfing**, which is when a patient is paid cash by an individual to illegally purchase pseudoephedrine from one or more pharmacies. These drugs are not for personal use but are illegally sold to individuals whose intent is to manufacture and sell methamphetamine. If three or four patients come into the pharmacy at one time to purchase such products, the pharmacist or technician should be suspicious and may elect to refuse the sale. Pharmacy personnel should be aware that there are limits on the amount of pseudoephedrine that can be sold per month. Therefore, it is critical that they are vigilant on tracking the sale of pseudoephedrine products, which may

FIGURE 7.1
Form for Recording Sales of Restricted Products Containing Pseudoephedrine

Pseudoephedrine Products Dispensing Record							
Purchaser's Name	Driver's License Number	Purchaser's Address	Date of Purchase	Product Name	Quantity Purchased	Dispensed by (Initials)	Purchaser's Signature

include the verification of medical need by the pharmacist. Violations of the state or federal law may result in the loss of the pharmacist's license or the business license of the pharmacy.

Emergency Contraceptives It has been estimated that up to 10% of women of child-bearing age may need emergency contraceptives sometime during their lives. Plan B and Next Choice are common examples of an emergency contraceptive drug that can be dispensed in most states without a prescription. However, federal laws require that the patient (or the patient's representative) be over age 17 (lowered from age 18 in 2009) in order to purchase the drug. Underage patients require a written prescription from a licensed prescriber.

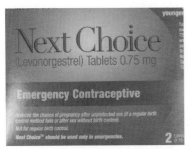

The "morning-after" pill is available to those over the age of 17 without a prescription. The pharmacist should counsel the patient on its proper use and side effects.

All patients purchasing Plan B should be counseled by the pharmacist on the appropriate use and expected side effects of this drug. The two-dose drug must be taken within 72 hours of unprotected sexual intercourse; the sooner the drug is taken the more effective it is. Efficacy is 75% to 90%. Some nausea may be expected with the high-dose hormone pills. As mentioned in Chapter 6, some pharmacists may object to selling drugs for emergency contraception on religious grounds; each state has laws governing actions for this moral dilemma.

Dietary Supplements

A **dietary supplement** can be a vitamin or mineral or an herbal product such as ginger, garlic, saw palmetto, glucosamine, or soy. Indications for some common dietary supplements are listed in Table 7.2 on the following page. Dietary supplements are sold in retail outlets and in health and wellness stores, as well as in pharmacies. Most consumers do not realize that dietary supplements are not regulated by the FDA in the same stringent manner as are OTC drugs. Scientific studies on the efficacy of these products are usually quite limited.

As you learned in Chapter 2, dietary supplements are primarily regulated by the Dietary Supplement Health and Education Act (DSHEA). The FDA does not approve dietary supplements; however, they must be *safe and accurately labeled*. In general, the label of a dietary supplement indicates "serving size" rather than dose and, compared with an OTC drug, offers limited information about the product. In fact, the amount of active ingredient in the supplement may not always match the labeled amount because of inconsistencies in quality control or product contamination. If the label contains an indication that has not been approved by the FDA, the FDA can act to remove the drug from the market. The FDA can also remove any dietary supplement that is deemed dangerous, which has occurred in the past with several "diet pills." The misuse of androgenic hormones as dietary supplements by amateur and professional athletes despite the health concerns associated with this practice is another example of the danger of unregulated products. As with the use of other OTC medications, it is important that the pharmacy technician not counsel customers regarding the appropriate use of dietary supplements unless directed to do so by the pharmacist.

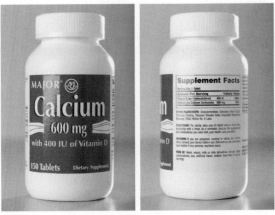

All vitamins and minerals are considered dietary supplements. However, the labels on these supplements provide less consumer information than the labels required for OTC drugs.

TABLE 7.2   Indications for Common Dietary Supplements

Dietary Supplement	Indication(s)
Calcium and vitamin D	Improves bone strength
Echinacea	Boosts the immune system
Garlic	Has an antibacterial and antiviral action; maintains healthy cholesterol
Ginger	Treats nausea, motion sickness, and morning sickness
Gingko	Improves memory; treats tinnitus and peripheral vascular disease
Glucosamine/chondroitin	Lessens joint pain
Melatonin	Treats insomnia, especially in shift workers or time zone travelers
Policosanol	Maintains healthy cholesterol levels
Omega-3 fatty acids (fish oil)	Lowers triglyceride levels
Red yeast rice	Maintains healthy cholesterol levels
Saw palmetto	Treats benign prostatic hypertrophy (BPH)
St. John's wort	Treats mild depression
Vitamin C	Treats the common cold
Zinc	Boosts the immune system; helps in the treatment of the common cold and wound healing

Medical Supplies

A community pharmacy sells disposable and durable medical supplies that may be needed by customers and their families. Some community pharmacies specialize in the sale or rental of **durable medical equipment (DME)**. DME includes hospital beds, wheelchairs, canes, walkers, crutches, prosthetics, orthotics, blood glucose meters, and so on. **Nondurable medical supplies** are consumable, disposable items that can only be used by one patient for a specific purpose; examples include diabetic supplies such as test strips and lancets.

Some pharmacies are licensed as medical suppliers, with the ability to provide direct Medicare Part B insurance coverage for many medical supplies and drugs for patients over age 65. These pharmacies must meet quality standards and accreditation requirements as set by the Centers for Medicare and Medicaid Services (CMS). In addition to DME equipment, medical and diabetic supplies, and nebulizer drugs, the pharmacy may also cover parenteral and enteral nutrition, home dialysis supplies, expensive injectable drugs for anemia and transfusion medicine, and drugs used for nausea and vomiting caused by chemotherapy.

Supplies to Manage Diabetes   The proper use of diabetic supplies is important in monitoring the blood glucose levels of a patient with diabetes. Maintaining these levels within an acceptable range delays or minimizes the development of long-term complications of diabetes and improves both the quality of life and life expectancy of the patient. Matching the specific needs of the patient with the proper equipment and supplies is an important responsibility of the pharmacist. In fact, many pharmacists acquire specialty training and certifications in this particular area. Pharmacy techni-

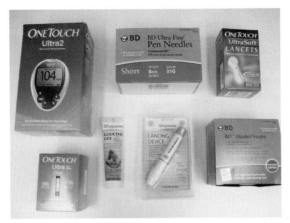

A patient who is diabetic is a frequent customer in the community pharmacy, with needs for glucose tablets and gel, lancets, alcohol wipes, and other supplies.

cians, as well, can now complete training, pass an examination, and become certified in patient education for diabetic patients. Such skills are considered valuable within the pharmacy and may enhance hourly pay. Even without this specialty training, technicians in community pharmacy are often called upon to assist patients in locating diabetic supplies, such as a glucometer, insulin syringes, pen needles, test strips, lancets, and alcohol wipes for skin cleansing.

Glucometer A glucometer, a DME device that measures blood glucose levels in diabetic patients, is available from several manufacturers in different sizes. Glucometers vary as to the amount of blood needed to make a reading, the time period necessary to provide the results of a reading, the memory capacity, and the ability to interface with a computer. These devices often can be purchased with a generous rebate that negates a majority of the original purchase price. Companies frequently upgrade their glucometers, so it is important for both the pharmacist and the technician to keep abreast of product changes.

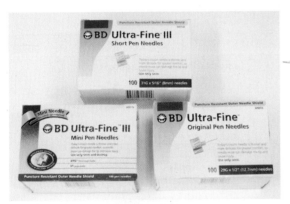

The technician can assist the patient who is diabetic in selecting the correct size and gauge of insulin needles.

Insulin Syringes Some patients who are diabetic require insulin syringes to self-administer their daily insulin shots. The policy for the sale of insulin syringes in a community pharmacy may vary by state in order to prevent diversion to potential illegal drug administration. Many pharmacies have a policy that no insulin syringes can be sold unless the patient is a proven diabetic or known customer of the pharmacy.

Insulin syringes and needles come in different sizes. Syringes are generally available in 0.3 mL, 0.5 mL, and 1 mL sizes depending on the dosage of the insulin prescribed. Instead of being marked in milliliters, the insulin syringe is marked in units in order to make the insulin administration more accurate. Most needles are "short" for easier and less painful injection under the skin rather than in muscle. Insulin syringes have needles already attached; the more portable insulin pens require a separate purchase of pen needles. As discussed in Chapter 4, the higher the gauge number of the needle, the smaller the width of the needle, potentially resulting in less pain at the injection site.

Pen Needles Needles for insulin pens are available in smaller sizes (½ inch or less in length) and with a needle gauge from 29 to 32. Needles are commercially available as original (12.7 mm or ½ inch), short (8 mm or ⅓ inch), mini (6 mm or ¼ inch, 5 mm or ⅕ inch), and nano (4 mm or ⅙ inch). The shortest needle with the least pain would be the 4 mm, 32-gauge needle to accompany the insulin pen.

Test Strips, Lancets, and Alcohol Wipes Disposable test strips are needed with the glucometer to test a diabetic patient's blood glucose levels. A test strip is the piece of paper on which the patient places a drop of blood after swabbing his or her finger and piercing it with a lancet or skin-piercing device. The test strip is then put into the glucometer for a blood glucose reading. Test strips are machine-specific and must be matched for the type of glucometer that the patient is using. Some bottles of test strips come with a computer chip (lot number) that must be inserted in the glucometer. Failure to replace this chip with a new bottle (different lot number) of test strips will lead to an error in the blood glucose readings. Test strips may be used from once daily up to six times daily and can be expensive if the patient does not have insurance coverage. A store brand glucometer and test strips will often result in a 50% savings to the patient. Prior to sale, the pharmacy technician should check the expiration date of the strips.

Insurance Coverage for Diabetic Supplies Insulin syringes and other diabetic supplies are sometimes covered by drug insurance or Medicare Part B if a prescription is written by the physician. If a patient is going to apply insurance coverage to the purchase of diabetic medical supplies, then it is important that the patient have a prescription from the prescriber indicating the ICD-9 (or ICD-10) diagnosis code and frequency of daily insulin injections and blood glucose testing. A **certificate of medical necessity** for diabetic supplies for each patient may need to be completed and signed by the prescriber (see Figure 7.2).

FIGURE 7.2
Certificate of Medical Necessity

If a physician writes a prescription and completes a certificate of medical necessity, then the cost of diabetic supplies may be partially covered by Medicare Part B or prescription insurance for some patients.

Patient Demographics	
Select Type of Diabetes ☐ Type 1 IDDM, Insulin-Dependent ☐ Type 2 NIDDM, Noninsulin-Dependent ☐ Type 2 NIDDMIR, Requires Insulin	**Indicates Diabetes Diagnosis** ICD-9 _ _ _ . _ _ ICD-9 _ _ _ . _ _ Type 1 Diabetic, ICD-9 must end in odd number. Type 2 Diabetic, ICD-9 must end in even number.

Number of Tests/Day	Required Supplies		
	Number of Test Strips	Number of Lancets	Healthcare Orders
☐ 1			
☐ 2			
☐ 3			____ test strips
☐ 4			____ lancets
☐ 5			____ glucometer(s)
☐ 6			____ lancet skin piercing device(s)
☐ 7			____ bottle(s) of control solution
☐ 8			
☐ 9			
☐ 10			
☐ 11			
☐ 12			
Provider Demographics with Date and Signature			

Test Kits In addition to blood glucose testing supplies, patients come to the pharmacy to purchase any number of test kits to help them monitor their health conditions. Some conditions that can be determined with these kits include:

- pregnancy
- ovulation cycle
- bladder infection
- high cholesterol
- illegal drug use
- human immunodeficiency virus (HIV) infection

The latter category—a test kit for HIV infection—is a relatively recent product. The increased availability and accessibility of an OTC test kit for HIV will hopefully result in the identification of an estimated 240,000 individuals who are unaware that they are infected with the virus. The FDA-approved test kit is called OraQuick and can be used at home to detect the presence or absence of the virus in the saliva. The mouth is swabbed and results are known within 20 minutes. Consumers should keep in mind that the test is not 100% accurate. It will rarely miss someone who is not carrying the virus but may miss 1 out of 12 patients infected with HIV. Patients who test positive on the OTC test must see their primary care providers for confirmatory testing. The manufacturer also provides a toll-free phone number for individuals to use in order to discuss their results with a trained staff member or to get a referral to a local center.

Occasionally, the pharmacy may need to special order a test kit for a customer. The pharmacy technician can help select and sell a test kit and can help the patient understand the kit's instructions.

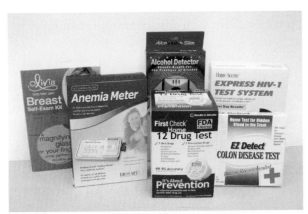

A typical community pharmacy sells many kinds of test kits. The pharmacy technician can assist the customer in selecting the best product to meet his or her needs.

General Medical Supplies Customers purchase several types of general medical supplies from a community pharmacy, and the pharmacy technician also assists with these transactions. Parents may need to purchase thermometers to check for fevers in their children. Patients with high blood pressure may need to purchase a sphygmomanometer for home use; the results can be recorded and brought to the physician's office on the next visit. Patients with asthma may need a spacer device to deliver inhaled medication more accurately or a peak flow meter to measure their expirations and assess severity of symptoms or benefit of therapy. Others may need wrist splints, back braces, bathroom accessories, nebulizer tubing and masks, and so on. Customers also need other disposable supplies such as bandages, gauze pads, adhesive tape, hydrogen peroxide, or isopropyl or rubbing alcohol to attend to their first-aid needs.

Automation in the Pharmacy

Automation plays an essential role in the everyday practice of community pharmacy. Computers, cash registers, bar code scanners, scales, and robotics are all examples of equipment that must be used and mastered by the pharmacy technician.

Computers

A **computer** is an electronic device used for inputting, storing, processing, and/or outputting information. In the community pharmacy, a computer is a critical tool needed for the safe and efficient dispensing of prescriptions and online billing. Consequently, pharmacy technicians need to have a working knowledge of computer hardware and basic keyboarding competency (minimum of 30 words per minute) in order to effectively perform their job responsibilities. Because software is often pharmacy-specific, technicians must learn their individual pharmacy's program during on-the-job training.

Computer Hardware In most small, independent pharmacies, the computer is a **smart terminal** that contains its own storage and processing capabilities. In larger pharmacies, including most drug chains, the technician or pharmacist may work at a **dumb terminal**, a computer device that contains a keyboard and a monitor but does not contain its own storage and processing capabilities. The terminal is connected to a **remote computer**—often a minicomputer or a mainframe at the company headquarters or home office—that stores and processes data such as patient information, prescription history, and insurance coverage.

Computer Software The software is designed to help the pharmacy technician process the prescription with both speed and accuracy. Pharmacy software systems vary widely among pharmacies, but most facilities use a software program application that allows one to enter, retrieve, and query patient records. This type of software is referred to as a database management system.

 Safety Note

Many pharmacy computer systems contain features that automatically warn of possible allergic reactions or adverse food or drug interactions based on information in the patient profile and on a database of known contraindications for given medications.

Capabilities of DBMS A **database management system (DBMS)** typically contains the patient profile, physician database, pharmacy drug inventory, and a directory of prescribers and insurance plans. For the patient profile, the system stores demographic, insurance, and prescription information on every patient. The DBMS allows the technician to scan a written prescription and enter new prescription information or retrieve refill information. Care must be taken to identify the correct patient, not only by name but also by date of birth.

Often the DBMS software is menu-driven or Windows-based, allowing the technician to choose fields or functions easily from a menu of options on the screen by typing a single keystroke or function key on the keyboard. The fields of information can be sorted or queried to meet the needs of the pharmacy or drug chain and may include the patient's name, address, phone number, and date of birth; the prescription's number, drug name, National Drug Code (NDC) number, dosage and quantity of drug, and number of refills; and the prescriber's name, address, phone number, and DEA number. Many systems also contain automatic warnings about possible allergic or other adverse reactions as part of the drug utilization review (DUR). These automatically generated warnings provide the pharmacist with an opportunity to review the prescriptions and the profile to minimize medication errors. Some software applications even provide a picture or description of the medication for a final visual check by the pharmacist in order to avoid medication errors.

Most of these database systems also print medication container labels and patient information sheets, and some specially designed systems are capable of tracking expenses and inventory reports, generating reports concerning controlled substances or patient insurance, performing special dosing calculations, and retrieving medical and pharmacy literature.

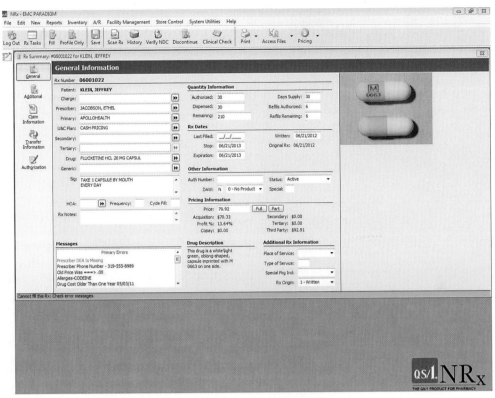

On-screen entry of patient and prescription data via a database management system (DBMS) is a valuable tool used by the pharmacy technician to easily and accurately process prescriptions.

Operation of DBMS A pharmacy software system accesses insurance plans via telecommunications, or linkups, to a remote computer via telephone lines, digital subscriber line (DSL), cable, or wireless connections in order to perform "real time" online billing. Wireless communications involve the transmission of data signals through the air via transmitters, receivers, and, often, cable and satellites. Wireless communications are critical for determining patient eligibility and online processing of prescription claims (discussed later in this chapter). Links to online insurance plans may also warn of potential errors with prescriptions previously dispensed at another pharmacy.

Because computers occasionally break down and are susceptible to such problems as power failures and surges, copies, or backups, of all data should be made by the pharmacist at regular intervals. A pharmacy may use a CD, a magnetic tape backup device, or remote storage to back up its prescription records, usually on a daily basis. Some computer systems automatically store prescription data.

Cash Register Management

In a community pharmacy, the pharmacy technician is often responsible for collecting payment that the patient owes at the point of sale (POS) to cover the cost of prescriptions and OTC drugs, vitamins, herbs, dietary supplements, medical supplies, and other store merchandise. The procedures for cash register management differ with each pharmacy. In larger pharmacies with multiple pharmacists, pharmacy technicians, and cash registers, it is not uncommon to have a sign-on and password code to assist in reconciling the receipts at the end of the day or shift. These pharmacies may also use bar-code scanning technology in concert with the cash register. The medication information

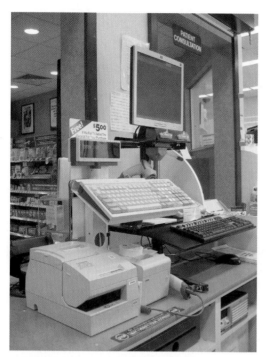

The workstation of the pharmacy technician often consists of a bar-code scanner, cash register, computer, and telephone.

sheet, as well as any nonprescription merchandise, can be scanned for pricing. When a prescription is scanned, the computer system may automatically prompt the technician to offer the patient counseling by the pharmacist. (Often, the pharmacist makes a note on the medication information sheet to initiate patient counseling.) Scanning of selected OTC items, such as pseudoephedrine products, Schedule V cough syrups, and contraceptive drugs (as discussed earlier), prompts a request for additional information from the patient, such as proof of age and identification to comply with federal and state laws. Finally, if the item is nonprescription, a sales tax is usually added.

Payment Options Customers may pay for prescriptions and other merchandise using cash, check, and various cards (including credit card, debit card, Flex card, and gift card). Regardless of the form of payment, the pharmacy technician should always present a **receipt**, or proof-of-purchase printout, at the conclusion of the purchase. Each payment option has a unique processing method; these payment methods are outlined in a pharmacy's training program.

Cash Cash transactions are fairly straightforward. The cash register usually calculates the amount of change needed. A given amount of change (varying with the size of the pharmacy) is provided at the start of the business day. Large bills, such as $50 and $100 bills, are usually placed under the change drawer to minimize mix-ups. The technician must become proficient in identifying counterfeit bills in denominations greater than $20.

Personal Check Some patients may elect to pay for their pharmacy purchases with a personal check. Procedures differ depending on the pharmacy. If the patient is not recognized as a regular customer, then the technician may need to ask for identification, such as a driver's license, and to transfer that information to the check. The amount of the check and the signature should always be verified. Checks written for a large amount (commonly greater than $100) may require documenting the driver's license number and/or approval of the store manager. In a nonautomated system, it is possible for the pharmacy to receive a check with insufficient funds to cover the bill. Most pharmacies have a policy on the additional cost of rebilling bad checks; in most cases, this higher cost acts as a deterrent. In some cases, the pharmacy may keep a list of customers from whom the technician is not allowed to accept checks.

Larger pharmacies may have a check reader connected to the cash register. The signed check is fed into the reader and the bank account is immediately accessed; in some cases, the check reader prints the entire check, ready for customer signature. If the account shows insufficient funds for the check, a prompt alerts the technician not to accept the check and to seek an alternate source of payment.

Card Transactions In addition to cash and check transactions, payments may be made using a credit, debit, Flex, or even a gift card. Scanning technology is usually available for the patient or the technician to swipe any type of card and follow the prompts. A **credit card** doesn't deduct the money directly but is a type of loan that is either paid off at the end of the month or accrues a finance charge. Depending on the policy of the pharmacy, patients may or may not need to sign for a credit card expense of less than $50. Some chain pharmacies have express pay options such that the credit card on file is automatically billed at the time of prescription filling.

A **debit card** is also a form of online cash payment; unlike a credit card, a debit card instantly deducts the cost of the purchase from the customer's bank account. A debit card purchase requires the customer to enter a confidential PIN number for account activation. A debit card can be used as a credit card if it is inconvenient for the customer to enter a PIN number, such as picking up prescriptions at the drive-thru pharmacy. The amount of the purchase should be verified prior to processing. Generally, these cards do not require a signature because the money is immediately transferred from the bank account. Credit and debit cards allow the option of the customer to request cash back after the claim is processed; cash-back options may be limited ($20 or less) or not available per store policy.

A **Flex card** is a medical credit card for prescription co-pays and select IRS-approved OTC items. The Flex card is cross-referenced with the bar code of the product so that coverage is determined immediately. This credit card option is available to customers with high deductible medical insurance plans. An individual contributes to a medical fund for out-of-pocket costs for medical and pharmacy co-pays as well as OTC drugs. The Flex card minimizes the need for submission of receipts, prevents delays in reimbursement, and offers tax advantages.

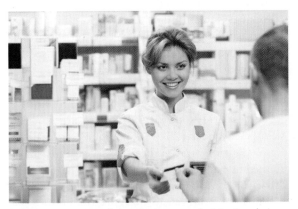

An important part of the pharmacy technician's role is to accept payment for pharmacy purchases in cash, check, or credit card from a customer.

Gift cards are handled similarly to credit, debit, and Flex cards, with the amount embedded in the bar code. With product or store coupons, as well as drug rebate forms, the technician must carefully review the requirements and expiration date before scanning. All credit card receipts (and coupons) are placed under the change drawer or in a separate, secure location for later reconciliation at the end of the day.

Other Payment Options Some small independent pharmacies allow their best customers to run a charge account and settle with the pharmacy at the end of the month. Personal charge accounts usually add to the overhead of the pharmacy because billing statements may need to be mailed out each month. If discretion is not used, then the pharmacy may have a lot of unpaid bills and uncollected debts, especially if store ownership is being transferred.

Cash Register Functions Occasionally, sales of prescription or nonprescription items are voided. This action may need to be completed for a variety of reasons: drugs may not be covered by insurance, the co-pay may be too high, or the merchandise may not be available at the same price as the customer assumed. In such cases, the sale must be voided and some record of the event must be recorded by the technician. In addition to voiding, a pharmacy technician may also be asked to verify the price of store items or, in some cases, may need to modify the price of prescription or nonprescription items. These functions can also be performed by using the cash register. If a patient is due a refund from a prior purchase, then a technician may need to obtain administrative approval from either the pharmacist or store manager before proceeding with the refund procedure.

Reconciliation of the Cash Register At the end of the business day, it is often the responsibility of the pharmacy technician to reconcile the cash, credit card receipts, personal checks, coupons, rebates, voided sales, and patient charges (if allowed) with the tape printout from the cash register. It is common to be off a few cents or dollars once in a while, but frequent or large discrepancies must be immediately brought to the attention of the pharmacist. In a chain pharmacy, one of the store managers may be responsible for reconciling the cash register, but technicians must be accountable for all customer receipts. The technician needs to understand that surveillance cameras are available in many pharmacies to protect the pharmacy from money loss or drug diversion.

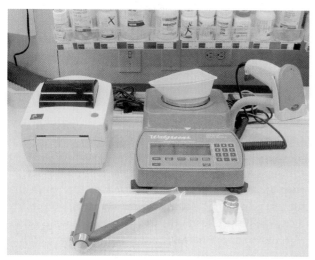

The use of a bar-code scanner and an automated counting machine allows for accurate, efficient processing of prescriptions in a community pharmacy.

Other Automation Tools Bar coding, weighing scales, and robotics are examples of automation tools that are more frequently being adopted in community pharmacies to improve efficiency and reduce medication errors. In Chapter 6, you learned the importance of bar-code scanning technology in the processing of prescriptions. This technology is used to compare NDC numbers during the filling process, during the final check by the pharmacist, and when the medication(s) is dispensed to the patient by the pharmacy technician.

In addition to bar-code scanners, some higher-volume pharmacies may use automated counting machines to facilitate the counting of large quantities (usually greater than 100) of tablets or capsules for medication orders. The pharmacy technician is trained to place 10 tablets or capsules on the machine. To reduce error, the counting machine takes into account the weight per unit of an individual tablet or capsule based on the 10 dosage units. However, the machine is not 100% accurate and should not be used to count prescription orders for controlled drugs. The counting machine must be calibrated and documented daily by the pharmacy technician; a known weight (for example, 200 g) is placed on the balance and the device is recalibrated if needed.

Many large-volume, independent community pharmacies are also adopting new technologies to improve both the speed and accuracy of counting out tablets and capsules from a stock bottle. One example of dispensing automation is the visual precision counting equipment from Eyecon. This technology is 99.99% accurate and documents and records the quantity of each prescription using scanner technology; it eliminates underfills and

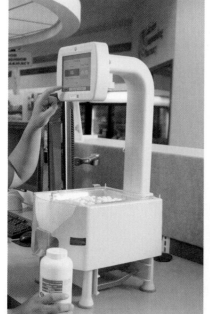

Eyecon® model 9400 shown courtesy of Avery Weigh-Tronix.

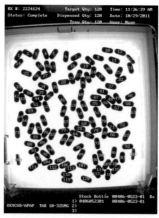

Many retail pharmacies are adopting innovative technologies to visually (rather than manually) count tablets and capsules. The equipment takes and records a snapshot of the placement of each tablet and capsule for each prescription.

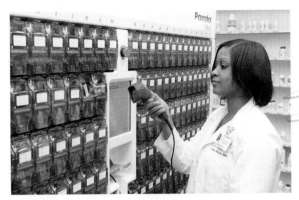

Parata Max® is a high-speed, high-accuracy automated dispensing system.

overfills and is sufficiently accurate to use with Schedule II prescriptions.

Some specially designed computer software programs, called "pharmacy management systems," manage a pharmacy's data, including dispensing operations, inventory control, billing, compliance with regulations, and more. The software can send filling orders directly to automated dispensing devices such as the Parata Max®, which labels, fills, caps, sorts, and stores prescriptions. Automation can improve dispensing efficiency by giving pharmacists more time to counsel patients, reduce costs, and improve accuracy to ensure fewer dispensing errors.

Inventory Management

The entire stock of pharmaceutical products on hand for sale at any given time in a community pharmacy is known as **inventory**. Community pharmacies must stock, or have ready access to, all drugs that may be written by the prescribers in their practice area. Unlike some businesses, however, a pharmacy may need to keep some very slow-moving drugs in stock as a service to a few customers. If the inventory is too tight, then the pharmacy frequently runs out of needed medication, causing either a potential loss of sale or an inconvenience to the patient, who must make another trip to the pharmacy when the inventory has been replenished.

Inventory value is defined as the total value of the drugs and merchandise in stock on a given day. In addition to prescription drugs, inventory includes OTC drugs, dietary supplements, medical supplies, and front-end merchandise. Inventory management of pharmaceuticals should be designed so that medications arrive shortly before they are dispensed and sold, to minimize shelf space needed and maximize cash flow. The primary purposes of inventory management are the timely purchase and receipt of pharmaceuticals and the establishment and maintenance of appropriate levels of materials in stock.

Several important issues with regard to inventory management include the following: how much inventory should be maintained, when inventory levels should be adjusted, and where inventory should be stored. Factors that bear on decisions regarding these issues include turnover of products, floor space allocation, design and arrangement of shelves, and demands on available refrigerator or freezer space.

Managing inventory is an important responsibility of the pharmacy technician. Restocking drug inventory, doing proper shelf labeling, locating stock, setting inventory reorder levels, rotating stock, and checking expiration dates are all important roles in the pharmacy. Checking for expired vitamins and herbs is especially important because they can lose their labeled potency quickly.

The pharmacy inventory must be carefully maintained to have an adequate but not excessive stock of drugs.

Purchasing, receiving, and inventory processes should be as uncomplicated as possible so as not to disrupt or interfere with the other activities of the pharmacy. Pharmacies must maintain a record of drugs and other supplies and merchandise purchased and sold in order to know when to reorder and when to adjust inventory levels of each item. The purchase and receipt of controlled drugs require additional procedures and documentation as discussed later in this chapter.

Purchasing

Purchasing is defined as the ordering of products for use or sale by the pharmacy and is usually carried out by either an independent or a group process. In independent purchasing, the pharmacist deals directly with a drug wholesaler regarding matters such as price and contractual terms. The wholesaler is the distributor of drug inventory from a local or regional warehouse. In group purchasing, a number of independent pharmacies work together to negotiate a discount for high-volume purchases and more favorable contract terms. The state pharmacy association may act as a facilitator for group purchasing, contracting for its members as a benefit.

The following three primary purchasing methods or systems are used in pharmacies:

- **Wholesaler purchasing** enables the community pharmacy to use a single source to purchase and receive numerous products from multiple manufacturers of brand and generic name pharmaceuticals. Some pharmacies use more than one wholesaler. Advantages of wholesaler purchasing include reduced turnaround time for orders, lower inventory and lower associated costs, and reduced commitment of time and staff. Disadvantages include higher purchase cost, occasional supply shortages (called *back orders*), and unavailability of some pharmaceuticals. The turnaround time for receipt of drug orders is usually the next day, with the possible exception of weekends and Schedule II drugs.

- **Just-in-time (JIT) purchasing** involves frequent purchasing in quantities that just meet supply needs until the next ordering time. JIT purchasing reduces the quantity of each product on the shelves and thus reduces the amount of money committed to inventory. However, such a system can be used only when supplies are readily available and pharmaceutical needs can be accurately predicted. Automation can enhance the accuracy of replacing needed inventory levels of drugs. In large chain pharmacies, a regional or centralized warehouse may provide once-weekly JIT purchasing; a local wholesaler is used for purchasing brand name and out-of-stock drugs that are needed the next day.

- **Prime vendor purchasing** involves an exclusive agreement made by a pharmacy for a specified percentage or dollar amount of purchases. Prime vendor purchasing offers the advantages of lower acquisition costs, competitive service fees, electronic order entry, and emergency delivery services. This type of purchasing is more common in hospital pharmacies.

The pharmacy technician plays a critical role in the purchasing of pharmaceuticals. Today, a variety of methods may be used for inventory management to determine when a product needs to be reordered. A small independent pharmacy may use a "want book" to record inventory that needs to be replaced; after a time, the technician has a good sense of how fast drug products move off the shelves and when they need to be reordered. Manual or automated inventory records based on usage and seasonal patterns may be used. For example, more antibiotics and cough and cold products may be purchased during the winter season. For fast movers, the purchase decision is often based on the most economic order quantity or best value (in other words, ordering capsules in a 1000 count size rather than 100 count size, or buying a case of antacid liquid rather than one or two bottles).

Larger pharmacies have software to automate the drug-ordering process, which can automatically generate purchase orders under predetermined conditions. An important goal of computerized inventory control is to reduce the time and staff required for inventory management, as well as to maintain an appropriate balance of adequate stock with adequate inventory turnover. Each time that drugs are purchased from the wholesaler, the product, quantity, and price are entered into the computer database. As each prescription is dispensed or as a customer purchases a nonprescription product, the computer system automatically adjusts the inventory record. Pharmacies usually establish an inventory range for each item (in other words, a maximum and a minimum number of units to have on hand). When the inventory drops to the minimum level, the item is purchased to restock the supply. This predetermined order point and the order quantity are based on the historical use of each drug. The following is an example of a calculation used to make inventory management decisions.

Example 1

The maximum inventory level for amoxicillin 500 mg capsules is 2000 capsules. At the end of the day, the computer prints a list of items to be reordered; the list indicates an inventory level of 975 amoxicillin capsules, the minimum quantity—and the point to reorder automatically is 1000 capsules. Has the automatic reorder level been reached? How many capsules should be ordered?

$$\text{maximum inventory} - \text{present inventory} = \text{amount sold}$$

$$2000 \text{ capsules} - 975 \text{ capsules} = 1025 \text{ capsules}$$

Because 1025 capsules sold is more than the minimum number needed to reorder automatically, the automatic reorder level has been reached. Two bottles of 500 mg capsules are ordered.

As discussed in Chapter 6, the technician also needs to consider special onetime orders for a specific patient, partial-fill prescriptions, and out-of-stock requests that occur during the day when placing an order. Most drug ordering occurs online, but telephoning a wholesaler may be needed for special or late-in-the-day orders. Special orders for seldom stocked injectable products may require additional delivery time if they are not in the wholesaler's inventory.

Occasionally, a pharmaceutical product is temporarily or permanently unavailable from a supplier. Drug shortages may be due to manufacturing quality control issues, FDA or voluntary drug recalls, expirations, or discontinuations. Pharmacy personnel should first determine the reason for the unavailability—for example, the drug is (1) on back order; (2) being recalled by the manufacturer; or (3) being discontinued. Then, the pharmacist should identify a therapeutically equivalent product if available and obtain permission to change the prescription from the medical office. Alternatively, the pharmacy could consider borrowing the drug from another pharmacy in the corporate chain. For any type of product exchange between pharmacies, personnel should refer to their facility's policy and procedure manual for the correct protocol for control and accountability. If a pharmacy does not have a certain medication, then it is common for personnel to check with a local competing pharmacy and transfer the prescription if such a pharmacy has the product in stock.

The pharmacy technician also has other inventorial responsibilities that are important to making the business of a community pharmacy successful. The technician is responsible for ordering and stocking necessary prescription supplies (various sizes of vials and bottles, medication and auxiliary labels, information sheets, measuring devices, paper). These supplies may or may not be available from the wholesaler and may require several days to receive if ordered directly from a manufacturer, so an adequate inventory must be kept on hand.

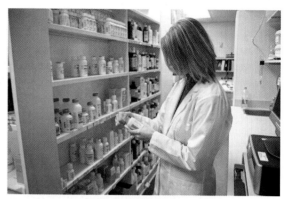

The pharmacy technician is responsible for ordering and stocking not only drug product inventory but necessary prescription supplies as well.

Receiving and Posting

The physical delivery of an order of products from a wholesaler, warehouse, or other pharmacy initiates a series of procedures known as **receiving**. As part of the receiving process, the pharmaceutical products must be carefully checked against the purchase order or requisition. The pharmacist or technician usually signs an invoice from a delivery representative, verifying the receipt of the number of totes or boxes delivered from the wholesaler. A separate invoice is required for the receipt of controlled substances. It is advisable for the pharmacist to check for intact seals and contents of totes containing controlled substances.

The contents of any shipment should be verified for name of product, manufacturer, quantity received versus quantity ordered, product strength, and package size. As discussed in Chapter 3, the NDC, a number assigned to every drug product, consists of three parts separated by dashes: The first part represents the number assigned to the manufacturer; the second part represents the drug entity (generic name and strength); and the third part indicates the package size of the drug. A drug ordered but not received should immediately be brought to the attention of the pharmacist, who can initiate the appropriate action.

When the inventory order is received from the wholesaler each weekday, it is important that the pharmacy technician "post" that order. **Posting** is the process of reconciling the invoice and updating inventory in the pharmacy product database. This process includes checking the newly received drug inventory for NDC numbers, expiration dates, and drug cost updates. Any large price increases should be brought to the attention of the pharmacist for verification. As part of the posting process, the pharmacy technician may affix stickers to the received unit stock bottles. These stickers document the wholesaler's item number and pricing information. Once the order from the wholesaler is posted, the drugs should immediately be

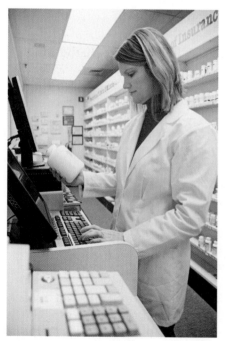

Pharmaceuticals in a shipment should be carefully checked by pharmacy personnel for NDC numbers, price updates, and expiration dates and then entered into the computer database.

appropriately stored—at room temperature, refrigerated, or frozen—depending on the requirements listed on the manufacturers' labels.

Each pharmacy has a policy for an acceptable range of product expiration dates. A typical requirement might be that products have expiration dates of at least 12 months from the date of receipt. After products are received and checked, they are placed in their proper storage locations and under proper storage conditions. New products may require new shelf labeling. An accepted method for stocking pharmaceuticals is to position the units of product with the shortest expiration dates where they will be the first units selected for use; this is known as "rotating the stock."

After posting and shelving inventory is complete, it is important for the pharmacy technician to initiate the prescription filling process for any OOS or partial-fill prescriptions from the day before. The prescription order is then processed, verified, and filled so that it can be available for the patient to pick up later that same day as promised. If possible, the patient should be notified that the prescription is now ready for pickup.

Handling Out-of-Stock and Partially Filled Medications

Most pharmacies maintain a limited drug inventory to remain profitable, so it is not uncommon to be either out of a prescribed medication or unable to completely fill a prescription order.

Out-of-Stock Medications A medication can go **out of stock (OOS)** if an uncommon specialty medication is ordered or if there has been a higher than normal demand for a certain prescription, such as an antihistamine during the allergy season. In the case of an OOS medication, options include:

- allowing the patient to take the prescription to another pharmacy
- borrowing the medication from another pharmacy
- ordering the medication for next-day delivery from the wholesaler

The patient may not be able or willing to wait until the next day to fill the prescription. As a service to the customer, the pharmacy technician should make a telephone call to a local pharmacy to see if the requested medication is in stock. If another store in the chain pharmacy is close by, the technician may be encouraged to call that pharmacy initially. Borrowing from another pharmacy is limited to stores within the same retail chain pharmacy (for example, Walgreens, CVS, or Rite Aid); medication may be available later that same day or early the next morning. Inventory levels must be adjusted and documented with all inter-store borrowing of pharmaceuticals per store procedure.

If a medication is ordered from the wholesaler, it typically can be received the next day. If the prescription is received on the weekend or late at night, the ordered medication may take two days before it arrives in the pharmacy from the wholesaler. The patient should be notified of an expected "promised date and time" when the OOS prescription can be filled.

Partial-Fill Medications Even when a drug is not out of stock, inventory may be insufficient to completely fill the prescription. Though policies may vary with the pharmacy, the pharmacy may provide the patient with a partial fill. A **partial fill** may provide a five-day supply of medication, which should be sufficient until the new drug inventory is received. The medication container label and patient information leaflet will indicate that a partial fill was dispensed.

Practice Tip

Many retail pharmacies now require pharmacy technicians to call customers when the remainder of a partial-fill medication is available. Technicians should check their pharmacy's Policy & Procedure manual for the protocol regarding partial fills.

In most cases, a partial fill of Schedule II drugs is not allowed. However, some states may allow the pharmacist to partial fill an emergency prescription under certain circumstances as discussed in Chapter 6. Pharmacy personnel should be aware that any emergency partial fill would void the remainder of the prescription. Receiving new inventory for a Schedule II drug may take 48 hours or longer because of required federal and state record keeping and paper trails. Many pharmacies have adopted a secure online ordering process to expedite orders for Schedule II drugs.

Drug Returns and Credits

Drugs may be returned to pharmacy stock or returned to the wholesaler for credit. This situation may occur if a patient does not pick up the filled medication within seven days after reminder calls and phone messages or if the patient may not need or be able to afford one or more of his or her filled medications. Consequently, the pharmacy technician must "reverse" or cancel the online insurance billing, store the prescription in the patient profile for possible future use, and return the stock to drug inventory. (Typically, pharmacy personnel cover or cross out the patient's name on the stock container before returning it to inventory.)

Product shortages, products that are damaged during shipment, or products that have been improperly shipped or stored, must be reported to the pharmacist immediately. Stringent laws regulate the return of pharmaceuticals to manufacturers, especially for controlled substances. In the case of a damaged or an incorrect shipment, the wholesaler should be notified immediately and authorization should be secured for the return of the defective shipment as soon as possible. A wholesaler may charge a restocking fee if the item(s) has not been returned in a specified number of days. The number of days that the pharmacy has to return pharmaceuticals depends on the contract. Typically, the products must be returned in two to four business days.

Drug Return Process The pharmacy technician is often responsible for handling drug returns to the wholesaler for credits of both prescription and nonprescription

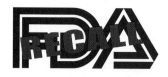

drugs. These returns may be because of drug overstocks, patient decline of medication pickup, soon-to-be-expired drugs, drug recalls by the drug manufacturer or FDA, reformulated drugs, drugs in new packaging, or drugs that are no longer manufactured. Drug returns must be in original stock bottles or unit-of-use packaging in their original condition.

Patient Decline of Medication If a patient declines to pick up a medication (such as the expensive diabetic drug Byetta), the pharmacy technician can return the medication to the wholesaler for credit, provided that the box is unopened and the medication container label can be removed without altering the packaging label. A return-for-credit form must be completed in duplicate by the pharmacy technician for all drugs returned to the wholesaler; the form lists the drug(s) and quantities to be returned for credit. The technician and the delivery driver from the wholesaler verify the contents of the tote and sign the credit form; the signature of the technician guarantees that the product was purchased directly from the wholesaler. The signature, under penalty of perjury, also states that the drugs have been stored, handled, and shipped by the customer in accordance with manufacturers' guidelines and all federal, state, and local laws. The tote is then sealed and returned to the wholesaler for credit, and the signed form is filed for future reference if necessary.

Expired Medications Pharmacy technicians must also check drug inventory for expired medications on a monthly basis or per store policy. They should remove all expired or near-expired (within three months) products from stock and return them to the wholesaler for partial credit. If a drug is past its expiration date, it can be returned to the wholesaler, but no credit will be issued to the pharmacy. This process of drug returns and credits often involves a lot of paperwork and is time-consuming; however, it is an important part of inventory management and business profitability.

Prescription medication vials returned to the pharmacy by the patient—even if unused and unopened—cannot, by federal law, be returned to stock once they have left the pharmacy. This law exists to protect patients from product tampering.

Safety Note

Prescription vials returned by the patient cannot be returned to stock, even if they are unopened.

Filled Prescriptions When both generic and brand name drugs exist, it is important for the technician to determine which type is written by the prescriber (DAW or dispense as written) or requested by the patient (generic or brand). To clarify this process, consider the following scenario: If a patient or prescriber requests Synthroid (a brand name drug) to be dispensed, and the pharmacy inadvertently dispenses levothyroxine (the generic form of the drug), two different procedures might ensue. If the drug did not leave the pharmacy, the prescription can be corrected and the drug can be returned to stock; it is generally kept in the medication container (with patient identifiers covered) rather than returned to a stock drug bottle in inventory. However, if the patient left the pharmacy, discovered the mix-up, and then returned to the pharmacy later, the generic drug can be returned and the correct medication dispensed but the generic must be discarded per pharmacy protocol.

If any medication or dispensing error was made by pharmacy personnel, the incorrect drug will be returned, the correct one dispensed, an apology by the pharmacist will be issued, and a reimbursement and credit will be made to the patient. Depending on the policy of the pharmacy, the cost of other returned drugs that have left the pharmacy, where no error occurred, may or may not allow a reimbursement to the patient. These drugs—even if unused and unopened—cannot be returned to inventory stock. Consequently, the pharmacy loses revenue. To minimize drug returns, the pharmacy technician should review the filled prescriptions with the patient at the time of pickup.

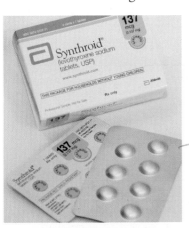

Thyroid is available as a brand-name drug (Synthroid) or as a generic drug (levothyroxine). A prescriber (or patient) may request the brand name. Before the medication is dispensed to the patient, the technician should be sure that the proper drug was dispensed.

Drug Recalls In the case of a drug recall, the patient can return the drug for credit or for a refund provided by the manufacturer. The pharmacy or store manager must generally approve a refund on all returned drugs. The refund may be issued using cash, credit, or a gift card for store merchandise, depending on the circumstances.

Inventory Requirements for Controlled Substances

The Controlled Substances Act (CSA) defines procedures for purchasing and receiving controlled substances in the pharmacy as well as the requirements for the inventory and record keeping of these drugs. Each pharmacy must register with the DEA in order to purchase and dispense controlled substances.

The FDA requires that all controlled-substance containers be clearly marked with their "schedule" on the product label. In light of that, pharmacy technicians should inspect containers for the schedule mark, which is an uppercase Roman numeral with or without a C symbol: II or C–II; III or C–III; IV or C–IV; and V or C–V. The symbol C and/or the Roman numeral must be at least twice the size of the largest letters printed on the label. If a bottle is too small to display the symbol or numerals, then the box and package insert must contain them. Symbols and/or numerals are not required on the containers of dispensed medications.

Schedule III, IV, and V Drugs In most pharmacies, the technician can order Schedule III–V medications. The pharmacist must, however, verify and sign the receipt for these drugs. Verification of the receipt involves comparing the invoice with the drug name, dosage, and quantity of physical inventory. Once the receipt is verified by the pharmacist, these drugs may be stored by the technician among the drug stock, usually alphabetically by brand or generic drug name. All Schedule III, IV, and V prescriptions and records, including purchasing invoices, are commonly kept separate from other records and must also be kept in a readily retrievable form.

Schedule II Drugs The processing of inventory for Schedule II controlled substances follows a strict protocol.

Purchasing The purchase of Schedule II controlled substances must be initiated and authorized by a pharmacist and executed on a DEA 222 form (see Figure 7.3). This form provides the record of any Schedule II substances sold or delivered to another DEA-registered dispenser. Ordering such drugs from a wholesaler may involve a wait of 48–72 hours because of the paperwork and special handling. Online ordering of Schedule II drugs is available to most community pharmacies, but it requires registration, user name, and password protection for each pharmacist. Online access to ordering allows next-day delivery in most cases. The pharmacist—not the technician—is legally responsible for the ordering of all Schedule II controlled substances, whether by submitting a DEA 222 form or ordering online. No Schedule II drugs can be borrowed from another pharmacy.

FIGURE 7.3
DEA 222 Form

This form must be completed and signed by the pharmacist for the ordering of all Schedule II controlled substances.

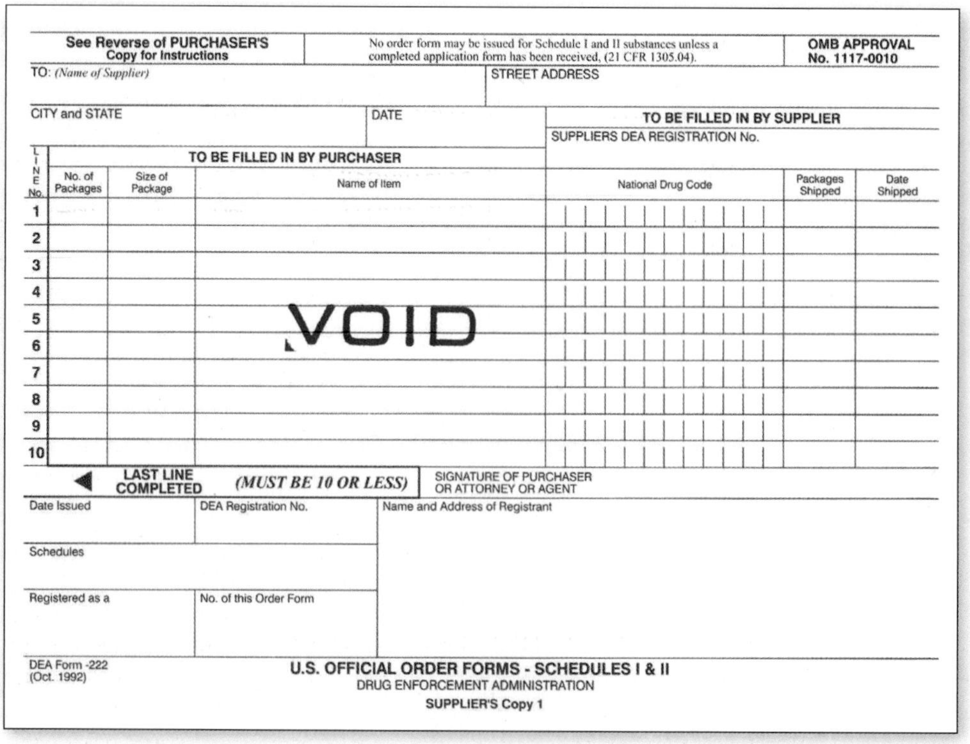
See Reverse of PURCHASER'S Copy for Instructions
No order form may be issued for Schedule I and II substances unless a completed application form has been received, (21 CFR 1305.04).
OMB APPROVAL No. 1117-0010
TO: (Name of Supplier)
STREET ADDRESS
CITY and STATE
DATE
TO BE FILLED IN BY SUPPLIER
SUPPLIERS DEA REGISTRATION No.
TO BE FILLED IN BY PURCHASER

LINE No.	No. of Packages	Size of Package	Name of Item	National Drug Code	Packages Shipped	Date Shipped
1						
2						
3						
4						
5			VOID			
6						
7						
8						
9						
10						

LAST LINE COMPLETED (MUST BE 10 OR LESS)
SIGNATURE OF PURCHASER OR ATTORNEY OR AGENT
Date Issued
DEA Registration No.
Name and Address of Registrant
Schedules
Registered as a
No. of this Order Form
DEA Form -222 (Oct. 1992)
U.S. OFFICIAL ORDER FORMS - SCHEDULES I & II
DRUG ENFORCEMENT ADMINISTRATION
SUPPLIER'S Copy 1

Receiving All Schedule II drugs should be received in a special tote with an unbroken seal. If the seal is broken, then the tote should not be accepted at delivery, and the wholesaler should be notified immediately. The pharmacist must break the seal on the tote and verify the contents with the invoice. After verification, the pharmacist must document the following information on the DEA 222 form: the date, the name and amount of Schedule II drugs received, and the corresponding NDC numbers. The pharmacist will post the Schedule II drug inventory to the database, including the NDC numbers, prices, and expiration dates. The pharmacist is responsible for the receipt and secure storage of all controlled drugs, but especially Schedule II drugs.

Inventory Many community pharmacies use a perpetual inventory to maintain close control of the Schedule II drug stock. A **perpetual inventory record** is a method of maintaining ongoing accountability for Schedule II medications on a tablet-by-tablet (or other dosage form) basis. Figure 7.4 shows an example of a perpetual inventory record. A perpetual inventory record documents each and every dosage of Schedule II drugs received and dispensed. This record includes product, dosage, quantity, date received or dispensed, prescription number, remaining inventory, and signature or initials of the pharmacist.

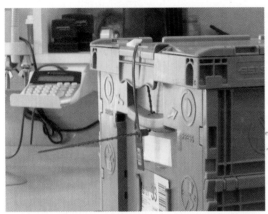

The seal on totes for controlled substances may only be broken by the pharmacist.

FIGURE 7.4
Perpetual Inventory Record

A perpetual inventory record accounts for each unit of a Schedule II drug dispensed or received.

Drug and Dose	Oxycodone 5 mg/325 mg APAP
Record Starting Date	01/02/201X
Record Starting Quantity	500

Prescription Number	Dispensing Date	Quantity Dispensed	Cumulative Total	RPh Initials
246734	01/03/201X	40	460	RJA
247981	01/06/201X	16	444	RJA
248103	01/07/201X	120	324	RJA
DEA 001234988	01/10/201X	+500	824	RJA
249008	01/12/201X	60	764	RJA

If allowed by the policy and procedures of the pharmacy, the technician will make entries on new inventory or prescription dispensing into this notebook. All entries should be co-initialed by the pharmacist. The correct drug, dosage, and quantity must be documented. Any discrepancies should be reported to the pharmacist; if the discrepancy cannot be resolved, then the pharmacist must contact the state drug inspector and the DEA.

There is a special policy and procedure for counting the inventory of controlled drug substances. A biennial (every two years) inventory of Schedule II drugs must be taken and reported to the DEA. Some states have even more stringent requirements, such as a yearly inventory. The date of the taking of an actual inventory should not vary by more than four days from the biennial inventory date. A copy of the controlled substances biennial inventory must be kept by the pharmacy with the original forwarded to the

DEA. The inventory record is completed by the pharmacist and must contain the following information for each controlled substance:

- name of the drug
- dosage form and strength
- number of dosage units or volume in each container
- number of containers

An exact unit count (number of tablets, capsules, patches, or milliliters) is required for all Schedule II drugs. For Schedules III, IV, and V substances, an estimated count and/or measure is permitted unless a container holds more than 1000 capsules or tablets. If the container has been opened, then an exact count is required.

Documentation The pharmacy must maintain complete and accurate records of all controlled substances. Receiving records include the signed and dated invoice and DEA order form, which must be filed together and readily retrievable for future inspection. The DEA requires that a complete paper trail of records be maintained for each Schedule II drug as the drug travels from manufacturer to wholesaler to the community pharmacy to the patient. The DEA 222 form documents the request from the manufacturer or wholesaler; the shipment receipt documents the delivery to the pharmacy; and the prescription documents the dispensing of the drug to the patient.

Tracking mechanisms exist by state and federal authorities to monitor the distribution of Schedule II drugs. If there is evidence of overprescribing by a physician, overdispensing by a pharmacy, or overselling of Schedule II drugs by a wholesaler, then the DEA—after a thorough investigation—has the authority to temporarily or permanently revoke the DEA license of that physician, pharmacy, or wholesaler.

All Schedule II prescriptions must be signed and dated by the pharmacist, kept separate from other prescription records, and be readily retrievable. Prescription records for all controlled substances must be maintained for a minimum of two years. Some states require holding records for five years. For legal purposes, most pharmacies keep all prescription records indefinitely.

Disposal Any disposal of a controlled drug must be witnessed, recorded, and signed by another pharmacist. In most cases, expired or defective formulations (broken tablets) of Schedule II drugs are saved for destruction on the next visit of the state drug inspector or returned to an authorized destruction depot after proper documentation is completed and filed.

Disposal of Syringes and Medications

Proper disposal of syringes and expired or unused medications is important in both the pharmacy setting and the home setting.

Pharmacy Disposal Guidelines The proper disposal of all "**sharps**" (needles, lancets, scalpel blades, and so on) in the pharmacy setting is critical not only to the safety of individuals but also to the prevention of communicable diseases such as hepatitis or HIV. For pharmacists who are administering vaccines, disposal of needles and syringes in a sharps container is mandatory. The sharps container should be placed in the pharmacy in a secure location away from children and, when full, should be sealed, labeled, and mailed according to pharmacy protocol.

Home Disposal Guidelines The proper disposal of expired or unused medications at home is important to the safety of patients, other individuals, and the environment.

Therefore, pharmacy personnel should discuss the proper disposal of medications with their patients. Flushing medication down the toilet is no longer recommended due to adverse effects on the environment. One option for the disposal of medications is to mix the medications with kitty litter or coffee grounds in a sealed plastic bag or can and place them in the trash. In addition, each pharmacy has a commercially available package for purchase in which medications (with the exception of controlled substances) can be safely mailed to a location where they are incinerated. Some local fire departments and waste management facilities may assist in disposing of medications in an environmentally friendly manner as well. Other methods for drug disposal can be found at www.paradigmcollege.net/pharm practice5e/drugdisposal.

Besides medications, the proper disposal of all "sharps" is a growing safety concern as more patients every year are self-administering injections (such as allergy shots, vitamin B_{12}, blood thinners, and hormones) while at home. Unfortunately, this increased patient use of sharps has resulted in an increase in improper waste disposal. According to the U.S. Environmental Protection Agency, up to 7.8 billion needles and syringes are improperly disposed of each year. A vast majority of these patients are diabetics who are administering insulin to treat their conditions. Proper disposal of sharps protects anyone from the risk of injury or infection who comes in contact with the trash. Pharmacy personnel should encourage patients to purchase a rigid, puncture-resistant, hard plastic sharps container to dispose of all sharps safely and should refer patients to www.paradigmcollege.net/pharmpractice5e/needledisposal for more information.

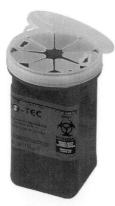

The proper disposal of insulin syringes in a sharps container is important to minimize the transmission of infectious diseases, even in the home.

Estimating Drug Inventory

Often, today's pharmacies have $150,000 to $300,000 or more in inventory on the shelves as drug products. If a chain has 10 stores in the region, then the amount of money in goods on the shelf adds up very quickly. Keeping medications on the shelf is a carrying cost to a pharmacy, and an excessive inventory can hinder cash flow and net revenue, tie up capital in inventory, incur wastage due to product expiration, and increase the likelihood of theft. Therefore, to minimize the cost of doing business, inventory levels must be adequate but not excessive, with a rapid turnover of drug stock on the shelf. Many pharmacies aim for an **inventory turnover rate** of approximately 12–24: That is, if the drug inventory turns over every month, the turnover rate is 12; if the drug inventory turns over every two weeks, the turnover rate is 24.

Although all of the transactions of drugs and products coming into and out of the pharmacy are carefully documented, the technician should, per store policy, occasionally take a physical count of the pharmacy's inventory. A counting of the items in stock is usually taken once or more each year, and the task is often assigned to a senior pharmacy technician or else it is outsourced to complete the project. An inventory value is used to determine average inventory and turnover rate and to make any necessary adjustments in stock levels. Adjustments may include returning a drug to a wholesaler, selling stock to another pharmacy, and lowering

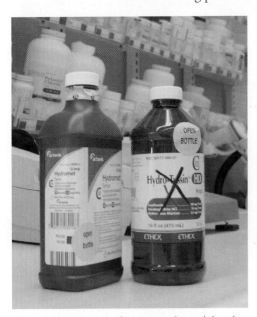

It is a common procedure to mark stock bottles with an "X" or to affix an "Open Bottle" label once the bottles have been opened. When the technician is counting inventory, an opened bottle is assumed to be half-full.

automatic restock levels. Whenever a pharmacy is in the process of being sold, an inventory is required and included in the purchase price.

When the inventory is counted, unopened bottles receive full credit. All opened bottles are assumed to be half-full for inventory purposes. Therefore, when filling a prescription, the pharmacy technician should make a note (usually an "X") on the stock drug bottle or cap (or affix an "Open Bottle" sticker) to indicate that the bottle has been opened. Similarly, stock drug bottles should not be overfilled. For example, the technician should not add 100 tablets of cyclobenzaprine to a stock bottle of 500 tablets; on inspection, the bottle would be counted as half-full (250 tablets), and the inventory would be underestimated by 350 tablets. For most expensive drugs, this overfilling practice undervalues inventory costs and, consequently, negatively impacts the financial status of the pharmacy.

Business Math Used in Pharmacy Practice

A community pharmacy operates under the same principles as any other business—it deals with expenses and receipts. In addition, like any other business, the pharmacy must make a **profit**. In other words, it must have more receipts than expenses in order to continue to provide customer services. One of the responsibilities of the pharmacy technician is to help ensure that inventory turns over and that the insurance reimbursements and receipts are greater than the expenses.

The technician often takes care of pricing in the pharmacy by billing online insurance, marking products up by a certain percentage over the acquisition cost, and marking products down by a percentage discount at other times. The successful pharmacy technician needs to master basic mathematical skills used in markup, discount, and average wholesale price. Understanding the terminology and mathematics used in community pharmacy is an important part of the pharmacy technician's job and can directly affect the profitability of the business.

Markup

Like all businesses, pharmacies purchase their products (in other words, drugs) at one price and sell them at a higher price. This difference is called the **markup**, but it is sometimes referred to as the **gross profit**. Prescription pricing is subject to governmental laws and regulations, as well as competition within the marketplace. Markup plays an important part in the pricing system. The markup is computed as follows:

$$\text{selling price} - \text{purchase price} = \text{markup}$$

The markup rate is expressed as a percentage and is calculated as follows:

$$\text{markup} \div \text{cost} \times 100 = \text{markup rate}$$

Example 2

One vial of Humulin regular insulin sells for $90 and costs the pharmacy $60. What is the markup and what is the markup rate?

The markup is computed as follows:

$$\text{selling price} - \text{purchase price} = \text{markup}$$

$$\$90.00 - \$60.00 = \text{markup}$$

$$\$30.00 = \text{markup}$$

The markup rate is computed as follows:

$$\text{markup} \div \text{cost} \times 100 = \text{markup rate}$$

$$\$30.00 \div \$60.00 \times 100 = \text{markup rate}$$

$$50\% = \text{markup rate}$$

Discount

Sometimes, a wholesaler offers an item to a pharmacy at a lower price. This reduced price is a **discount**. Often this discount may be passed on to the consumer, or it may help offset expenses and low reimbursements from insurance. The pharmacy may offer the consumer a discount, or a deduction from what is typically charged, as an incentive to purchase an item, especially on a nonprescription product or store merchandise. Discount and discounted purchase price are calculated with the following formulas:

$$\text{total purchase price} \times \text{discount rate} = \text{discount}$$

$$\text{total purchase price} - \text{discount} = \text{discounted purchase price}$$

Example 3

Assume that the pharmacy purchases five cases of hydrocortisone 1% cream at \$100 per case. If the account is paid in full within 15 days, then the supplier (wholesaler) offers a 15% discount on the purchase. What is the total discounted purchase price?

Begin by calculating the total purchase price.

$$\text{quantity of product} \times \text{cost per unit} = \text{total purchase price}$$

$$5 \text{ cases} \times \$100.00/\text{case} = \$500.00$$

Next, calculate the discount for payment within 15 days.

$$\text{total purchase price} \times \text{discount rate} = \text{discount}$$

$$\$500.00 \times 0.15 = \$75.00$$

Finally, to obtain the discounted price, subtract the discount from the original price.

$$\text{total purchase price} - \text{discount} = \text{discounted purchase price}$$

$$\$500.00 - \$75.00 = \$425.00$$

Average Wholesale Price Applications

The **average wholesale price (AWP)** of a drug is an *average* price that wholesalers charge the pharmacy for a given drug, dose, and package size. Usually, third parties reimburse a pharmacy based on the AWP less a discount that has been agreed on in a negotiated contract. Therefore, the pharmacy has an incentive to purchase a drug at a price that is as far below its AWP as possible. Drugs are sold below AWP via group purchasing, volume discounts, contracts, and rebates from manufacturers. The AWP is used to calculate a prescription reimbursement with the following formula:

$$\text{prescription reimbursement} = \text{AWP} + \text{percentage} + \text{dispensing fee}$$

Example 4

Actos comes in a quantity of 90 tablets and has an AWP of $150. The pharmacy has an agreement with the supplier to purchase the drug at the AWP minus 15%. The insurer is willing to pay the AWP plus 5% plus a $3 dispensing fee. A patient on this insurer's plan purchases 30 tablets for $55.50. How much profit does the pharmacy make on this prescription?

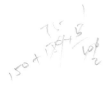

Begin by calculating the amount of the discount.

$$\$150.00 \times 0.15 = \$22.50$$

Use the discount to calculate the purchase price of the drug.

$$\$150.00 - \$22.50 = \$127.50$$

Therefore, the pharmacy can purchase 90 tablets for $127.50.

The insurance company pays the pharmacy AWP plus 5%.
(Note that 5% = 0.05.)

$$\$150.00 + (\$150.00 \times 0.05) = \$150.00 + \$7.50 = \$157.50$$

Using the insurance reimbursement of $157.50 for 90 tablets, calculate the reimbursement for 30 tablets.

$$(\$157.50 \div 3) + \$3.00 \text{ (dispensing fee)} = \$52.50 + \$3.00 = \$55.50$$

Compare this to the pharmacy's cost of 30 tablets.

$$\$127.50 \div 3 = \$42.50$$

Therefore, the pharmacy's profit on 30 tablets is:

$$\$55.50 - \$42.50 = \$13.00$$

Health Insurance

Health insurance is coverage of incurred medical costs such as physician visits, laboratory costs, and hospitalization. In the past, this medical coverage was primarily limited to hospitalizations and emergency room (ER) visits with a 20% deductible; health

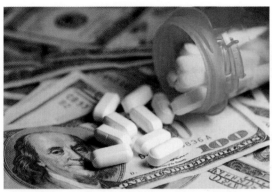

The cost of health care in general, and medications in particular, has outpaced the cost of inflation. Technicians must become knowledgeable in prescription drug insurance plans.

insurance would cover the remaining 80% of the hospital or ER costs. A patient had to pay cash for each physician visit and at the time of picking up a prescription.

Today, the cost of health care and health insurance is far outpacing the rate of inflation. These escalating costs have forced government insurance programs (such as Medicaid and Medicare) as well as private insurance companies to adjust their coverage. In fact, without major changes, the future solvency of the Medicaid and Medicare insurance programs is questionable for private healthcare coverage. Without major changes, the cost of premiums and co-payments will continue to skyrocket.

Businesses have also had to reassess the healthcare plans that they offer to their employees. Many small employers, for example, elect not to provide health insurance coverage for their workers because they can't absorb the high costs of healthcare plans. Those companies that do offer healthcare coverage to their employees have had to increase their employees' co-payments and deductibles and decrease or eliminate the coverage for many services.

The rising costs of health care have also contributed to the growing pool of uninsured individuals. For these individuals—as well as those who work part time or those who are underinsured by their employers—the cost of private health insurance is prohibitive.

In recent years, federal and state governments have attempted to provide health insurance for their citizens. The passage of the Affordable Care Act of 2010 became the first step in a plan to provide comprehensive health insurance coverage, including preventive care and affordable healthcare options, to individuals. This legislation also provides insurance to those individuals with preexisting health problems who have been denied coverage in the past. The passage of this legislation was a topic of intensive debate among government officials, including a subsequent challenge concerning the constitutionality of the law that was heard by the Supreme Court. The Court upheld the law, although healthcare policy continues to be on the political agenda and on the minds of U.S. citizens as the competitiveness of the country's global markets are threatened by the rising cost of healthcare benefits for employees and retirees.

Prescription Insurance Plans

Today, most patients have health and prescription drug insurance coverage from a private insurance company through their employer or from the state government (Medicaid) or federal government (Tricare, Medicare). Many Medicare patients may have additional supplemental insurance to cover medical and/or prescription expenses. The most recent data is available from the IMS Institute for Healthcare Informatics in its report "The Use of Medicines in the United States: Review of 2011" and can be seen in Figure 7.5 on the following page. To gain an understanding of the significance of these statistics, just 30 years earlier, 100% of prescriptions were paid for in cash.

The number of prescription medications and their costs have risen dramatically over the past 30 years as well. According to "Trends in Retail Prescription Expenditures" by S.W. Schondelmeyer and J. Thomas III (www.paradigmcollege.net/pharmpractice5e/retailprescriptions), in 1990, 1.47 billion prescriptions were dispensed, and the average cost of a prescription was $6.62. Today, more than 4 billion prescriptions are dispensed, and the average cost of a prescription is more than $80.

FIGURE 7.5
U.S. Prescription
Drug Insurance
Coverage

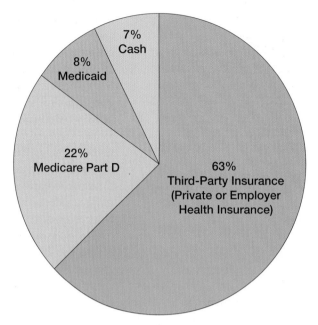

7%
Cash

8%
Medicaid

22%
Medicare Part D

63%
Third-Party Insurance
(Private or Employer
Health Insurance)

Most insurance companies—including Blue Cross/Blue Shield, Aetna, United Health, some Medicaid, and all Medicare Part D plans—elect to outsource the administrative processing of drug claims to a pharmacy benefits manager. A **pharmacy benefits manager (PBM)** is a company that provides such service by administering the prescription drug benefits and pharmacy reimbursements for many insurance companies. Common examples of PBMs who agree to process drug claims for insurance companies include Express Scripts International (ESI), Caremark, and PAID. A large health insurance company such as Aetna and Humana may process their own prescriptions in-house.

Several important terms for the pharmacy technician to understand are related to prescription insurance plans. The **deductible** is an amount that must be paid by the insured before the insurance company will consider paying its portion of the medical and medication cost. This annual deductible is commonly $100 to $3000 and usually starts with the first of the calendar year. A **co-payment (co-pay)** is the flat amount that the patient is to pay for each prescription; co-pays vary by both drug (generic vs. brand) and insurance company. The higher-cost premium plans may have no or a lower deductible and co-payment. **Coinsurance** is a percentage-based plan in which the patient must pay a certain percentage of the prescription price. This plan is not as common as the deductible and co-pay insurance arrangements. The deductible, co-pay, or coinsurance are all methods by which an insurance company tries to control healthcare costs.

With the exception of Medicaid (low income, disabled) and Tricare (military), most patients with prescription insurance pay a monthly premium for prescription drug coverage that may or may not be subsidized by their employer. A PBM controls costs through generic prescribing, formularies, prior authorizations (PAs), and tiered pricing, as well as lower reimbursements to community pharmacies. The very survival of a pharmacy depends on its ability to contain drug costs.

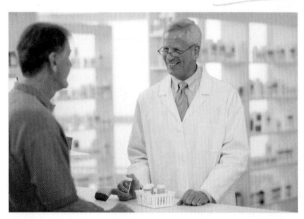

Pharmacy personnel may discuss insurance coverage with patients to help them understand their medication expenses.

Private Insurance Most patients have **private insurance** either through their employer during their wage-earning years, or as retirees of large companies. During working years, the health insurance costs are subsidized by the employer as a benefit to the full-time employee; during retirement years, the retiree is typically required to pay a higher premium depending on age and health status. An individual can also purchase private drug insurance, but it is very expensive without the group purchasing power of a large employer. A wide variety of private insurance plans are available, ranging from premium to more basic plans, and their costs reflect the coverage provided. An employer commonly offers a health maintenance option (HMO); costs are generally lower but not all providers or pharmacies are covered and the preferred drug list (see section below on this topic) is commonly restricted to generic drugs.

Co-Payments Private health insurance usually includes some combination of individual and family deductible and co-payment (commonly referred to as co-pay) per prescription. In some cases, a patient may have a **dual co-pay**: one co-pay for brand name drugs and a lower co-pay for generic drugs (for example, $40 for brand names and $10 [or lower] for generics). These co-pays are for each drug. A more common drug insurance plan of today is the use of a tiered co-pay. The **tiered co-pay** has an escalating cost for a generic, a preferred brand, and a nonpreferred brand. For preferred medications, the patient pays a lower co-pay than for a nonpreferred drug that has a higher co-pay or is not covered at all. For example, a PBM may elect to cover the generic drug simvastatin for the treatment of high cholesterol, which incurs a co-pay of, perhaps, $10. However, the co-pay for Crestor (the preferred brand name drug) may be $40, and the co-pay for Livalo (the nonpreferred brand name drug) may be $60. Patients should understand that most insurance plans only cover a 30-day supply of a brand name medication in a community pharmacy and a 90-day supply if a mail-order pharmacy is used, regardless of how the prescription was written. Even with drug insurance coverage, a patient commonly pays five or six co-pays at the time of each refill with medications for high blood pressure, diabetes, and high cholesterol. Depending on the insurance plan and formulary status of the medications, the patient may need to pay $100 to $250 or more per person per month in out-of-pocket expenses, in addition to monthly insurance premium expenses.

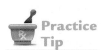

Practice Tip

At times, pharmacy technicians may need to contact prescribers to discuss therapy options for patients who cannot afford a high-cost medication that has been ordered.

Preferred Drug List Patients are often provided with their insurance company's **preferred drug list (PDL)** and are encouraged to share the list with their physicians so that these medications may be selected whenever possible. Often, prescribers do not know or do not remember which drug is on which PBM formulary, so the patient—or the pharmacist or the technician acting as the patient's advocate—may need to discuss therapy options with the prescriber or PBM, especially if drug affordability is an issue. To complicate matters, these formulary listings for each PBM are constantly changing.

Medicaid **Medicaid** subsidizes the cost of health care, including drugs, for indigent and disabled citizens of each state who meet age and income eligibility requirements. Pharmacy technicians should understand that each state has its own policies, procedures, and regulations on the reimbursement of prescription drugs for patients who are eligible for Medicaid. Eligibility for Medicaid is frequently renewed by the state and checked online by the pharmacy each time that a prescription is processed.

Most community pharmacies sign a contract to agree to provide prescription benefits to this disadvantaged population according to the terms of that state. With very few exceptions, OTC drugs as well as prescriptions that are filled in a state other than the state in which the patient resides are not covered by Medicaid. Some states may have a formulary of acceptable drugs that they cover; other states provide a maximum number of prescriptions (usually five) that can be covered in any single month. The co-pays for covered prescriptions will vary with the state and the age of the patient (generally, $0.00 co-pay for children and $0.50 to $4.00 co-pay for adults). Not all medications are covered. Some states may limit the number of prescriptions allowed per month.

The state reimbursement rate to pharmacies is generally **usual and customary charges**. This term means that the pharmacy cannot charge the state more for the same prescription dispensed to a patient with private insurance. Thus, the pharmacy must avoid agreeing to nonprofitable contracts with PBMs because patients eligible for Medicaid add more financial loss to the balance sheet. For example, in 2012, Walgreens decided not to accept a "lowball" contract from Express Scripts International (ESI); without a contract, patients with prescription insurance from ESI (Blue Cross/Blue Shield, Tricare, Anthem, Wellpoint) no longer had coverage if their prescriptions were processed at Walgreens. Later in the year, Walgreens and ESI resolved their contractual differences.

Many states outsource their drug coverage to PBMs because of the rising nature of drug costs and shrinking state tax revenues. In Georgia, for example, an eligible patient may be covered by Medicaid, AmeriGroup, Peach Care, or Wellcare. Each of these state plans for approved low-income patients has different requirements. Insurance coverage frequently changes once or twice during the year to another PBM without notice to the patient or issuance of a new insurance card. During the process of online drug claims, the new insurance coverage information may be provided and identified by the experienced technician.

Some community pharmacies elect not to accept Medicaid coverage because of low reimbursement, delays or errors in receipt of payment, and challenges on legitimate drug claims from accounting audits. The pharmacy can receive stiff financial and civil penalties for intentional or unintentional errors in billing.

Tricare Tricare is a federal health and prescription drug insurance plan that is available to active and retired members of the military and their families. The program has generous coverage of drug costs, with relatively low co-pays for generic and brand name drugs. The prescription co-pays may differ depending on active or inactive status in the military. This insurance plan usually covers a 90-day supply of medication from any community pharmacy.

ESI is the PBM that processes most of the prescriptions from Tricare patients; in 2011, co-payments were increased with little or no notice to military patients, their families, or retirees. The pharmacy technician had to explain why the co-payment increased at the time of dispensing.

Medicare Once a patient is age 65, he or she is eligible for Medicare and, subsequently, receives a red, white, and blue insurance card. Medicare mainly covers some percentage of costs for hospitalizations and ER visits. A patient will pay for Medicare by automatic deductions from their monthly Social Security checks. With few exceptions (diabetic supplies, nebulizer drugs, some vaccines), Medicare does not cover prescription drugs. Most patients require the additional coverage (and costs) of supplemental coverage for doctor visits and prescriptions.

Medicare Advantage Patients over age 65 are also eligible for Medicare Advantage (Medicare Part C), which is a combination of both health and prescription insurance from the same provider. This insurance has "first dollar coverage" with no deductible, unlike other insurance programs. Approximately 25% of all Medicare patients opt for this program. In the past, this insurance program has included incentives such as coverage for eye and hearing examinations, glasses, hearing aids, and gym memberships. Under the Affordable Care Act of 2010, the government subsidies for these additional benefits will be phased out or included as an option at an additional cost.

Medicare Part D The Medicare Prescription Drug, Improvement, and Modernization Act (MMA) of 2003, also called **Medicare Part D**, offers eligible patients the option to add drug insurance to their existing health coverage at an additional monthly charge to their current Medicare (Part B) premium. In addition to patients over age 65, patients with chronic kidney disease and those who are "dual eligible" for Medicare and Medicaid (usually disabled patients) are covered under the plan. More than 40 million patients who are eligible for Medicare have taken advantage of this insurance program. If patients opt not to enroll when eligible at age 65, then the monthly cost may be higher if they decide to join in the future.

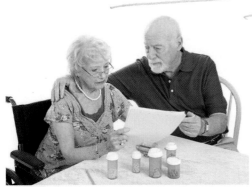

Each year, Medicare-eligible patients have an "open enrollment" period to change their drug insurance program. The pharmacy technician can often assist them in clarifying insurance options.

In this voluntary program, a patient (including retirees) may elect to continue current drug coverage through his or her existing supplemental health insurance or employer or to select an insurer participating in the Medicare Part D program in his or her state. Older adults can choose from several insurance plans that are available in each region of the country, and pharmacy personnel can direct patients to www.paradigmcollege.net/pharmpractice5e/Medicare to obtain more information about the program. The plan has special provisions for low-income seniors and provides catastrophic coverage for all patients who develop serious medical conditions requiring expensive drug treatments.

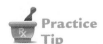

Practice Tip

As a customer service, pharmacy personnel should direct patients who are approaching age 65 to obtain information about Medicare Part D and its benefits. Information can be found online or by discussing options with the pharmacist.

Medicare Part D is complex, with many choices for coverage. Each plan has its advantages and disadvantages, and each has a different list of lower-cost, *preferred* drugs. Most plans cover all or most of the cost for generic drugs. Preferred and non-preferred formulary drugs are subject to a tiered co-pay. If a patient has a brand name product with a high co-pay, the pharmacy technician should alert the pharmacist, who may suggest a lower-cost alternative. If financial hardship exists, many prescribers are willing to change to a less expensive product.

Each patient who enrolls in Medicare Part D can expect to save an average of 25% to 30% from annual out-of-pocket cost of prescriptions. For example, in some plans, a $320 deductible must be paid before the patient is eligible for benefits. After the deductible is met, patients pay an average of 25% of the cost for their new and refilled prescriptions until the total drug costs (from out-of-pocket and insurance) reach approximately $3000. From $3000 to approximately $7700, patients are responsible for the increased cost of their medications. This gap in coverage is what patients and the media refer to as the **donut hole**. Patients are often shocked by the reality of drug costs when in the donut hole. In light of that, the government has provided subsidies via rebates and discounts of 50% on brand name drugs and 14% on generic drugs when the patient is in the donut hole. Once approximately $7700 in drug costs have been reached in the calendar year, the patient only pays 5% of the cost of the medications. The premium and the annual drug costs are adjusted annually with inflation. Pharmacy personnel should be aware that the Affordable Care Act of 2010 has a provision to eliminate the donut hole by 2019.

Prescription Insurance Patient Needs To best serve the needs of this older adult patient population, pharmacy technicians should become knowledgeable of drug insurance coverage and, along with pharmacists, should provide education and guidance as needed. Individual drug regimens will determine the most appropriate plan for patients. To help them make their selections, pharmacy personnel should also recommend to patients to research their options on the Internet and to seek guidance from family members.

Workers' Compensation In addition to PBMs representing commercial insurers such as Medicare, Tricare, and Medicaid, some patients may present prescriptions that are to be billed to **workers' compensation** (commonly referred to as *workers' comp*). Workers' comp provides insurance to cover medical care and compensation for an employee who is injured in the course of employment, in exchange for a waiver of the employee's right to sue his or her employer. Though the insurance is administered by state governments, the claim is processed through a PBM and paid for by the employer. The patient will have no insurance card, so the information must be gleaned from written information that the patient presents or from communication with an assigned caseworker.

The pharmacy must have a contract with a third-party PBM that is providing reimbursement to the pharmacy for the workers' comp claim. Depending on the pharmacy, there may be contracts for one or more workers' comp PBMs. On a prior authorization (PA) rejection for a workers' comp case, the caseworker or adjuster is called instead of the medical office to seek approval of the claim from the employer.

To process workers' comp insurance, the patient must present certain information to the pharmacy technician so that it can be entered into the patient profile. In addition to PBM information, the social security number, date of injury, and the name of the business compensating the patient must be entered. The initial data entry may take additional time and require a telephone call to a caseworker to verify information and drug coverage.

A workers' comp claim is generally entered as a secondary insurer (assuming that the patient has other drug insurance coverage); the coverage is based on the extent and severity of the injury and typically ranges from 3–12 months. Drug coverage is usually limited to specific classes of drugs that are needed to treat the injury. For example, if back pain is the primary symptom, analgesic and back spasm medication may be covered, but antibiotics for a sinus infection would not be covered. For covered drugs, the patient pays no co-pay.

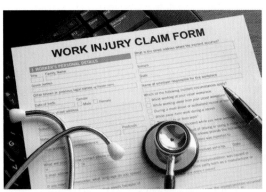

A pharmacy technician must gather additional information to process each workers' comp prescription claim.

Pharmacy technicians should become familiar with the policy and procedure for handling workers' comp claims at their pharmacy. The patient may have multiple claims to process; some drugs may be billed to the primary insurer and selected approved claims sent to the workers' comp PBM.

Coordination of Benefits Processing a claim through both a primary and a secondary insurer is known as **coordination of benefits (COB)**. In this scenario, a patient's claim is processed to the primary insurer. If the drug is not covered or if a co-pay exists, then the technician must bill the secondary insurer. Patients who have both primary and secondary insurance are called "dual eligible." For example, a disabled patient may have primary coverage from Medicare Part D and secondary coverage from Medicaid.

Coordination of benefits also occurs when a patient presents a coupon from the medical office for a prescription. The coupon is processed like drug insurance, and all pertinent information must be entered into the patient database. The coupon generally covers part or all of the co-payment from the primary insurance. If the patient has no drug insurance, the coupon will reduce the cost by a set amount. In nearly all cases, the coupon is for an expensive brand name medication.

The online processing of coordination of benefits depends on the type of software that a pharmacy uses. The co-payment cost to the patient is determined, and the COB is documented and filed. The technician must carefully review the coupon to note the processing requirements—for example, coupons may require activation or rebates to be made directly to the customer rather than online billing by the pharmacy. Patients with government drug programs such as Medicare Part D, Tricare, or Medicaid are not eligible for a coordination of benefits with a coupon reimbursement.

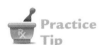

Uninsured There are more than 50 million adults and children in the United States, or more than 16% of the population, who do not have any type of health or drug insurance. This situation is often due to unemployment or underemployment. For example, if an individual works part-time (generally less than 32 hours per week), he or she is not eligible for employer-provided health benefits. In fact, some small businesses are currently exempt from offering a health insurance benefit even to their full-time employees.

To assist those who are **uninsured**, prescribers and pharmacy personnel should work together to identify the most common low-cost generic prescription for the required disease or illness. Some pharmacies may even advertise a list of "free" or low-cost ($4) prescriptions. These medications are known within the trade as "loss leaders"; the retailer may choose to lose or break even on drug costs if the lowered prices entice consumers to visit the store and buy more groceries or merchandise.

Drug Discount Cards and Coupons As a benefit to uninsured patients and others, some pharmacies offer a prescription savings club card that is available for individuals or families (including pets). Other patients use a drug discount card or present a coupon from their physicians to partially cover or discount the cost of the medication. There are many drug discount cards available in the mail or distributed as a fundraiser. The conditions for the discount card or coupon (including expiration date, amount of drug allowed, and so on) must be carefully reviewed by the pharmacy technician. Some discount cards or coupons can only be used if no additional insurance claim is processed or if no government insurance (Medicaid, Medicare, Tricare) is available; in other words, there is no coordination of benefits between government insurance programs and manufacturer coupons. Other drug discount cards do not reimburse the pharmacy. If the discount card is processed by the pharmacy, then the technician enters the bank identification number (BIN), subscriber identification number, and group number information from the coupon into the patient profile, akin to other insurance plans.

Drug discount and prescription club cards offer more savings for the patient when used for generic drugs rather than brand name medications. As with manufacturer coupons, patients on any government insurance program are ineligible for enrollment in a store discount drug program.

Other options for a patient without health insurance include free or low-cost charity clinics voluntarily staffed by doctors, nurses, and pharmacists; most urban areas have one or more community health centers that are subsidized by the federal government and through private grants and foundations. Costs for all health care are based on patients' needs and income levels.

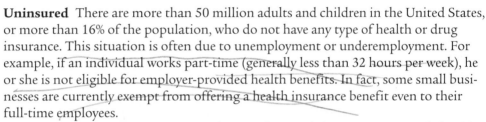

Practice Tip

Starting in 2014, many of these uninsured individuals will be covered under the Affordable Care Act. This expanded coverage will likely increase the workload of pharmacy personnel.

Receiving and Entering Insurance Information

For pharmacy technicians, learning the ins and outs of various insurance plans as well as their interface with the pharmacy's software package is a challenging task—second only to learning the generic and trade names of drugs. Experienced pharmacy technicians can greatly assist the pharmacist and the patient by making the drug insurance claim process a success. The procedures to bill online PBMs are similar—but not identical—whether the billing is to private insurance, the federal government (Medicare, Tricare), or state government plans (Medicaid). Typically, pharmacies have annual renewable contracts with most plans, but some plans—especially those out-of-state—may not be covered.

If the customer has drug insurance, then he or she should carry a prescription insurance card containing the following information: the name of the primary insured person, the insurance carrier, a group number, a nine-digit cardholder identification number, information on coverage of dependents, an effective date, and—sometimes—the amount of the co-pay for generic and brand name prescriptions. The technician must carefully review the prescription insurance card and identify the name of the insurer and the PBM servicing that plan. In addition to the patient information mentioned earlier, the technician should locate the BIN and processor control number (PCN), user number or person code, and group number of the plan on the insurance card. The BIN and PCN allow the technician to identify the correct PBM. Some insurance cards do not list a PCN, making the technician's job a little more difficult. The patient's relationship to the cardholder (spouse, child, and so on) is the person code and is often required for processing the online claim. For example, in Figure 7.6, the mother is the primary cardholder for the four children; "Fast RX" is the PBM or prescription processor; and "Central Healthcare" is the insurance plan provider.

An important responsibility of the technician is to update the prescription drug insurance plan in the pharmacy database.

FIGURE 7.6
Parts of an Insurance Identification Card

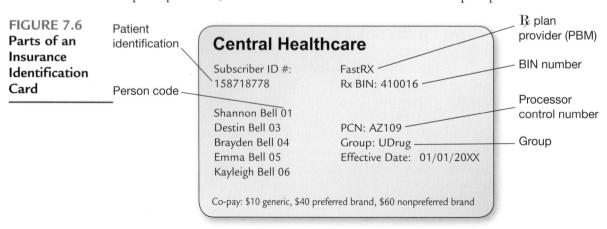

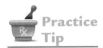

Practice Tip

Pharmacy technicians can provide an important customer service by helping patients sort out their insurance cards while explaining their coverage.

For every new patient or for any new changes in insurance coverage, the pharmacy technician must request this information and enter it into the patient profile. If the cardholder's employment status has changed recently, then the drug insurance may have expired. Some patients have more than one insurer, in which case the primary and secondary insurer ("dual eligibles") should be designated.

Receiving and entering insurance information can be a challenging task for pharmacy technicians. There are thousands of drug insurance plans with several major PBMs that process their prescription claims. In addition, the information on insurance cards is not standardized or always accurate, making the job of online processing and billing prescriptions difficult. Technicians may also need to spend time with customers who are confused or overwhelmed by the various healthcare cards they possess.

Processing Prescription Claims

Identifying and processing insurance claims are very important steps and are key to the profitability of a pharmacy. The prescription drug insurance information entered into the patient profile allows online adjudication from the pharmacy to a third-party PBM as the new prescription (or refill) is being processed. **Online adjudication** refers to using wireless communications to process prescription claims for private insurance, as well as Medicaid and Medicare Part D drug insurance. This action usually takes less than 30 seconds during the prescription-filling process and can save the pharmacy a great deal of time and paperwork when it is performed properly. When the prescription is billed to a PBM, the pharmacy is immediately notified as to what amount it should charge the patient for the co-payment and what amount the pharmacy will be reimbursed. If the cost is not covered, the patient may need to meet a deductible first, or the drug may simply not be covered under the insurance plan. It is common for many plans to list the amount saved by insurance coverage on the medication information sheet that accompanies the dispensed medication.

The customer should know that his or her co-pay and drug coverage are determined by the insurance plan, not by the pharmacy. If the pharmacy accepts the insurance plan, the process of online billing is similar among all pharmacies, and the co-pays are identical, regardless of where the prescription is filled. With drug insurance, a patient may go to any pharmacy to get his or her prescriptions filled; the only differences are location, hours of operation, and quality of service.

Potential Processing Errors The technician should be aware of several potential errors that can occur when processing a prescription claim. One such error can occur if there are discrepancies between the name on the patient's insurance card and the name in the insurance database. For example, Rick Smith may be in the insurance database as Charles R. Smith, and if a technician tries to process a drug claim under Rick Smith, it will be denied with the error message "unmatched recipient." This is important to remember for all insurance, but especially for Tricare, which covers uniformed service members, military retirees, and their dependents.

Another common processing error on insurance can occur if either the pharmacy or the insurance company has the incorrect date of birth. Even if the pharmacy has the correct date of birth, if the date does not match the one in the PBM database, the claim will not be approved. To correct this error, the technician must call the PBM, verify the birth date, and enter the incorrect date in the patient profile in order to process the claim. The patient (or parent) must then call the insurance company to correct the dates and then advise the pharmacy on his or her next visit to update the corrected birth date in the patient profile.

If the drug claim is not processing (in other words, causing an error message), then the pharmacy technician should take another look at the ID numbers. Many plans may use letters preceding the ID number, e.g., XYZ1199A2883; some insurance plans require the letters, but some do not. Letters in the middle of the ID number are commonly required. Tricare uses the social security number as the ID number for both retired military personnel and their dependents. To make matters more complicated, the group number on the prescription card may be incorrect or missing (some plans do not require a group number).

Some insurance plans (or pharmacy software) require a two-digit or three-digit person code to follow the ID number, but some do not. For example, the husband may be there to pick up a prescription, but his wife is the primary insured under the plan; his nine-digit ID number may be 119922883-02 (or 002), whereas his wife may have the same ID number but a different person code of 01 (or 001). Dependent children may be 03, 04, 05, and so on. Most Medicare Part D and Medicaid programs have a patient-specific ID number without a user number.

The notation "refill too soon" may be another reason that a claim cannot be processed. Most insurance plans allow refills to be processed if the request is within five to seven days of the patient's depletion of medication, but some plans are more restrictive. If the refill involves a controlled substance, then the pharmacist may not allow early refills (even if insurance does), depending on the policy at the community pharmacy.

Another claim processing error may be because the pharmacy technician entered the incorrect number of days' supply of medication into the patient profile. The prescription may have been written for a 90-day supply of Lipitor but only 30 days are covered. Calculating the number of days' supply for creams, ointments, and gels is difficult, but it can be estimated—depending on the size of the tube (usually 15 g, 30 g, 45 g, or 60 g), the application site (face, arm, body, and so on), and the frequency of application.

Calculating Medication Quantity and Days' Supply

As discussed previously, preparing a drug claim for online billing and processing includes entering specific information about each prescription filled, including the medication quantity and days' supply of medication. **Days' supply** is the time that a given amount of prescribed medication lasts. If the information submitted is incorrect, then the claim may be denied, or—if audited—the pharmacy may not be reimbursed for the medication. Thus, calculating days' supply of medication accurately is an important skill.

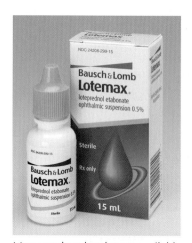

Many eyedrop bottles are available in various volumes. The correct bottle to dispense is dependent on the prescriber's directions—for example, the number of drops per day, the instillation of the drops in one eye or both eyes, etc.

Certain drug formulations, such as otic and ophthalmic solutions and suspensions, are a bit more challenging to calculate when determining days' supply (see Table 7.3). For example, a pharmacy may receive a prescription for Lotemax with the sig "Place 2 drops in each (OU) eye qid for 14 days with 1 refill." The technician must learn that 20 drops of solution is equal to 1 mL, so a 10 mL bottle will contain 200 drops. If the patient is taking 16 drops of medication daily for 14 days, they will need 224 drops (16 drops/day × 14 days). A 5 mL bottle would not provide a sufficient quantity (100 drops), and neither would a 10 mL bottle (200 drops). A 15 mL bottle (such as the one shown here) would provide more than a sufficient amount to fill the prescription. If the technician entered 10 days, then the claim may be rejected or challenged in an audit. Notice that 1 mL of an otic or ophthalmic suspension formulation is 20% less or equivalent to 16 drops; the number of days' supply and thus insurance billing will differ if the suspension is prescribed.

TABLE 7.3 Medication Volume Equivalences

Medication	Equivalences	
Otic/ophthalmic solution	1 mL	20 drops
Otic/ophthalmic suspension	1 mL	16 drops
MDI asthma	1 canister	200 inhalations
Nasal sprays for allergies	1 bottle	120 doses
Insulin (NovoLog, Humulin, Lantus, and so on)	10 mL vial	100 units/mL or 1000 units/vial

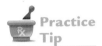

Practice Tip

When calculating days' supply, pharmacy technicians should know that 1 mL of ophthalmic solution is equivalent to 20 drops.

For some prescriptions, dispensing the exact days' supply is not practical. For example, a pharmacy may receive a prescription for cefdinir (Omnicef) antibiotic suspension with a sig "Give 1 teaspoonful daily for 10 days." The total volume is 50 mL (5 mL/day × 10 days), but the smallest bottle of cefdinir suspension is 60 mL. Insurance plans recognize that there will be 10 mL of wastage and approve the claim. In this circumstance, the technician should add the statement "Discard remainder after 10 days" to the medication container label.

The following examples show how to calculate medication amounts and days' supply for actual prescriptions.

Example 5

A prescription is received for Ciprofloxacin 500 mg and the sig "Take one tablet twice daily. Quantity: 28." What is the medication amount and the days' supply?

$$\text{days' supply} = 28 \text{ tablets} \div 2 \text{ tablets/day} = 14 \text{ days}$$

Example 6

A prescription is received for Augmentin 600 mg/5 mL with the sig "Give ¾ teaspoonful twice daily for 10 days." Augmentin is available as a generic in 75 mL, 100 mL, and 150 mL. What is the days' supply? What size bottle should be used? How much dispensed product will be unused?

Step 1. Calculate volume taken in each dose by converting ¾ teaspoonful to milliliters (abbreviated as mL). Because 1 tsp = 5 mL,

$$\frac{3}{4} \text{ tsp/dose} \times 5 \text{ mL/1 tsp} = 3.75 \text{ mL/dose}$$

Step 2. Calculate the amount of drug prescribed per day.

$$2 \text{ doses/day} \times 3.75 \text{ mL/dose} = 7.5 \text{ mL/day}$$

Step 3. Determine the number of days the prescription should last. According to the prescription, the days' supply is 10 days.

Step 4. Calculate total volume needed.

$$7.5 \text{ mL/day} \times 10 \text{ days} = 75 \text{ mL}$$

Step 5. Select the bottle size from the available stock and determine how much product will remain after the patient takes the prescribed amount. Because Augmentin comes in 75 mL, 100 mL, and 150 mL bottles, the 75 mL bottle will be selected. Because the bottle amount equals the prescribed amount, none of the drug will be left over.

$$75 \text{ mL/dispensed amount} - 75 \text{ mL/prescribed amount} = 0 \text{ mL}$$

Example 7

The pharmacy receives a prescription for Augmentin 400 mg/5 mL. The prescription states "Give 1 tsp tid for 7 days." Medicaid insurance does not cover this strength but will cover Augmentin 600 mg/5 mL. If the substitution to the insured strength is made, what will the new sig be? Augmentin suspensions are available in 50 mL, 75 mL, and 100 mL bottles. Which bottle will be dispensed and how much should remain after seven days?

Step 1. Calculate the volume of Augmentin 600 mg/5 mL needed to provide the prescribed dose of 400 mg tid. Set up a ratio comparing the prescribed dose to the insured product.

$$\frac{x \text{ mL}}{400 \text{ mg}} = \frac{5 \text{ mL}}{600 \text{ mg}}$$

$$\frac{(400 \text{ mg}) \, x \text{ mL}}{400 \text{ mg}} = \frac{(400 \text{ mg}) \, 5 \text{ mL}}{600 \text{ mg}}$$

$$x \text{ mL} = 3.333 \text{ mL, rounded to } 3.33 \text{ mL}$$

The sig must be changed to read "Take 3.33 mL 3 times daily for 7 days."

Step 2. Calculate volume needed per day.

$$3.33 \text{ mL} \times 3 \text{ doses/day} = 9.99 \text{ mL/day, rounded to } 10 \text{ mL}$$

Step 3. Calculate the total volume needed for the days' supply.

$$7 \text{ days} \times 10 \text{ mL/day} = 70 \text{ mL}$$

Step 4. Use the 75 mL volume of the 600 mg/5 mL Augmentin. Approximately 5 mL will remain after 7 days and should be discarded. Because of the 3.33 mL dose, a measuring device should be included with the prescription. If you incorrectly chose the 100 mL size, then more product would be wasted and the claim may not be processed. During an audit, the pharmacy may not be reimbursed for dispensing more medication than necessary. (Some overage is allowed by insurance.)

Example 8

A prescription is written for Hydrocodone/APAP in a strength of 5 mg/500 mg #90 with the sig "Take 1 to 2 tablets every 4 to 6 hours prn pain" with one refill. How many days will the dispensed medication last?

Step 1. Calculate the maximum number of tablets taken each day. If the patient takes 2 tablets every 4 hours, 12 tablets could be taken in a day. However, you will learn with experience that the maximum safe amount for this drug is 8 tablets per day.

Step 2. Assuming the patient takes 8 tablets per day, calculate the days' supply for the 90 tablets dispensed.

$$90 \text{ tablets} \div 8 \text{ tablets/day} = 11.25 \text{ days, or } 11 \text{ days}$$

This means that the prescription cannot be refilled—or the claim processed—prior to 11 days from the date of initial dispensing.

Example 9

A prescription is written for Cortisporin Otic suspension with the sig "Place 4 gtt AS qid for 5 days." This product is available as a generic in package sizes or volumes of 5 mL and 10 mL. Assuming there are 16 gtt in 1 mL, how much medication is dispensed to fill the prescription?

Step 1. Because the available stock is in milliliters (mL), convert the prescribed units of measure, drops (abbreviated as gtt), to milliliters (mL).

$$4 \text{ gtt/dose} \times 1 \text{ mL/16 gtt} = 0.25 \text{ mL/dose}$$

Step 2. Calculate the amount of drug used per day.

$$0.25 \text{ mL/dose} \times 4 \text{ doses/day} = 1 \text{ mL/day}$$

Step 3. Calculate the amount of drug needed to complete the prescribed therapy.

$$1 \text{ mL/day} \times 5 \text{ days/therapy} = 5 \text{ mL/therapy}$$

Because the product is available as a 5 mL size, which meets the needs of the prescription, the 5 mL size should be dispensed. If the 10 mL size were dispensed, then the insurance claim would not be accepted, and the pharmacy would not be reimbursed.

Example 10

A prescription is written for 30 g of Lotrisone Cream with the sig "Apply to affected area tid" with one refill. How many days will the prescribed medication last?

Estimate may be seven days or longer; it would depend on the area being covered (for example, arm, leg, or trunk). Asking the patient can assist in making this estimate. After this time, the medication can be refilled and billed online to insurance.

Example 11

A prescription is received for 2 vials of Novolin N with the sig "Inject 40 units under the skin in the morning and 25 units in the evening" with prn refills. Insulin is available in 10 mL vials (or 1000 units per 10 mL). How many days will the prescribed medication last?

Step 1. Calculate the total daily dose of insulin.

$$40 \text{ units/morning} + 25 \text{ units/evening} = 65 \text{ units/day}$$

Step 2. Calculate the number of days' supply that 2 vials will satisfy. Each vial contains 1000 units of insulin.

$$2 \text{ vials} \times 1000 \text{ units/vial} = 2000 \text{ units}$$

$$2000 \text{ units} \div 65 \text{ units/day} = 30.769 \text{ days, or } 30 \text{ days' supply}$$

If you mistakenly put 60 days' supply (30 days for each vial), then the initial claim will be processed; however, the patient will not be able to get a needed refill after 30 days without calling the insurance provider to change and correct the original claim.

Example 12

A prescription is received for Cialis 20 mg #30 with no refills and the sig "Take as directed 1 hour prior to sexual intercourse." What is the medication amount and days' supply?

A pharmacy technician may, at first, conclude that the ℞ is written for 30 tablets, so it must be 30 days' supply. But, after submitting the insurance claim, the claim is denied. Although each PBM may differ, insurance may cover only 5 tablets for 30 days. The technician should then question whether the prescriber meant to write a prescription for Cialis 5 mg #30—a prescription that is for daily use and represents a 30-day supply. If in doubt, the technician should follow up on the discrepancy by contacting the prescriber's office for verification.

Step 1. After verification, the technician should update the prescription entry in the computer with 5 tablets and 30 days' supply and re-submit the claim to the insurance company.

Step 2. The technician should then explain to the patient that insurance only covers 5 tablets dispensed for a $30 co-pay. Consequently, the patient has the option of purchasing the remaining 25 for cash (at a cost of more than $300). Explain to the patient that he can get 5 refills of 5 tablets each month because the total quantity written on the prescription was 30 tablets.

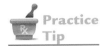

Practice Tip

Assuming the role of patient advocate in insurance claims may be time-consuming for the pharmacy technician but fosters patient trust as well as pharmacy loyalty.

Resolving Prescription Drug Claims, Audits, and Charge-backs

Billing policies and procedures differ from pharmacy to pharmacy and from customer to customer. In a majority of cases, billing involves direct online transactions between the pharmacy and the customer's insurance plan. A claim is processed, and the patient cost of the prescription is determined if the patient is eligible.

If a claim cannot be resolved, then the pharmacy technician should call the toll-free number on the back of the patient's insurance card to try to clear up the issue. Assuming the role of patient advocate in insurance claims may be time-consuming for the technician but fosters patient trust as well as pharmacy loyalty. The pharmacy technician often has to be empathetic toward a patient who does not fully understand why his or her medications are so expensive but not covered—or only partially covered—by the insurance company. Clearly, much can go wrong when the technician is processing a drug claim. The technician should have a personal notebook to make entries for future reference, including helpful tips and shortcuts, on the various insurance plans.

Prior Authorization When a medication is not covered by drug insurance, or when the prescriber decides that the patient must have a medication that is not on the PBM's formulary, the prescriber's nurse may have to call the PBM to obtain **prior authorization (PA)** for the prescription to be covered properly. For example, if a patient's cholesterol cannot be controlled with lovastatin (a generic cholesterol drug) and the patient suffers an adverse reaction to Crestor (the preferred brand cholesterol drug), then the PBM would, in most cases, approve drug coverage and a lower co-pay for Livalo ($40 as opposed to $60 in this example). The pharmacy sends a PA request to the prescriber, whose representative contacts the insurance company to determine whether coverage will be approved (and for how long) or whether an alternative drug must be prescribed. Or, for example, if Nexium is prescribed for heartburn but not covered by insurance, the prescriber may elect to change the order to generic omeprazole rather than pursuing approval of the PA. Pending legislation in some states would allow the pharmacist to act on behalf of the prescriber and the patient in resolving PAs.

Medications without Insurance Coverage Cases exist in which the medication selected by the physician and needed by the patient is not covered by the insurance under any circumstances. This lack of coverage applies to newly marketed innovative drugs that are extremely expensive; drugs that promote weight loss and sleep; certain medications for anxiety or nervous disorders; certain cough syrups for adults; vitamins; and drugs that have less costly alternatives or that are available as OTC drugs. If a question about coverage arises, then having a photocopy of the patient's insurance card on file, with the appropriate (toll-free) contact phone numbers, is helpful. If insurance denies coverage, the patient has the right to appeal; most patients are unaware of this right, but the process requires the completion of a lot of paperwork and is exceedingly slow. In most cases, the patient pays cash or uses a discount card if eligible.

Insurance Fraud Filing a false claim is considered insurance fraud and subject to potential civil and criminal penalties as well as termination of employment. For example, a pharmacy technician cannot dispense a medication to a patient and then post or bill the insurance three days later; the patient must return in three days to pick up the medication after the insurance has been accepted. Any prescription or processing error, such as an incorrect quantity or days' supply, results in a rejection of the claim and, consequently, no reimbursement to the pharmacy. The importance of the technician in accurately billing third-party prescriptions has a definite impact on the profitability of the pharmacy.

Medication Audits A pharmacy is subject to medication audits from any insurer. An **audit** is a challenge on a reimbursement from a PBM or insurance provider on a prescription claim that has been previously processed. These challenges can be from prescriptions that were processed three to six months earlier. Audits are intended to reduce fraud and waste; however, as in any business, customer service must be balanced with profitability.

The audit challenge is commonly conducted via the mail, but, occasionally, insurance representatives personally investigate past claims on-site. The pharmacy technician investigates the validity of the claim and must resolve the issue within two weeks of receipt of the challenge. If the audit challenges are not resolved in a timely manner, then the pharmacy forfeits all reimbursement to those claims resulting in a revenue loss. The following are examples of potential audit challenges:

- A patient was "not eligible" for prescription coverage on the date of the claim.
- The days' supply of the tablets, capsules, eardrops/eyedrops, or antibiotic suspension was entered incorrectly; for example, a prescription for the migraine drug Imitrex 100 mg #9 should be entered as a 30-day supply, not as a 9-day supply.
- Initials from the pharmacist on phone or transfer prescriptions or the signature of the patient (or their representative) may be missing; the patient "attestation" signature is considered proof that the prescription was dispensed; Medicaid requires signatures and hard copies or computer copies to be kept on file for the audit.
- On an "as directed" prescription, the frequency of the insulin dose or blood glucose check was not determined by a call to the prescriber's office; therefore, the days' supply of medication may be incorrect.
- Documentation was not provided on the original prescription for large quantities dispensed or the verification of larger-than-normal doses prescribed.
- If a patient (not a prescriber) requests a brand name medication, then the order must be entered as a DAW2 (brand requested by patient) order; or, if the prescriber does not specify "brand necessary" on the prescription, a generic is prepared by pharmacy personnel, and then the patient requests that the brand name drug be dispensed, the order must be entered as a DAW2.

Charge-Backs A **charge-back** is a rejection of a prescription claim by a PBM or insurance provider that must be investigated and, if possible, resolved by the pharmacy technician. A charge-back could occur for a number of reasons:

- The certificate of medical necessity form for diabetic supplies was not completed properly for a Medicare Part B claim or a signed renewal from the doctor was not obtained.
- Online processing was not functioning due to an Internet malfunction, and it was determined later on that a patient was ineligible for drug insurance benefits.
- The primary insurance of a "dual eligible" patient was not billed.
- A prescription was filled too soon (based on days' supply) or filled at another pharmacy.

The technician must verify that the patient received the prescription and check the original copy of the prescription and patient profile to resolve any inconsistencies.

Chapter Summary

- The pharmacy technician has an important role in helping with the business operations of the pharmacy.
- The technician has an important responsibility in assisting customers in locating needed OTC drugs, dietary supplements, and medical supplies.
- Some OTC drugs—such as Schedule V cough syrups, decongestants containing pseudoephedrine, and Plan B contraceptives—require specific procedures prior to sales.
- The technician can assist the diabetic patient who needs syringes, needles, test strips, glucometers, and related medical supplies.
- The technician must be competent in all cash register management functions, including sales by cash, check, credit card, debit card, and Flex card.
- The technician's responsibilities in inventory management include the purchasing, receiving, and return of drugs; the technician must understand these responsibilities in order to run a profitable pharmacy.
- Purchasing, receiving, taking inventory, and record keeping of controlled substances require specific legal paperwork procedures.
- Calculating the markup on the products and computing any discounts are often the responsibilities of the technician.
- Understanding the concept of average wholesale price (AWP) is necessary for billing insurance companies.
- A basic knowledge of both computer and mathematical skills is necessary for the technician to manage pharmacy business functions successfully.
- The technician must have an understanding of various private and government insurance programs and the knowledge to process online claims for prescriptions successfully.

Key Terms

audit a challenge on a reimbursement from a PBM or insurance provider on a prescription claim that has been previously processed

average wholesale price (AWP) the average price that wholesalers charge the pharmacy for a drug

certificate of medical necessity form to be completed and signed by the prescriber for Medicare Part B insurance payment for diabetic supplies

charge-back a rejection of a prescription claim by a PBM or an insurance provider that must be investigated and resolved

coinsurance a percentage-based insurance plan in which the patient must pay a certain percentage of the prescription price

computer an electronic device for inputting, storing, processing, and/or outputting information

coordination of benefits (COB) online billing of both a primary and a secondary insurer

co-payment (co-pay) the amount that the patient is to pay for each prescription as determined by insurance

credit card a method of online payment that is a type of loan, either paid totally at the end of the month or partially with a finance charge added

database management system (DBMS) an application that allows one to enter, retrieve, and query records

days' supply the duration of time (number of days) a dispensed medication will last a patient; required on drug claims submitted for online insurance billing

debit card a method of online cash payment that instantly deducts the cost of the purchase from the customer's bank account

deductible an amount that must be paid by the insured before the insurance company considers paying its portion of a medical or drug cost

dietary supplement a category of nonprescription drugs that includes vitamins, minerals, and herbals that are not directly regulated by the FDA like OTC drugs

discount a reduced price

donut hole insurance coverage gap in Medicare Part D programs by which the patient must pay a higher portion of the cost of the medication; to be phased out by 2019

dual co-pay insurance coverage in which a patient pays one co-pay for brand name drugs and a lower co-pay for generic drugs

dumb terminal a computer device that contains a keyboard and a monitor but does not contain its own storage and processing capabilities

durable medical equipment (DME) medical equipment such as hospital beds, wheelchairs, canes, or crutches that may be covered under Medicare Part B insurance

Flex card a medical and prescription insurance credit card

gross profit the difference between the purchase price and the selling price; also called *markup*

health insurance coverage of incurred medical costs such as physician and emergency room visits, laboratory costs, and hospitalization

inventory the entire stock of products on hand for sale at a given time

inventory turnover rate the amount of time the average drug inventory will be replaced during a 12-month period; most pharmacies replace inventory every two to four weeks

inventory value the total value of the entire stock of products on hand for sale on a given day

just-in-time (JIT) purchasing frequent purchasing in quantities that just meet supply needs until the next ordering time

markup the difference between the purchase price and the selling price; also called *gross profit*

Medicaid a state government health insurance program for low-income and disabled citizens

Medicare Part D a voluntary insurance program that provides partial coverage of prescriptions primarily for patients who are eligible for Medicare

nondurable medical supplies consumable, disposable items that can only be used by one patient for a specific purpose

online adjudication real-time insurance claims processing via wireless telecommunications

out of stock (OOS) a situation in which the pharmacy does not have the prescribed drug in inventory

over-the-counter (OTC) drug a medication that the FDA has approved for sale without a prescription; another name for a *nonprescription drug*

partial fill a situation in which the pharmacy cannot completely fill the prescribed quantity written on the prescription

perpetual inventory record a record that accounts for each unit of Schedule II drug dispensed or received

pharmacy benefits manager (PBM) a company that administers drug benefits for many insurance companies

posting the process of reconciling the invoice and updating inventory at time of receipt

preferred drug list a formulary provided by an insurance company that indicates preferred prescription generic and brand name drugs and their corresponding co-pays

prime vendor purchasing an agreement made by a pharmacy for a specified percentage or dollar amount of purchases

prior authorization (PA) approval for coverage of a high-cost medication or a medication not on the insurer's approved formulary, obtained after a prescriber's office calls the insurer to justify the use of the drug; must be obtained before the drug is dispensed by the pharmacy in order to be covered by insurance

private insurance coverage for medical or prescription costs provided by an employer or purchased by an individual

profit the amount of revenue received that exceeds the expense of the sold product, services, and overhead

purchasing the ordering of products for use or sale by the pharmacy

receipt a printout that is a proof of purchase

receiving a series of procedures for accepting the delivery of products to the pharmacy from a wholesaler or centralized warehouse

remote computer a minicomputer or a mainframe that stores and processes data sent from a dumb terminal

Schedule V drug a medication with a low potential for abuse and a limited potential for creating physical or psychological dependence; available in most states without a prescription

sharps any needle, lancet, scalpel blade, or other medical equipment that could cause a cut or puncture

smart terminal a computer that contains its own storage and processing capabilities

smurfing a practice that occurs when a patient is paid cash by an individual to illegally purchase pseudoephedrine from more than one pharmacy

tiered co-pay insurance coverage in which the patient has an escalating cost or co-pay, depending on whether the filled prescription is a generic drug, a preferred brand name drug, or a nonpreferred brand name drug

Tricare a federal government health insurance program for active and retired military personnel and their dependents

uninsured patients with no insurance who must pay out-of-pocket for medical and/or prescription costs

usual and customary charges the total cost of dispensing a prescription to the general public; a pharmacy cannot bill government insurance programs more than the usual and customary charge

wholesaler purchasing the ordering of drugs and supplies from a local or regional vendor who delivers the product to the pharmacy on a daily basis

workers' compensation insurance provided for a patient with a medical injury from a job-related accident; also called *workers' comp*

Checking Your Understanding

To check your comprehension of this chapter's key concepts, read the following multiple-choice questions and then record your answers on a separate sheet of paper. Write your answers as modeled in these examples: 1d; 2c; 3b; *etc.*

1. Dietary supplements are regulated by
   a. the FDA.
   b. the DSHEA.
   c. the CDC.
   d. state laws.

2. Diphenhydramine (Benadryl) capsules are regulated by
   a. the FDA.
   b. the DSHEA.
   c. the CDC.
   d. state laws.

3. A computer software application that can enter, retrieve, and query patient records is a(n)
   a. spreadsheet.
   b. word processing system.
   c. database management system (DBMS).
   d. Internet browser.

4. Processing of prescriptions to insurance is done by
   a. using wireless telecommunications.
   b. completing a universal claim form.
   c. telephoning the insurance company.
   d. using a patient's Flex card.

5. A PBM is best described as a(n)
   a. insurance company.
   b. company that contracts with several insurance companies.
   c. drug wholesaler.
   d. prime vendor.

6. If an insurance company has three different co-pays for each class of medications, then its payment structure is best described as
   a. average wholesale price.
   b. out-of-pocket.
   c. tiered co-pay.
   d. dual co-pay.

7. Who is eligible for Medicare Part D?
   a. patients with incomes below the poverty line
   b. disabled patients
   c. any patient eligible for Medicare
   d. retired military personnel and their families

8. How do most independent community pharmacies maintain their daily inventory of drugs?
   a. purchasing directly from the drug manufacturer
   b. purchasing using the Internet
   c. purchasing from a local wholesaler
   d. borrowing from the hospital pharmacy

9. A DEA 222 form must be used to order and receive which controlled substance?
   a. Schedule II
   b. Schedule III
   c. Schedule IV
   d. Schedule V

10. The average price that wholesalers charge a pharmacy for a medication is also called
    a. AWP.
    b. usual and customary.
    c. markup.
    d. discount.

11. If a patient is prescribed gabapentin 300 mg po tid #270, what would you record as the "days' supply"?
    a. 30 days
    b. 60 days
    c. 90 days
    d. 6 months or 180 days

12. A prior authorization or PA is best described to the patient as a situation in which
    a. the prescriber must be contacted in order for the pharmacist to substitute a generic drug.
    b. the pharmacy must dispense a brand name drug.
    c. the patient must meet an insurance deductible before insurance will cover the drug.
    d. insurance requires the prescriber to justify the need for a particular drug.

13. To successfully process a prescription claim, insurance requires the patient ID number or user number, processor control number (or PCN), group number, and the _____

a. BIN.
b. NPI.
c. DEA.
d. pharmacy license number.

14. Which of the following patients is eligible to use a coupon or drug discount card?
    a. uninsured
    b. Medicare Part D
    c. Medicaid
    d. Tricare

15. Safe disposal of syringes and needles using a sharps container is necessary to prevent transmission of HIV and
    a. tetanus.
    b. hepatitis.
    c. influenza.
    d. pneumonia.

Reinforcing Your Learning

To build on your understanding of the topics in this chapter, complete the following enrichment activities.

1. Create a diagram outlining the steps from receipt of a prescription through online adjudication. What key pieces of information are needed from the patient and the insurance card to process the claim?

2. Solve the following business math problems:
   a. Eyedrops with antihistamine are purchased in cases of 36 dropper-dispensed bottles. The pharmacy desires a markup of $1.75 per bottle. The purchase price is $111.60 per case. What is the selling price per bottle?
   b. Identify the markup and the selling price of an oral antibiotic suspension that costs the pharmacy $15.60 per bottle and has a markup rate of 25%.
   c. A month's supply of an asthma tablet costs the pharmacy $24.80, and the selling price is $30.75. Calculate the markup rate.

   d. Van Ingen's Drug Shop purchases two cases of hydrocortisone cream at $100 per case. The invoice specifies a 15% discount if the account is paid in full within 15 days. What is the total discounted price of the two cases?
   e. In question *d*, each case contains 24 tubes of cream. You are to mark up each tube by 20% based on the discounted cost. What is the selling price per tube?
   f. A prescription is written for a tube of ointment. The AWP is $62. Grimm's Pharmacy purchases the tube at AWP, and Erickson's Pharmacy purchases the tube at AWP minus 10%. The insurer reimburses at AWP plus 2% plus a $1.50 dispensing fee. How much profit does each pharmacy make?

g. Sinus tablets have an AWP of $37.50 per 50 tablets. The Corner Drug Store dispensed prescriptions for a total of 300 sinus tablets during May. They were purchased at AWP minus 15%. The insurer reimburses at AWP plus 1.5% plus a $2 dispensing fee. Fifteen prescriptions of 20 tablets each were filled that month. How much profit was made?

h. Review Garcia's Drug Shop Inventory below and calculate the necessary purchases to reestablish maximum inventory. Write your answers in the *Purchased* column.

Garcia's Drug Shop Inventory

Drug	Maximum Level	Dispensed Today	Minimum Level	Current Inventory	Purchased
Eucerin cream, jars	10	1	3	3	
Amoxicillin, capsules	4500	500	4000	2400	
Eyedrops, bottles	24	4	4	4	
Nystatin oral solution	1000 mL	100 mL	200 mL	400 mL	
Viscous lidocaine, bottles	600 mL	300 mL	200 mL	100 mL	

3. Calculate the days' supply for insurance billing on each of the following prescriptions.

a.
R_X
Ventolin MDI #1 (200 inhalations per MDI)

Sig: 1 spray q6 h prn wheezing

c.
R_X
Gentamicin Ophthalmic Solution 5 mL

Sig: 2 gtts OD qid for 7 days

b.
R_X
Nasonex Nasal Spray #1 (120 sprays per canister)

Sig: 2 sprays in each nostril daily for allergies

d.
R_X
Cefdinir 250 mg/5 mL 60 mL

Sig: 1 tsp po qd for 10 days

4. There are many patients with diabetes—both young and old—that must be careful of sugar (and alcohol) content in their liquid prescriptions as well as in their OTC products. Visit a community pharmacy and identify two or three sugar-free cough or cold OTC products that would be safe to recommend to a parent with a young child who is diabetic. What information is found on the OTC label?

Thinking on Your Feet

To gain practice in handling challenging situations in the workplace, consider the following real-world scenarios and then use the guiding questions to help you formulate your responses.

1. An elderly patient who is a regular customer at your pharmacy is very confused upon hearing that you cannot fill his prescription for Dexilant due to a "prior authorization." In terms understandable to the patient, how would you describe the problem? What is the process for resolving a PA? What alternatives exist?

2. Mr. Pavlovich approaches the pharmacy counter and wants to pick up his Cialis 20 mg prescription. He hands you a drug coupon that he obtained at his doctor's office to help defray the cost of his expensive prescription. When you tell him that you cannot honor the coupon, he becomes upset. What are some reasons why you cannot honor or process the drug coupon?

3. You receive a prescription for insulin pen needles from Mrs. Thao. The prescription asks the pharmacy to dispense 31 gauge 5/16 inch needles. When you check the pharmacy stock, you find a supply of 31 gauge needles in 8 mm and 5 mm sizes. Which size should be dispensed to Mrs. Thao: the 8 mm or the 5 mm? What determined your selection choice?

Acquiring Field Knowledge

To expand your knowledge of pharmacy practice, explore the following online activities that focus on research and information retrieval.

Reminder: *As you navigate the Internet, remember to exercise caution and good judgment when evaluating information. A thoughtful review of online text should take into consideration the following factors: the creator and sponsors of the website, the intended audience, the credentials of the authors and contributors, the reliability and validity of the posted information, the frequency of updates to the site, and the ease of navigation for a range of user skill levels.*

1. Because patients often have difficulty understanding how their prescription insurance plans work, pharmacy technicians working in a retail setting should be familiar with various terms related to health insurance. Sharing this knowledge with patients provides clarity for them on their insurance coverage and shows your willingness to serve as a patient advocate for prescription drug benefits. To check your understanding of insurance terminology, research the following terms online and define them in words that would be easily understood by a customer of your pharmacy.
   a. major medical insurance
   b. Medicare, Parts A, B, C, and D
   c. Medicaid
   d. deductible
   e. co-pay
   f. coinsurance
   g. preferred vs. nonpreferred brand
   h. pharmacy benefits manager (PBM)
   i. usual and customary
   j. dual and tiered co-pays

2. Go to www.paradigmcollege.net/pharmpractice5e/glucometers. Compare the cost and features of brand-name glucometers stocked in a community pharmacy. Which would you recommend and why? What are the advantages and disadvantages of a store or generic brand glucometer? Then compare the cost of test strips that go with each meter. What is the average cost of a month's supply of strips (box of 100)?

3. Many individuals in the United States have undiagnosed diabetes. To protect your own health and to educate your patients about the warning signs of the disease, visit www.paradigmcollege.net/pharmpractice5e/diabetestest. Take the diabetes risk test to determine your susceptibility for the disease, and encourage your family members, friends, and patients to do the same.

Sampling the Certification Exam

To provide you with practice for the Certification Exam, read the following questions that have been patterned after the test format and then record your answers on a separate sheet of paper. Write your answers as modeled in these examples: 1d; 2c; 3b; etc.

1. A physical inventory of controlled substances in Schedule II must be done
   a. daily.
   b. monthly.
   c. yearly.
   d. every two years.

2. What is the name for the general cost of doing business?
   a. overall cost
   b. income
   c. overhead
   d. professional handling

3. The term used to describe having more receipts than expenses is
   a. turnover.
   b. profit.
   c. markup.
   d. dispensing fee.

4. Which of the following products must be sold behind the pharmacy counter?
   a. Next Choice
   b. Aleve
   c. Monistat 3
   d. condoms

5. Purchasing that is done frequently in quantities to meet demand until the next ordering time is called
   a. direct purchasing.
   b. prime vendor purchasing.
   c. JIT.
   d. DUR.

6. Which is an advantage to monitoring inventory?
   a. an increase in expired products
   b. a decrease in capital that is tied up
   c. an increase in the risk of diversion
   d. an increase in shelf space needed

7. When checking in an order from a wholesaler, which document should be used for verification of the order?
   a. invoice
   b. want book
   c. purchase order
   d. last 24-hour usage

8. When stocking pharmaceuticals received from the wholesaler, pharmacy technicians should always place products with the shortest expiration dates
   a. behind other stock.
   b. on the counter.
   c. in front of the other stock.
   d. next to the other stock.

9. Insulin needles for subcutaneous administration are typically
   a. 28 gauge.
   b. 22 gauge.
   c. 18 gauge.
   d. 15 gauge.

10. To combat methamphetamine abuse, state and federal laws restrict the sale of
    a. codeine-containing cough syrups.
    b. insulin syringes.
    c. pseudoephedrine.
    d. guaifenesin (Robitussin).

Nonsterile Pharmaceutical Compounding

8

Learning Objectives

- Define the term *compounding*, describe common situations in which compounding is required, and identify rationale and examples of nonsterile compounding.

- Discuss the impact of the Food and Drug Administration Modernization Act (FDAMA) of 1997 on the practice of a compounding pharmacy.

- Understand the distinction between a manufactured product and a compounded nonsterile preparation.

- Define the regulatory role of the state board of pharmacy.

- Identify quality standards for nonsterile compounding contained in USP Chapter <795>, including product selection and beyond-use or expiration dating.

- Review and follow the components of good compounding practices in the pharmacy.

- Discuss reasons and process for accreditation of specialty compounded pharmacies.

- Understand the minimum training and attire requirements for pharmacy technicians in a compounding pharmacy.

- Distinguish the components and purpose of a master control record from a compounding log.

- Define the term *percentage of error* and understand how the concept relates to accuracy in the compounding pharmacy.

- Identify and describe the function of the equipment used for the weighing, measuring, and compounding of pharmaceuticals.

- Explain the proper techniques for weighing pharmaceutical ingredients, measuring liquid volumes, and compounding nonsterile preparations.

- Define the various terms used for comminution and blending of pharmaceutical ingredients.

- Examine the techniques by which solutions, suspensions, ointments, creams, powders, suppositories, and capsules are prepared.

- Understand and calculate common mathematical problems that occur in a compounding pharmacy.

- Identify the steps that are necessary in the compounding process.

- Compare reimbursement procedures of a compounding pharmacy and a retail pharmacy.

- Identify references with a specialty focus on compounding.

STUDY PARTNER

Preview chapter terms and definitions.

Since early civilization, compounding has always been an important part of the art and science of pharmacy practice. Pharmacists routinely prepared (i.e., compounded) a majority of all prescriptions from raw pharmaceutical ingredients. They used their combined understanding of botany, chemistry, and herbology to produce medications to treat a variety of healthcare disorders. This practice continued for centuries until the emergence of modern, large-scale pharmaceutical manufacturing in the twentieth century. In fact, before 1950, it has been estimated that 80% of all prescriptions required compounding by the pharmacist. As the use of automation became more widespread, the need for compounding in the community pharmacy setting waned, and the role of the pharmacist shifted from creating and dispensing medications to mainly dispensing medications.

However, recent trends indicate that the practice of compounding may be on the upswing. Today, approximately 30 to 40 million prescriptions are compounded in

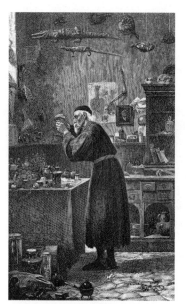

In the Middle Ages, most medications were compounded by the "apothecary" from herbs.

the United States each year, which accounts for about 1% of prescriptions dispensed. Because many high-volume chain pharmacies (and even most independent pharmacies) do not have the time, space, equipment, or expertise for compounding, a growing number of independent community pharmacies are initiating or specializing in compounding services. Community pharmacists and their technicians are increasingly being called upon to prepare a recipe or compounded preparation in doses or strengths for human or veterinary use. To engage in this practice, pharmacy technicians must have advanced training and experience in compounding and devote the majority of their workday performing precise calculations and mixing ingredients rather than communicating with patients.

In light of this growing trend, this chapter examines the compounding of nonsterile preparations or products that are not commercially available—a process known as *extemporaneous compounding*. Because nonsterile pharmaceutical compounding is a pharmacy specialty, this practice has a unique set of supplies, techniques, and terminology that accompany this task. In addition, like other areas of pharmacy practice, nonsterile pharmaceutical compounding also is governed by specific federal and state laws, regulations, and standards. Pharmacy personnel in a community pharmacy may perform these compounding procedures and therefore must have a good understanding of this specialty area.

Sterile and Nonsterile Compounding

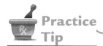

Practice Tip

Pharmacy technicians should have a clear understanding of the difference between mixing and compounding. Mixing a commercially available product (such as a powdered antibiotic) with a compatible solvent per manufacturer's instructions in order to make an oral product is *not* considered pharmacy compounding.

Compounding is defined as the process in which a pharmacist uses bulk ingredients to prepare a prescribed medication that treats a specific patient's medical condition. The compound is made according to a prescription or recipe by a licensed prescriber who individualizes the appropriate quantity and dosage form for his or her patient. The compounding of a medication is ordered because a pharmaceutical product that meets the patient's needs is not commercially available. Compounding may be sterile or nonsterile.

Sterile Compounding

Sterile compounding is the process of using aseptic technique to prepare sterile solutions, or solutions that are free of microorganisms, for parenteral products or ophthalmic preparations. Most sterile compounding is

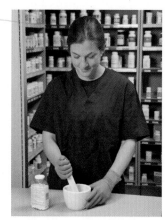

A pharmacy technician mixes a compounded nonsterile preparation. Compounding, or the art of pharmacy, involves combining patient-specific medications.

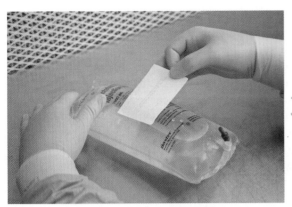

The pharmacy technician labels a CSP before administration to the patient.

performed in the "clean room environment" of a hospital pharmacy, but this process also commonly occurs in specialty compounding, home healthcare, and nuclear pharmacies. Sterile compounding must be performed under strictly controlled environmental conditions to minimize the risk of contamination of the compounded sterile preparations (CSPs). Introduction of any microorganisms into the CSP could lead to life-threatening infections for patient recipients.

Because CSPs are administered parenterally, these products are prepared under strict federal and state board of pharmacy regulations. There must be documentation not only for product stability but also for sterility. To that end, an incubator may be used to culture products, surfaces, or air for microbial contamination; most growth of microorganisms, if present, occurs in the first 48 hours, but the CSP is checked again after two weeks of in-house sterility testing for slower-growing microorganisms. Pharmacy personnel should also be aware that most CSPs do not contain a preservative; consequently, these products have a brief beyond-use date of 24–72 hours due to sterility rather than stability concerns.

The guidelines for sterile compounding—including a clean room environment, correct aseptic technique, and specialized equipment and training—are further discussed in Chapter 10.

Nonsterile Compounding

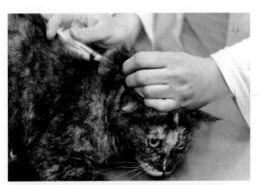

Compounding pharmacies often prepare a drug in a special formulation for a pet.

Safety Note

Products compounded for veterinary use cannot be used in humans.

Nonsterile compounding is used in the preparation of commercially unavailable drug formulations (such as capsules, tablets, ointments, creams, solutions, suspensions, powders, and suppositories) from bulk ingredients in the community pharmacy. Dentists and physicians (especially dermatologists and gynecologists) often prefer to individualize their prescriptions for their patients. Physicians from hospice care, or care for the terminally ill, and pain management clinics often use the services of a compounding pharmacy to meet specific patient needs as well. In addition, veterinarians frequently require the compounding expertise of pharmacists in order to fulfill the unique medication requirements of their animals. To that end, nonsterile compounding allows medications to be catered to an animal's species and size.

Possible Scenarios for Nonsterile Compounding To gain a better understanding of the circumstances in which nonsterile compounding is performed in the pharmacy setting, here are some possible scenarios:

- A medication dose that is smaller than any dose that is commercially available may be ordered by a prescriber for pharmacy compounding. This situation commonly occurs with pediatric medications. For example, a prescription might call for 10 mg per dose of a medication, but that medication is available only in unscored tablets containing 30 mg of the active ingredient. To match the 10 mg prescribed dose, the pharmacist might have to pulverize, or triturate, the tablets and then mix the resultant powder with an inactive powder to fill 10 mg capsules.

- A medication typically available in a solid dosage form might have to be prepared in another dosage form, such as a liquid, suspension, or suppository, for administration to a patient who cannot or will not swallow the solid form or is experiencing severe nausea. For example, tablets may need to be triturated using a mortar and pestle, with a suitable suspending agent added.
- A commercially unavailable dose or dosage form of a medication may need to be prepared for a veterinary application, such as a thyroid medication for a cat.
- An oral compound preparation with an unpleasant bitter taste might have to be prepared in a more palatable, flavor-masking syrup base to ensure compliance by a pediatric patient.
- A topical gel formulation may be prepared for a patient whose oral medication has had adverse effects (such as ulcers) on the stomach.
- A medication for a patient with allergies may be available only in commercial forms containing preservatives, colorings, or other ingredients; therefore, an alternative medication without the unwanted ingredients needs to be prepared.
- A dosage form other than those commercially available may be desired to customize the rate of delivery, rate of onset, duration or site of action, or other pharmacokinetic properties of the drug. Postmenopausal women may have differing needs for hormone replacement therapy than commercially available fixed-dose tablets. These patients also may be concerned about side effects of the hormones. A compounded mixture of hormones, in a cream or gel formulation, can be individualized to relieve a patient's symptoms and minimize the risk of side effects.

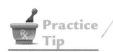
Practice Tip

The abbreviation *qs* means "a quantity sufficient up to the necessary amount."

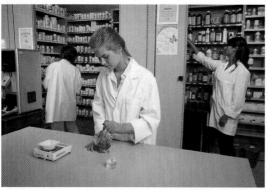

Pharmacy technicians may prepare nonsterile compounds in both a retail or a compounding pharmacy.

Role of the Technician in Nonsterile Compounding The pharmacy technician often assists the pharmacist in the time-consuming and labor-intensive task of weighing, measuring, mixing, and preparing products for pharmaceutical compounding; checking and ordering quality inventory ingredients; and maintaining a clean work environment. Any compounding tasks undertaken by the technician must, in any case, be directly supervised (in the same room) and checked by the pharmacist. The equipment and techniques utilized by the pharmacy technician to prepare nonsterile preparations are discussed later in this chapter.

Laws, Regulations, and Standards

More and more independent community pharmacies are dedicating their practice to sterile and nonsterile compounding. If a community pharmacy compounds both sterile and nonsterile preparations, then all necessary federal and state laws and regulations, United States Pharmacopeia (USP) guidelines, and standards must be followed. State regulations vary, but nationwide professional organizations including the International Academy of Compounding Pharmacists (IACP), the American Pharmacists Association (APhA), the American Society of Health-System Pharmacists (ASHP), the National Community Pharmacists Association (NCPA), and the USP work in concert with the state authorities to ensure the safe and legal practice of pharmacy compounding. Community pharmacies that exceed minimum standards in their compounding practices may become accredited and recognized for the quality of their compounded preparations. (For more detailed information on the accreditation process, see the "Accreditation" section later in this chapter.) Pharmacy personnel should also be aware that compounding pharmacies are allowed to advertise their services, but not the compounding of specific preparations.

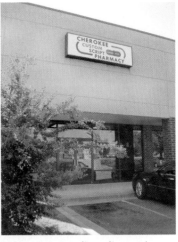

Many compounding pharmacies are specialized and prepare and dispense only nonsterile prescriptions.

Food and Drug Administration Modernization Act of 1997

Before 1997, there were no specific federal or state laws governing the practices of pharmacy compounding; thus, the distinction between manufacturing and compounding was not defined. The Food and Drug Administration Modernization Act (FDAMA) of 1997—an amendment to the FD&C Act—serves to clarify the status of pharmacy compounding. This legislation allows pharmacists to compound nonsterile (and/or sterile medications) for an individual patient if these medications meet established USP standards. The amendment distinguishes compounding from manufacturing practices and provides three major exemptions under which compounded products will not be viewed as new and unapproved drugs. The major provisions state that compounded products need not follow the requirements for drug adulteration, misbranding, and new drug approval as manufactured products do. In other words, compounding pharmacies are not required to follow current good manufacturing practices (CGMPs), to adhere to product labeling regarding directions for use, or to submit drug approval applications. Public health concerns are minor when mass production is not involved. The compounder can typically control quality if drug products are prepared in small quantities. These exemptions are not meant to undermine the safety and efficacy of compounded products; rather, they are based on the assumption that compounded products are typically used for a small group of patients with specific medical needs.

Compounding Regulations Like retail pharmacies, compounding pharmacies must be licensed by both the federal government (including a license by the Drug Enforcement Administration if the pharmacy is dispensing controlled substances) and the facility's state board of pharmacy. The oversight of compounding pharmacies is a function of the state board of pharmacy; however, for situations in which significant violations or manufacturing practices are identified, the Food and Drug Administration (FDA) cooperates with state authorities for inspections and follow-up actions.

Compounding a preparation that is commercially available is generally prohibited. If a compound is requested by a provider, the medication is typically prepared for the individual patient once the prescription is received at the pharmacy. However, pharmacies are allowed to prepare excess product, a practice called **anticipatory compounding**, as long as quantities are reasonable. These excess compounded preparations must be labeled with a lot number and beyond-use dating (discussed later in this chapter). For example, a prescription may call for #30 rapid-dissolving hormone tablets, but the mold to compound this dosage form has the capability to make #96 tablets. Thus, #30 tablets are dispensed and the remaining #66 tablets are appropriately labeled and stored for a refill or for a future prescription.

Federal laws also have an impact on those pharmacies specializing in making the prescription product in bulk in advance and selling it to other pharmacies or healthcare professionals. If a community pharmacy is selling compounded products directly to healthcare professionals or to out-of-state pharmacies rather than to individual patients, then the facility must apply for a manufacturing license. A manufacturing license requires additional regulations, procedures, and quality-control checks. In addition, a community pharmacy that sells a compounded preparation to an out-of-state pharmacy may also have to apply for a pharmacy license in the state involved in the transaction. It is not feasible for most small compounding pharmacies to comply with these requirements. A recent example of the importance of these additional regulations was the 2012 outbreak of fungal meningitis from epidural injections of a contaminated corticosteroid. This product was prepared in a compounding pharmacy and distributed to many states.

USP Chapter <795>

As mentioned earlier, compounding pharmacies are not required by law to follow current good manufacturing practices (CGMPs). To address this concern, the USP has developed standards to enhance patient safety and to protect pharmacists from litigation involved in both nonsterile and sterile compounding. The *USP Pharmacists' Pharmacopeia*, an official publication whose guidelines are a mainstay for pharmacists and pharmacy technicians, devotes a chapter to each type of compounding: USP Chapter <795> provides the protocol for nonsterile compounding, and USP Chapter <797> (discussed at length in Chapter 10) outlines the regulations for sterile compounding. Although USP is not affiliated with any governmental agency, the FDA elects to use and enforce USP standards in the inspection of compounding pharmacies. Many states have adopted these regulations as well.

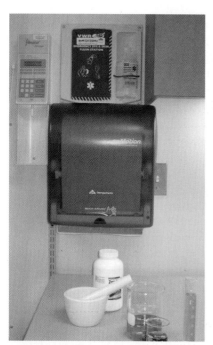

Beakers, graduated cylinders, and a mortar and pestle are frequently used equipment in measuring and preparing nonsterile compounds.

To grasp compounding regulations, pharmacy personnel need to understand the distinctions among several key terms. Pharmaceutical manufacturers such as Eli Lilly and Merck produce **manufactured products**, whereas pharmacies produce **compounded preparations**. USP Chapter <795> states that a pharmacy must meet minimum standards to ensure a high-quality compounded preparation. In lieu of CGMP, a pharmacy must follow **good compounding practices (GCPs)** as outlined in Table 8.1. The pharmacist and the pharmacy technician share the responsibility to ensure that all compounded products are prepared using GCPs.

Nonsterile Compounding Environment

The USP standards focus on written policies and procedures for adequate space and equipment, quality control, pharmacist verification of source ingredients, and patient counseling. Quality control includes not only the use of high-grade pharmaceutical ingredients for compounding but also the training of personnel, the maintenance of the compounded preparation's stability and consistency, the safeguards for calculation errors, and the documentation of beyond-use dating of compounded preparations.

General Facility Requirements A nonsterile compounding facility must have adequate space and storage as well as appropriate equipment that must be properly maintained, used, calibrated, and

TABLE 8.1   USP Good Compounding Practices

Components of GCPs	Standards
Facility	A designated area with adequate space and a separate area for sterile compounding
Personnel	Staff members with education, training, and proficiency in this specialized area; compounders must wear protective clothing
Equipment	Appropriate design, size, and space of balances and measuring devices; equipment must be cleaned and calibrated
Ingredient selection	Only high-grade chemicals; ingredients are used and stored appropriately
Compounding process	Each step reviewed, with final check by the pharmacist
Packaging and storage	All ingredients and containers properly labeled
Controls	Quality control programs implemented by the pharmacist
Labeling of excess product	Labels showing quantity and lot number
Beyond-use dating	Stability (and sterility in some cases) of preparation after compounding reflected in beyond-use dating
Records and reports	Documents including master control, compounding, equipment maintenance, and ingredients records
Patient counseling	Discussion with patient on the safe administration and storage of the compounded preparation

cleaned. The space must meet high cleanliness standards, have sufficient ventilation, and have counters that are free from potential contaminants. The compounding area itself should be free of dust-collecting overhangs, such as ceiling pipes and light fixtures; have an eyewash station in case of accidental contact or exposure to a hazardous chemical; and provide access to refrigeration equipment. The work surface should be a nonshedding surface that is level, smooth, and free of cracks. The staging area of the work surface should only contain the equipment and pharmaceutical ingredients needed for the compounding process. With that in mind, pharmacy personnel should be reminded that no food items should be stored or consumed in the staging area. Equipment must be placed in areas where air currents will not interfere or compromise the accuracy of the delicate digital balance. All chemicals or products should be properly labeled with expiration or beyond-use dating, and Material Safety Data Sheets should be available. (For more information on these data sheets, see Chapter 11.)

If coupled with a dispensing pharmacy, the nonsterile pharmacy must be physically separate. If the pharmacy also prepares sterile preparations, a separate clean room environment (see Chapter 10) must be utilized.

Safety Note

A certificate of analysis provided by the American Chemical Society ensures that an ingredient is a high-grade, purified product.

Product Inventory The quality of the ingredients is important when compounding a product that is both efficacious and safe. USP Chapter <795> specifies that only USP or National Formulary (NF) pharmaceutical-grade (as opposed to chemical-grade) ingredients should be used. Pharmacy personnel must secure a high-grade, purified product that is accompanied by filing a certificate of analysis (indicating that it is certified by the American Chemical Society).

Sources for Bulk Ingredients The pharmacist typically makes the decision about what source is used for ingredients—both active and inactive—in compounded preparations. The decision is based on cost, quality, and purity of product. The reputation of the manufacturer and the support that the manufacturer provides also influence the choice of products selected for use in the compounding pharmacy. Many large-volume compounding pharmacies use their membership with the Pharmaceutical Compounding Centers of America (PCCA) as a primary source of product because these centers have been certified after undergoing extensive research and scientific testing. PCCA also provides a reputable source for new compounding recipes as well as information and research on compatibility and stability of prepared or new compounds.

Often, the pharmacist must balance the higher cost of PCCA source ingredients with other lower-cost sources that also provide certified USP- or NF-grade ingredients. Pharmacists should have more than one source of quality ingredients, in case of a shortage, back order, or drug product recall. Table 8.2 contains a representative list of sources of bulk product and contact information for the pharmacy technician. On request, any manufacturer of bulk ingredients will provide a certificate of analysis for any of their products.

TABLE 8.2 Bulk Product Contacts

Organization	Phone Number	Web Address
PCCA	800-331-2498	www.pccarx.com
Perrigo (Paddock Labs)	866-634-9120	www.perrigo.com
Fagron	800-423-6967	http://fagron.us/
Medisca Inc.	800-932-1039	www.medisca.com
Letco Medical	800-239-5288	www.letcoinc.com

Note: The phone numbers and web addresses of these organizations were accurate as of this printing.

Storage of Bulk Ingredients Ingredients are commonly ordered by the technician two or three times per week, depending on volume and inventory of the compounding pharmacy. The ingredients are received the next day from one of several overnight mail services and properly recorded and stored by the technician. A **Material Safety Data Sheet (MSDS)** needs to be filed by the technician for all bulk chemicals or drug substances that are stored in the pharmacy. The MSDS contains important information on hazards and flammability of chemicals and procedures for treatment of accidental ingestion or exposure. Hazardous chemicals must be stored separately in the drug inventory. (For more detailed information on the MSDS, including expected 2015 changes, refer to Chapter 11.)

Bulk ingredients are typically stored in tight, light-resistant containers at room temperature. If the technician or pharmacist is unsure about temperature requirements, then he or she should refer to the USP or NF compendia. The technician should always check expiration dates prior to mixing any ingredients listed in the master control record, or compounding recipe. The technician should always list the source of ingredients and the NDC number on the compounding log,

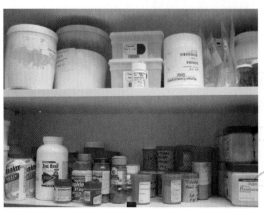

Bulk ingredients must be stored under proper temperature and labeled with expiration dating.

especially if the manufacturer of any bulk ingredient has recently changed. The master control record and the compounding log—two important procedural documents—are discussed in detail later in this chapter.

Controlled Substances Inventory If the compounding pharmacy receives prescriptions for hospice care or pain management patients, then it may be necessary to compound controlled substances. As expected, the procedures and record keeping for Schedule II compounds are much more detailed and extensive. Each and every milligram of the narcotic must be accounted for on the compounding log and deducted from inventory. As with Schedule II prescriptions in the community pharmacy, the pharmacist is accountable and typically prepares such compounded preparations. Controlled substances inventory must be in locked storage accessible only to the pharmacist, and prescriptions for Schedule II drugs must be filed separately. The written manual of the pharmacy should outline the exact procedures to follow in order to meet state and federal regulations.

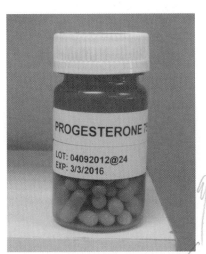

Excess nonsterile compounds must be labeled with drug name, lot number, and expiration dating and stored in a suitable container.

Beyond-Use Dating USP Chapter <795> (nonsterile preparations) and USP Chapter <797> (sterile preparations), as well as the process of accreditation, require a written policy and procedure for **beyond-use dating**, or the expiration date of compounded preparations based on stability and temperature storage conditions. For nonsterile compounding facilities, USP Chapter <795> provides specific guidelines on beyond-use dating that must be followed by pharmacy personnel. One of these guidelines includes documentation of product stability. **Stability** is defined as the extent to which a product retains the same properties and characteristics that it possessed at the time of preparation. Some allowable variation (typically, +/−2%) is to be expected. Stability includes physical properties (appearance, taste, uniformity, dissolution, and suspendibility) and chemical properties (potency).

Pharmacy personnel must be aware that beyond-use dating is initiated at the time of compounding, not at the time of dispensing. Therefore, compounded medications should be prepared as close to the time of patient dispensing as possible. USP Chapter <795> provides estimates for beyond-use dating. For example, a refrigerated aqueous solution or suspension has a beyond-use date of 14–30 days. Solids such as tablets and capsules and nonaqueous solutions have a beyond-use date of six months or less, depending on the ingredients making up the compound. All other formulations are labeled with a 30-day, beyond-use date or duration of therapy, whichever date is earlier.

Determining the beyond-use date for a prescription having two or more active or inactive ingredients with varying expiration dates is a bit trickier. In this situation, if a manufacturer or bulk drug is used, the beyond-use date is determined by taking 25% of the remaining expiration date or six months, whichever date is earlier. If dates differ among ingredients, then the earliest date is always used. Examples 1 and 2 demonstrate the calculation of beyond-use dating for two nonsterile preparations.

Practice Tip

Pharmacy technicians should understand the distinction between a beyond-use date and an expiration date: A *beyond-use date* is a term that applies to compounded preparations, whereas an *expiration date* is a term that applies to manufactured products.

3 months 6/4

Example 1

A low-dose pediatric capsule of a blood pressure medication is combined with a filler agent on March 30, 2014, with the following drug sources and expiration dates:

Drug	Drug Source	Expiration Date
Lisinopril	Manufacturer	July 2014
Suspending agent	Bulk chemical	October 2015

What should the beyond-use date be?

The labeled date should be April 30, 2014. This is 25% of the four months that elapse between the date that the compound was made (March 30, 2014) and the expiration date of the manufactured drug (considered to be July 31, 2014). If a pediatric suspension of the compound was prepared, the beyond-use date would have been 14 to 30 days, regardless of the expiration of the individual ingredients.

Example 2

A bioidentical cream is formulated with two different hormones on March 30, 2014, with the following drug sources and expiration dates:

Drug	Drug Source	Expiration Date
Hormone A	Bulk chemical	July 2015
Hormone B	Bulk chemical	October 2015

What should the beyond-use date be?

In this case, both ingredients are bulk chemicals. The labeled date should be July 31, 2014, or 25% of the earlier expiration date of Hormone A. If Hormone A had an expiration date of October 2015, then the beyond-use date is September 30, 2014, or a maximum of six months after the product was formulated.

The integrity of the final compounded preparation must be verified by scientific research if other beyond-use dating is used. If the compounding pharmacy has verifiable data from the PCCA or an outside analytical laboratory to extend the beyond-use dating, then the preparation can be dispensed. The cost of testing each compounded preparation would be prohibitive for a small compounding pharmacy. Thus, conservative beyond-use dating guidelines in USP Chapter <795> are most often used. The technician should always check with the pharmacist to be sure that the labeled beyond-use dating is in accordance with the standards.

Accreditation Compounding pharmacies have the necessary equipment, space, and expertise to prepare compounded prescriptions safely. In light of that, many compounding pharmacies are currently seeking national accreditation to protect their

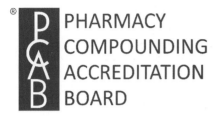

PHARMACY COMPOUNDING ACCREDITATION BOARD

patients and their businesses from legal challenges and to differentiate their practices from those of other pharmacies. The organization responsible for accreditation is the **Pharmacy Compounding Accreditation Board (PCAB)**. The primary role of the PCAB is to provide quality and safety standards for compounding through voluntary accreditation. The pharmacy must agree to follow specified principles as well as meet all standards for both nonsterile (USP Chapter <795>) and sterile (USP Chapter <797>) compounded preparations in order to receive a "seal of accreditation." An accredited compounding pharmacy provides a higher standard of care and a competitive advantage in the marketplace.

Continuous quality improvement (CQI) is a process of written procedures in the PCAB standards designed to identify problems and recommend solutions. As part of CQI procedures of an accredited compounding pharmacy, there is a monthly or quarterly spot check of the technician's work. A random product is selected and sent to an outside analytical lab for analysis and exact measurement of the components. The product generally must be +/– 2% of the potency of the individual ingredients. If the steps in a procedure were not followed or if the technician needs additional training as a result of the analysis, then the corrective action must be documented and dated by the pharmacist.

Regulations for Pharmacy Personnel

Pharmacy technicians who want to work in compounding pharmacies must obtain special certification and undergo advanced training in the preparation of these various products. In addition, these technicians must don certain attire when performing nonsterile compounding.

Certification of Pharmacy Technicians

Both pharmacists and pharmacy technicians require special training and certifications to work in a compounding pharmacy. In addition to successfully passing a broad national certification examination (discussed in detail in Chapter 14), the technician who aspires to work in a compounding pharmacy must complete mini-certifications and laboratory training in nonsterile and sterile (if preparing parenteral preparations) compounding. The knowledge and skills necessary to pass these specialty certifications are commonly developed as workshops and labs by the PCCA. Certifications by all technicians and specialty training may be necessary to attain or maintain PCAB accreditation of the pharmacy.

Nonsterile Compounding Attire

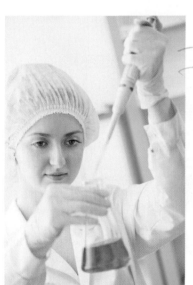

A pharmacy technician must wear a lab coat, gloves, and a hairnet when preparing nonsterile products in a compounding pharmacy.

Before weighing, measuring, mixing, and preparing ingredients in a compounding pharmacy, pharmacy personnel must don the proper attire. These attire requirements are provided in the USP *Pharmacists' Pharmacopeia* as well as in a facility's policy and procedure (P&P) manual. Understandably, the required attire for nonsterile compounding—outlined in USP Chapter <795>—is less rigid than the attire for sterile compounding. Generally, the minimum requirements for nonsterile compounding include clean protective clothing, a hairnet, a long lab coat, and disposable gloves. If hazardous chemicals are used, then eye goggles, a mask, and double gowning may be necessary.

USP Chapter <795> also specifies that all personnel must wash their hands before performing nonsterile compounding procedures. Personnel should use a liquid antimicrobial soap and rub their hands briskly for a minimum of 15 seconds. When finished scrubbing, they should rinse their hands well, dry them with paper towels, and dispose the used towels in a waste receptacle. After completion of the compounding procedure, personnel should dispose of their gloves and wash their hands again.

Documentation of Nonsterile Compounding

Compounding is done with a receipt of a prescription and in accordance with specific, documented instructions or a recipe. Documentation of all active and inactive ingredients, as well as the procedures for proper sequencing and mixing, is crucial in preparing a high-quality preparation. All calculations for the amounts of individual ingredients must be made initially by the pharmacist, double-checked by the pharmacy technician, and verified by the pharmacist after the preparation has been compounded.

Master Control Record

The compounding of a medication requires the addition and mixing of several necessary ingredients. The compound requires a formula (or recipe) before the technician can begin to prepare the product. After a prescription has been received by the pharmacist, the instructions for making the compound are retrieved or developed by the pharmacist. This recipe is called a **master control record**, which is available either in the computer database or as a hard copy on recipe-like cards stored in a file box. Figure 8.1 is an example of a computerized master control record.

FIGURE 8.1
Computerized Master Control Record

This master control record was created using PCCA's PK software.

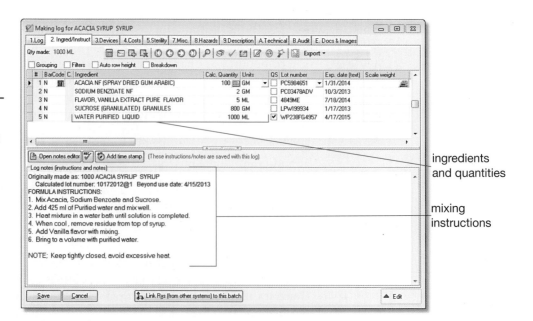

The master control record is prepared (for a new compound) and reviewed by the pharmacist or provided by a subscriber compounding service such as PCCA's CompounderLab™ from PK Software. The pharmacist uses his or her best professional judgment to assess the safety and suitability of compounding the prescription, as well as its intended use, especially on new orders for which a recipe must be created. Physicians are open to suggestions from the pharmacist to improve the quality or safety of their compounding prescriptions.

The master control record lists the drug's name, strength, and dosage form; the ingredients and their quantities; and the sequencing and mixing instructions. Because of wastage, the master control record usually accounts for some overage in the weights of all of the ingredients needed. This record also includes recommended beyond-use dating and storage and labeling requirements. (To view other examples of master control records, refer to Figures 8.8 and 8.9.)

Compounding Log

From the master control record, a printed **compounding log** is generated for each prescription. The compounding log is unique for each prescription and is thus intended for a specific patient. The pharmacist uses the compounding log to complete the initial mathematical calculations and documents those calculations on the print-out. The pharmacist also identifies on the log any special equipment for the technician to use when compounding the preparation. This compounding log is then turned over to the pharmacy technician to initiate the preparation of the product. A computer-generated copy of the log, called the **prescription record**, is also stored and is thus retrievable for future refills.

The compounding log lists the following information:

- patient name
- date of compounding
- Rx number
- Master Control Record number
- names of all ingredients of the compounded preparation and their individual expiration dates
- amount needed
- quantity made
- manufacturer
- wholesaler source
- NDC number
- assigned lot number
- initials of the pharmacist and compounding technician

An example of a manual compounding log (see Figure 8.2 on the following page) lists the ingredients and directions for compounding a preparation called Magic Mouthwash. This formula has many variations in different regions of the country and is commonly compounded in many community pharmacies. The mouthwash product is an example of a basic compound that is prepared by mixing together ingredients of commercially available liquids or suspensions to make a new product.

FIGURE 8.2
**Compounding
Log**

This record
is for Magic
Mouthwash, a
commonly made
formula.

Patient Name _____ Date Prepared _12/2/201X_____

Rx # _____ Master Control Record # _____

Compounding Formula for Magic Mouthwash

Ingredient Name	Amount Needed	Manufacturer	NDC #	Lot #	Expiration Date	Prepared By	Checked By
Lidocaine 2% viscous	60 mL	Hi-Tech	50838-0775-04		12/10/201X		
Diphenhydramine 12.5 mg/mL	60 mL	Walgreens	00363-0379-34		07/12/201X		
Mylanta, generic	60 mL	Qualitest	00603-0712-57		03/12/201X		
Nystatin suspension	60 mL	Qualitest	00603-1481-58		09/11/201X		
Total quantity	240 mL						

Prepared by _____

Approved by _____

Date _____

Directions _____

Auxiliary Labeling: SHAKE WELL

_____

Example 3

Using 10% oral viscous Lidocaine to make Magic Mouthwash, how many milligrams in 1 mL of 10% viscous Lidocaine?

Because a 1% concentration = 10 mg/mL, a 10% concentration = 100 mg/mL.

Calculations in the Compounding Pharmacy

The pharmacy technician practicing in a compounding pharmacy must have a thorough knowledge of mathematical conversions and a good aptitude for performing calculations accurately. Although the pharmacist is legally responsible for overseeing the compounding process and for checking all calculations made by the technician, a double check by the technician of both the pharmacist's initial calculations and those contained in the master control record is strongly recommended to minimize medication errors. All measurements and mathematical calculations must be documented and reviewed by the pharmacist during the final check of each compounded preparation. Examples illustrating how a technician uses calculations in a compounding practice are provided throughout this chapter.

Equipment for Weighing, Measuring, and Compounding

A myriad of equipment is used in a specialty compounding pharmacy for measuring, mixing, and molding. Large pieces of equipment that may be utilized include a convection oven to create rapid-dissolving tablets, pellets, and suppositories; an autoclave to sterilize metal instruments and glassware; and, for quality control, an incubator to test compounded preparations for bacteria. Smaller devices used in the compounding process include different types of balances, graduated cylinders and pipettes, mortars and pestles, various beakers and flasks, ointment mills and slabs, and molds.

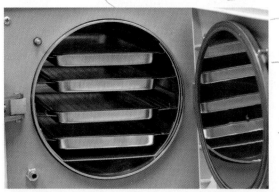

Heat autoclaves are often used in compounding pharmacies to sterilize metal instruments or glassware.

In addition, the technician must ensure that all materials needed for proper packaging and labeling of the end product are available. Storage of ingredients and final products must also be considered. Freezers and refrigerators are required for some compounded preparations, and pharmacy technicians must monitor and document their temperatures, as well as room temperatures, on a daily basis in order to maintain the stability of the stored products.

Nonsterile compounding requires pharmacy personnel to exercise care at each step of the process: Any error in weighing or measuring ingredients could result in serious drug toxicity for the patient recipient, and improper mixing or molding may result in a poor quality preparation and/or a product that is not pharmaceutically elegant.

Measuring Devices for Solids

Accurately weighing ingredients is one of the most essential parts of the compounding process and a technique that is crucial for the technician to learn. A technician must continually practice to feel confident and comfortable with weighing products on various prescription balances.

Many types of balances and weights are used to weigh pharmaceutical ingredients accurately in order to produce a quality and safe compounded preparation. The type of balance that a pharmacy utilizes is based on the volume of pharmaceutical compounding and the cost of the balance. To operate any type of balance in a community or compounding pharmacy, personnel must become familiar with the device's calibration of weights. The following balances are frequently seen in the pharmacy setting.

Two-Pan Balances Two types of two-pan balances are used to weigh ingredients in nonsterile compounding: a Class III prescription balance and a counterbalance.

Class III Prescription Balance A **Class III prescription balance**, formerly known as a *Class A prescription balance*, is a common fixture in most pharmacies—a throwback to the days in which extensive compounding was a routine task in community pharmacies. The Class III prescription balance is a two-pan balance with a capacity of 15 to 120 grams. This balance can be used to weigh small amounts of material and has a sensitivity requirement (SR) in the range of +/–6 mg. This SR range means that a 6 mg weight moves the indicator on the balance by one degree. To maintain an acceptable error of <5%, no less than 120 mg should be measured on such a balance. The Class III prescription balance is sufficiently accurate for infrequent compounding in a community pharmacy.

The correct technique for weighing ingredients with a Class III prescription balance is demonstrated in Figure 8.3. Variations in technique could easily result in a small but serious error, resulting in a subtherapeutic or even toxic dose of medication. Weighing the exact amount prescribed is essential because the product cannot be easily checked for content once mixed. A pharmacist must inspect the weight measurements of all ingredients that the technician has weighed using this type of balance.

FIGURE 8.3   Weighing with a Class III Prescription Balance

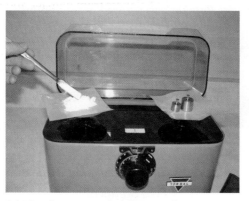

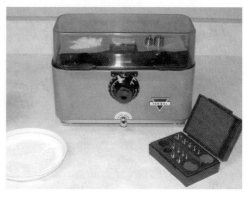

(a) The pharmacy technician transfers a substance to the scale.

(b) The final measurement is taken with the lid closed.

Counterbalance   Like a Class III prescription balance, a **counterbalance** also contains two pans, but this device is used for weighing larger amounts of material, up to about 5 kg. It has an SR range of +/−100 mg. Because of its lesser sensitivity, a counterbalance is not used in prescription compounding but rather for tasks such as measuring bulk products—for example, Epsom salts. A weighing boat (discussed in the following section) may be used to contain the large quantities of bulk ingredients to be measured.

Pharmaceutical Weights for Two-Pan Balances   Weights are used for both measurement and calibration of equipment. When using a two-pan balance, a standardized set of **pharmaceutical weights** is used to offset the ingredient weight. Weights are generally made of polished brass and may be coated with a noncorrosive material such as nickel or chromium. Sets contain both metric and apothecary weights. (For information about the metric and apothecary measurement systems, see Chapter 5.) Typical metric sets contain gram weights of 1, 2, 5, 10, 20, 50, and 100 g, which are conically shaped, with a handle and flattened top. Fractional gram weights (for example, 10, 20, 50, 100, 200, and 500 mg) are also available. These weights are made of aluminum and are usually flat, with one raised edge to facilitate being picked up using forceps. Avoirdupois weights of 1/32, 1/16, 1/8, 1/4, 1/2, 1, 2, 4, and 8 oz may also be used.

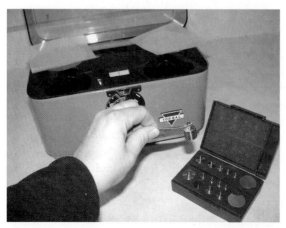

Weights should be transferred using forceps and should not be touched with bare skin. Moisture or oils affect their accuracy.

Handling and Storage of Weights   Pharmacy technicians should exercise care when handling pharmaceutical weights. When grasping and transferring weights, technicians should use forceps, not their fingers. A **forceps** is an instrument used for grasping and holding small objects. Forceps are used for picking up smaller weights and transferring them to and from measuring balances to avoid transferring moisture or oil from the fingers to the weights. Over time, moisture and oil can change the fixed quantity of the weights and become a potential source of error in preparing small doses, such as for pediatric patients. Because forceps are only used with lighter weights, technicians typically use a cloth to handle larger weights. During the transfer process, pharmacy personnel should avoid touching, contaminating, or damaging the weight.

Weights should always be placed on a weighing paper or powder paper. **Weighing paper** is placed on the pans to protect the balances from damage and to avoid contact between pharmaceutical ingredients and the metal trays. Typically, glassine paper is used. Glassine paper is a thin paper that has been coated with a nonabsorbent paraffin wax. The paper on each balance pan should be of exactly the same size and weight, and the edges of the paper on the pan may be folded upward to hold the ingredient to be weighed. The weighing paper must be weighed prior to adding the ingredient to be measured and should be discarded after each measurement to prevent contamination. To weigh larger quantities of chemicals, a plastic **weighing boat** should be utilized. This boat should also be weighed before beginning the measuring process.

Weights come in a container in which they should be stored when not in use. Proper storage of weights maintains their stated values.

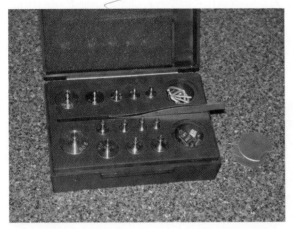

This set of pharmacy weights shows metric weights in the front row and apothecary weights in the back row.

Digital Electronic Analytical Balance A **digital electronic analytical balance** uses a single pan and is easier to learn to use and more accurate than a Class III prescription balance or a counterbalance. However, electronic balances tend to be much more costly ($1000 or more) and are typically used in large-scale or dedicated pharmacy compounding labs and hospitals. Electronic balances generally do not need to use pharmacy weights. The sensitivity of an electronic balance is in the range of +/−2 to 30 mg, depending on the balance. Weighing various bulk ingredients is more efficient and accurate compared with the two-pan balances.

Operating an Electronic Balance An electronic balance should be placed on a secure, level, nonvibrating surface, at waist height. It must be perfectly level, both side to side and front to back. Leveling is often the most time-consuming process for beginners. The levelness should be checked often throughout the day if the balance is heavily used. The area where the balance is placed should be well lit and free from air current drafts, dust, corrosive vapors, or high humidity that might affect the ingredients or the weight measurements. In fact, electronic balances are usually enclosed on all four sides to minimize any air current impacts during the weighing process.

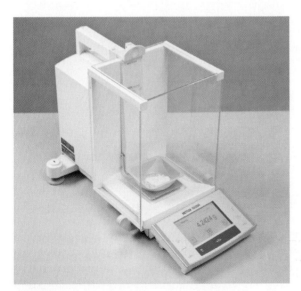

A digital electronic balance is very accurate, with a capacity of 100 g or more and a sensitivity as low as +/−2 mg.

Prior to use, the electronic balance should be warmed up for 30 minutes after the AC adapter is plugged in, and then it should be calibrated. The calibration process must be documented each day. Similar to two-pan balances, pharmacy personnel should use weighing papers or boats when weighing ingredients. Personnel should also avoid spilling materials onto the balance itself and, in the event of a spill, should wipe it up immediately with the balance in the locked position. Following an inadvertent spill, a staff member should recalibrate the balance. To avoid damaging this sensitive instrument, pharmacists and technicians should be advised to not place materials onto the balance while it is released (or unlocked), which can result in a sudden, forceful drop of the pan.

Many electronic balances produce a hard-copy printout of the weights of the individual ingredients that the technician has measured; some advanced balances allow bar code scanning of the drug chemicals. This printout is then attached to the compounding log for the pharmacist to check the final compounded preparation. A pharmacist or an experienced certified technician may need to check the technician's weighing technique after initial training, especially if no printout for the weights of ingredients is available. The procedure for measuring an ingredient with an electronic balance is outlined in Table 8.3.

TABLE 8.3   Steps for Using an Electronic Balance

1. Locate the zero point, including the weight of the weighing or powder paper.
2. Place a small amount of chemical or drug to be measured (from the compounding record) onto the paper on the pan, using a spatula to transfer it.
3. Once a nearly precise amount of material has been transferred to the pan, a very small adjustment upward can be made by placing a small amount of material on the spatula, holding the spatula over the paper, and lightly tapping the spatula with the forefinger to knock a bit of the substance onto the pan; this is done with the balance unlocked and the balance beam free to move.
4. Read the digital weight measurement.
5. Lock the balance before removing the measured substance.

Balances and Percentage of Error   In the compounding pharmacy, percentages are used in determining the possible **percentage of error**, or the acceptable range of variation above and below the target measurement of a bulk ingredient. Percentage of error is based on the least weighable quantity of an ingredient(s) to compound a safe preparation.

Allowances are made for a certain percentage of error over or under the target measurement in the weighing of compound preparations. The percentage of error within this range is not consequential in most cases. Pharmacy balances are generally very accurate; however, knowing the margin of error or sensitivity of a particular balance is important. Most balances are marked with their degree of accuracy. When any substance is weighed, the scale will appear to have measured correctly. However, too small a sample may have an unacceptable margin of error.

Most compounded nonsterile preparations—such as tablets, capsules, ointments, creams, and gels—are prepared in larger quantities than the original prescription from the physician, especially if refills are written. For example, instead of preparing 30 capsules of a medication each month, the master control record or recipe may call for preparing a minimum quantity of 100 capsules to be made. The reasons include both the costs in terms of personnel preparation time and a lower percentage of error in the measuring and mixing of ingredients. The stock bottles for the excess product must be labeled with quantity, lot number, date compounded, and beyond-use dating, as well as the initials of the pharmacist and compounding technician. The technician must check the stock medication on the shelf monthly for expiration dates or as specified in the pharmacy's P&P manual.

If a substance was weighed or measured incorrectly and an instrument is available to remeasure the amount in question more accurately, then the percentage of error can be determined. This can be found by using the following formula:

$$\frac{\text{amount of error}}{\text{quantity desired}} \times 100 = \text{percentage of error}$$

In this equation, the amount of error is the difference between the actual amount and the quantity desired, or

$$\text{actual amount} - \text{quantity desired} = \text{amount of error}$$

Safety Note

Pharmacy technicians should always work within the acceptable percentage of error range of their equipment.

For example, a new brand of vitamins claims to have a range of 9% bioavailability of a national brand of 1000 mg vitamin C. The range of error is +/-90 mg or 910 mg to 1090 mg. This is 9% less and 9% more than the labeled amount of 1000 mg. Compounded nonsterile preparations must have an error range less than 5%.

Measuring Devices for Liquids

Liquid volumes are often much easier to measure than solid ingredients that must be weighed on balances. To perform **volumetric measurement**, pharmacy personnel can choose from a wide variety of glassware that is designed to measure—not mix—liquids. These containers include graduated cylinders, pipettes, oral syringes, and droppers.

Graduated Cylinders A **graduated cylinder** is a glass or polypropylene flask used for measuring liquids. The flasks come in two varieties: conical and cylindrical. Both kinds of graduated cylinders are available in a wide variety of sizes, ranging from 5 mL to more than 1000 mL. These cylinders are calibrated in both metric and apothecary units (in other words, cubic centimeters).

A general rule of thumb is to always select the device that yields the most accurate volume. Conical graduates have wide tops and narrow bases and taper from the top to the bottom. Cylindrical graduates are more accurate and have the shape of a uniform column. Selecting a container that is at least half full during measurement, or using the smallest device that holds the required volume, is considered good practice.

Choosing the appropriate-sized cylindrical graduate is important to the accurate measurement of liquids.

TABLE 8.4 Measuring Liquid Volumes

1. Choose a graduated cylinder with a capacity that equals or very slightly exceeds the total volume of the liquid to be measured. Doing so reduces the percentage of error in the measurement. In no case should the volume to be measured be less than 20% of the total capacity of the container. For example, 10 mL of liquid should not be measured in a graduated cylinder exceeding 50 mL in capacity. The closer the total capacity of the container is to the volume to be measured, the more accurate the measurement will be.

2. Note that the narrower the column of liquid is in the graduated cylinder, the less substantial any reading error will be. Thus, for very small volume measurements, a pipette is preferable to a cylindrical graduate, and, for larger measurements, a cylindrical graduate is preferable to a conical graduate, and a conical graduate may be preferable to a glass beaker.

3. Pour the liquid to be measured slowly into the graduated cylinder, watching the level of the liquid in the container as you do so. If the liquid is viscous, or thick, then you should attempt to pour it toward the center of the container to avoid having some of the liquid cling to the sides.

4. Wait for liquid clinging to the sides of the graduated cylinder to settle before taking a measurement.

5. Read the level of the liquid *at eye level* and read the measure at the bottom of the meniscus (see Figure 8.4).

6. When pouring the liquid out of the graduated cylinder, allow ample time for all of the liquid to drain. Depending on the viscosity of the liquid, more or less clings to the sides of the container. For a particularly viscous liquid, some compensation or adjustment for this clinging may have to be made.

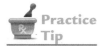
Practice Tip

Pharmacy technicians need to remember that milliliters (abbreviated as mL) and cubic centimeters (abbreviated as cc) are equivalent and interchangeable terms of liquid measurement.

FIGURE 8.4 Meniscus

Liquid in a narrow column usually forms a concave meniscus. Measurements should be taken at the bottom of the concavity when read at eye level.

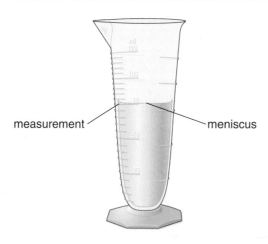

measurement · meniscus

Using a Graduated Cylinder When measuring liquid volumes in a graduated cylinder, be sure that the cylinder is on a flat surface before following the procedure outlined in Table 8.4. Step 5 of the procedure instructs the technician to read the volume measurement at the bottom of the meniscus. A **meniscus** is the half-moon–shaped or concave appearance of the upper surface of a liquid (see Figure 8.4). As the illustration shows, the level of the liquid in the graduated cylinder is slightly higher at the edges; therefore, pharmacy technicians should not measure the level by looking down on the container. Rather, technicians should measure the level of the liquid at eye level and should note the measurement at the *bottom* of the meniscus. The transfer of viscous liquids such as syrups, propylene glycol, mineral oil, and glycerin may take as long as 60 seconds before an accurate measurement of the meniscus can take place.

Pipettes A **pipette** is a long, thin, calibrated hollow glass tube (similar to a glass straw) that is used for accurate measurement and transfer of small volumes of liquid. The types of pipettes include a one-volume-only transfer pipette (for measuring a volume of liquid such as 10 mL), a calibrated pipette (for measuring precise, multiple volumes of liquid), and a micropipette (for measuring a very small volume of liquid). To use a pipette, pharmacy personnel should attach a pipette filler or rubber bulb to

Safety Note

When measuring liquids with a graduated cylinder, pipette, oral syringe, or dropper, always use the smallest size that can contain the volume to be measured. Doing so minimizes your percentage of error in measurement.

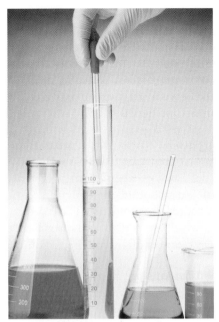

the end of the pipette. This attachment works like a suction device by cautiously drawing up the liquid. The use of this attachment is particularly important when drawing up a hazardous substance such as an acid.

Oral Syringes and Droppers Oral syringes (or hypodermic syringes without a needle) may also be used to measure small or large quantities of liquids. Oral syringes are more accurate than a cylindrical graduated cylinder, especially when measuring thick, viscous liquids. Droppers can be used to transfer small volumes of liquid; the dropper must be calibrated because the drop size will differ among various liquids.

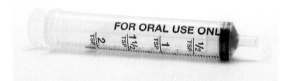

A suction device is used on a pipette to withdraw hazardous liquids.

An oral syringe provides an accurate measurement of viscous liquids.

Supplies for Mixing and Molding Ingredients

Pharmacy personnel use specific supplies to mix liquid and solid ingredients during the compounding process. These supplies include a mortar and pestle, various beakers and flasks, and an ointment mill. With the exception of an ointment mill, these basic supplies are commonly found in community pharmacies and are used for the occasional measuring of ingredients for a compounded nonsterile preparation.

Mortar and Pestle The **mortar and pestle** is widely used in the compounding of both liquid and solid ingredients. These familiar devices come in glass, porcelain, and Wedgwood varieties, and pharmacy personnel select a particular type based on the compounding process at hand. A coarse-grained porcelain or Wedgwood mortar and pestle set is used for triturating (or pulverizing) crystals, granules, and powders; a glass mortar and pestle, with its smooth surface, is preferred for mixing liquids and semisolid dosage forms such as creams, ointments, and gels. A glass mortar and pestle also has the advantage of being nonporous and nonstaining.

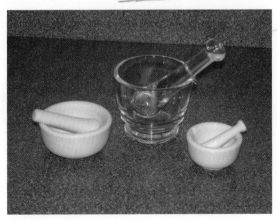

An electric mortar and pestle is often used in a high-volume compounding pharmacy to reduce particle size and to mix the pharmaceutical compound more thoroughly after the weighing and manual manipulation of ingredients with a spatula. Such equipment can mix at a low rate (50 revolutions per minute or RPMs) or a high rate (2500 RPMs). This equipment can be calibrated to a specific product if necessary, but it generally produces a pharmaceutically elegant cream or ointment after three minutes of constant automated mixing.

The mortar and pestle are used to mix or grind substances.

Beakers and Flasks Glass beakers and Erlenmeyer flasks such as those that you may have used in the chemistry lab are available in various sizes and are considered **nonvolumetric glassware**. These beakers and flasks can only approximate larger volumes of liquids (usually eight fluid ounces or more); consequently, the containers are not used when an exact measurement of liquid is required. Their role is to store, contain, and mix liquids. To aid the transfer of liquids contained in this glassware, pharmacy technicians should use plastic or glass funnels or sieves.

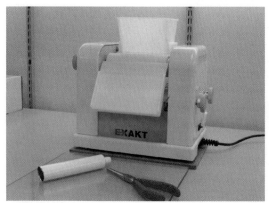

The use of an ointment mill will produce a more elegant end product.

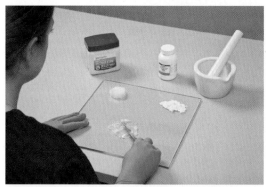

An ointment slab is used to prepare specialized prescriptions for creams and ointments.

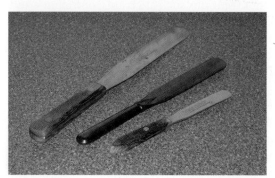

Spatulas are a common tool in a compounding pharmacy.

Ointment Mill A three-roller ointment mill mixes and greatly reduces the particle size of ingredient powders used to compound a dermatological ointment or cream preparation. The result is a smoother, more pharmaceutically elegant end product for consumer use. The speed of the rolling or milling is easily controlled, and the rollers can be removed for easy cleaning after each preparation.

Ointment Slab An **ointment slab**, also known as a *compounding slab*, is a plate made of ground glass that has a flat, hard, nonabsorbent surface ideal for mixing topical compounds. In lieu of a compounding or ointment slab, compounding may be performed on special disposable nonabsorbent parchment paper, which is discarded after the compounding operation has been completed.

Spatula A **spatula** is an instrument used for transferring solid pharmaceutical ingredients to and from weighing pans. This instrument is also utilized for various compounding tasks, such as preparing ointments and creams, loosening material from the surfaces of a mortar and pestle, and transferring the compounded preparation into its final container. A spatula may be made of stainless steel, plastic, or hard rubber. Hard rubber spatulas are used when corrosive substances, such as iodine and mercuric salts, are handled. Spatulas must be thoroughly cleaned before each use.

Molds and Presses Molds are needed to make rectal and vaginal suppositories or oral rapid-dissolving tablets and troches. Aluminum metal molds come in a variety of cavity sizes and can fill up to 100 cavities at one time. Common ingredient doses are in the range of 1 g to 2.5 g.

A pellet press is used to compound an implantable urethral pellet of medication. Hot plates may also be occasionally used to assist in melting down powders or mixing ingredients with various solvents in order to make suppositories, pellets, or rapid-dissolving tablets.

Containers for Packaging

Various sizes of prescription bottles, capsule vials, suppository boxes, ointment jars, and special delivery units must be available to contain and store compounded preparations. Most products will be in amber-colored vials or bottles or other ultraviolet (UV) light-protected packaging to prevent premature degradation of the products. Specialized packaging is needed for certain compounds. For example, rapid-dissolving tablets may need individualized blister packaging similar to many unit-dose products in the hospital pharmacy. Hormones in a cream or gel formulation are often dispensed to consumers in many pharmacies in an oral syringe, with the dosage calibrated to milliliters on the syringe. Another method that is used to apply topical hormone creams is the Topi-CLICK delivery system.

Topi-CLICK Delivery System Topi-CLICK is an easy-to-use, unique delivery system for topical creams. Well-accepted by physicians and patients, the patented, metered-dose applicator delivers a topical treatment of gel or cream (in this case, hormone cream). The unit is made of UV-blocking plastic and can hold up to 35 mL. Depending on the dose, the Topi-CLICK applicator may provide one to three months of medication. To operate, patients twist the base a quarter turn (one click) to move the plunger, thus delivering a given amount (0.25 mL per click) of medication in a topical base. Depending on blood levels, the patient dose may be one or more clicks per day. For patients on more than one hormone, the units are color-coded to limit errors. To promote compliance, Topi-CLICK provides an integrated applicator pad so topicals do not have to be applied by hands. The hand is a great absorber; therefore, when using hands as the applicator, patients are rubbing a percentage of the topical treatment into their hands rather than applying the cream to the prescribed treatment area. Using the hands can also increase the chances of others accidentally being exposed to someone else's prescription when holding or shaking hands. Overall, the Topi-CLICK delivery system helps promote patient compliance and has accuracy unmatched by the traditional tube delivery method.

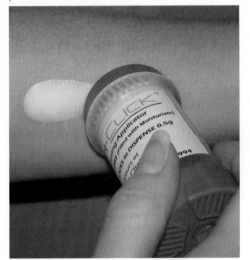

Most compounded tablets and capsules for future dispensing must be stored in amber light-protected vials.

Topi-CLICK is a patented delivery system to dose hormone creams and gels accurately.

Techniques for Mixing Compounded Drugs

Before preparing a drug for compounding, the technician should gather the master control record, ingredients, equipment, glassware, packaging material, and mixing directions. Providing adequate and uninterrupted time to the person who is compounding the prescription is also very important to minimize measurement or calculation errors.

After the technician has accurately weighed or measured out the individual ingredients in a compounded prescription, he or she must learn the best technique to mix the active and inactive ingredients for a tablet, capsule, cream, ointment, gel, suppository, or other dosage formulation. The mixing directions should include the need for diluting and sequencing the addition of ingredients. The best technique for mixing a given set of compounded medications should be included in the master control record or suggested by the experienced compounding pharmacist.

Comminution and Blending

Comminution is the act of reducing a substance to fine particles. **Blending** is the act of combining two substances. Techniques for comminution and blending include trituration, levigation, pulverization, spatulation, sifting, tumbling, and the use of the geometric dilution method. With repetition and experience, the technician can become more proficient in the preparation of a high-quality, pharmaceutically elegant compounded preparation.

Trituration The process of rubbing, grinding, or pulverizing a substance to create fine particles is called **trituration**. Using minimal pressure, pharmacy personnel typically rotate the pestle rapidly within the mortar to grind the ingredients. As discussed previously, various types of mortar and pestle sets are available for different ingredients. When mixing solids and liquids, reducing the particle size of the solid by gently heating the liquid (if the liquid is stable or nonvolatile) on a hot plate generally makes the solid dissolve faster and more uniformly. In addition, there will be less precipitation or clinging together of the solute into particles of unacceptably large size. To gain a better understanding of trituration in the compounding process, refer to Figure 8.5.

Trituration is also used when a potent or hazardous drug is mixed with a diluent powder. A **diluent powder** is an inactive ingredient that is added to the active drug when compounding a capsule.

At first, equal amounts of the potent drug and the diluent are triturated with a mortar and pestle. When these are thoroughly mixed, more of the diluent is added, equal to the amount already in the mortar. This process is continued until all of the diluent is incorporated into the compound.

Levigation The **levigation** technique is typically used when reducing the particle size of a solid during the preparation of an ointment. A levigating agent—such as castor oil, glycerin, or mineral oil—is slowly added to the ingredients in a glass mortar or on an ointment slab to wet (not dissolve) the insoluble chemicals. This tiny amount of levigating agent forms a paste. The amount of levigating agent added to the final preparation depends on the desired consistency and is included in the compounding log or record. The resulting paste is then triturated with a pestle or metal spatula to further reduce the particle size and then added to an ointment base. One example of levigation is adding glycerin to reduce the particle size of bismuth subnitrate.

Pulverization In nonsterile compounding, **pulverization** by intervention is the process of reducing the size of particles in a solid with the aid of an additional ingredient in which the substance is soluble. A volatile solvent such as camphor, alcohol, iodine, or ether is often used for this process. The solvent is added per mixing directions on the master control record, and then the mixture is triturated. The solvent is permitted to evaporate so it does not become part of the final product.

Spatulation The process of combining and mixing substances by means of a spatula, generally on an ointment slab or tile, is called **spatulation**. This technique is effective when mixing fine-particle powders.

Sifting In nonsterile compounding, **sifting** is a process not unlike the sifting of flour in baking. This process blends or combines powders using a wire mesh sieve. Pharmacy personnel select the mesh size based on the particle size needed. The powder is poured through the sieve, and a rubber spatula is used to force the powder through the sieve and onto the glassine paper.

FIGURE 8.5 Preparing a Solution for Sparky the Dog

(a) A pharmacy receives a prescription from a veterinarian to compound a preparation for Sparky the dog. This illustration shows the compounding log for this prescription.

(b) To prepare this medication, the pharmacist follows the steps in Table 8.3 for weighing the product (potassium bromide).

(c) Next, the product is placed in a mortar to be triturated and combined with the beef flavoring.

(d) The ingredients are mixed, but more trituration is needed to get the particles to a more even texture.

(e) The pharmacist uses a wall-mounted source of distilled water (also used to reconstitute antibiotic powders) to add to the veterinary mixture.

(f) The mixed and triturated ingredients are put into an amber bottle, using a glass funnel. Then, the bottle is shaken well and labeled.

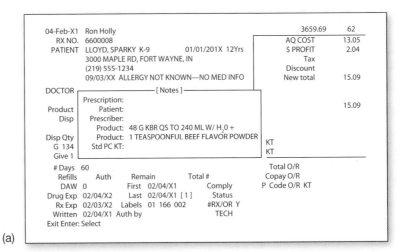

(a)

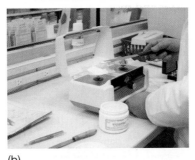

(b)

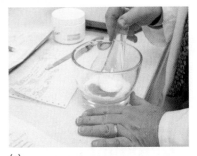

(c)

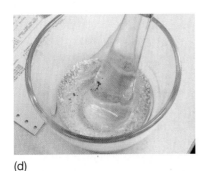

(d)

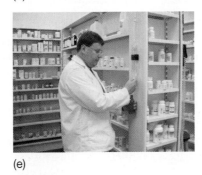

(e)

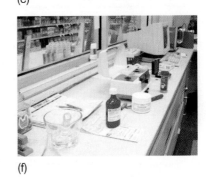

(f)

Tumbling The **tumbling** technique can also be used to mix powders. Pharmacy personnel place the powders being combined into a container such as a resealable plastic bag or a glass bottle and "tumble" or rotate the container to mix the ingredients well. An inert coloring agent may be added to ensure adequate mixing of the ingredients. This technique is frequently used when combining hazardous substances.

Geometric Dilution Method Often, a mortar and pestle is used to combine or blend more than one drug using a **geometric dilution method**. In this method, the pharmacy technician places the most potent ingredient, which is most likely the ingredient that occurs in the smallest amount, into the mortar first. Then, he or she adds an equal amount of the next most potent ingredient and mixes well. The technician continues in this manner by adding, each time, an amount equal to the amount in the mortar, until successively larger amounts of all the ingredients are added. Any residual amount of any ingredient should then be added and mixed well.

The same concept can be used when mixing incompatible or insoluble liquids. When mixing two liquids, a possible precipitation of solutes within the liquids can sometimes be avoided by making each portion as dilute as possible before mixing the liquids together.

Example 4

A prescription is received to prepare a compound for three ingredients in a ratio of 1:1:6 = 80 g. How much of each of the three ingredients is needed?

$$A = 10 \text{ g}$$
$$B = 10 \text{ g}$$
$$C = 60 \text{ g}$$

$$1:1:6 = \text{total of 80 g}$$

$$10 \text{ g} : 10 \text{ g} : 60 \text{ g} = 80 \text{ g}$$

The total amount of the preparation equals 80 g, with ingredient C added at six times the amount of ingredients A and B.

Compounding of Specific Formulations

In nonsterile compounding, powders, tablets, capsules, solutions, suspensions, ointments, creams, lotions, and suppositories are all compounded with various ingredients pursuant to a prescription and directions contained in the master control record.

Powders

In earlier times, the pharmacist commonly prepared prescription medicines in the form of **powders**. Often, the pharmacist dispensed powders that were measured, mixed, divided into separate units, and placed on pieces of paper. These pieces of paper were then folded and given to the patient. This dispensing method is all but obsolete in current pharmacy practice. The few exceptions are the individually wrapped over-the-counter (OTC) BC powder and Goody's Headache Powder. In Eastern medicine practice, fresh herbs are still prepared in wrapped paper packets and sold in Chinese herb shops.

Powders dispensed in bulk amounts have the disadvantage of leading to inaccurate dosing. For example, Metamucil is an example of a bulk powder used as an OTC fiber supplement in which the "approximate" dose may be one teaspoonful of powder added to a glass of water or orange juice. For many drugs, the dose of the medication must be more exact.

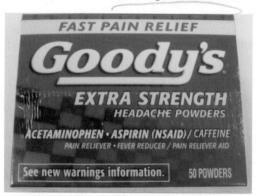

Goody's Headache Powder dates back to 1932 when pharmacist Martin "Goody" Goodman compounded his own formulation to treat the headaches that were common among tobacco and textile factory workers in North Carolina.

Types of Powders Most active and inactive bulk ingredients come in powder form to make a compound. To a layperson, a powder is any finely ground substance. To a pharmacist, a powder is a finely divided combination, or admixture, of drugs and/or chemicals ranging in size from extremely fine to very coarse. Official definitions of powder size include very coarse (No. 8 powder), coarse (No. 20 powder), moderately coarse (No. 40 powder), fine (No. 60 powder), or very fine (No. 80 powder), according to the amount of the powder that can pass through mechanical sieves made of wire cloth of various dimensions (for example, No. 8 sieves, No. 20 sieves, and so on).

Mixing of Powders Powders are combined and mixed by a variety of means, including trituration, spatulation, sifting, and tumbling in a container. The mixing process can also be accomplished using automated equipment.

Example 5

A prescription is received to prepare a gel or cream formulation using 30 g of Ketoprofen 10%, 30 g of Gabapentin 10%, and 30 g of Lidocaine 3%. Calculate the amount of each bulk ingredient needed and then prepare the compound.

Step 1. Determine how many grams of each bulk ingredient are needed.

Ketoprofen
$$10\% \times 30 \text{ g} = 3 \text{ g of Ketoprofen needed}$$

Gabapentin
$$10\% \times 30 \text{ g} = 3 \text{ g of Gabapentin needed}$$

Lidocaine
$$3\% \times 30 \text{ g} = 0.9 \text{ g, or } 900 \text{ mg of Lidocaine needed}$$

Step 2. Weigh out these amounts of each medication.

Step 3. Mix these powders, add a sufficient amount of propylene glycol to dissolve them, and then add the powdered glycol mixture to a gel or cream base formulation to make 90 g of final product.

Tablets and Troches

A tablet may be compounded in a traditional compression formulation; however, a rapid-dissolving tablet or a troche is typically compounded in a special contained hood to minimize airborne contamination. The compounding of tablets requires a single-punch tablet press to blend active and inactive ingredients (or excipients). Pharmacy personnel weigh the powders and place them in a die; then they lower the handle to compress the ingredients and form the tablets. Compression tablets are rarely compounded in most pharmacies; this process requires expensive equipment, expertise, and labor-intensive preparation. It is often easier to pulverize compression tablets and use them in the compounding of a capsule or suspension formulation.

Rapid-Dissolving Tablets Rapid-dissolving tablets (RDTs) are a unique tablet formulation that can be prepared in a specialty compounding pharmacy. These tablets disintegrate rapidly and dissolve on the tongue within 30 seconds. In addition to the active ingredient, a base, sweetener, and flavoring agents are used in the process. After the powders of the active and inactive ingredients are mixed, they are placed in a special Teflon mold (using a rubber spatula only, no metal) and then baked in a convection oven for a specified period. After cooling, the compound is then packaged and labeled in a blister pack for consumer use. Hormones such as estrogen, testosterone, and thyroid may be prepared as RDTs.

Troches Troches are small, circular lozenges that contain active medication. In addition to active ingredients, troches commonly include a base such as polyethylene glycol, suspending agents, sweeteners, and flavorings. These medication lozenges are dissolved in the mouth (or vagina, in some cases) rather than being swallowed. Troches are well-absorbed because the lining of the mouth (and vagina) is thin and rich in blood supply. An example of a prescription-only troche formulation is the antifungal drug clotrimazole; however, troches are also used to deliver bioidentical hormones (twice daily) and pain-relieving medications.

Capsules

A capsule is a solid dosage form consisting of a gelatin shell that encloses the medicinal preparation, which may be a powder, granule, or liquid. The hard shells of capsules are made of gelatin, sugar, and water and consist of two parts: (1) the body, which is the longer and narrower part, and (2) the cap, which is shorter and fits over the body. In some cases, capsules have an interlocking design (marketed as Snap-Fit), with grooves on the cap and the body that fit into one another to ensure proper closure (see Figure 8.6). Hard-shell capsules come in standard sizes indicated by the numbers 5, 4, 3, 2, 1, 0, 00, 000 (from smallest to largest). The largest capsule, size 000, can contain about 1000 mg of medication; the smallest, size 5, contains about 100 mg (see Figure 8.7).

Most hard-shell capsules are meant to be swallowed whole; however, some capsules are intended to be opened so that their contents can be sprinkled on food or in drink. Therefore, patients should be advised as to which administration method should be used with their medications. They should also be warned that opening and ingesting the contents of certain capsules can adversely affect the controlled-release properties of certain medications and may upset the stomach.

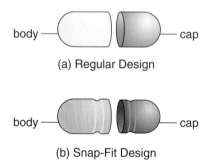

(a) Regular Design

(b) Snap-Fit Design

FIGURE 8.6 Types of Hard-Shell Capsules

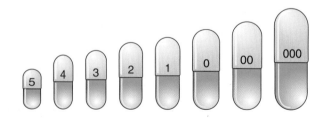

FIGURE 8.7 Hard-Shell Capsule Sizes

The sizes in which hard-shell capsules are available range from 5, the smallest, to 000, the largest.

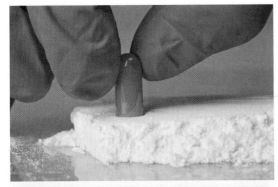

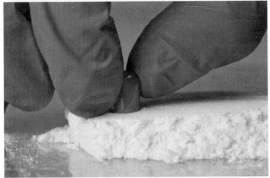

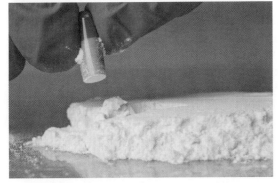

In the punch method for extemporaneous filling of capsules, the body of the capsule is filled by "punching" it into a cake of the powder. The filled capsule is then weighed to verify the dose.

Filling Capsules Nonsterile compounding of ingredients for capsules is often done to provide unusual dosage forms, such as those containing less of an active ingredient than is readily available in commercial tablets or capsules. For example, in order to create an oral capsule in a pediatric dose that is not commercially available, the pharmacist might have to pulverize, or triturate, commercially available tablets, mix the resultant powder with a diluent powder, and use that powder mixture to fill capsules. This diluent powder provides bulk and stability to the capsule.

Punch Method When hand-filling a capsule with powder, a pharmacist or technician may use the **punch method**. First, the number of capsules to be filled is counted. Then the powder is placed on a clean surface of paper, porcelain, or glass and formed into a cake with a spatula. The cake should be approximately ¼ to ⅓ the height of the capsule body. The body of the capsule is then punched into the cake repeatedly until the capsule is full. The cap is then placed snugly over the body. Granules are generally poured into the capsule body from a piece of paper.

Capsule Machine A capsule machine with multiple metal plates may be used to replace the one-at-a-time punch-and-fill method; a capsule machine can make 100 capsules within a short period.

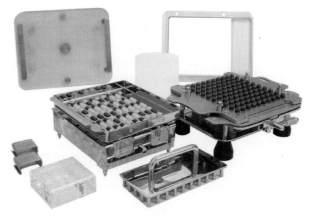

ProFiller 1100 is a 100-hole capsule-filling system used in compounding pharmacies.

Example 6

Nystatin powder has an activity of 100,000 units/g. How many milligrams of nystatin would you use in each capsule if the final preparation is supposed to be 1,500,000 units per capsule?

Step 1. Convert 100,000 units/g to units/milligram.

$$100{,}000 \text{ units/g} \times 1 \text{ g}/1{,}000 \text{ mg} = 100 \text{ units/mg}$$

Step 2. Determine the amount of milligrams needed in each capsule using the ratio-proportion method.

$$\frac{x \text{ mg}}{1{,}500{,}000 \text{ units}} = \frac{1 \text{ mg}}{100 \text{ units}}$$

$$\frac{(\cancel{1{,}500{,}000 \text{ units}}) \, x \text{ mg}}{\cancel{1{,}500{,}000 \text{ units}}} = \frac{(\cancel{1{,}500{,}000 \text{ units}}) \, 1 \text{ mg}}{100 \, \cancel{\text{units}}}$$

$$x \text{ mg} = 15{,}000 \text{ mg}$$

Solutions

As defined in Chapter 4, a solution is a liquid dosage form in which the active ingredients are dissolved in a liquid vehicle. The vehicle that makes up the greater part of a solution is known as the *solvent*. The ingredient (medication) dissolved in the solution is known as the *solute*. Solutions may be aqueous (made with water), alcoholic, or hydroalcoholic. Hydroalcoholic solutions contain both water and alcohol, which may be needed to dissolve some solutes. Solutions are prepared by dissolving the solute in the liquid solvent or by combining or diluting existing solutions. Colorings or flavoring agents may be added to solutions for appearance or improved palatability or taste; for example, a syrup—known as *Syrup NF*—can be made by combining 85 g of sucrose with 100 mL of purified water.

Otic solutions are a commonly requested preparation in a compounding pharmacy. An example of a recipe or master control record for an otic solution to remove ear wax is shown in Figure 8.8.

FIGURE 8.8
Master Control Record for Otic Solution Compound

Compound Title
urea and hydrogen peroxide otic solution

Compound Ingredients
carbamide peroxide ....6.6 g
glycerin, as much as necessary to total ....100 mL

Compounding Procedure
Dissolve the carbamide peroxide in sufficient glycerin to volume; then package and label. A beyond-use date of up to six months can be used for this preparation.

Suspensions

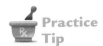

Practice Tip

Regardless of their apparent stability, all suspensions should be dispensed with an auxiliary label stating "Shake Well."

In a suspension, as opposed to a solution, the active ingredient is not dissolved in the liquid vehicle but rather is dispersed throughout it. An obvious problem with suspensions is the tendency of the active ingredient to settle. To avoid settling of the insoluble drug, a suspending agent is added after vigorous trituration or grinding of the tablets into a powder. Such suspending agents include tragacanth, acacia, and carboxymethylcellulose (CMC). Still, the auxiliary medication label "Shake Well" should always be affixed to a suspension container.

Many pediatric suspensions that are commercially unavailable can be prepared in the pharmacy from adult tablets or capsules. A good example is compounding a suspension of captopril for a pediatric patient under age six. The drug is only available in 12.5 mg, 25 mg, 50 mg, and 100 mg oral tablets. The pediatric dose is approximately 0.2 mg/kg. For a patient weighing 10 kg (22 lb), the dose is 2 mg. Tablets must be crushed, and a suitable suspending and flavoring agent must be identified for stability and palatability.

Another example is calculating a dose for the cardiovascular drug Coreg for a pediatric patient. See the example below for a step-by-step explanation of the compounding process.

Example 7

A prescription for a pediatric patient calls for 60 mL of a suspension of Coreg at a concentration of 5.5 mg/mL. Coreg is not available commercially as a suspension, but only as tablets in strengths of 3.125 mg, 6.25 mg, 12.5 mg, and 25 mg. How would you compound this prescription?

Step 1. Determine how many milligrams of Coreg are needed to compound this prescription using the ratio-proportion method.

$$\frac{x \text{ mg}}{60 \text{ mL}} = \frac{5.5 \text{ mg}}{1 \text{ mL}}$$

$$\frac{(60 \text{ mL}) \, x \text{ mg}}{60 \text{ mL}} = \frac{(60 \text{ mL}) \, 5.5 \text{ mg}}{1 \text{ mL}}$$

$$x \text{ mg} = 330 \text{ mg}$$

Step 2. Determine the tablet sizes and number of each that must be crushed or ground up with a mortar and pestle to equal approximately 330 mg.

$$12 \text{ tablets} \times 25 \text{ mg/tablet} = 300 \text{ mg}$$

$$2 \text{ tablets} \times 12.5 \text{ mg/tablet} = 25 \text{ mg}$$

$$1 \text{ tablet} \times 6.25 \text{ mg/tablet} = 6.25 \text{ mg}$$

300 mg + 25 mg + 6.25 mg = 331.25, which is close to the desired 330 mg

Step 3. After crushing the tablets, 60 mL of suspending agent is slowly added to the pulverized tablets; a small amount (usually ½ to 1 dropperful) of flavoring agent is added; and then the product is labeled with beyond-use dating and the following instructions: "Shake Well" and "Refrigerate."

The point (and rate) at which the suspending agent is added in the mixing procedure can be crucial. Therefore, the technician must always remember to add the ingredients in the proper order, according to the formula or recipe contained in the master control record. Flavoring agents may sometimes be incompatible with the active ingredient because of pH or acid/base balance. Many vendors provide flavoring vehicles that have been proven to be safe and effective in children for compound preparations as well as commercially available reconstituted antibiotic suspensions.

Ointments, Creams, and Lotions

Ointments, creams, and lotions are semisolid dosage forms that are meant for application to the skin.

Ointments As you may recall from Chapter 4, an ointment is a water-in-oil (w/o) emulsion that is occlusive, greasy, and not water-washable. The properties of "ointment" bases such as lanolin, petrolatum, and Aquaphor vary in their degree of occlusiveness, emolliency, water washability, and water absorption. An occlusive ointment base has the ability to hold moisture in the skin and is best used when additional hydration is needed, such as for a patient with dry skin. An emollient base has the ability to soften skin, such as in bath oils. White petrolatum is an example of a lipophilic base with high occlusive and emollient properties. Most ointment bases are commercially available from a wholesaler or pharmacy compounding vendor and are best prepared using water-repellent plastic equipment.

Creams A cream is an oil-in-water (o/w) emulsion that is nonocclusive, nongreasy, and water-washable. Water washability and absorption relate to cosmetic appearance such as vanishing creams. Polyethylene glycol is an example of a water-soluble base.

Lotions A lotion is a liquid suspension or oil-in-water emulsion used topically in areas of the body such as the scalp, where a lubricating effect is desirable.

Example 8

How much Nitro-bid 2% ointment is required to make 100 g of a 0.2% ointment?

Nitro-bid is commercially available as a 2% ointment, but the prescription calls for a 0.2% ointment. The desired concentration is one-tenth or 10% of the commercially available product. Mix 10 g of 2% Nitro-bid (10% of 100 g) ointment with approximately 90 grams of ointment base to make a final preparation of 100 g of 0.2% ointment.

In this example, you could also use the alligation method discussed in Chapter 5, with 2% Nitro-bid combined with 0% active ingredients of the ointment base.

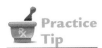

Practice Tip

Pharmacy technicians must remember that a 1% concentration equals 10 mg/mL and a 20% concentration equals 200 mg/mL. This conversion is often used to make sterile preparations in the hospital and in the home health-care environment.

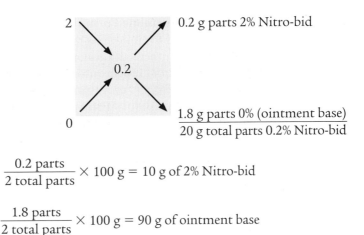

$$\frac{0.2 \text{ parts}}{2 \text{ total parts}} \times 100 \text{ g} = 10 \text{ g of 2\% Nitro-bid}$$

$$\frac{1.8 \text{ parts}}{2 \text{ total parts}} \times 100 \text{ g} = 90 \text{ g of ointment base}$$

Compounding Ointments, Creams, and Lotions Dermatologic therapies may call for combining existing ointments or creams. Most ointments and creams are prepared via mechanical incorporation of materials, levigation, or mixing in a mortar and pestle. When an ointment slab and spatula are used (spatulation), the edge of the spatula should press against the slab to provide a shearing force, which allows for a smoother preparation. A cream and lotion are best prepared using glass equipment.

In other cases, the dry ingredients of an ointment or a cream may have to be triturated, or reduced to a fine powder, in a mortar and pestle before being added to the ointment or cream base. This trituration process is necessary to avoid a gritty, nonuniform appearance of the preparation. For example, when placing a powder into an ointment or a cream, adding the powder in small amounts and constantly working the mixture in with the spatula or pestle result in a pharmaceutically elegant product. An electric mortar and pestle or automated ointment mill can be used if available to maximize the mixing of ingredients and to improve the appearance of the final preparation.

If mixing three or more ingredients to the ointment or cream base, then adding them sequentially using the geometric dilution method (discussed earlier in this chapter) rather than mixing them all together is important; this allows for more drug stability and a more pharmaceutically elegant end preparation.

An example of a topical compound can be seen in the master control record shown in Figure 8.9.

**FIGURE 8.9
Master Control Record for Topical Compound**

Compound Title
ketoprofen 10% and ibuprofen 2.5% in pluronic lecithin organogel

Compound Ingredients

ketoprofen ....10 g

ibuprofen ....2.5 g

lecithin:isopropyl palmitate 1:1 solution...............................22 mL

Pluronic F127 20% gel qs to total ....100 mL

Compounding Procedure

Mix the ketoprofen and ibuprofen powders with propylene glycol to form a smooth paste. Incorporate the lecithin:isopropyl palmitate solution and mix well. Add sufficient Pluronic F127 gel to volume and mix using high-shearing action until uniform. Package and label.

Compounding Hormone Formulations Gynecologists in particular are requesting more compounded formulations to individualize hormone treatments for their patients. Many commercially available hormones are available in a fixed-dose, oral synthetic formulation. **Hormone replacement therapy (HRT)** consists of some combination of estrogen, progestin (female), and androgen (male) to relieve specific postmenopausal symptoms. **Estrogen replacement therapy (ERT)** consists of female hormones and is sometimes used in postmenopausal women and premenopausal women who have had complete hysterectomies. However, many women have concerns about the long-term safety of taking oral synthetic hormones. With that in mind, more specialists are prescribing compounded cream and gel formulations for their patients. These compounded preparations of bioidentical hormones attempt to match the individual requirements for women. (Men, as well, are also prescribed these compounded hormone formulations to treat male hormone deficiencies.)

Table 8.5 lists the most common abbreviations for the various estrogen hormones contained in a compound prescription. The dose is often based on symptoms, clinical observations, and laboratory analyses of serum, saliva, or urine levels. During the hormone therapy treatment, a woman maintains a symptom diary so that the dose can be fine-tuned if necessary. A compounded cream or gel formulation may release the active ingredients more slowly and provide more long-lasting relief (less peaks and valleys) than a commercially available oral preparation. Because the various hormones in a topical formulation do not have to be eliminated through the liver like an oral tablet, it is much safer to use, although the long-term effects are unknown. Even with topical hormone compounds, the risk vs. benefit must be assessed by the physician on an annual basis.

TABLE 8.5   Abbreviations on Bioidentical Hormone Compound Prescriptions

Bioidentical Hormone	Abbreviation	Percentage
Estrone	E1	100%
Estradiol	E2	100%
Estriol	E3	100%
Biestrogen	E3/E2	80%/20%
Triestrogen	E3/E2/E1	80%/10%/10%

Suppositories

As mentioned in Chapter 4, suppositories are solid dosage forms that are inserted into the body's orifices, generally the rectum or the vagina (less commonly, the urethra). They are composed of one or more active ingredients placed into one of a variety of water-soluble bases (such as glycerinated gelatin and polyethylene glycol) or oleaginous bases (such as cocoa butter and hydrogenated vegetable oil). These dosage forms melt or dissolve when exposed to body heat and fluids. Compounding high-quality suppositories typically requires the skills of a highly experienced pharmacy technician or a pharmacist.

Suppositories are produced by molding and by compression. The preparation of suppositories involves melting the base material, adding the active ingredient(s), and pouring the resultant liquid into a mold. (When using an aluminum metal mold, a light coating of lubricant such as mineral oil or glycerin must be applied prior to filling the mold.) Each cavity of the mold should be filled slowly and carefully ensuring that no air bubbles are entrapped in the cavity. To prevent layering in the suppositories, the pouring process should not be stopped until all the cavities have been filled. Once filled, the mold should be allowed to congeal or solidify at room temperature. Upon dispensing the suppositories, pharmacy personnel should advise patients to refrigerate the medication to minimize premature melting of the active ingredients.

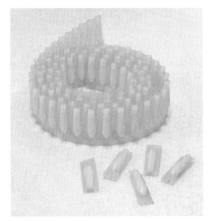

Disposable suppository molds are commonly used to dispense and shape suppositories.

The Compounding Process

 Safety Note

Compounding should never be rushed.

Each step of the compounding process is checked and initialed by the pharmacist and pharmacy technician. The technician should double-check the calculations by the pharmacist and those contained in the master control record. Any calculations completed by the technician should be written on the compounding record and checked by the pharmacist. A printout of the weight of each ingredient from an electronic digital balance is usually attached to the compounding record or log sheet for pharmacist verification so that each weight in the preparation of the compound can be double-checked. It is also important to document the beyond-use date of a prepared compound.

Table 8.6 summarizes the 14 steps required by USP Chapter <795> to compound a nonsterile preparation. These steps, or something similar, should appear in the P&P manual for the compounding pharmacy. If these steps are followed on each and every compound prescription, then the quality and efficacy of the preparation will be maximized and the risk of medication error minimized. Following these steps also minimizes legal liability and ensures continuing accreditation status.

The following sections discuss further the proper selection of medication containers, labeling, record keeping, and cleanup requirements, as well as the final check process by the pharmacist and the counseling of the patient. Issues related to insurance coverage for compounded products are discussed at the end of this section.

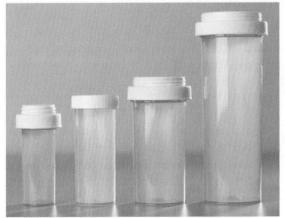

Compounded tablets and capsules should be dispensed in UV light-protected containers.

Selecting Medication Containers

With so much emphasis on chemical stability, it is important for the pharmacy technician to select the appropriate container to extend the beyond-use dating as much as possible. Standards for packaging the most common compounds are provided by USP in the *Pharmacists' Pharmacopeia* (see under Reference Sources for the Compounding Pharmacy). For tablets and capsules, amber-colored prescription vials are used to protect the product from light. Ointments and creams may be placed in white ointment jars in various sizes. Suppositories and pellets may be

TABLE 8.6   Steps in the Compounding Process

1. The pharmacist judges the suitability of the prescription to be compounded in terms of safety and intended use.

2. The pharmacist retrieves and reviews the master control record in the computer.

3. The pharmacist prints out a compounding record or log sheet for the technician to make the nonsterile preparation.

4. The pharmacist performs all necessary mathematical calculations and identifies the necessary equipment for the technician; the technician double-checks all calculations.

5. A medication container label is typed or created by the computer software using information in the compounding log. The label includes the following:
   a. patient name
   b. physician name
   c. date of compounding
   d. name of preparation
   e. internal ID or lot number
   f. beyond-use date
   g. initials of compounding technician and pharmacist
   h. directions for use, including any special storage conditions
   i. any additional requirements of state or federal law

6. The pharmacy technician uses appropriate protective clothing and hand-washing technique.

7. The technician gathers all necessary active and inactive ingredients, as well as prepares and calibrates any necessary equipment.

8. The technician weighs and adds all ingredients for the preparation, initials each step, and adds documentation (such as source and NDC number) to the compounding record.

9. The technician stores the medication in a suitable container.

10. The technician affixes the medication label to the proper container.

11. The pharmacist reviews the compounding record (with the printout of the weights of all ingredients) and medication container label and assesses appropriate physical characteristics of the preparation, such as any weight variations, adequacy of mixing, clarity, odor, color, consistency, and pH.

12. The pharmacist signs and dates the compounding log record and/or prescription, files the records (computer entry and printed copy), and places the compounded preparation in a storage bin for patient pickup or mails the preparation to patient.

13. The technician cleans all equipment thoroughly and promptly, reshelves all active and inactive ingredients, and properly labels and stores any excess preparation.

14. The pharmacist counsels the patient at the time of pickup.

dispensed in cardboard boxes. As mentioned earlier in the chapter, bioidentical hormone creams are often packaged using the Topi-CLICK delivery system.

Labeling and Cleanup

After the compounding operation, the preparation must be labeled with a medication container label containing all information for the consumer as required by the governing laws and regulations of the state and federal government. The ingredients of the compound and the amounts of these ingredients should be clearly stated on the medication container label. The label should also include beyond-use dating (often labeled "discard after"), the lot number, and the date of the compounding. If commercial products are used, then the brand or generic drug names should be listed on the medication container label. No abbreviations of active drug ingredients should be used (in the rare event that the drug must be identified in an emergency). If Topi-CLICK is used, the medication container label can be directly affixed to the delivery system.

The prescription balance, when not in use or in transit, should be placed in the locked position and covered, and weights must be placed back in their original container. Balances must be cleaned after each use, with documented daily calibration. Once the compounding operation is completed for each product, equipment and the work area should be thoroughly cleaned, and ingredients should be returned to their proper storage areas. The technician must pay special attention to correct cleanup disinfectants and procedures to minimize cross-contamination and potential allergic reactions.

Many active pharmaceuticals and bulk ingredients used in compounding are considered hazardous chemicals. This designation may reflect chemical ignitability, corrosivity, reactivity, or toxicity. These chemicals are prepared in very small doses in compounded preparations and thus are not generally considered to be hazardous. If state regulations allow, these compounds can be labeled and mailed without special precautions if proper storage conditions can be maintained.

Any expired or discarded product containing a hazardous chemical should be placed in a sealed container in a designated biohazard container (not the wastebasket) per written policy and procedure. After the contents have been verified and signed off by the pharmacist, an outside vendor takes receipt and discards the materials per state and federal regulations.

Final Check by the Pharmacist

The pharmacist is legally responsible for checking the final product, including ensuring that the correct master control record was used, that mathematical calculations were accurate on the compounding record, and that printouts on all weighed ingredients (if available) were verified. The medication container label must also be checked. A careful record of the compounding operation—including ingredients and amounts of ingredients used, the preparer of the compound, and the name of the supervising pharmacist—should be kept.

Finally, the pharmacist checks the **pharmaceutical elegance** (or how the product looks) by performing a physical inspection of the preparation. The pharmacist uses his or her knowledge and experience to review the adequacy of mixing, odor, color, consistency, and pH (acid or base balance) if necessary. The pharmacist initials the compounding record and the label and places the product under proper storage conditions for future pickup or mailing to the patient.

After the product is prepared by the technician and checked by the pharmacist, a printed copy of the compounding record is filed with the original prescription, for later retrieval or recall if necessary. Prescriptions are filed and maintained in accordance with state, federal, and other legal regulations. Easy retrievability is important if there is a drug recall of any ingredients in the compounded prescription or if an adverse effect occurs in the

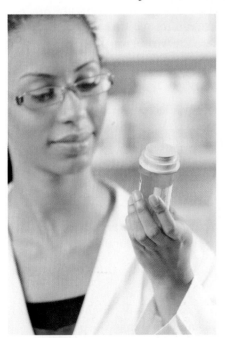

As with any prescription, the pharmacist must provide a final check of the medication and label before dispensing to the patient.

patient. In addition to printed copies of the formula and prescription, most records are stored on a CD or hard drive of the computer on-site or, preferably, through an off-site vendor.

Patient Counseling by the Pharmacist

The pharmacist should communicate to the patient that his or her prescription has been individually prepared and compounded pursuant to a prescription. In addition, the sig or directions from the prescriber compounded preparation information must be typed on the medication container label. The patient should be aware of all the ingredients contained in the compound prescription and their expected therapeutic and potential adverse effects.

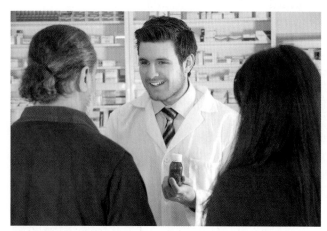

Counseling by the pharmacist on proper use, storage, and beyond-use dating is important on any compounded preparation.

The pharmacist must be sure that the patient understands how to take the medication, especially if an unusual delivery system is used. For example, how does the dosage compare to the milliliters or cubic centimeters on a syringe or to the clicks on a Topi-CLICK? How is this delivery device primed or how often does it need to be primed? The pharmacist should demonstrate how the medication should be applied—for example, on one arm and rubbed in by the other for 15 to 20 seconds.

As with all prescriptions, the technician must offer pharmacist counseling to all patients regarding compounded preparations. Patients must be counseled on the proper storage conditions for the compounded preparation as well as labeling requirements, especially if they will be using the medication beyond the labeled dating. A written medication information sheet may be printed by the pharmacy software or developed internally within the pharmacy.

Reimbursement

Insurance generally does not cover the cost of a compounded preparation. This lack of coverage is a major reason for the growth of specialized compounding pharmacies, as insurance denials have had a major impact on the profits of independent community pharmacies. The patient cost for a compounded medication is based on the time and experience of the pharmacist and technician rather than on the costs, which are usually minimal, of the active and inactive ingredients. Most compounded prescriptions take a minimum of 30 to 60 minutes to prepare.

Patients pay out-of-pocket for compounded preparations; with proper forms completed (and a lot of patience), they may be reimbursed by their insurance at a later date. A compounding pharmacy provides the patient with all necessary information regarding the compounded preparation on a Universal Claim Form (UCF) so that the patient can bill insurance. This information includes the NDC numbers and cost of each ingredient as well as time necessary to prepare. The success of reimbursement for a compounded medication may be greater if the patient, rather than the pharmacy, submits the claim billing a third-party insurer.

Reference Sources for the Compounding Pharmacy

Nonsterile compounding requires specialty training, certification, and experience. In addition to receiving advice from the supervising pharmacist, the pharmacy technician can refer to standard reference works on the subject, such as *Remington: The Science and Practice of Pharmacy* by Gennaro, and from the following sources:

- Professional Compounding Centers of America (PCCA)
- United States Pharmacopeia (USP)
- *Secundum Artem: Current & Practical Compounding Information for the Pharmacist*
- International Academy of Compounding Pharmacists (IACP)

As discussed earlier in the chapter, PCCA is a source supplier of high-quality USP- and NF-grade pharmaceutical ingredients. Membership entitles the compounding pharmacy access to the master formulas that have been developed and proven safe and effective over the years. The PCCA also holds national and regional educational and certification seminars in sterile and nonsterile compounding for both pharmacists and pharmacy technicians. PCCA is also a source of pharmacy software as well as marketing, business, and clinical consultations.

As discussed in Chapter 2, the USP is a private, nongovernmental organization that is responsible for setting standards, such as USP Chapter <795>, that are recognized by the government (FDA) and by private organizations such as the PCAB for accreditation. The USP has published a *Pharmacists' Pharmacopeia*, which is a reference for pharmacy personnel involved in sterile and nonsterile compounding; this reference is also available online. This text includes approved monographs for more than 120 compounded preparations, as well as all necessary guidelines and standards for the safe preparation, packaging, and storing of many compounded prescriptions.

Pharmacy technicians who are interested in nonsterile compounding practice are encouraged to visit the Paddock Labs website (www.paradigmcollege.net/pharmpractice5e/paddocklabs), a website that has been acquired by the Perrigo Company. There, technicians can view archived articles from the past 25 years under the title "Compounding" for helpful information in the *Secundum Artem* series. Another helpful local source of information for the compounding community pharmacist and technician is a hospital pharmacy, especially a pediatric hospital pharmacy, where a pharmacist may have a needed recipe or formula and has experience compounding and flavoring formulations for neonates, infants, and pediatric patients.

The International Academy of Compounding Pharmacists is a political action group; membership is open to both pharmacists and pharmacy technicians. The group's mission is to promote and advance personalized medication solutions for patients. In addition, the organization keeps compounding pharmacy personnel alert to legislative challenges that have an impact on their profession. For example, the FDA has suggested in the recent past that all compounded preparations should be considered new drugs and thus subject to undergoing a new drug application process similar to the requirements for pharmaceutical manufacturers. If such legislation were passed, then compounding pharmacies—the embodiment of a long-standing tradition that lies at the heart of pharmacy practice—would cease to exist. Keeping attuned to changes in the pharmaceutical industry is essential to fulfilling the responsibilities of practicing safe and effective patient care.

Chapter Summary

- Nonsterile compounding is used today to prepare medications in strengths, combinations, or dosage forms that are not commercially available.
- Pharmacies must follow good compounding practices as outlined in USP Chapter <795>.
- Product quality for bulk ingredients is important in compounding a high-quality product.
- Beyond-use dating is the assignment of an expiration date on a compounded preparation that meets USP guidelines or is supported by independent scientific research.
- Many specialty compounding pharmacies seek national accreditation for marketing and reimbursement.
- Pharmacy technicians often need additional training and certification to practice in a compounding pharmacy.
- Minimum proper attire includes a long lab coat, hairnet, and disposable gloves.
- The master control record and the compounding log document that the correct ingredients, equipment, and technique have been used to prepare a quality preparation for a legal prescription.
- The compounding log documents the patient-specific prescription.
- Calculations for individual ingredients and the final compounded preparation must be double-checked by the pharmacist.

- Instruments for extemporaneous compounding include the Class III prescription or electronic balances, pharmaceutical weights, forceps, spatulas, weighing papers, compounding or ointment slab, parchment paper, mortar and pestle, graduated cylinders, and pipettes.
- Mortars and pestles are available in glass, Wedgwood, and porcelain varieties. Graduates are available in various sizes in both conical and cylindrical shapes, the latter being the more accurate.
- Proper technique and use of the correct measuring devices are crucial when weighing and measuring pharmaceutical ingredients.
- Several techniques are used for the comminution and blending of ingredients.
- Geometric dilution is utilized when mixing potent or toxic ingredients.
- Compounding is used to prepare tablets, capsules, powders, solutions, suspensions, ointments, creams, lotions, and suppositories according to a formula contained in the master control record.
- The compounding process includes selecting the most appropriate medication container, affixing a label, keeping accurate prescription records, and cleaning up.
- The pharmacist is legally responsible for the final check of the compounded prescription and for counseling the patient.
- Nonsterile compounding is an art to be learned under the tutelage of an experienced pharmacist.

Key Terms

anticipatory compounding the preparation of excess product (besides an individual compound prescription) in reasonable quantities; these preparations must be labeled with lot numbers

beyond-use dating the documentation of the date after which a compounded preparation expires and should no longer be used

blending the act of combining two substances using techniques such as spatulation, sifting, and tumbling

Class III prescription balance a two-pan balance used to weigh material (120 g or less) with a sensitivity rating of +/–6 mg; also known as a *Class A prescription balance*

comminution the act of reducing a substance to small, fine particles using techniques such as trituration, levigation, and pulverization

compounded preparation a patient-specific medication prepared on-site by the technician, under the direct supervision of the pharmacist, from individual ingredients

compounding the process of preparing a medication for an individual patient from bulk ingredients according to a prescription by a licensed prescriber

compounding log a printout of the prescription for a specific patient, including the amounts or weights of all ingredients and instructions for compounding; used by the technician to prepare a compounded medication for a patient

continuous quality improvement (CQI) a process of written procedures designed to identify problems and recommend solutions

counterbalance a two-pan balance used for weighing material up to 5 kg with a sensitivity rating of +/–100 mg

digital electronic analytical balance a single-pan balance that is more accurate than Class III balances or counterbalances; it has a capacity of 100 g and sensitivity as low as +/–2 mg

diluent powder an inactive ingredient that is added to the active drug in compounding a tablet or capsule

estrogen replacement therapy (ERT) treatment consisting of some combination of female hormones

forceps an instrument used to pick up small objects, such as pharmacy weights

geometric dilution method a process that uses a mortar and pestle to gradually combine several drugs and inactive ingredients

good compounding practices (GCPs) USP standards in many areas of practice to ensure high-quality compounded preparations

graduated cylinder a flask used for measuring liquids

hormone replacement therapy (HRT) therapy consisting of some combination of estrogen and progestin (female) and androgen (male) hormones

levigation a process usually used to reduce the particle size of a solid during the preparation of an ointment

manufactured products products prepared off-site by a large-scale drug manufacturer

master control record a recipe for a compound preparation that lists the name, strength, dosage form, ingredients and their quantities, mixing instructions, and beyond-use dating; many recipes available from PCCA

Material Safety Data Sheet (MSDS) a document that contains important information on hazards and flammability of chemicals used in compounding and procedure for treatment of accidental ingestion or exposure

meniscus the moon-shaped or concave appearance of a liquid in a graduated cylinder; used during the measurement process

mortar and pestle equipment used for mixing and grinding pharmaceutical ingredients

nonsterile compounding the preparation of a medication, in an appropriate quantity and dosage form, from several pharmaceutical ingredients in response to a prescription written by a physician; sometimes referred to as *extemporaneous compounding*

nonvolumetric glassware a beaker or flask that is not calibrated and cannot be used to accurately measure liquids; its use is limited to store, contain, and mix liquids with other bulk ingredients

ointment slab a flat, hard, nonabsorbent surface used for mixing compounds; also known as a *compounding slab*

percentage of error the acceptable range of variation above and below the target measurement; used in compounding and manufacturing

pharmaceutical elegance the physical appearance of the final compounded preparation

pharmaceutical weights measures of various sizes made of polished brass, often used with a two-pan prescription balance; available in both metric and apothecary weights

Pharmacy Compounding Accreditation Board (PCAB) an organization that provides quality and safety standards for a compounding pharmacy through voluntary accreditation

pipette a long, thin, calibrated hollow tube used for measuring small volumes of liquids

powders preparations in the form of fine particles

prescription record a computer-generated version of the compounding log that documents the compounding recipe for a specific prescription and patient

pulverization the process of reducing particle size, especially by using a solvent

punch method a method for filling capsules in which the body of a capsule is repeatedly punched into a cake of medication until the capsule is full

rapid-dissolving tablet (RDT) a tablet that disintegrates rapidly (within 30 seconds) on the tongue

sifting a process used to blend powders through the use of a sieve

spatula a stainless steel, plastic, or hard rubber instrument used for transferring or mixing solid pharmaceutical ingredients

spatulation a process used to blend ingredients; often used in the preparation of creams and ointments

stability the extent to which a compounded product retains the same physical and chemical properties and characteristics it possessed at the time of preparation

sterile compounding the preparation of a parenteral product in the hospital, home healthcare, nuclear, or community pharmacy setting; an example is an intravenous antibiotic or an ophthalmic solution

trituration the process of rubbing, grinding, or pulverizing a substance to create fine particles, generally by means of a mortar and pestle

troche a small, circular lozenge that contains active medication

tumbling a process used to combine powders by placing them in a bag or container and shaking it

volumetric measurement a calibrated graduated cylinder or pipette that accurately measures liquids

weighing boat a plastic container used to weigh large quantities of chemicals

weighing paper a special paper that is placed on a weighing balance pan to avoid contact between pharmaceutical ingredients and the balance tray; also called *powder paper*

Chapter Review

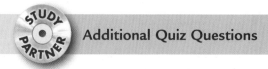

Additional Quiz Questions

Checking Your Understanding

To check your comprehension of this chapter's key concepts, read the following multiple-choice questions and then record your answers on a separate sheet of paper. Write your answers as modeled in these examples: 1d; 2c; 3b; *etc.*

1. Beyond-use dating is the expiration date of
   a. the manufactured product.
   b. a compounded preparation.
   c. the individual ingredients.
   d. pharmacy technician certification.

2. The most accurate balance used in a compounding pharmacy is a
   a. Class III prescription balance.
   b. Class A prescription balance.
   c. counterbalance.
   d. digital electronic analytical balance.

3. An alternative to the ointment slab is
   a. weighing paper.
   b. parchment paper.
   c. a graduated cylinder.
   d. a pipette.

4. A Class III prescription balance is unlocked, temporarily, when the technician
   a. adds weighing papers to the trays.
   b. adds pharmaceutical ingredients to the trays.
   c. moves the balance from one place to another.
   d. checks a measurement.

5. When measuring the amount of liquid in a graduated cylinder, read the level of the liquid at eye level and read the level of the meniscus from the
   a. top.
   b. bottom.
   c. back.
   d. front.

6. When using the geometric dilution method, the most potent ingredient (typically, the one that occurs in the smallest amount) is placed into the mortar _____ of the compounding process.
   a. at the beginning and end (split evenly)
   b. at different stages
   c. at the end
   d. at the beginning

7. The process of using a mortar and pestle to pulverize an ingredient into very fine particles is called
   a. trituration.
   b. levigation.
   c. spatulation.
   d. tumbling.

8. When preparing a nonsterile compound, pharmacy personnel should wash their hands with an antimicrobial soap
   a. before donning a sterile gown, shoe covers, a hair cover, and a face mask.
   b. before and after the preparation of each compound.
   c. before each compounding process.
   d. after each compounding process but only if toxic ingredients are utilized.

9. The punch method is used for filling
   a. capsules.
   b. rapidly dissolving tablets.
   c. suppositories.
   d. caplets.

10. An appropriate auxiliary label for all liquid suspensions is
    a. "Take with food."
    b. "For topical use only; do not swallow."
    c. "Shake well before using."
    d. "May cause drowsiness."

11. Which of the following compounds is an example of a water-in-oil emulsion?
    a. lotion
    b. cream
    c. suppository
    d. ointment

12. The accrediting body for compounding pharmacies is the
    a. PCCA.
    b. PCAB.
    c. FDA.
    d. USP.

13. Which of the following types of bulk ingredients *cannot be used* in a nonsterile compound for humans?
    a. chemical-grade ingredients
    b. USP-grade ingredients
    c. NF-grade ingredients
    d. high-grade, purified products

14. The calculated, beyond-use date for various nonsterile compounds is based on storage conditions and
    a. sterility.
    b. stability.
    c. pharmaceutical elegance.
    d. container packaging.

15. The accepted range for percentage of error for the final weight of a nonsterile compounded preparation is
    a. +/-1%.
    b. +/-2%.
    c. +/-5%.
    d. +/-10%.

Reinforcing Your Learning

To build on your understanding of the topics in this chapter, complete the following enrichment activities.

1. Practice using a Class III prescription balance and a mortar and pestle to prepare the following amounts of ingredients:
   - 2.75 g ground cinnamon
   - 8.5 g sugar
   - 7.5 g ground nutmeg
   - 1.5 g allspice
   - 2.5 g triturated anise seed or clove

   Combine the ingredients and use the punch method to fill capsules with this "pumpkin pie spice" compound. What size of capsule should be used? How many capsules will this fill?

2. Compare and contrast employment in a compounding pharmacy and a retail pharmacy. Examine the following elements: facilities and equipment, skills training, job responsibilities, certifications, personnel attire, patient contact, health insurance processing, and types of calculations.

3. Your pharmacy has several sizes of graduated cylinders available for your use, including 30 mL, 60 mL, 120 mL, 240 mL, 500 mL, and 1000 mL. Select the most appropriate size to measure the following volumes:
   - 45 mL
   - 75 mL
   - 125 mL
   - 450 mL
   - 550 mL
   - 890 mL

4. The art of compounding uses a unique language, and you have been asked to define the following terms to a pharmacy student who is visiting your pharmacy. Keeping your audience in mind, provide a simple, concise definition for the following terms:
   - levigate
   - punch method
   - triturate
   - spatulation
   - diluent
   - tumbling
   - geometric dilution
   - comminution

5. You are to dispense 453 mg of a powder. The original measurement is 453 mg. When you double-check the amount using a more accurate scale, the actual amount is 438 mg. What is the percentage of error of the first measurement?

Thinking on Your Feet

To gain practice in handling challenging situations in the workplace, consider the following real-world scenarios and then use the guiding questions to help you formulate your responses.

1. A patient has arrived at the pharmacy where you work. She has a prescription for a compound that your pharmacy often makes. You are very busy and will not be able to get to this compound for at least one hour. Frustrated from waiting so long at the physician's office, the patient is now frustrated that you cannot prepare her prescription immediately. What do you tell her? Explain why special compounded prescriptions take longer than other prescriptions. Write out your response.

2. A patient presents a prescription for a compounded hormone cream, which is then dispensed in a Topi-CLICK applicator. How would you describe this delivery system to a patient who is unfamiliar with this type of product? Be specific in your response.

3. A dermatologist has prescribed a topical cream for a patient's chronic eczema. You are instructed to weigh 80 g of a cream base for a topical compound. Your error range is +/–3%. What are the least and most acceptable amounts within this error range?

4. A prescription is received at your pharmacy for 8 ounces of Magic Mouthwash containing the ingredients lidocaine, diphenhydramine, Mylanta, and Nystatin (see Figure 8.2). What information is needed to be written down in the compounding log? Calculate the beyond-use date for this Magic Mouthwash compound.

Acquiring Field Knowledge

To expand your knowledge of pharmacy practice, explore the following online activities that focus on research and information retrieval.

1. Go to www.paradigmcollege.net/ pharmpractice5e/hazardousdrugs to access the publication *Secundum Artem*. Read the compounding requirements and procedures for hazardous drugs and compare this pharmacy protocol with the compounding protocol of nonhazardous drugs. Record the similarities and differences and present your findings in a written report.

2. Visit the PCAB website at www .paradigmcollege.net/pharmpractice5e/ accreditation. Click on the "For Pharmacists" tab at the bottom of your screen, and locate four advantages of PCAB accreditation. Then click on the "Find an Accredited Pharmacy" tab at the top of your screen and use the pull-down menu to enter the name of your state. Doing so will pull up a list of the compounding pharmacies accredited in your state. If one accredited pharmacy is nearby, visit the facility and speak with a pharmacist or pharmacy technician about the impact of accreditation on the pharmacy, its personnel, and its customers.

3. Conduct an Internet search for "Magic Mouthwash" prescriptions and list all of the ingredients you can find in the various formulations.

Sampling the Certification Exam

To provide you with practice for the Certification Exam, read the following questions that have been patterned after the test format and then record your answers on a separate sheet of paper. Write your answers as modeled in these examples: 1d; 2c; 3b; etc.

1. The federal standards used to regulate the extemporaneous compounding of nonsterile preparations are provided in
   a. USP Chapter <795>.
   b. USP Chapter <797>.
   c. the Food, Drug, and Cosmetic Act.
   d. the Orphan Drug Act.

2. When preparing 10% hydrocortisone ointment, a nonsterile compound, the compounding log
   a. is not necessary.
   b. only requires the name of the compounded preparation and the name of the compounder.
   c. reflects the compounding process, including ingredients and their amounts, the name of the compounder, and the name of the supervising pharmacist.
   d. is the recipe for how to make a compounded preparation.

3. Disposable molds are commonly used to prepare
   a. hormonal creams.
   b. suppositories.
   c. transdermal patches.
   d. timed-release capsules.

4. What size of a hard-shell capsule is the smallest?
   a. 000
   b. 0
   c. 1
   d. 5

5. Which term describes the guidelines that govern nonsterile compounding?
   a. good manufacturing practices
   b. good compounding practices
   c. acceptable manufacturing practices
   d. good mixing guidelines

6. When using a Class III prescription balance, where do you place the substance being weighed?
   a. on the left pan
   b. on the right pan
   c. on the compounding slab
   d. in the center of the single pan

7. The master control record contains
   a. the original prescription.
   b. the recipe with all the ingredients and mixing directions.
   c. the beyond-use dating of all active and inactive bulk ingredients.
   d. the cost of the final compounded preparation.

8. Training for pharmacy technicians to work in a compounding pharmacy is provided by the
   a. FDA.
   b. USP.
   c. PCAB.
   d. PCCA.

9. Which balance is best to use when measuring large quantities of bulk ingredients?
   a. Class A prescription balance
   b. digital electronic analytical balance
   c. counterbalance
   d. Class III prescription balance

10. Which number powder is most in need of pulverization to finer particles with a porcelain mortar and pestle?
    a. 8
    b. 20
    c. 60
    d. 80

Unit

3

Institutional Pharmacy

Hospital
Pharmacy Practice

9

Learning Objectives

- Describe the classifications and functions of a hospital and its organizational framework.

- Identify the roles of major hospital committees that impact pharmacy.

- Describe the role of the Institutional Review Board in approving investigational drug studies.

- Explain the functions of a hospital pharmacy department.

- Describe the roles and responsibilities of the director of pharmacy, pharmacist, and pharmacy technician in a hospital pharmacy.

- Describe the types of medication orders and the order entry system.

- Understand the unit dose dispensing system and the unit dose cart used in hospital pharmacy practice.

- Identify the advantages and disadvantages of a unit dose vs. a robotic drug distribution system.

- Explain the proper procedure for preparing, labeling, and repackaging of medications.

- Identify the process of medication filling and dispensing in a hospital pharmacy.

- Describe specialty services, such as intravenous admixtures and total parenteral nutrition.

- Discuss the advantages of an automated floor stock system for medication, including narcotics.

- Describe the purpose and advantages of an electronic medication administration record.

- Discuss the role of automation and inventory control in the hospital.

- Understand inventory management of pharmaceuticals, including drug-bidding, ordering, receiving, and storage processes.

- Explain the major role of the Joint Commission in establishing accreditation standards for hospitals.

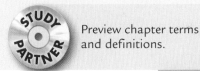

Preview chapter terms and definitions.

Hospital pharmacy practice has a unique organizational structure, set of tasks and responsibilities for personnel, and medication filling and distribution system. Pharmacy technicians who work in this practice setting *must be certified* and have specialized education and training in such areas as oral and parenteral unit-of-use medications, unit dose medications, repackaging, floor stock, narcotic inventory, intravenous (IV) admixtures, and chemotherapy. Even more so than community pharmacy practice, hospital pharmacies rely on the use of automation in medication ordering, filling, distribution, and patient bedside drug administration. Pharmacy personnel must be familiar with these advanced technologies that have made a significant impact on reducing medication errors.

This chapter provides an overview of hospital pharmacy practice, including regulatory controls and standards, and outlines the role and responsibilities of pharmacy technicians in providing safe, effective patient care.

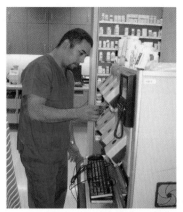

Automation—large and small—is increasingly being adopted in hospital pharmacies to improve efficiency and reduce medication errors.

Hospital Functions and Organization

A hospital is a facility that provides emergency, trauma, surgical, and medical services to a community. Hospitals perform several major functions, as outlined in Table 9.1, and are often classified by a set of defining characteristics, including:

- bed capacity
- patient population (children's hospital vs. geriatric facility)
- type of service (general vs. specialized)
- affiliation (university or teaching hospital vs. a private or nonteaching hospital)
- ownership (state-owned vs. community-owned, government vs. nongovernment)
- length of stay (short-term care [less than 30 days] vs. long-term care [more than 30 days])
- financial status (for-profit vs. not-for-profit)

TABLE 9.1   Functions of a Hospital

The major functions of a hospital include:
- diagnosis and testing (laboratory, X-ray, and so on)
- treatment and therapy, including surgical intervention
- patient processing (including admissions, record keeping, billing, and planning for postdischarge patient care)
- promotion of public health and wellness through programs such as smoking cessation, weight loss, peer support, and so on
- preventive health initiatives such as mammographies, blood pressure readings, and cholesterol screenings
- training healthcare professionals
- conducting research studies that add to the sum of medical knowledge

Organizational Framework

Quite often, hospitals establish an organizational structure that mimics a corporate framework. A president, or chief executive officer (CEO), runs the hospital and reports to a board of directors. The CEO guides the overall direction and long-range planning of a hospital and—depending on bed size and scope of services—may supervise several vice presidents who preside over various departments in the hospital. For example, a

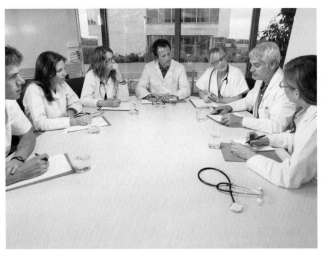

Members of the P&T committee meet primarily to discuss drug formulary changes as well as review medication error reports.

vice president of patient care typically oversees departments such as laboratory, medical records, rehabilitation, respiratory care, social services, and pharmacy. Other vice presidents may oversee medicine, nursing, and finance departments. In larger hospitals, a chief operating officer (COO) may supervise hospital operations and direct departmental vice presidents.

Hospital Committee Structure

An extensive committee structure is needed to support the functions of a hospital. The main committees relating to pharmacy include the Pharmacy and Therapeutics (P&T) Committee, the Institutional Review Board (IRB), and the Infection Control Committee. (The important role of the Infection Control Committee is discussed in Chapter 10.)

Pharmacy and Therapeutics Committee In the hospital setting, the **Pharmacy and Therapeutics (P&T) Committee** meets on a monthly or quarterly basis to review medication guidelines and issues pertinent to patient care. The committee's responsibilities include:

- reviewing, approving, and revising the hospital's drug formulary
- maintaining the drug use policies of the hospital
- reviewing studies on the appropriate use of drugs within the hospital
- studying investigational drugs for hospital use
- monitoring medication error reports (including computerized adverse drug event monitoring)

The P&T Committee is typically composed of several members of the medical staff, as well as representatives from the hospital and nursing administration. The director of pharmacy and a drug information pharmacist often represent the pharmacy department on the P&T Committee. The director of pharmacy often acts as the secretary and is responsible for recording and disseminating the minutes of the meeting; the drug information pharmacist is responsible for researching and making unbiased drug formulary recommendations to the committee. A pharmacy technician may also represent the pharmacy department on this committee by lending support to the data collection role and audits of the drug information pharmacist.

Drug Formulary As mentioned earlier, the P&T Committee reviews, approves, and revises the hospital's **drug formulary**, or an accepted list of approved drugs used in that hospital. Most hospitals have adopted a formulary system based on providing the most effective medications while limiting patient and hospital costs. Drug formularies do not exist in the community pharmacy setting with the exception of some managed care organizations such as Kaiser Permanente.

If a medical staff member wants the P&T Committee to consider a new drug to be added to the hospital's drug formulary, then he or she must complete and submit an extensive medication application form. The drug information pharmacist then reviews this initial information and completes an independent search of the medical literature. The cost, advantages, and disadvantages of the new drug are then compared with an existing formulary drug, and these findings are presented to the entire committee for their consideration.

At times, formulary approval may be restricted to a specific medical service. For example, a new, high-cost antibiotic with limited indications and high resistance patterns may be restricted to the Infectious Disease Service. A physician not on this service is prohibited from writing a prescription for this new antibiotic (and the pharmacy cannot fill this medication order) unless the order is approved and signed or co-signed by an infectious disease physician.

If a physician writes a new medication order for a *nonformulary drug*—or a drug that is *not* on the approved list—then he or she may need to justify to the chairperson of the P&T Committee or to an attending physician the necessity of such a drug for this particular patient.

Medication Error Reports The P&T Committee reviews all medication error reports that are relayed from the drug information center of the hospital pharmacy. (For more information on this center, refer to the section titled "Hospital Pharmacy Department.") The drug information center collects and analyzes reports from pharmacy, nursing, and medicine. These adverse drug events are easily tabulated through the use of pharmacy automation, such as electronic health records. When the committee reviews a medication error report, the focus is not to fix blame, but to identify and correct the system's problem so that the error does not recur.

Institutional Review Board The **Institutional Review Board (IRB)**—also known as the Human Use Committee—typically meets on a monthly basis to review the use of investigational drugs or procedures in the hospital setting and to provide appropriate safeguards for its patient population. An **investigational drug** is defined as a drug (or an indication for an approved drug) that is being used in clinical trials and has not yet been approved by the Food and Drug Administration (FDA) in the general population. This committee consists of representatives from medicine, pharmacy, nursing, and hospital administration, as well as a consumer member.

Clinical Research Investigational Study Any clinical research investigational study requires approval by the IRB before enrollment can begin. The investigator usually submits an application outlining the goals of the study and the participating patient population, including the number of subjects, their ages, and their healthcare status (i.e., patients vs. healthy volunteers). The investigator must also submit an **informed consent**, or a document written about the study in terms that are understandable to laypersons. The informed consent for the study must specify the risks vs. the benefits, reimbursement (if any), and follow-up responsibilities and procedures in case of an adverse event. Both the investigator and the IRB must meet federal and state regulations that apply to clinical research investigational study.

The IRB protects the patient by ensuring both adequate knowledge of the risks of the study and confidentiality of medical information. Adverse events must be reported to the IRB, which reevaluates the approval of the study if necessary. Special procedures exist for neonates, pediatric patients, underage women of childbearing age, and patients with mental health problems. The IRB protects patient confidentiality for participation in investigational studies; access to patient-specific medical information must be stated explicitly in the application and protocol. Most commonly, patients are assigned a subject number (separate from their hospital number) to maintain anonymity. Investigational data may be collected, collated, and sent outside the hospital to a government agency or private sponsor; however, the individual patient's identity and medical data must remain protected. Patient confidentiality is discussed in more detail in Chapter 13.

Hospital Pharmacy Department

A hospital pharmacy department occupies a central location that is readily accessible to the emergency room and to elevators to the patient care units and surgical

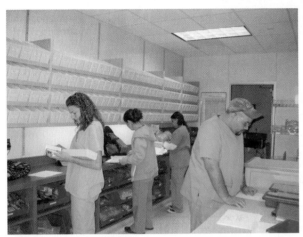

Hospital pharmacy technicians often work at multiple workstations.

suites. The pharmacy is also in close proximity to a central storage area for bulk items such as boxes of IV solutions and IV sets. The interior layout typically has several designated areas, including unit dose cart filling, repackaging, narcotic and investigational drug storage, and preparation of sterile products. Aside from the typical pharmacy equipment, hospital pharmacies may also have unit dose carts for each patient care unit, repackaging equipment, IV infusion pumps, and laminar airflow cabinets for the safe preparation of compounded sterile preparations and chemotherapy products.

Specialized Services

A large community or university hospital's on-site pharmacy department is typically staffed 24 hours a day, 7 days a week and provides a number of specialized services. These services encompass medication preparation and delivery (including chemotherapy and antibiotics), IV additive programs such as total parenteral nutrition (TPN), investigational drug storage and control, and a drug information center. The drug information center in the pharmacy is often responsible for investigating, evaluating, and recording medication errors and adverse drug reactions and reporting the results to the P&T committee.

Unlike a community pharmacy, a hospital pharmacy setting is less chaotic. Whereas community pharmacy staff members have quite a bit of external communication (patients at the counter and drive-thru window; phone calls from patients, healthcare personnel, and insurance companies; cashiering), hospital pharmacy personnel have minimal interaction with the public and communicate mainly with physicians, nurses, and other staff members. There are few phone calls (most communications are transmitted via computer) and no prescription insurance issues.

Hospital Pharmacy Personnel

A hospital pharmacy staff is typically composed of a director of pharmacy, additional associate or assistant directors of pharmacy (for larger hospitals), pharmacists, and pharmacy technicians. A large city hospital usually staffs 10 or more pharmacists and pharmacy technicians per day shift. In addition, larger hospitals may have both pregraduate

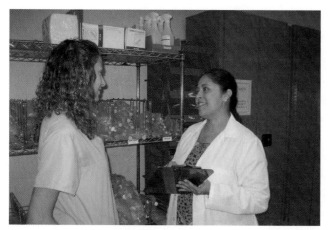

The director of pharmacy is responsible for overseeing the drug distribution and specialized services within the hospital.

pharmacy interns and postgraduate residents. In a small rural hospital, one or two full-time pharmacists and technicians, plus part-time pharmacists, may make up the entire pharmacy staff. No matter the size of the staff, the overall roles and responsibilities of hospital pharmacy personnel remain the same.

Director of Pharmacy

Appointed by hospital administrators, the **director of pharmacy** is the pharmacist-in-charge who oversees the day-to-day operations of the hospital pharmacy department. The director's office is located within the pharmacy for frequent contact with pharmacists and pharmacy technicians. This individual assumes many responsibilities such as managing the pharmacy budget; hiring, evaluating, and firing personnel; developing a strategic vision (long-term planning); complying with all federal and state regulations and laws; and establishing policies and procedures to conform with hospital policies and accreditation standards. The director of pharmacy generally reports to a vice president for professional or patient care services (or similar title) and works closely with the director of nursing and the chief of staff in medicine to provide high-quality patient care.

Key Responsibilities The director of pharmacy has a number of key responsibilities that affect the overall operation of the hospital pharmacy, including the establishment of pharmacy services, budget, and the pharmacy's Policy & Procedure (P&P) manual.

Determining Pharmacy Services The director determines the level and scope of pharmacy services, including:

- type of medication distribution systems
  - unit dose cart exchange for medication delivery vs. floor stock system
  - frequency of unit dose cart exchanges (twice daily, daily, or less often)
  - use of automated robotic dispensing system
  - centralized vs. decentralized narcotic inventory control system
  - presence of an IV admixture program including preparation of hazardous agents such as cancer chemotherapy drugs
  - in-house TPN or nutrition service vs. off-site preparation or outsourcing
- service availability (24 hours a day, 7 days a week—or less)
- source of pharmaceutical inventory, including the process of bids, contracts, and purchase orders
- pharmacy protocol in providing medications and supplies in emergency codes
- instructional support for pharmacy residents and interns
- provision of specialty services
  - satellite or small pharmacies located on a patient care unit within the hospital
  - decentralized pharmacists
  - clinical pharmacists making rounds with physicians and monitoring patients
  - consultation service for pharmacokinetics or individual patient dosing
  - drug information center or service staffed by pharmacy personnel
  - presence or absence of a drug formulary
  - outpatient or discharge pharmacy service vs. outsourcing space to a retail pharmacy

Several of these pharmacy services, including medication distribution systems and pharmaceutical inventory, are discussed more in depth later in this chapter.

Planning and Monitoring the Budget The director of pharmacy is responsible for submitting a budget and monitoring that approved budget. A vast majority of the budget is for the purchase of pharmaceuticals; the director has little or no control over this portion of the budget. Drug budgets, in particular, can be difficult to predict, especially one to two years in advance. Newer, more expensive drugs or biotechnology may come into the marketplace to replace lower-cost alternatives, or a new Transplant Service may be implemented in the hospital, requiring the use of expensive immuno-suppressive drugs. Consequently, the budgetary impacts of new drugs and hospital services must be continually assessed by the director of pharmacy.

Budgetary restrictions on services may result in the outsourcing of distribution or clinical services. For example, a smaller hospital pharmacy may contract with an IV admixture or nutrition service outside the hospital to formulate and deliver products to the hospital. A hospital may also contract with a local community pharmacy to lease space and provide outpatient pharmacy services in the hospital. In any case, safety and quality of care must never be compromised; all state and federal guidelines and accreditation standards must be followed even if some pharmacy services are outsourced to others.

The budget also affects the staffing of the hospital pharmacy. The director of pharmacy bases staffing needs on projected census (hospital bed occupancy) as well as hours of operation and scope of services. All personnel must pass criminal background checks before hiring due to access to pharmaceuticals—in particular, narcotics. Other ancillary personnel that the director may hire include administrative support staff, part-time professional staff, and pharmacy interns and residents. The hospital's human resources department generally advertises for personnel positions and screens candidates; however, the director of pharmacy makes the final decision when pharmacy staff is hired.

Developing the Policy & Procedure Manual The director of pharmacy oversees the development of the hospital pharmacy's **Policy & Procedure (P&P) manual**. A P&P manual is a written, step-by-step set of instructions for pharmacists and technicians alike on all operations within the pharmacy department. These policies and procedures are written in accordance with state and federal laws. The manual is updated frequently and mandated for institutional accreditation. All pharmacy personnel are required to follow these outlined policies and procedures. Technician supervisors may be involved in developing and updating P&P items that are directly related to pharmacy technicians.

Hospital Pharmacist

In Chapter 6, you learned the roles and responsibilities of pharmacists in general, as well as the specific functions of a pharmacist in the community pharmacy setting. Pharmacists who work in hospital practice share several of these functions but also have a unique set of responsibilities that cater to the needs of a different patient population. Hospital pharmacists must have an extensive knowledge of medications to consult with physicians, interns, residents, and nurses. For that reason, pharmacy personnel must keep up-to-date on drugs moving into and out of the market, including high-potency sterile drugs that are rarely, if ever, dispensed in a community pharmacy. In addition, hospital pharmacists must have the skills necessary to compound sterile products for extremely ill patients and to prepare (and document) emergency medications that are needed in "code blues."

Many larger hospital pharmacies also have specialty trained clinical pharmacists on staff in such areas as internal medicine, pediatrics, surgery, nutrition, and pharmacokinetics. These pharmacists may assist prescribers in ordering TPN solutions or in dosing high-risk medications. Clinical pharmacists also work closely with the medical and nursing staff to resolve medication issues and improve the quality and safety of patient care.

Hospital pharmacists typically wear name tags with their white lab coats so that they are easily recognizable in the hospital pharmacy setting.

Major Responsibilities The responsibilities of a hospital pharmacist include:

- entering medication orders into the computer
- assisting in medication cart fills and the preparation of sterile products
- closely monitoring narcotic drug usage on each patient care unit
- ordering necessary pharmaceuticals, products, and supplies
- checking all pharmacy technician work including cart fills, repackaging, and sterile products
- providing necessary drug information to physicians and nurses
- monitoring and maintaining automated systems in the pharmacy and patient care units
- assisting in cardiopulmonary resuscitation (CPR) codes
- dispensing any investigational drugs and completing the necessary documentation
- completing and documenting detailed medication histories on all newly admitted patients
- providing medication counseling for patients discharged from the hospital
- investigating all medication error reports
- representing the pharmacy department on select hospital committees

Hospital Pharmacy Technician

Since the 1960s, the role and responsibilities of the pharmacy technician in the hospital practice setting have dramatically expanded. Technicians now play a key role in preparing and delivering the right drug at the right dose by the right route to the right patient at the right time. Just as in the community pharmacy setting, all work must be checked and verified by the pharmacist.

Technicians who work in hospital practice typically wear scrubs in a designated color. This attire protocol has been implemented by many hospitals in response to a movement to quickly identify hospital personnel in the event of an emergency. Wearing similarly colored scrubs also helps to identify pharmacy technicians who deliver medications to patient care units. For those technicians preparing sterile or potentially toxic products, additional protective hospital garb is required to maintain the sterility of the products and to protect pharmacy personnel from exposure to toxic chemicals. (Detailed information on this protective garb is presented in Chapters 10 and 11.) Lastly, hospital pharmacy technicians in most states must wear a name tag.

Key Responsibilities To maintain flexibility in scheduling, each technician is trained to perform all major functions within the pharmacy department. To accomplish this training, technicians rotate through these functions, which include filling the unit dose cart, stocking the medication dispensing units, preparing IV admixtures in a clean room environment, monitoring inventory and narcotic control in both the

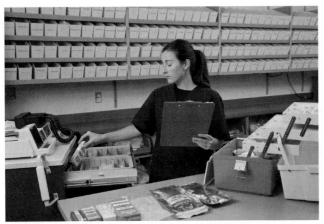
The pharmacy technician is responsible for replacing floor stock as well as filling medications for the unit dose cart.

pharmacy and on the nursing unit, and stocking the crash cart. These specific responsibilities are discussed in detail later in this chapter.

Filling the Unit Dose Cart Pharmacy technicians are responsible for filling the unit dose cart—a cart that supplies oral medications to the nursing units. This procedure is done after pharmacist verification of the medication orders for each patient. In hospital pharmacy practice, medication orders replace the prescriptions that are used in community pharmacy. (For more on medication orders, see the section titled "Hospital Medication Orders and Order Entry" later in this chapter.) Oral medications are commonly dispensed as an individualized unit dose in a patient-specific drawer of a unit dose cart that is delivered to the nursing unit. Unlike a 30-day or 90-day supply of medication dispensed in the community pharmacy, a hospital pharmacy typically dispenses enough medication for a 12- to 72-hour window.

If a unit dose is not commercially available, the technician may be involved in a nonsterile compounding or repackaging operation. Many pharmacies are adopting robotic technology to provide efficient work flow and eliminate errors in medication cart filling.

Stocking the Medication Dispensing Units Another responsibility of pharmacy technicians is restocking the automated locked dispensing units that are located on each nursing unit. The technician is often responsible for checking for expired drugs, adjusting inventory levels, and transporting necessary medications (IV solutions, narcotics, prn drugs, etc.) to the nursing unit. The technician must ensure that all medications are labeled and stored properly, including refrigerated items.

Preparing IV Admixtures The pharmacy technician's involvement in the aseptic preparation of parenteral products, including TPN and hazardous drugs, is a major difference from community pharmacy practice. To perform these sterile compounding procedures, technicians must comply with specific United States Pharmacopeia (USP) Chapter <797> standards, including donning protective garb; working in a clean room environment; adhering to aseptic technique protocol during product preparation, transfer, and cleanup; monitoring environmental quality control; and following proper storage guidelines for compounded preparations. (For more information on this segment of hospital pharmacy practice, refer to two subsequent chapters: Chapter 10, "Infection Control," which discusses the importance and use of aseptic technique, and Chapter 11, "Compounding Sterile Products and Hazardous Drugs," which discusses the techniques and procedures used in the preparation of parenteral medications and the proper handling and disposal of hazardous agents.)

Monitoring Inventory and Narcotic Control Inventory control in the pharmacy is an important task for the pharmacy technician. The ordering, receiving, and proper storage of medications—including narcotics and investigational drugs—are critical to the operations of the pharmacy and to safe patient care.

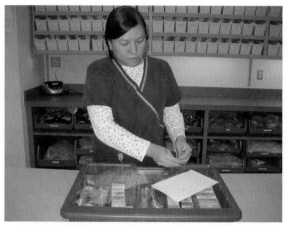

Filling the Crash Cart Restocking the drug **crash cart**, a mobile cart that holds necessary drugs for an emergency code such as a "Code Blue," is typically a task delegated to technicians in a hospital pharmacy department. This cart may be housed in the pharmacy, on a nursing unit, or in the emergency department.

The pharmacy technician checks expiration dating and replaces drug stock in the hospital's many crash carts.

Training and Certification The complex environment of a hospital pharmacy department requires highly trained pharmacy technicians, and the learning curve for these technicians may be three months or longer to develop the necessary skills for this position. These technicians often specialize in one area such as unit dose, robotics, floor stock, IV admixtures, TPN or chemotherapy preparation, inventory control, or staff training and development. In larger hospitals, there may be different grade levels and specialization within the pharmacy depending on skills and experience. For example, in some hospital pharmacies, a senior pharmacy technician may have additional administrative responsibilities and may supervise other technicians in their daily responsibilities.

All technicians working in a hospital pharmacy must also be certified. In fact, many hospitals will only hire certified technicians with hospital experience. Those technicians who specialize in IV admixture services require additional certification and training. Staff development and training in all areas is important and must be documented with annual updates. In addition to on-the-job training, pharmacy technicians working in a hospital practice setting must study and carefully follow their pharmacy's P&P manual.

Inventory Management

As mentioned earlier, one key responsibility of the pharmacy technician is managing inventory. Up to 70% of the budget of a hospital pharmacy department is spent on pharmaceuticals. Budgetary planning and an accurate inventory tracking system are extremely important responsibilities of the pharmacy staff. To that end, many hospital pharmacies have assigned inventory management to a senior pharmacy technician. That individual assumes the position of a buyer and is therefore responsible for preparing contracts and bids, ordering pharmaceuticals, and receiving shipments of these ordered items. These technician duties are performed under the supervision of the director of pharmacy.

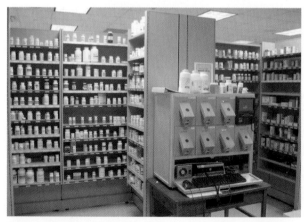

Drug inventory—including oral drugs, injectables, and IV fluids—comprise a majority of the department budget and must be carefully monitored.

Automation greatly assists the pharmacy department in meeting and adjusting a budgetary goal. In addition to pharmaceuticals, the budget often includes IV solutions, sets, and pumps, as well as various other medical supplies. Storage space in a hospital pharmacy is often limited, so having sufficient inventory without shortages is important to providing good patient care. Similar to the community pharmacy, hospital pharmacy personnel usually perform a physical inventory of their drugs annually.

Bidding and Purchasing of Pharmaceuticals

Pharmacists must ensure that their patients receive the highest quality pharmaceuticals at the lowest cost. In many large hospitals, the pharmacist may develop specific criteria that serve as the basis for a confidential, sealed bid process, which includes prime vendor wholesalers and manufacturers of drugs and IV solutions.

Drug-Bidding Process The inventory control technician may be responsible for collecting information necessary for the drug-bidding process. For example, the technician may be asked to estimate the annual usage for the antibiotic Zosyn in its many dose formulations or to estimate the number of cases of dextrose 5% in water (D_5W) that may be used next year. An accurate estimation of the number of units of formulary drugs for the next calendar or fiscal year must be determined.

The drug-bidding process is competitive, especially in large hospitals where hundreds of thousands of units of some products may be used each year. Most accepted bids "lock in" the medication cost for one year. Changing manufacturers of generic medications (or switching from brand name drugs to generics) too often may cause confusion for the pharmacist, nurse, and physician because the color, shape, or packaging may differ from that of previously stocked medications. If the hospital operates an outpatient community pharmacy, many states require a separate bidding process and a separate physical inventory.

The bid contract on IV solutions may be for a longer period (typically, five years) because switching IV solutions and sets requires the re-education of nursing personnel to these changes, and completing this task on a yearly basis is neither feasible nor cost-effective. Plus, constant fluctuation of IV solutions and equipment increases the risk of medication administration errors.

Ordering of Pharmaceuticals

Once bids and purchasing contracts are finalized, an important responsibility of the inventory control technician is ordering pharmaceuticals. Most hospital pharmacies order their pharmaceuticals from a prime vendor wholesaler (such as McKesson Provider Technologies or Cardinal Health) and their IV solutions and administration sets directly from a medical device company (such as Baxter or Hospira). Automation from software provided by the wholesalers— as well as internal automation used by the hospital and pharmacy department—makes inventory management more accurate and less costly.

The pharmacy technician may use a handheld bar-code scanner to manage inventory in the pharmacy.

Nonformulary Drugs Occasionally, a nonformulary drug must be purchased from a wholesaler (or community pharmacy) if prescribed and approved for use within the hospital. Depending on hospital policy, the patient receiving the medication may be charged by the hospital for the bulk purchase (for example, a quantity of 100 tablets or capsules). That nonformulary drug may be repackaged into a unit dose or placed at the patient's bedside per the physician's orders. At discharge, any remaining medication would then be returned to the patient.

Drugs Borrowed from Other Facilities At times, a hospital pharmacy may need to borrow a medication from another corporate member hospital, a community hospital, or a community pharmacy. In that situation, the hospital's P&P manual should outline the process, and the borrowed drug should be returned when the next shipment is received from the wholesaler. The reconciliation of each facility's inventory is settled at the end of the month. Careful documentation with proper signatures is needed in the rare event that controlled substances are borrowed between institutions to provide a paper audit trail.

Safety Note

Pharmacy refrigerators are designated for medication storage. No food items are allowed to be stored alongside these medications.

Receiving and Storage of Drug Inventory

Once the drugs ordered from the wholesaler are received, the order must be checked against the invoice of the wholesaler or pharmaceutical manufacturer. Any discrepancies in the order must then be resolved. The inventory control technician should inspect the order for completeness as well as for any potentially damaged goods. If items are missing or damaged, the technician should not accept the receipt of these items. Pharmaceuticals should be properly stored on inventory shelves or placed in the pharmacy refrigerator or freezer. Storage guidelines for pharmaceuticals can be found in the attached product package inserts or by consulting pharmaceutical references such as the *American Hospital Formulary Service* or the *Physicians' Desk Reference (PDR)*.

Special Handling of Certain Pharmaceuticals

Two types of pharmaceuticals require special consideration in inventory control: controlled substances and investigational drugs.

Controlled Substances The Controlled Substances Act (CSA) defines ordering inventory, filing, and record-keeping requirements for controlled substances. As in the community pharmacy, the purchase of Schedule II controlled substances must be authorized by a pharmacist and executed on the Drug Enforcement Administration (DEA) 222 form as discussed in Chapter 7. Hospital pharmacy personnel must also conduct a physical inventory of Schedule II substances every two years, per DEA regulations. Any destruction of Schedule II drugs must be witnessed and documented in the pharmacy department records.

Investigational Drugs As discussed earlier in the chapter, all investigational drug studies must be approved by the IRB, or the Human Use Committee. Investigational drugs require special ordering, handling, and record-keeping procedures by the pharmacy technician. These drugs must be maintained in a secure and separate area

Schedule II drugs and investigational drugs must be stored in a locked cabinet, safe, or vault with a transparent paper trail.

of the pharmacy until a valid written medication order is received from the primary physician investigator. In most of these research studies, the drug is not labeled with a name or strength but is packaged and labeled with a lot number and expiration date. If an adverse reaction occurs, it must be reported by the nurse or pharmacist to the primary physician investigator. Depending on the severity of the reaction, the investigational drug may need to be "unblinded" and reported to the IRB.

Performing Daily Inventory Responsibilities

Whereas the inventory control technician is primarily responsible for purchasing and ordering medications, all pharmacy technicians assist in receiving and storing the ordered items from the wholesaler. Medications must be stored under proper conditions on designated shelves, in the refrigerator, or in the freezer. The temperatures of refrigerators and freezers in the centralized pharmacy and the nursing units must be checked (in degrees centigrade) and documented per hospital policy. Plastic bags of IV solutions must be removed from boxes and wiped down before placement in the IV storage area to keep the room clean and free of dust. Technicians should also check all special orders (medications not routinely stocked in the pharmacy) on a daily basis for out-of-stocks in case a patient needs a newly received medication from the wholesaler.

Rotating Inventory As in the community pharmacy, stock on the shelves must be rotated so that the most recent inventory is not used first. In the pharmacy and in the patient care units, all technicians should periodically document inspections for expired drugs, including opened multi-dose vials of sterile water. Automation may alert the technician to lot numbers of drugs that will soon be out-of-date. Inventory turnover is rapid and expired drugs rarely are found.

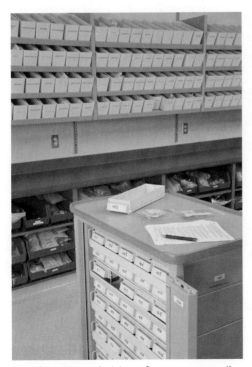

The pharmacy technician often must reconcile why medications were returned in the unit dose cart and not administered to the patient.

Processing the Returned Unit Dose Cart When the unit dose cart is returned to the pharmacy, all patient cassette drawers are checked by the technician and emptied. Any medications returned in the unit dose cassette drawer must be credited back to the patient; this includes both scheduled and *prn* medications. This can be a labor-intensive process. Unit dose medications may not be administered to the patient for a variety of reasons. For example, a patient may be undergoing a procedure such as an X-ray at the time medication is scheduled, cannot take oral medications before surgery by the physician's order (NPO or nothing by mouth), or may have become nauseous, so an oral medication was changed to an injectable or a suppository dosage form.

Although a dose may have been skipped intentionally, it may also have been missed accidentally and not administered by the nurse. Some pharmacy departments use the medications remaining in the cart's patient cassette drawer after an exchange as a quality assurance tool: Remaining medications may prompt an investigation into why the medications were missed. The pharmacy technician plays a crucial role in bringing missed doses of scheduled drugs such as antibiotics to the attention of the pharmacist. He or she may also be asked to conduct an investigation as to why the medication dose was not given to a patient.

Restocking Automated Equipment A perpetual inventory is maintained for most medications (especially all controlled, investigational, and expensive drugs) in the computerized inventory database. A designated technician may be assigned to restock or "feed the robot" with a replacement inventory of frequently used medications. Another technician may be responsible for restocking the automated medication dispensing system (AMDS) in each nursing unit and checking or adjusting inventory levels as needed. Though medications are stored on the nursing units, the Joint Commission holds the pharmacy department accountable for monitoring the safety, security, and inventory of the AMDS.

Patient care units send reports, sometimes called out-of-stock reports, to the hospital pharmacy throughout the day requesting selected drug inventory to be replaced. Some automated systems allow centralized access of inventory levels by a computer in the pharmacy. These automated systems optimize inventory control by minimizing costs and out-of-stock items.

Transporting and Tracking of Narcotics Pharmacy technicians are often responsible for transporting narcotics to the nursing units after the shipment order has been received and the pharmacist has adjusted the inventory. Depending on hospital policy, the exchange of narcotics from the pharmacy technician to a nursing staff member requires documentation, including the names of both parties and the narcotics being delivered. Automation has simplified the narcotic inventory and tracking records without increasing the risk of drug diversion.

Pharmacy technicians are also responsible for reporting to the pharmacist any unusual increases in the use of controlled substances on any nursing unit. A pharmacist may also be responsible for checking and reconciling the narcotic inventory records, especially if discrepancies cannot be resolved; discrepancies must be immediately resolved with the nurse supervisor by the end of the nursing shift.

The pharmacy technician is responsible for delivering narcotics to each nursing unit; the inventory must be checked and signed off by the nursing supervisor.

Checking for Drug Recalls Another inventory responsibility of technicians is the retrieval of any medications that are subject to FDA or drug manufacturer recall. This recall notice may come from the wholesaler or from a letter sent to the director of pharmacy. To perform a drug recall, the technician compares the lot number of the drug in the recall notice or letter with the inventory in pharmacy storage. Typically, a form indicating drug, strength, amount, and lot number is completed, signed, and returned to the wholesaler (or drug manufacturer) with the drugs for credit. Returns of Schedule II drugs are rare and must be recorded on a special DEA 106 form by the pharmacist.

Hospital Medication Orders and Order Entry

A prescriber's order for medication for a patient arrives at the hospital pharmacy in a different format than the prescription form that is commonly seen in the community pharmacy setting. This form is called a medication order, and it is typically sent to the central hospital pharmacy via an electronic transmission (computerized prescriber order entry). However, the medication order may also be delivered to the pharmacy via a personal delivery, fax, phone order, or a pneumatic tube system from a nursing unit.

Medication Order

As mentioned earlier, a prescription that arrives in a hospital pharmacy is in the form of a **medication order**. Medication orders are commonly written in the patient's

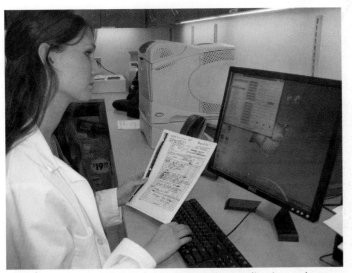
Pharmacists often are responsible for entering medication orders into the computer database in a hospital pharmacy.

medical chart or record, which is a legal document that contains the patient's demographics and room number as well as all orders written by the medical staff. These orders include medications, nursing assessments (vital signs, nursing notes, and medication administration times), laboratory and radiology results, and consultations from nutritionists and other specialists. Unlike a community pharmacy, most medication orders are entered into the computer by the hospital pharmacist.

Types of Medication Orders There are several kinds of medication orders, including an admitting order, a stat order, a daily or continuation order, a standing order, and a discharge order. These orders are discussed below.

Admitting Order An **admitting order** is written by the physician upon patient admission to a hospital. The order may be written in the emergency department or in a patient's room. This type of medication order may contain drugs prescribed and taken before admission and suspected diagnoses; requests for lab tests or radiology exams; instructions for the nursing staff; medication orders, including the notation of drug allergies; and the patient's dietary requirements (see Figure 9.1 on the following page). An admitting order also contains a list of the medications, including dosages and dosing intervals, that the patient has been taking at home. These medications, called *home medications* or *meds*, may be continued by the physician by writing "Continue home meds" on the order. The pharmacy will then dispense new prescriptions for these medications for hospital administration. If these prescribed medications are approved nonformulary drugs, the medications may be assigned over to the pharmacy for use in the cart fill or may be given to the patient to keep at the bedside for self-administration, depending on hospital policy. For the latter, the patient's physician must write an order for "Bedside medications," which alerts nursing and pharmacy personnel to this directive. At discharge, any remaining "at bedside" medications are returned to the patient. All formulary and nonformulary controlled drugs must be sent to the pharmacy and individually dispensed per cart fill and accounted for in the nursing administration record.

FIGURE 9.1
Admitting
Order

DATE	HOUR	PHYSICIAN'S ORDERS
9-1-201X		Admit to: Dr. Chung
		Diagnosis:
		1. lower abdominal pain with history of diverticulitis
		2. asthma
		3. chronic back pain
		4. anxiety
		Condition: fair
		Vitals: per routine
		Labs: chem 12, electrolytes, ABG
		X-ray: lungs
		Allergies: codeine, Floxin, Biaxin, PCN, Ceclor, doxycycline
		Diet: clear liquids, low salt, 1800 kcal/day
		IVFs: NS @ 125 mL per hour
		Meds: Phenergan 25 mg IV q6 h prn nausea/vomiting
		Levaquin 500 mg IV daily
		Levsin 0.125 mg po tid
		zolpidem 10 mg po hs prn sleep
		carisoprodol 350 mg po tid prn muscle spasm
		Advair 250/50 1 puff bid
		montelukast 10 mg po daily
		Lorcet 10/500 po bid
		famotidine 40 mg po bid
		albuterol 0.083% 1 unit via nebulizer q6 h prn
		Nasonex 2 sprays in each nostril daily
		sertraline 100 mg 2 tabs po daily

Stat Order A **stat order** is an emergency order that is typically called in or sent electronically to the pharmacy. This type of order must receive priority attention and, consequently, must be immediately input into the pharmacy database and filled. After a final verification from the pharmacist, the medication is then sent to the patient care unit by the pharmacist or technician for patient administration.

Daily and Continuation Orders A **daily order** is a new medication order written daily by a physician after every patient examination. Most hospitals have a policy that a physician must review, approve, and rewrite all daily medication orders at least weekly; this is called a *continuation order*. Continuation orders are also written for those patients that transfer from one unit of the hospital to another. Continuation medication orders for antibiotics may need to be checked and renewed on a more frequent basis per hospital policy.

Standing Order A **standing order** is a medication order in which the same set of medications and treatments applies for each patient who receives a similar treatment or surgery. The physician may then sign this preprinted order or slightly modify the standing order by adding or deleting items before signing the form. Postoperative (postop) orders written after surgery are often examples of standing orders.

Discharge Order A **discharge order** is an order that provides take-home instructions for a patient who is being discharged from the hospital. This order includes all prescribed medications and dosages. Prescriptions are commonly written for a seven-day or one-month period until the patient's follow-up visit with his or her primary care physician or specialist.

Inputting of Hospital Medication Orders

Hospital pharmacy personnel may receive copies of medication orders for individual patients written by their physicians or transmitted via computerized prescriber instructions (see section below titled "Computerized Prescriber Order Entry"). Regardless of being handwritten or computer-generated, these hospital orders may include the individual patient's diagnosis, allergies, diet, activity level, vital signs, requested radiology images and lab tests, and medications (both routine scheduled and *prn* oral drugs as well as parenteral medications).

The pharmacist or experienced pharmacy technician must review all written hospital orders to determine which ones are for medications that must be input into the pharmacy computer database. The pharmacist verifies the accuracy of the transcription with the original physician medication order before any medication is sent to the patient care unit, or released for nurse administration on the unit.

Computerized Prescriber Order Entry As with other areas of the healthcare system, such as e-prescribing in the community pharmacy setting, the use of automation and electronic health records (EHRs) is becoming increasingly commonplace in hospitals of all sizes. EHRs are interactive and allow multiple healthcare providers to share patient information. To that end, patient management software, called **computerized prescriber order entry (CPOE)**, is being acquired in hospitals for the electronic entry of prescriber instructions for several departments, such as laboratory, radiology, physical therapy, dietary, and pharmacy. For the latter department, these instructions include patient medication orders. Using CPOE software, a key feature of an EHR, provides the following benefits to members of the healthcare team:

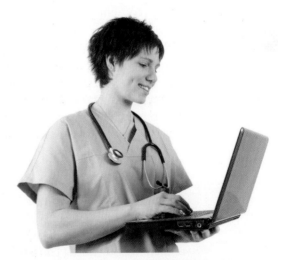

The use of electronic health records gives healthcare practitioners immediate access to patients' medical records and allows for coordination of patient care.

- immediate access to patients' medical records
- streamlined workflow processes
- improved documentation
- enhanced coordination of patient care
- clear communication with other healthcare personnel

Currently, more than 25% of hospitals have adopted CPOE to maintain their patients' health records, and the end result has been improved patient care and safety. Adoption has been delayed in many facilities due to high costs for initial implementation and maintenance, adequate time and costs for training staff, resistance by prescribers to embrace change, and the complexities of converting existing department-specific software to standardized, hospital-wide software. To accelerate the CPOE adoption process, the American Recovery and Reinvestment Act (ARRA) of 2009, a government stimulus program, included provisions and financial incentives for the adoption of health information technology (i.e., EHRs) in hospitals.

Pharmacy Department and CPOE For the pharmacy department in particular, CPOE adoption provides efficient medication order completion (orders sent directly to the pharmacy), allows for prescriber order entry from off-hospital sites, and results in a simplification of inventory ordering and the posting of patient hospital charges.

More importantly, the implementation of CPOE has led to dramatic improvements in medication safety. Using this software program avoids any transcription errors that may result from the interpretation of a prescriber's handwriting (the number one preventable error). In addition, the built-in features of the program provide safeguards to the medication filling and dispensing process. These safeguards include error-checking functions to identify duplicate drugs, incorrect doses, and laboratory test results that may impact choice of drug or dose. All of these associated benefits have helped to reduce the incidence of medication errors. In fact, for those hospitals that have implemented CPOE, preliminary studies have demonstrated that the medication error rate has decreased 80% in some facilities. In addition, CPOE may prevent as many as 3 million medication errors a year, which cost the healthcare system an estimated $81 billion. In combination with the use of state-of-the-art automation technologies such as robotic and floor stock dispensing systems and electronic medication administration records (eMARs), the possibility of medication errors can be virtually eliminated.

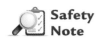

Safety Note

All computerized software, including CPOE, EHRs, and eMARS, must protect patient privacy.

Hospital Pharmacy Inpatient Drug Distribution Systems

Hospitals use an **inpatient drug distribution system** to dispense medications to patients. In this system, a 12- to 72-hour supply of individual doses of medication is prepackaged or specially prepared and sent to each patient care unit. These medication doses are then administered by the nurses on that unit. The inpatient drug distribution system in many hospital pharmacies is composed of unit dose, IV admixture, and TPN services. Pharmacy technicians are actively involved in these pharmacy services as well as in monitoring and transporting the inventory of floor stock drugs and narcotics sent to each nursing unit. (The latter two tasks will be discussed later in the chapter.)

Most medications in the hospital pharmacy are prepared in a "unit of use" format—that is, an individually prepared drug and dose that is labeled for a specific patient. To that end, many hospital pharmacies are moving toward the use of robotics to assist in the accurate filling of medication orders and to computerized compounders to prepare TPN solutions. Individual medication orders for IV admixtures are prepared by specially trained and certified pharmacy technicians in a sterile, clean room environment.

Unit Dose Dispensing System

Beginning in the early 1960s, hospitals have implemented a unit dose drug distribution system for dispensing medications. A **unit dose** is an amount of a drug prepackaged for a single administration. In other words, it is an amount of medication in a dosage form that is ready for administration to a particular patient at a particular time. Unit dose is an important part of the inpatient drug distribution system, and its use streamlines the medication distribution process.

Unit Dose Formulations Most common oral medications—such as tablets, capsules, and some liquids—are commercially available in a unit dose formulation. Unit dose labels include the following information, at minimum:

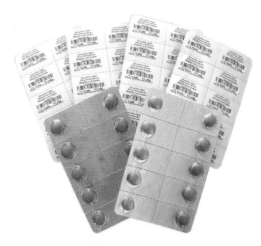

A unit dose is an individually prepared medication and dose for a specific patient. The lot number (on the labeling) from the manufacturer is needed in case of a drug recall. A bar code is often used for scanning in the pharmacy or patient care unit.

- generic or brand name of the drug
- strength of the dose
- bar code of the product
- manufacturer's name, lot number, and expiration date from packaging
- expiration date

Each unit dose is actually a separate prescription or medication order.

Unit Dose Cart Unit dose medications are distributed to the nursing units via a unit dose cart. A **unit dose cart** is a movable cart that contains removable cassette drawers that house medications. Typically, the cart has two sets of drawers: one for use on the patient care unit and a replacement for filling the next cart exchange medication orders. These drawers are maintained by the pharmacy technician. Unit dose carts are typically exchanged after the scheduled morning dose administrations. When not in use, the unit dose cart is locked on the nursing unit for security.

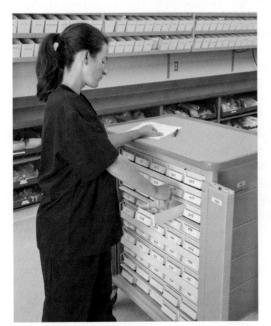

A unit dose cart has individually labeled drawers that contain medications for patients assigned to a designated patient care unit.

Each cassette drawer of the unit dose cart is labeled with a specific patient's name and room number. Typically, a patient's drawer is designated for that patient until the patient is discharged from the hospital or transferred to another patient care unit. Each drawer of the cart contains a unit dose or prepackaged medication and medication container labels, which are created using information from the computer-generated list. Medications are usually provided for 24 hours, although smaller hospitals may exchange patient drawers less frequently.

Benefits of the Unit Dose System The unit dose drug distribution system offers several benefits for patients, healthcare personnel, and the hospital. These benefits offset the higher packaging costs and labor-intensive activity that is involved in utilizing this drug distribution system.

Streamlined Work Flow Process With the drug formulation already prepared, nurses on the patient care unit simply administer the medication to the patient, rather than preparing the dose from multiple-dose containers. This process allows the nursing staff more time to perform other patient care responsibilities.

Decreased Medication Errors The unit dose system decreases the likelihood of medication errors because the bar codes placed on the unit dose medications offer an additional safety check before administration of the medications. If a medication does not scan correctly at the patient's bedside, then the wrong medication has been dispensed and the error is detected before patient administration. In many hospitals, the bar code on the patient wristband is compared with the bar code on the medication to further reduce the risk of a medication error.

Increased Medication Security A unit dose system places all necessary oral medications, including prn medications, in a patient-specific cassette drawer. Each nursing unit has its own unit dose cart that is locked at all times for added security when not in use by the nurse administering medications. The administration of each dose for each patient must be documented in a hard copy in the medical chart or in an electronic nurse administration record.

Safety Note

Only unopened unit doses can be returned to stock. For ease of reuse, the unit doses are labeled with the name of the drug, its strength, and the expiration date.

Reduced Medication Wastage In the unit dose system, unused medications can be returned to inventory in their original, unopened packages and reused.

Increased Cost-Effectiveness Using a unit dose system provides an easier method for the hospital accounting department to maintain patients' accounts (including charges and credits). Each medication dose filled is billed to the patient's account. Any unused medication returned to the pharmacy gets credited back to the individual patient's account by the pharmacy technician or pharmacist. If the packaging is not compromised and the expiration date still valid, the medication can then be reused.

Patient Costs of the Unit Dose System The pharmacy technician must understand that the cost of one dose of medication is proportionately higher in a hospital than one dose from a retail pharmacy. A patient is typically charged for each dose administered; the cost may include pharmacy, nursing personnel, and hospital overhead costs in addition to the cost of the drug and unit dose packaging. Consequently, a dose of Tylenol in the hospital may cost $5 or more for each tablet.

Repackaging Medications into Unit Doses

Because manufacturers do not prepare all drugs in a unit dose form and because individual medication orders may call for nonstandard doses, the pharmacy technician often needs to repackage medications. A **medication special** is a single dose preparation made for a particular patient. Oral tablet, capsule, or liquid medication specials are examples of drug formulations that are typically prepared and packaged in a unit dose form. The process of creating patient-specific unit doses is labor intensive and is often the responsibility of a designated pharmacy technician.

Large hospital pharmacies may use a variety of time- and cost-saving devices to assist in the preparation of medications such as automated high-speed packaging machines for oral medications and an automated liquid-filling apparatus (for example, PACMED from McKesson). Typical unit dose manual packaging includes heat-sealed ziplock bags, adhesive-sealed bottles, blister packs, and heat-sealed strip packages for oral solids, as well as plastic or glass cups, heat-sealable aluminum cups, and plastic syringes labeled "For Oral Use Only" for oral liquids. The packaging provides an airtight and light-resistant delivery system to ensure physical stability of the drug.

Labeling and Documentation of Repackaged Medications Repackaged medications must be carefully labeled. In addition to labeling, it is also important—and legally required—to carefully record and document information about the medications that have been repackaged in the hospital pharmacy. Repackaging includes bar codes for bedside scanning. The repackaging documentation is made using the **repackaging control log** (see Figure 9.2). Note that the pharmacy technician who completed the repackaging, as well as the pharmacist who checked the medications, must initial the log.

High-volume repackaged drugs may be prepared for use with the automated robotic dispensing system. Additional information may be required for repackaged drugs, depending on hospital policy, state guidelines, and accreditation standards. Multiple drugs may be repackaged and listed on the log sheet. The pharmacist must check the stock bottle from which the pharmacy technician obtained the medication, the unit dose medication container label, and the packaging and labeling of the final product before it is added to the unit dose cart.

 Safety Note

As in the community pharmacy, the technician in the hospital pharmacy works under the direct supervision of the pharmacist.

 Safety Note

Expiration dates and lot numbers must be included on all repackaged medications.

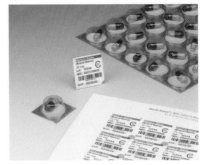

Labeling of unit doses that have been repackaged in the hospital pharmacy should include the drug name, strength, dosage form, manufacturer, lot number, and beyond-use dating.

Copyright 2013 Medi-Dose, Inc. All Rights Reserved. Used with Permission.

FIGURE 9.2
Repackaging Control Log

Repackaging Control Log
Department of Pharmaceutical Services

Date Repackaged	Pharmacy Lot Number	Drug Name, Strength, and Dosage Form	Manufacturer and Lot Number	Expiration Date	Quantity Packaged	Initials	
						Prep. By	Approved By

Processing Medication Orders Using the Unit Dose System

Medication orders that have been received by the hospital pharmacy and entered into the pharmacy database are filled on a regular basis until the patient is released from the hospital. Figure 9.3 on the following page shows examples of medication orders for hospital patients. Most hospitals have adopted a drug formulary system to control inventory costs; if a nonformulary drug is ordered, the P&P manual of the hospital pharmacy must be consulted. Often, the drug is purchased from a wholesaler and charged to the patient. If a hospital pharmacy is not open 24/7, the P&P manual outlines the process for securing a new medication order after hours or on the weekends.

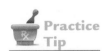 **Practice Tip**

The *NPO* designation indicates that nothing be given by mouth. This directive is typically ordered for patients before surgery.

Using a Cart Fill List After the medication order(s) is entered into the computer database, a patient-specific **unit dose label** is created and includes the name of the patient; the name and strength of the medication; the frequency, route, and time of

FIGURE 9.3
Medication
Orders

Patient Name	Order	Room #
Jessica Shirley	labetalol 200 mg IV q8 h	825
	Phenergan 25 mg IV q6 h prn	
	D5 ½ NS 20 mEq KCl at 50 mL/h	
	NPO after 12M	
Bobbie King	gentamicin 20 mg IV q8 h	432
	baby powder	
	ASA gr V po q6 h	
Roscoe Mack	Nitrostat SL prn	503
	Capoten 25 mg po STAT, then bid	
Megan Mills	10,000 units heparin IV STAT	407
	gentamicin 60 mg IVPB tid	
	Bentyl 10 mg po tid prn	
Shannon Bell	continue Rocephin 1 g IV q24 h	335
	continue Zithromax IV 500 mg q24 h	

FIGURE 9.4
Unit Dose
Label

℞ Javier Lopez   Room 535
    #10051948
    ciprofloxacin 500 mg PO
    Q12 H   1700   0500

FIGURE 9.5
Cart Fill List

℞ Amina Ali   Room 532
    #06051957
    cyclobenzaprine 10 mg PO
    Q12 H   0800   2000
    ibuprofen 800 mg PO
    Q6 H   0000 0600 1200 1800
    zolpidem 10 mg PO
    HS   2200

    Irma Elmore   Room 638
    #12121926
    trazodone 100 mg PO
    Q HS   2200
    sertraline 100 mg PO
    QAM   0900

    Patrice Anderson Room 714
    #11121956
    amoxicillin-clavulanate 875 mg PO
    TID   0800   1400   2200
    morphine sulfate 10 mg IM
    Q6 H   0000 0600 1200 1800

administration; and the bar code (see Figure 9.4). A printout of all **patient profiles** in the hospital results in a daily **cart fill list** (see Figure 9.5). This list identifies the unit dose and/or repackaged medications and the administration times needed by each patient in the hospital. Labels are then printed for each drug for each patient before the technician begins the unit dose cart fill process.

The cart fill list is usually printed each morning by the pharmacy technician to prepare doses to be sent to the patient care unit (assuming that the medication is not in automated floor stock, a separate situation that will be addressed later in this chapter). In many hospitals, the medication filling of unit dose preparations is limited to infrequently used medications not on floor stock inventory or those that are not commercially available. If not on floor stock, the technician must estimate the number of doses

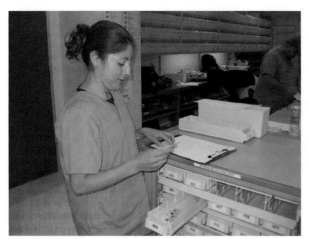

Pharmacy technicians are responsible for daily cart fills with unit dose packaged medication for each patient.

needed for a *prn* medication. For example, if a prescriber orders Zofran 4 mg po q6 h prn, a maximum of four doses may be needed in any 24-hour period.

Each hospital has a standard time for various dose administrations, such as q4 h, q6 h, q8 h, q12 h, hs, bid, tid, and qid. As discussed in Chapter 5, hospitals commonly use 24-hour time (military time) for scheduled dose administration times. For example, if a patient is prescribed Penicillin VK 500 mg po q6 h, the doses may be administered at 0600, 1200, 1800, and 0000. If the hospital is on a 24-hour cart exchange, the pharmacy technician would place four doses of medication and their accompanying labels in the patient specific drawer of the unit dose cart. If the patient is receiving other medications, those unit doses and labels would also be stored in the drawer. Once the cart is delivered to the nursing unit, the nurse must verify (often using bar codes) the medication before administration and documentation in the patient record.

If an order is received after the unit dose cart has already been delivered to the floor, then the pharmacist or pharmacy technician supplies sufficient medication until the next cart exchange. For example, if Zantac 300 mg q8 h (0600, 1400, 2200) is ordered at 1300, then two doses need to be delivered for the 1400 and 2200 dose administrations, and a third dose is placed in the patient's unit dose cart drawer for the next morning. A total of three doses is needed until the next cart exchange.

Filling Unit Dose Orders The technician fills the medication order at a designated **pick station**, or an area of the inpatient pharmacy with frequently prescribed formulary drugs in commercially available unit dose packaging. These medications are then placed in the unit dose drawers. Unlike these formulary drugs, Schedule II, III, and IV substances are not dispensed in a unit dose cart per hospital policy. Instead, they are obtained from the narcotics cabinet or the locked and secure automated floor stock system in which documentation of each dose for each patient is made by the nurse. This restriction minimizes illegal drug diversion.

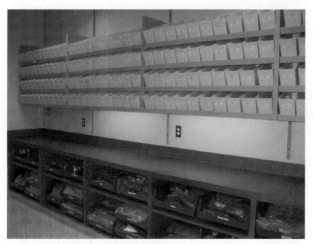

Mirror image pick stations are used by pharmacy technicians to fill the unit dose cart.

As more hospitals turn to sophisticated robotic dispensing and nursing unit floor stock systems, the traditional unit dose system will be used less frequently in pharmacy practice.

Robotic Dispensing System

Many medium- to large-size hospital pharmacies use a centralized automated robotic dispensing system to fill unit dose orders. The goal is for all hospital pharmacies of any size to adopt automation technology in place of a unit dose distribution system within the next decade. This automated medication dispensing system is integrated with hospital and pharmacy software and stores more than 1,000 of the most frequently prescribed medications. Similar to a vending machine, this automated dispensing system can hold most of a hospital's drug inventory of these selected drugs for three days and can accommodate all dosage forms—tablets, capsules, prepackaged unit dose liquids, patches—even those items requiring refrigeration. For security reasons, there are no controlled substances stored in the robot. Robotic dispensing is sometimes done off-site due to space requirements, and the facility that houses this technology is often centrally located to serve several area corporate hospitals, much like a mail-order warehouse.

Operation of the Robot After a medication order is written (or entered into the computer) and checked by the pharmacist, the robot takes over. Using bar-code technology, the robot can pick, count, package, label, store, and dispense the medication. In addition, the robot can process drug returns, credits, inventory reordering, and record keeping. A robotic arm uses suction and pneumatic tubes to pull the medication and transfer it to a collection area where it is then packaged into an envelope or dispensed onto a tray for proper placement by the technician onto a unit dose cart.

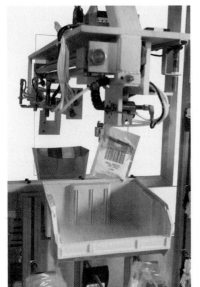

A robotic device fills prescriptions using the downloaded prescription orders and bar-coded unit dose medication packages.

Some automated systems have the capability to assist in the compounding of sterile preparations. The robot selects the vial by bar code, adds the proper amount of diluent, withdraws the correct dose, and then injects the drug into an IV bag or places the drug into a syringe for later administration by the nurse. There is no "touch contamination" and, with proper cleaning and maintenance of the equipment, the end product should be free from microorganisms.

All medications for the next cart exchange are prepared and placed in a patient-specific tray. They are then packaged in an envelope or a plastic bag and labeled with the patient's name, the drug name and dose, the medication administration time, and an identifying bar code. The technician scans the bar code of the computer-generated unit dose label and/or envelope as a final check before the medication order is placed in the unit dose cassette drawer. The technician may deliver any needed unit doses to the patient care unit. Nurses can scan the bar code of the drug and the bar code of the patient bracelet for error-free medication administration. The use of this bar-code technology at the patient's bedside is known as **bar-code point-of-care (BPOC)**.

Benefits of the Robotic Dispensing System There are many advantages to using automation for dispensing medications in the hospital setting.

Decreased Medication Errors Dispensing medications is a labor-intensive process with more than 10 discrete steps required from physician order entry to nurse administration of the drug at the patient's bedside. For large hospitals that administer more than 10,000 individual doses to patients each day (with 10 steps for each of these doses), the possibility of medication errors is obvious. Indeed, medication errors represent 21% of all medical errors in the hospital, are responsible for the deaths of 7,000 patients annually, and result in injuries to thousands of individuals. These errors amount to a conservative estimate of $3.5 billion per year.

In light of those statistics, one-third of medium- and large-size hospital pharmacies currently use ROBOT-Rx automation for medication dispensing, and half of these hospitals have also adopted BPOC technology. Used in combination with CPOE and BPOC technologies at the patient's bedside, ROBOT-Rx automation in these hospitals has resulted in an accuracy rate near 100% for more than 350 million dispensed doses, according to McKesson, the manufacturer of this pharmacy robotics system.

Reduced Pharmacy Workload Using robotic dispensing has been estimated to reduce pharmacist workload by 90% and pharmacy technician workload by 72%. Automation allows the pharmacist to redirect his or her efforts to more patient care and allows the pharmacy technician to shift from time- and labor-intensive preparation of unit doses to repackaging, inventorying floor stock and the robot, and preparing IV admixtures.

Increased Long-Term Cost Savings The high short-term costs associated with the robotic dispensing system (which amount to approximately $1 million) are substantial but thought to be offset by the long-term cost savings. Cost savings may be realized in staff efficiencies, improved productivity, fewer medication errors, and less litigation and settlement costs. In the future, such automation may become the standard of care for the hospital pharmacy community.

Intravenous Admixture Service

Nearly all hospital pharmacies provide an **intravenous (IV) admixture service** (also known as an IV additive service or IV add for short). This service is responsible for the safe and accurate preparation of many parenteral medications, including antibiotics, thrombolytics (or clot busters), nutrition, and cancer chemotherapy. Parenteral medications are administered directly into the bloodstream; therefore, these solutions must be sterile, or free from contaminants. The preparation of sterile parenteral products by the hospital pharmacy is a high-priority safety standard in all hospitals.

Preparation of Parenteral Medications To prepare parenteral medications, pharmacy personnel typically reconstitute or dissolve the medications in sterile water or normal saline (salt) solution. These medications are then administered to patients by IV infusion over several hours. Other IV medications are prepared in small-volume mini-bags that, when administered by nursing personnel, are piggybacked or connected to the tubing of patients' existing large-volume IV infusions. Intravenous piggyback (IVPB) solutions are discussed in more detail in Chapter 11.

Parenteral medications are prepared by specially trained pharmacists and pharmacy technicians in a sterile, germ-free "clean room" work environment in the hospital pharmacy. IV admixture personnel must follow strict aseptic protocol set forth by USP Chapter <797>, including the donning of sterile garb and the use of aseptic technique, during the preparation of these sterile IV medications. The medications are prepared in a horizontal laminar airflow hood, which ensures a contaminant-free environment for the procedure. Some potentially hazardous drugs—such as those used for cancer chemotherapy—require special handling. To prepare these caustic medications, pharmacy personnel must don protective clothing and use a specialized hood in the clean room.

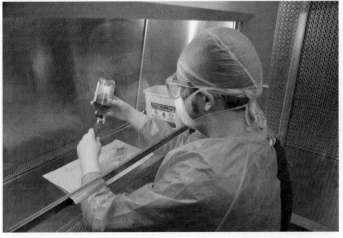

A pharmacy technician preparing chemotherapy drugs must be specially trained, wear protective garb, and work in a vertical laminar airflow hood.

Total Parenteral Nutrition Service

Many hospital pharmacies have a **total parenteral nutrition (TPN)** service as a part of the IV admixture service. A TPN service is often staffed by a team of hospital personnel, including a certified physician, nurse, nutritionist, and pharmacist. In most hospitals, however, it is the responsibility of specially trained and certified technicians in the pharmacy department to prepare the TPN solution under the direction and supervision of experienced and trained pharmacists. These pharmacists typically have advanced training and certification in TPN and are often members of an interdisciplinary TPN team. Their role on this team is to assist in writing individualized medication orders and to monitor patients' drug response.

Preparation of TPN A TPN is a specially formulated IV parenteral solution that provides for the entire nutritional needs of a patient who cannot or will not eat. Recipients of TPN include patients of all ages in both hospital and home healthcare settings. Like parenteral medications, TPN is administered directly into the patient's vein (in this case, via a central line); therefore, the solution must be sterile. TPN must also be contaminant-free because the solution may be hanging at room temperature for up to 24 hours.

A TPN solution may contain more than 20 ingredients, including amino acids, carbohydrates, fats, sugars, vitamins, electrolytes, and minerals. To improve efficiency, reduce calculation errors, and lower intensive labor costs, many large hospitals use an **automated compounding device (ACD)** to prepare multiple TPN solutions. With so many additives and calculations and multiple entries into a sterile IV solution, the need for a reliable, programmable, automated device to reduce medication errors and contamination is readily apparent. USP Chapter <797> guidelines specify that the hospital pharmacy must ensure both the accuracy and the precision of ACDs. The accuracy of the volume and the weight is verified by performing test trials using sterile water for injection for comparison.

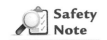
Safety Note

The accuracy of the ACD must be continually monitored by both the technician and the pharmacist.

A validated chemical analysis of all ingredients of a TPN is usually outsourced to a laboratory with the proper equipment. The precision of the ACD is important, especially when adding electrolytes such as potassium chloride, which can be toxic. Daily records on calibration must be kept by the technician and reviewed by the pharmacist at least weekly. The testing, monitoring, and surveillance of ACDs are outlined in the written P&P manual of the hospital pharmacy department.

Smaller hospitals may elect to outsource their TPN preparations to a larger hospital pharmacy or an off-site pharmacy. In this situation, the physician order for TPN is received by the pharmacy, reviewed and verified by the pharmacist, and then forwarded to the larger hospital or outsourced pharmacy. The off-site pharmacy is responsible for the preparation, beyond-use dating, verification, labeling, and transport of the final product. The director of the hospital pharmacy must be assured that the off-site pharmacy meets all state and federal laws and regulations as well as adheres to the standards set by the USP and the Joint Commission.

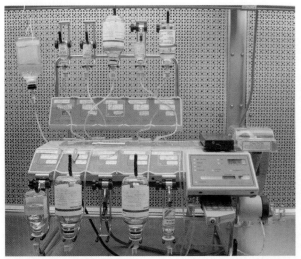
The ACD is used to mix multiple additives more accurately in a TPN nutritional solution for adults and children.

Nursing Unit Drug Administration and Documentation

Aside from the hospital's pharmacy department, medications can also be obtained through a secured floor stock medication delivery system. In this system, the medication order is still received at the pharmacy and approved by the pharmacist, but nursing personnel can retrieve the ordered medications from floor stock on the nursing unit. Floor stock may include common oral drugs, IV solutions, and controlled drugs such as oral and parenteral narcotics. The administration of the medications to the patient must be documented in the patient's medication administration record (MAR) and nursing notes.

Floor Stock

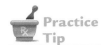
Practice Tip

The medical abbreviation *prn* comes from the Latin term *pro re nata*, which means "according to circumstances" or "as needed."

Floor stock is an inventory of frequently prescribed drugs that is stored on the patient care unit rather than delivered by a unit dose cart. Historically, floor stock was limited to selected drugs used on a *prn* or as needed basis and included mainly over-the-counter medications. Ointments, creams, eardrops, and eyedrops—considered bulk items—were also commonly supplied as floor stock and placed at the patient's bedside upon request of a physician's order.

Floor Stock and Automated Medication Dispensing Systems Today, automation is playing a major role in drug distribution on the nursing unit. With the advent of a decentralized **automated medication dispensing system (AMDS)**, such as AcuDose-Rx (McKesson) and Pyxis MedStation (CareFusion), floor stock now consists of frequently used medications, including controlled substances and IV fluids, that meet the needs of a particular patient care unit. The maximum restock and minimum reorder levels for each drug on each unit are set by the pharmacy department.

An AMDS uses touch screen technology to match each dose in the floor stock system with a patient specific medication order. The software highlights the status of each medication order, indicates the exact location of the prescribed floor stock medication, and then records the time and initials of the nurse who retrieves and administers the medication. An AMDS is designed to interface with the pharmacy's computer information system and the hospital's EHR system.

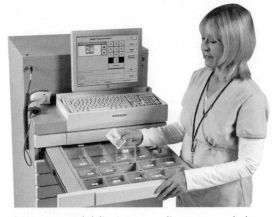
This automated delivery system dispenses stock drug items on the patient care unit.

Benefits of Floor Stock AMDS The floor stock AMDS is an extension of the unit dose delivery system and offers several advantages for patients, healthcare personnel, and the hospital. These benefits offset the high equipment cost that is involved in implementing this drug distribution system.

Decreased Medication Errors The use of AMDS reduces the incidence of medication errors. In one study at Beloit Memorial Hospital in Beloit, Wisconsin, the Pyxis AMDS reduced medication errors by 93%. Each dose for each patient must be accounted for each time by the nurse. The bar codes of the drug from the AMDS and patient wristband are scanned before drug administration.

Secure Medication Storage The drawers of an AMDS can be set up for various security levels such as *prn* medications, frequently used drugs, and controlled substances. This medication distribution system also has varying levels of access for hospital personnel, with parameters set for pharmacists, pharmacy technicians, nursing supervisors, and nurses. The security and accountability incorporated in the AMDS provides a strong deterrent to illegal drug diversion and medication theft of controlled substances.

Streamlined Work Flow The use of an AMDS streamlines the medication distribution process, thus allowing nursing personnel to administer medications in a more timely manner. For pharmacy personnel, this automated drug distribution provides them with more time to complete necessary centralized pharmacy technician tasks such as filling the unit dose cart, ordering and replenishing drug inventory within and outside the pharmacy, and repackaging and preparing IV sterile products. By having the most frequently needed medications on each nursing unit, there are fewer telephone calls and interruptions of daily activities.

Improved Tracking of Medications An AMDS documents each step of the medication dispensing and administration process, including the distribution of narcotics. This system also tracks all medications by type of drug, dose, patient, and caregiver, as well as captures all charges for dispensed medications.

Narcotics

As in the community pharmacy, all Schedule II controlled substances in a hospital pharmacy must be secured in a locked cabinet or safe, whether stored in the pharmacy or in an AMDS in the patient care unit. Narcotics are commonly included in the floor stock inventory of each patient care unit in the hospital, though type and quantity may vary by unit. A careful audit trail must exist to account for each dose of each controlled substance to comply with strict regulations established by the DEA. The date and time that the narcotic is administered to a specific patient must be verified with the medication order, nursing administration record in the patient chart, and a **Schedule II drug administration record**. An example of such a hard copy form is provided in Figure 9.6. This record is a balance of each remaining dose of narcotic and may be manual or automated.

In the now archaic manual systems, the controlled drug administration record was reconciled at the end of each nursing shift. The names of the prescribing physician and the nurse administering the medication were recorded, as well as the amount of drug given. If any amount of drug was wasted (or any amount of drug destroyed), then the record had to be witnessed and signed by another healthcare professional. The nurse supervisor and pharmacist had to reconcile each dose of each narcotic drug administered in the hospital.

Narcotics and Automated Inventory Systems Today, automated narcotic inventory systems provide increased security and tracking of controlled substances. For example, the NarcStation, an automated system by McKesson, provides a compatible software tracking system using state-of-the-art bar-code technology to maintain the record keeping, reporting, and transaction date for all controlled substances from the wholesaler to the patient. This system allows separate reporting for Schedule II, III, and IV drugs to meet DEA and state and federal requirements.

FIGURE 9.6
Schedule II
Drug
Administration
Form

SCHEDULE II DRUG ADMINISTRATION FORM				
Drug Demerol	**Strength** 100 mg	**Quantity** 25	**Form** ☐ Tablet ☐ Capsule ☑ Injection ☐ Liquid	**Control Number** A 3735
Issued By Andy Saul		**To Station** CCU		**Date Issued** 10/10/201X
Received By (Nurse in Charge) David Anderson				**Date Received** 10/10/201X

Date	Time	Patient Name	Room No.	Medication	Dosage Given	Wasted	Physician	Administered By	BAL
10/11/201X	0550	Martelli	CCU	Demerol	100 mg		Schnars	Lynch	24
10/12/201X	1245	Singh	CCU	Demerol	100 mg		Fields	Bond	23
10/14/201X	1625	Kappel	CCU	Demerol	90 mg	10 mg	Serrao	Richards	22
10/15/201X	1130	Gehrig	CCU	Demerol	75 mg	25 mg	Aicher	Fibich	21

RECORD OF WASTE AND SPOILAGE					
Dose No	**Date**	**Amount**	**Explain Wastage**	**Signature #1**	**Signature #1**
	10/15/201X	25 mg	defective syringe	*Updegraff*	*Anderson*

Automated systems provide real-time reports and immediate access to information that identifies trends in narcotic usage in a patient care unit. Using NarcStation, the time for reconciling inventory is reduced by more than 90%. The audit trail both deters and detects potential drug diversion and greatly aids in regulatory compliance.

Medication Administration Record

When a nurse administers any medication—oral, IV, or *prn*—it is recorded in the patient's medical record on a form called a **medication administration record (MAR)**. Each record is patient-specific and includes a medication order number; the names of all drugs, doses, routes of administration, administration times, and start and stop dates; and special instructions for the hospital staff. The exact administration time for each dose of each drug is recorded and initialed by the nurse on the MAR. A separate listing in the MAR is kept for *prn*, or as needed, drugs. An example of an MAR is included in Figure 9.7 on the following page.

Technology has also been developed to help nurses document the administration of drugs accurately and quickly. An **electronic medication administration record (eMAR)** legibly documents the administration time of each drug to each patient using bar-code technology at the patient's bedside. The Horizon Admin-Rx (McKesson) is one example of a commercially available eMAR software application that helps reduce medication errors and improve nursing productivity. This software provides an online clinical flow sheet documenting the patient's history, vital signs, medication profile and administration, and nursing care comments. The software also

FIGURE 9.7 Medication Administration Record (MAR)

Patient Name: Wanda Han   **Physician:** Arnold   **Allergies:** Codeine sulfate

Hospital ID: 5522103   CCU   **Diagnosis:** (1) Gastroenteritis,

Gender: F   (2) Renal failure

Age: 46

Order No.	Medication	Start	Stop	Days 0700 to 1859	Nights 1900 to 0659
433800	PANTOPRAZOLE SOD IV 40 MG IVP EVERY 24 HOURS	09/10 0800 OCW	12/09 0800	0800	
435135	VANCOMYCIN-AV 1 GRAM SODIUM CHLORIDE AV 0.9% 250 ML IVPB EVERY 24 HOURS, INFUSE OVER 60 MIN	09/11 0800 OCW	09/18 0800	0800	
448842	DEMEROL 100 MG IM EVERY 4 HOURS	09/12 1000 PLH	12/11 1000	0800 1200 1600	2000 0000 0400
448891	ENOXAPARIN INJ 40 MG/0.4 ML SC ONCE A DAY	09/12 1000 PLH	12/11 1000	1000	
449100	NEUTRA-PHOS 1 PACKET PO TWICE A DAY MIX CONTENTS WITH 2.5 OZ OF WATER OR JUICE STIR WELL AND GIVE PROMPTLY	09/12 1000 PLH	12/11 1000	1000	2200
458037	CHLORDIAZEPOXIDE HCL CAP 25 MG PO EVERY 8 HOURS WARNING: DOSE IS 50 MG = 2 CAPS	09/13 1400 RGC	09/20 1400	1400	2200 0600

provides real-time warnings and alerts on all new, changed, or canceled medication orders before administration. In addition, the eMAR software provides an additional safeguard requiring the nurse to check both the new physician medication order and the pharmacist verification of that order.

Many hospitals have adopted an eMAR software system, and pharmacy technicians should be familiar with this medication documentation process.

eMAR Process In hospitals using an eMAR system, patients are given bar-coded wristbands to wear that confirm their identities and the prescribed medications, and that link healthcare personnel to their eMARs. To implement the eMAR process, each patient's medication orders are input by the physician into a handheld computer device at the patient's bedside. Once a physician inputs the order, it is electronically transmitted to the hospital pharmacy. After the medication order is checked and verified by the

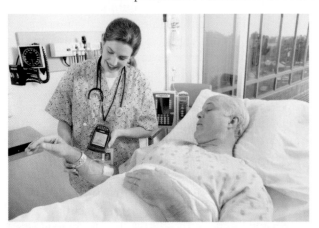

Using BPOC technology, the nurse can verify the drug to be administered with the patient wristband, thus reducing potential errors.

pharmacist, the order is then filled by the pharmacy technician (or robot), and sent to the patient care unit (or retrieved from floor stock). During medication administration times, the nurse compares all new medication orders with the physician's computerized entries. Once the order is confirmed, the nurse scans his/her ID badge as well as the bar code on the patient's wristband. The nurse compares the scanned bar code to the bar code on the medication (from pharmacy or floor stock). If the numbers match, the nurse can proceed with the medication administration. Using this BPOC technology reduces the potential for medication errors because of the software's embedded safeguards.

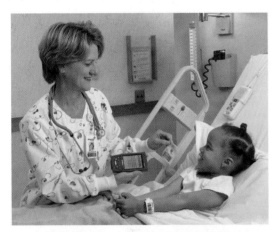

Automation and bar-code scanning technologies on the patient care unit reduce errors in medication administration. The right drug and the right dose must be delivered to the right patient.

Benefits of eMARs The adoption of eMARs in hospitals enhances communication among healthcare team members and ensures that the five rights of medication administration—right patient, right drug, right dose, right route, and right time—are met. In conjunction with the use of other automation in the hospital setting—such as CPOE, robotic filling of medication orders, automated floor stock systems, and BPOC—medication errors are minimized. Another advantage to using these advanced technologies lies in meeting documentation guidelines established by federal and state regulations as well as accreditation standards established by the Joint Commission. (For more on accreditation standards, see the following section titled "Joint Commission.")

Hospital Accreditation

Every hospital seeks initial accreditation and reaccreditation by the Joint Commission to receive reimbursement from Medicare, Medicaid, and private insurance. To receive accreditation, standards for high-quality care and patient safety must be followed in every hospital department, including the pharmacy.

Joint Commission

The **Joint Commission** is an independent, not-for-profit organization that sets and measures the standards for quality and safety of health care through an accreditation process. The end result of this process is to provide better health care and quality of life for patients and to lower healthcare costs. The Joint Commission accredits more than 19,000 hospitals, home healthcare systems, and long-term care facilities. **Accreditation** is like a *Good Housekeeping* stamp of approval; it means that the hospital has met specific standards for both quality and safety. If approved, accreditation is for three years.

The Joint Commission acts as a patient and healthcare advocate, making sure that a hospital is following the appropriate standards and procedures. The organization evaluates a hospital's performance in specific areas, compares that performance against the defined standards, and then awards a hospital accreditation status if the hospital meets or exceeds those standards. These evidence-based standards of care used as part of the accreditation process are developed in consultation with healthcare experts, providers, and researchers.

All departments, including the pharmacy, need to have an up-to-date P&P manual, as required by the Joint Commission. In addition, all pharmacy personnel, including pharmacy technicians, should be trained and updated on all policies and procedures outlined in the manual. Annual documentation of such training is required. The percentage of technicians who are certified may be used as a surrogate measure of competency or adequate staffing.

Conducting an On-Site Survey The inspection of a hospital for pending Joint Commission accreditation, sometimes referred to as a *survey*, requires an extensive, multiday, on-site visit. The inspection is conducted by a survey team that is composed of healthcare professionals who are extensively trained, certified, and educated in quality-related performance evaluation.

The survey team makes an unannounced, random visit to a hospital to conduct its evaluation. The evaluative process is not meant to be punitive but to assure patients that all standards are being met or improvements are being instituted for the hospital to be in compliance. For example, if a hospital pharmacy has received multiple budget cuts that may compromise the quality of care or the level of safety of its procedures, then the Joint Commission survey team has the authority to require prompt corrective action by hospital administration.

During the visit, the survey team evaluates the hospital's performance, reviews the P&P manual to check for compliance with quality and safety standards, and may interview hospital personnel. In addition to the evaluation, the Joint Commission offers education and guidance to improve the hospital's overall performance. The survey team generally provides a summary report to the hospital administrative staff and employees. The final accreditation report is available on the Joint Commission's website for review by any consumer or healthcare professional.

In addition to Joint Commission standards, the hospital pharmacy must comply with all federal and state laws and regulations with oversight provided by the state board of pharmacy. Most federal and state agencies for Medicare and Medicaid patients, as well as private insurance, require Joint Commission accreditation for reimbursement of services provided by the hospital.

Setting Quality of Care Standards The Joint Commission has National Quality Improvement Goals, which provide standards for quality of patient care in select patient populations. The Joint Commission requires hospitals to report on the key indicators of quality of care in areas such as heart attack, heart failure, community-acquired pneumonia, and surgical infection rates.

During the accreditation visit, the survey team requests a number of medical charts to randomly review for compliance with national quality standards of care. For example, in assessing the hospital performance for the care of the heart attack patient, the following medication- and health-related factors are evaluated, measured, and compared with those at other hospitals that have been accredited by the Joint Commission:

- use of aspirin, prescribed on arrival and at discharge because it decreases the risk of recurrent blood clots and improves survival
- use of certain heart drugs, called *beta blockers*, within the first 24 hours and at discharge to minimize damage to the heart
- timely use of thrombolytic or clot-buster therapy within 30 minutes of arrival to reduce heart muscle damage

- timely use of percutaneous coronary intervention (PCI) or balloon angioplasty for heart blockage within 120 minutes of arrival
- use of certain heart drugs, called *angiotensin-converting enzyme inhibitors (ACEIs)* or *angiotensin receptor blockers (ARBs)*, at discharge if the patient has a diagnosis of heart failure
- documentation that the physician discussed smoking cessation programs with patients who smoke
- comparison of rates of inpatient mortality for heart attack patients

The performance is compared with that of other hospitals of similar size that are accredited by the Joint Commission. Comparative analysis is performed at a national and state level and is made available to employers and patients. For example, inappropriate antibiotic use could lead to an increase in surgical site infections, resistance patterns within the hospital, and healthcare costs. Hospitals would make it a high priority to correct any performance deficiencies that would otherwise risk accreditation.

Establishing Safety-Related Standards The Joint Commission's safety-related standards involving the hospital pharmacy include reconciling a patient's medication profile upon admission to the hospital with medication orders, improving safety of medication use and drug infusion pumps, and reducing the risk of hospital-acquired infections. These standards address a number of significant patient safety issues, including the implementation of patient safety programs, the response to adverse events when they occur, and the prevention of accidental harm. Medicare no longer reimburses hospitals for the additional cost of treating preventable medication errors, injuries, and infections, so a strong economic incentive exists. Medicare also no longer reimburses for preventable hospital readmissions within 30 days. The Joint Commission's role in establishing safety standards is further discussed in Chapter 12.

Safety Note

Approximately 50% of the Joint Commission standards relate directly to safety.

Chapter Summary

- The hospital is a complex organization.
- The P&T Committee is primarily responsible for making the final decision on the medications included in the hospital's drug formulary.
- The IRB is responsible for protecting the patient in investigational studies undertaken in the hospital.
- The director of pharmacy is the chief executive officer of the pharmacy department and is responsible for its safe and efficient operation.
- Automation is widely used in the hospital pharmacy to fill inpatient and outpatient medication orders, prepare IV and TPN solutions, document floor stock and medication administration, and manage inventory.
- The pharmacy technician assists in ordering, purchasing, and receiving medications.
- Hospital pharmacies carry out a number of unique activities, such as managing the unit dose drug distribution system; repackaging; maintaining floor stock, including narcotics; and providing IV admixture and TPN services.
- In the hospital setting, a prescription is called a *medication order*; it is written as an admitting, stat, daily, continuation, standing, or discharge order.

- Technology such as CPOE, robotics, and BPOC has significantly reduced the risk of medication errors.
- A unit dose drug distribution system saves money and also reduces the chance of medication errors.
- A cart fill list is used by the technician to fill medication needs for a hospitalized patient.
- The pharmacy technician is often responsible for preparing repackaged units of medications that are not commercially available in unit dose packaging.
- Most hospitals today have an extensive automated floor stock dispensing system, consisting of frequently used unit dose drugs as well as narcotics and IV solutions.
- An IV admixture service may reduce the risk for medication dosage and calculation errors and product contamination.
- Many hospital pharmacies have a centralized TPN service in which electrolytes and vitamins are added to a variety of IV nutrition solutions.
- An eMAR is used by a nurse to document the administration time of each medication to each patient.
- The Joint Commission sets and measures the standards for quality and safety of health care in hospitals through an accreditation process.

Key Terms

accreditation the stamp of approval of the quality of services of a hospital issued by the Joint Commission

admitting order a medication order written by a physician on admission of a patient to the hospital; may or may not include a medication order

automated compounding device (ACD) a programmable, automated device to make complex IV preparations such as TPNs

automated medication dispensing system (AMDS) a secure, locked storage cabinet of designated drugs on a nursing unit whose software can track the dispensing and administration of each dose of medication to each patient

bar-code point-of-care (BPOC) the use of automation scanning by a nurse at a patient's bedside to minimize medication administration errors

cart fill list a printout of all unit dose profiles for all patients

computerized prescriber order entry (CPOE) the process of having a prescriber use a handheld device at a patient's bedside to enter and send medication orders to the pharmacy

crash cart a mobile cart that holds necessary drugs for an emergency CPR code

daily order a medication order written by a physician to continue treatment; similar to a refill of medication

director of pharmacy the chief executive officer of the hospital pharmacy department

discharge order an order written by a physician that provides take-home instructions, including prescribed medications and doses, for a discharged patient

drug formulary a list of approved medications for use within the hospital; this list is approved by the P&T Committee

electronic medication administration record (eMAR) a record that documents the administration time of each drug to each patient, often using bar-code technology

floor stock medications stocked in a secured area on each patient care unit

informed consent written permission by the patient to participate in an IRB-approved research study in terms understandable to the lay public

inpatient drug distribution system a pharmacy system to deliver all types of drugs to a patient in the hospital setting; commonly includes unit dose, repackaged medication, floor stock, and IV admixture and TPN services

Institutional Review Board (IRB) a committee of the hospital that ensures that appropriate protection is provided to patients using investigational drugs; sometimes referred to as the Human Use Committee

intravenous (IV) admixture service a centralized pharmacy service that prepares IV and TPN solutions in a sterile, clean room work environment

investigational drug a drug used in clinical trials that has not yet been approved by the FDA for use in the general population, or a drug used for nonapproved indications

Joint Commission an independent, not-for-profit organization that sets the standards by which safety and quality of health care are measured and accredits hospitals according to those standards

medical chart a legal document that contains a patient's demographics and room number as well as all orders written by the healthcare team

medication administration record (MAR) a form in the patient's medical chart used by nurses to document the administration times of all drugs

medication order a prescription written in the hospital setting

medication special a single-dose preparation not commercially available that is repackaged and made for a particular patient

patient profile the documentation that provides the information necessary to prepare the unit doses, including patient name and location, medication and strength, frequency or schedule of administration, and quantity for each order

Pharmacy and Therapeutics (P&T) Committee a committee of the hospital that reviews, approves, and revises the hospital's formulary of drugs and maintains the drug use policies of the hospital

pick station an area of the inpatient pharmacy that houses frequently prescribed formulary drugs in commercially available unit dose packaging, thus allowing efficient medication cart filling

Policy & Procedure (P&P) manual a written, step-by-step set of instructions for pharmacists and technicians alike on all operations within the pharmacy department

repackaging control log a form used in the pharmacy when drugs are repackaged from manufacturer stock bottles to unit doses; the log contains the name of the drug, dose, quantity, manufacturer lot number, expiration date, and the initials of the pharmacy technician and pharmacist

Schedule II drug administration record a manual or electronic form on the patient care unit to account for each dose of each Schedule II narcotic administered to a patient

standing order a preapproved list of instructions, including specific medications and doses, commonly written after surgery or a procedure

stat order a medication order that is to be filled and sent to the patient care unit immediately

total parenteral nutrition (TPN) a specially formulated parenteral solution that provides nutritional needs intravenously to a patient who cannot or will not eat

unit dose an amount of a drug that has been prepackaged or repackaged for a single administration to a particular patient at a particular time

unit dose cart a movable storage unit that contains individual patient drawers of medication for all patients on a given nursing unit

unit dose label directions for use on a patient-specific medication order

Chapter Review

 Additional Quiz Questions

Checking Your Understanding

To check your comprehension of this chapter's key concepts, read the following multiple-choice questions and then record your answers on a separate sheet of paper. Write your answers as modeled in these examples: 1d; 2c; 3b; etc.

1. A formulary is a
   a. list of approved drugs available through a hospital pharmacy.
   b. description of the contents and pharmacological characteristics of manufactured drugs.
   c. master control record for nonsterile compounding.
   d. set of formulae for preparation of common parenteral admixtures.

2. Patient confidentiality for participation in investigational studies is a function of the
   a. P&T Committee.
   b. Infection Control Committee.
   c. Institutional Review Board (IRB).
   d. Joint Commission.

3. A medication special is
   a. a supply of medication prepared for a hospital patient care unit.
   b. a single dose oral preparation that is prepackaged by the technician.
   c. the average recommended dose for an adult male.
   d. the dose recommended by the United States Pharmacopeia (USP).

4. A function unique to hospital pharmacy practice is
   a. maintaining drug treatment records.
   b. ordering and stocking medications and medical supplies.
   c. dispensing and repackaging medications.
   d. preparing sterile parenteral hazardous drugs.

5. The Joint Commission is primarily interested in patient safety and
   a. quality of care.
   b. patient satisfaction.
   c. the reduction of hospital costs.
   d. drug information services.

6. Which of the following is not a key responsibility of the director of pharmacy?
   a. determining the level and scope of pharmacy services
   b. planning and monitoring the budget for pharmaceuticals
   c. establishing the hospital's drug formulary
   d. developing the pharmacy's Policy & Procedure manual

7. In the hospital, a prescription is commonly referred to as a(n)
   a. medication order.
   b. MAR.
   c. protocol.
   d. floor stock medication.

8. When the pharmacy technician receives a *continuation* order, the medication should be sent to the nurse
   a. immediately.
   b. within the next one to two hours.
   c. at the next shift change.
   d. the next morning.

9. Physical inventory of Schedule II drugs in the hospital pharmacy is usually conducted every
   a. month.
   b. six months.
   c. year (annually).
   d. two years.

10. The provision of the entire nutritional needs of a patient by means of IV infusion is known as a(n)
    a. eMAR.
    b. CPOE.
    c. ACD.
    d. TPN.

11. Medication errors can be virtually eliminated by use of all of the following technologies *except*:
    a. robotic dispensing systems.
    b. computerized prescriber order entry.
    c. bar-code scanning technology at the patient's bedside.
    d. computer-generated daily cart fill list.

12. AcuDose Rx is an example of a commercially available
    a. TPN service.
    b. automated floor stock dispensing system.
    c. centralized pharmacy inventory system.
    d. pediatric dosing algorithm.

13. Accreditation of hospitals by the Joint Commission is generally for
    a. 1 year.
    b. 2 years.
    c. 3 years.
    d. 5 years.

14. A medication order is received by the pharmacy as "NPO." What does that medical term mean?
    a. nothing by mouth
    b. as needed
    c. send immediately
    d. no medication allergies

15. Returns of Schedule II drugs to the wholesaler must be made on what DEA form?
    a. 106
    b. 222
    c. special invoice signed by both the technician and pharmacist
    d. a letter signed by the pharmacist and notarized

Reinforcing Your Learning

To build on your understanding of the topics in this chapter, complete the following enrichment activities.

1. Write a complete description, without using abbreviations, of the following medication orders.

Patient Name	Order	Room #
1. Trevor Millen	ascorbic acid 500 mg po daily	230
	Basaljel po prn ac and hs	
	Toradol 10 mg po q4-6 h	
	Demerol 50 mg IM q4 h prn	
2. Tara Anderson	Lunesta 3 mg po q hs	311
	Zyrtec 1 tsp po q hs	
	MOM 30 mL po tid prn	
	Humalog 70/25 30 units subcutaneously in AM ac and 20 units in PM ac	
3. Kali Shaddy	atorvastatin 40 mg po q hs	402
	Dulcolax 5 mg po q24 h	
	hydrocodone 5/500 1-2 tab q6 h prn pain	
	amoxicillin 1 g IVPB q6 h	
	gentamicin 80 mg IVPB q8 h	
	D$_5$ ½ NS 1L @ 125 mL/h	
4. Wesley Elmore	atenolol 100 mg q am	321
	MOM 10 mL po q pc	
	Colace 150 mg po hs	
	Ativan 2 mg IM 2 h prior to surgery	
5. Matthew Young	Minitran 0.2 mg/h apply q am; remove in 12 h	401
	Fleet prep kit ut dict 1 h prior to colonoscopy	
	acetaminophen 650 mg po q4 h	
	Cipro 500 mg IVPB q12 h	
	NS 500 mL with KCl 20 mEq @ 100 mL/h	

2. Medication errors make up 21% of all hospital errors and contribute to the premature deaths of more than 7,000 patients annually. List four ways your hospital could reduce its medication error rate and liability.

3. Communicating in the hospital setting often means working with a variety of healthcare providers outside the pharmacy department. Understanding what roles they play in patients' health care is essential to effective communication. What duties do each of the following positions have in the hospital?
   a. hospitalist
   b. anesthesiologist
   c. registered nurse
   d. licensed practical nurse
   e. housekeeping aide
   f. social services worker
   g. respiratory therapist
   h. phlebotomist
   i. medical lab technician

Thinking on Your Feet

To gain practice in handling challenging situations in the workplace, consider the following real-world scenarios and then use the guiding questions to help you formulate your responses.

1. The time is 0945 hours. You receive medication orders for the following: Vancomycin 1 g IV infusion q6 h *stat*. When should the first dose be sent to the nursing unit and what times should future doses be sent?

2. Helena Angelopoulos is admitted to the hospital at 1800 Saturday evening with the following medications: pravastatin 40 mg hs, levofloxacin 500 mg PO q AM, Zantac 300 mg PO q12 h, Phenergan 25 mg q6 h prn, and morphine 10 mg IM q4 h prn. Which medications should be sent to the nursing unit tonight? Which medications will be dispensed and administered by the nurse from the Pyxis MedStation, and which medications—including their doses—will be in the unit dose drawer for Sunday morning administration? (Assume your hospital pharmacy delivers the unit dose cart once daily every morning.)

3. You receive a new prescription for an expensive antibiotic from a hospitalist. The drug cannot be dispensed as is because it is in "restricted status" as a nonformulary drug. How do you resolve this issue?

Acquiring Field Knowledge

To expand your knowledge of pharmacy practice, explore the following online activities that focus on research and information retrieval.

Reminder: *As you navigate the Internet, remember to exercise caution and good judgment when evaluating information. A thoughtful review of online text should take into consideration the following factors: the creator and sponsors of the website, the intended audience, the credentials of the authors and contributors, the reliability and validity of the posted information, the frequency of updates to the site, and the ease of navigation for a range of user skill levels.*

1. Visit the website of the American Society of Health-System Pharmacists at www.paradigmcollege.net/pharmpractice5e/WhitePaper. Search for the document titled "White Paper on Pharmacy Technicians 2002: Needed Changes Can No Longer Wait." Review the paper; then interview a hospital pharmacy technician and see what has changed over the past decade and what issues remain to be resolved.

2. Go to www.paradigmcollege.net/pharmpractice5e/unitdose and conduct a search on unit dose drug distribution systems. Identify nine advantages of a unit dose drug system over alternative distribution systems.

3. Pharmacy technicians working in a hospital setting are often responsible for repackaging drugs into a unit dose package. Go to www.paradigmcollege.net/pharmpractice5e/repackaging and search for "Single Unit and Unit Dose Packages of Drugs." Identify and describe in detail the seven parts of a label for a repackaged drug.

4. The Joint Commission focuses on patient safety. In the hospital pharmacy, patient safety includes the prevention of medication errors. Go to www.paradigmcollege.net/pharmpractice5e/mederrors. Under the Topics tab, highlight "Sentinel Event—Sentinel Event Alert" and then click on "Sentinel Event Data—Event Type by Year." Look for year trends in medication errors from 1995 to the present.

5. Go to www.paradigmcollege.net/pharmpractice5e/abbreviations and conduct a search for The Official "Do Not Use" List of Abbreviations. Interview a hospital pharmacy technician to determine which of these "nonapproved" abbreviations remains in common use.

Sampling the Certification Exam

To provide you with practice for the Certification Exam, read the following questions that have been patterned after the test format and then record your answers on a separate sheet of paper. Write your answers as modeled in these examples: 1d; 2c; 3b; etc.

1. The Pharmacy and Therapeutics (P&T) Committee's primary function is to
   a. formulate policies pertaining to pharmaceutical use in the hospital.
   b. establish job descriptions for hospital employees.
   c. review investigational drug research and publish articles.
   d. establish care plans for the treatment of disease states.

2. Crash carts in a hospital contain medication and equipment for
   a. patients' daily use.
   b. emergency use.
   c. physician use.
   d. sterile product preparation.

3. A Pyxis MedStation is an example of a(n)
   a. pneumatic delivery system.
   b. prepackaging device.
   c. automated medication dispensing system.
   d. automated compounding device.

4. A medication order for ampicillin 1 g IVPB q4 h is started at 0600. When will the next two doses be given?
   a. 1200, 1800
   b. 1000, 1400
   c. 0900, 1300
   d. 0800, 1200

5. If a product on formulary is not available from the manufacturer in unit dose packaging, the technician should
   a. recommend it be taken off of the formulary.
   b. order bulk and repackage in unit dose packaging.
   c. order bulk and send bulk package to the floor for patient use.
   d. interchange with a therapeutic equivalent drug that is available in unit dose packaging.

6. An Institutional Review Board (IRB) is responsible for approving the
   a. drug formulary.
   b. hospital's policy and procedures.
   c. use of investigational drugs.
   d. hiring of the director of pharmacy.

7. An example of an emergency medication order is a(n)
   a. stat order.
   b. standing order.
   c. discharge order.
   d. automatic stop order.

8. What percent of medication errors can be reduced with adoption of CPOE?
   a. 10%
   b. 30%
   c. 50%
   d. 80%

9. The amount of drug prepackaged for single administration to a patient is called a(n)
   a. IV additive.
   b. unit dose.
   c. floor stock.
   d. eMAR.

10. A TPN is best defined as
    a. an antibiotic added to one liter of IV solution.
    b. an oral packaged medication special not available commercially.
    c. a special nutritional parenteral solution.
    d. an IV nitroglycerin solution used to relieve chest pain in the intensive care unit.

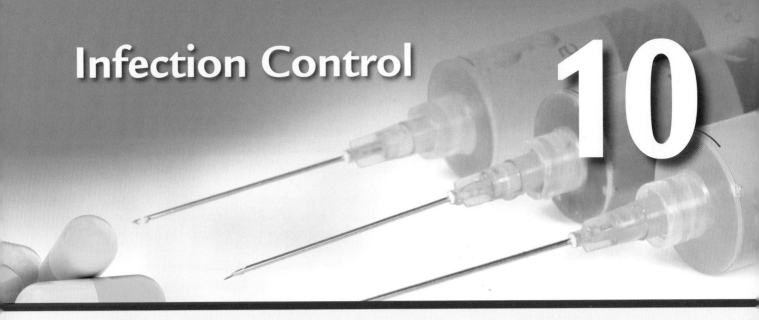

Infection Control

10

Learning Objectives

- Explain the role of pathogenic organisms in causing disease.

- Distinguish among bacteria, viruses, fungi, and protozoa.

- Discuss the advantages and disadvantages of various forms of sterilization.

- Identify common modes of contamination and preventive measures that can be taken to reduce or eliminate these risks.

- Discuss the guidelines set forth by the Centers for Disease Control and Prevention that address preventing the transmission of infectious agents in the hospital.

- Understand the distinction between hand-washing and hand-hygiene practices and the importance of these practices in infection control.

- Discuss the importance of vaccinations for healthcare workers.

- Discuss the USP Chapter <797> guidelines for sterile compounding and aseptic technique.

- Identify procedures to minimize airborne contamination during the compounding of sterile preparations.

- Contrast a manufactured sterile product with expiration dating vs. a compounded sterile preparation with beyond-use dating according to USP Chapter <797> guidelines.

- Apply contamination risk level designations and appropriate beyond-use dating for compounded sterile preparations.

- Identify the role of the Infection Control Committee within a hospital.

- List Universal Precautions that protect hospital employees.

Preview chapter terms and definitions.

H ospitals, home healthcare pharmacies, and some compounding pharmacies prepare compounded sterile preparations (CSPs), or medications that are created by mixing one or more sterile products using aseptic technique. These products are created in a strictly controlled sterile environment and are prepared by highly trained pharmacy personnel using aseptic technique. To gain insight into this type of pharmacy practice, pharmacy personnel must have a general understanding of **microbiology**, or the study of microorganisms; the germ theory of disease; various sources of contamination; and the processes of sterilization and aseptic technique. Awareness of infection control procedures is critical during sterile compounding; consequently, this chapter also discusses several key

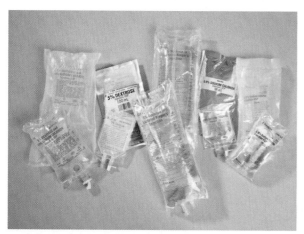

Medications are added to various IV solutions to make a compounded sterile preparation.

organizations that provide and enforce guidelines for the aseptic preparation of CSPs: the Centers for Disease Control and Prevention (CDC), the United States Pharmacopeia (USP), and an individual hospital's Infection Control Committee (ICC). The CDC provides recommendations on infection control; the USP publishes guidelines on the aseptic preparation of CSPs that have been adopted by accrediting organizations as national standards; and the ICC ensures the implementation of the USP guidelines.

For pharmacy technicians working in the hospital setting, a good understanding of infection control procedures is critical. Patients with severe disease may have a compromised immune system and, consequently, may be more susceptible to serious and sometimes life-threatening infections. In addition, microorganisms have a greater ability to adapt and become resistant to potent antibiotics in a hospital setting. In light of those facts, it is important for pharmacy personnel to understand how infection spreads and how hospitals can employ special infection control practices to limit the possibility of contamination. Any breach in aseptic protocol increases the risk for the development of serious healthcare-associated infections (HAIs), which can lead to patient mortality.

The Development of the Germ Theory of Disease

Until relatively recently, the causes of illness—especially infectious diseases—were not fully understood. Diseases were attributed to evil influences, and knowledge of their causative factors progressed slowly over the centuries.

Seventeenth-Century Scientists

Several European scientists made important advances in understanding the microscopic world of one-celled organisms, or microbes, in the seventeenth century. The Dutch merchant Anton van Leeuwenhoek made the first crude microscope and, in 1673, confirmed what many of his predecessors had theorized for centuries: the existence of a microculture of organisms. He called these organisms "animalcules" (meaning "little animals"), a name that has since been changed to **microorganisms**. Although Leeuwenhoek observed microorganisms, the Englishman Robert Hooke used a microscope to observe the walls of dead plant cells. Hooke called the pores between the walls "little cells." His discovery of cell structure marked the beginning of cell theory.

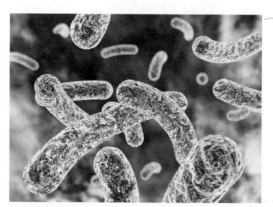

Anton van Leeuwenhoek's discovery of microorganisms led other scientists to explore the connection between microorganisms and disease.

Until the second half of the seventeenth century, it was generally believed that some forms of life could arise spontaneously from matter. This process was known as **spontaneous generation**. People thought that toads, snakes, and mice could be born from moist soil, that flies could emerge from manure, and that maggots could arise from decaying flesh. In 1668, the Italian physician Francesco Redi was the first to demonstrate that maggots could *not* arise spontaneously from decaying meat by conducting a simple experiment in which jars containing meat were left open, sealed, or covered with a fine net. Redi showed that maggots appeared only when the jars were left open, allowing flies to enter to lay eggs.

Important Discoveries of Jenner and Pasteur

As discussed in Chapter 3, Edward Jenner discovered the principle of immunization against disease in 1798. He noticed that milkmaids who had caught cowpox from cows were subsequently immune to contracting smallpox from humans. By infecting healthy individuals with cowpox, Jenner successfully inoculated them against smallpox. However, because microorganisms had not yet been identified as disease-causing agents, the reasons behind the success of Jenner's immunizations were not fully understood.

The French research scientist Louis Pasteur was instrumental in proving the connection between microorganisms and disease. Pasteur theorized that the fermentation process was caused by the growth of microorganisms in the liquid, not by spontaneous generation, which was the common belief at the time. In 1861, he put his theory to the test. Pasteur filled several short-necked flasks with beef broth and boiled ham. Some flasks were left open and allowed to cool. In a few days, these flasks were contaminated with microbes. The other flasks, sealed after boiling, remained free of microorganisms. His experiment demonstrated that microorganisms are present in the air and that they can contaminate seemingly sterile solutions. His research also revealed that the air itself does not spontaneously give rise to microbial life.

Pasteur also noted that microorganisms can contaminate fermenting beverages. In his time, the quality of winemaking was inconsistent. One year the wine was sweet, but the next year it was sour. No uniform method had been discovered to ensure the same quality year after year. Employing methods used in his broth experiment, Pasteur conducted research with grape juice. He discovered that if grape juice was heated to a certain temperature, cooled, and treated with specific yeast, then the wine would be more consistent year after year. Based on his discovery, Pasteur developed a process to kill most bacteria and mold in milk called **pasteurization**. To his credit, pasteurization is still used today.

Beverage contamination led Pasteur to conclude that microorganisms infected animals and humans as well. The idea that microorganisms cause diseases came to be known as the **germ theory of disease**. Pasteur, the originator of the theory, designed experiments to prove it. The germ theory also led Pasteur and other scientists to link the activity of microorganisms with physical and chemical changes in organic materials.

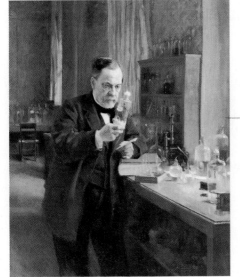
Pasteur demonstrated that microorganisms are present in the air and can infect animals and humans.

Medical Advances of Lister and Koch

Joseph Lister, an English surgeon, built on Pasteur's work and applied it to human medicine. Lister knew that carbolic acid (or phenol) killed bacteria, so he began soaking his surgical

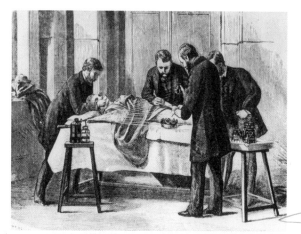

Lister used a mist of carbolic acid to disinfect the operative area during surgery.

dressings in a mild carbolic acid solution to prevent infection. He also developed other antiseptic protocol for his surgical procedures, including aseptic hand-washing and gowning procedures. Lister's sterile practices formed the basis of aseptic technique, which was widely and quickly adopted and is still in use in hospitals and pharmacies. His sterile surgical techniques significantly reduced postoperative infections and saved thousands of lives.

In 1876, German physician Robert Koch advanced the study of microbiology by defining a series of steps, known as *Koch's postulates*, that could be taken to prove that a certain disease was caused by a specific microorganism. Koch's theory was based on his discovery of rod-shaped bacteria in cattle that had died from anthrax. He cultured the bacteria in artificial media and used them to infect healthy animals. When these animals became sick and died, Koch isolated the bacteria in their blood, compared the two sources of the bacteria, and found them to be the same. His research led the way for other scientists to link 20 types of bacteria to specific diseases by the close of the nineteenth century.

Microorganisms

Microorganisms are classified according to type (bacterium, virus, fungus, or protozoan) as well as function (nonpathogenic vs. pathogenic).

Types of Microorganisms

Microorganisms such as bacteria, viruses, fungi, and protozoa are mainly single-celled living organisms and can be found in every habitat on the planet. Specific characteristics of each type are discussed below.

Bacteria A **bacterium** is a type of small, single-celled microorganism. Bacteria can exist in three main forms when viewed under the microscope (see Figure 10.1): spherical (i.e., cocci), rod-shaped (i.e., bacilli), and spiral-shaped (i.e., spirochetes). In the microbiology lab, after Gram staining, some bacteria are identified as either Gram-positive (blue or purple) or Gram-negative (red). Normal human skin is colonized by several bacteria. Bacteria cause a wide variety of illnesses, such as food poisoning, strep throat, ear infections, rheumatic fever, meningitis, pneumonia, tuberculosis, and conjunctivitis.

FIGURE 10.1
Characteristic Bacterial Shapes

(a) Round cocci

(b) Rodlike bacilli

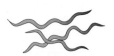

(c) Spiral-shaped spirochetes

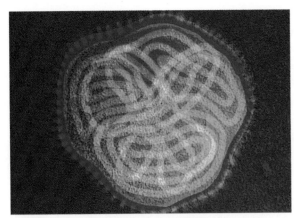

An electron micrograph of a virus. The virus is much smaller than a bacterium and can be viewed only with an electron microscope. It does not have all of the components of a cell and requires other living cells to replicate itself.

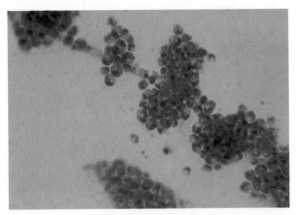

This photomicrograph of the fungus *Candida albicans* indicates its multicellular structure.

Viruses A **virus** is a tiny microorganism that consists of little more than a bit of genetic material enclosed by a casing of protein. Viruses need a living host in which to reproduce, and after replicating, these organisms cause a wide variety of illnesses and diseases, including colds, polio, mumps, measles, chicken pox, shingles, influenza, hepatitis, and human immunodeficiency virus (HIV).

Fungi A **fungus** is a parasite that lives on organisms by feeding on living or dead organic material. Fungi reproduce slowly by means of spores. Spores are microscopic reproductive bodies that can develop into molds, mildews, mushrooms, yeasts, or plants that travel through the air. Some molds are the source of antibiotics such as penicillin. Other fungi are implicated in topical conditions such as athlete's foot, ringworm, or vaginal yeast infections, or in more serious systemic fungal infections deep within the body, which can be potentially life threatening.

Protozoa A **protozoan** is a microscopic organism made up of a single cell or a group of more or less identical cells. Protozoa live in water or as parasites inside other creatures. Examples of protozoa include paramecia and amoebas. Amoebic dysentery, malaria, and sleeping sickness are examples of illnesses caused by protozoa.

Functions of Microorganisms

As mentioned earlier, microorganisms can either be nonpathogenic (harmless or beneficial) or pathogenic (harmful).

Nonpathogenic Microorganisms The majority of microorganisms are, surprisingly, beneficial. Some, in fact, perform essential functions, such as creating by-products that are used to formulate medicines, ferment wine, fix nitrogen in the soil, and help the body break down various food substances. For example, yogurt consists of good bacteria that can reestablish normal flora or the bacteria typically found in the gastrointestinal (GI) tract and reduce diarrhea that may be a side effect of antibiotics.

Pathogenic Microorganisms Pathogenic microorganisms, on the other hand, have led to widespread illness and disease throughout the world.

Epidemics and Pandemics Thousands of pathogenic, or disease-causing, microorganisms have been the scourge of humankind since the beginning of civilization. These microorganisms have been the catalysts of epidemics and pandemics, killing millions of people worldwide. An **epidemic**, according to the CDC, is the increased incidence of a particular disease in a given area or among a certain group of people over a specific period. If an epidemic spreads beyond the borders of a country and affects a sizable population of several other countries, the occurrence is called a **pandemic**. Throughout history, many pandemics have killed millions of people. Some of the most notable pandemics include:

- bubonic plague, a disease caused by bacteria and spread by the fleas of diseased black rats. This pandemic killed 25 million people throughout Europe and Asia during the fourteenth century.
- smallpox, a disease caused by a virus and spread through close contact with others. This disease killed thousands of its victims (mainly children) in seventeenth-century Europe and is responsible for the deaths of more than 300 million people in the twentieth century alone.
- cholera, a disease caused by bacteria and spread through contaminated food or water. There have been seven pandemics of cholera since the nineteenth century, killing millions of individuals on five continents.
- influenza (Spanish flu), a disease caused by the H1N1 virus. This 1918 pandemic killed more than 25 million people worldwide, including 650,000 in the United States, and there are

During the bubonic plague of the fourteenth century, doctors wore full-body garb to protect themselves from the disease. This garb included a leather hat, a mask that covered the entire head, a beak that held pungent herbs to purify the "bad air," a full-length heavy robe coated in wax, leather breeches, and leather gloves and boots.

concerns that a reactivation of this virus could create another pandemic in the near future.

Current Antimicrobial Medications Knowledge of disease transmission, preventive healthcare measures, and advances in medication therapy have had a significant impact on patient outcomes and mortality rates in recent times. Many antimicrobial medications—including antibiotics, antivirals, and antifungals—are effective in killing or neutralizing pathogenic microorganisms. However, many microorganisms can adapt and become resistant to medications. This resistance can be caused by overprescription of antibiotics by prescribers or by incorrect administration of prescribed antimicrobials by patients. The development of antibiotic-resistant bacteria has led to the rise of superbugs, a growing, worldwide healthcare concern.

Sources of Contamination

Harmful microorganisms, especially bacteria, are everywhere in large numbers. However, these microbes cannot cause an infectious disease unless they are transmitted. Unfortunately, this transmittal process is easily accomplished through various modes, including touch, air, and water.

In the hospital pharmacy setting in particular, pharmacy technicians who are preparing CSPs for patient administration must be keenly aware of these modes of microorganism transmission during the preparation of these products. Bacteria or other contaminants can be introduced easily onto a sterile object or device or into a sterile solution. Administration of a contaminated intravenous (IV) solution into a surgical patient or into a patient with a compromised immune system can cause a serious infection or, possibly, death. Therefore, technicians preparing CSPs need to implement preventive measures to reduce or eliminate contamination via touch, air, or water.

Touch

Safety Note

Touch contamination is the most common and dangerous source of contamination when preparing CSPs. Therefore, pharmacy personnel who are preparing sterile products must strictly follow aseptic protocol.

Millions of bacteria live on skin and hair and under nails. Therefore, properly scrubbing the hands and fingernails and following strict aseptic procedures are important to reduce the number of bacteria on the hands before handling and preparing sterile materials. Touching is the most common method of contamination and the easiest to prevent. In addition to frequent hand washing, the use of disposable gloves can minimize touch contamination.

Air

Microorganisms are commonly found in the air, in dust particles, and in moisture droplets. For that reason, sterile materials should be prepared in a designated area in which the number of possible contaminants is maintained at a low level. Special equipment, called a laminar airflow hood or workbench, can control airflow and minimize contamination; this equipment is discussed later in this chapter.

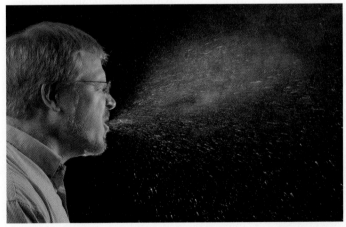
Sneezing causes air contamination by emitting thousands of microorganisms in tiny water droplets.

Water

Even tap water is not completely free of microorganisms. Moisture droplets in the air, especially after a sneeze or cough, often contain harmful microbes. Sterile materials should not be contaminated by exposure to droplets of tap water or other sources of contaminated moisture. A pharmacy technician assigned to prepare sterile products with a common cold should notify the pharmacist supervisor; often a change in work functions for that day is recommended. Protective plastic shields on equipment and the use of face masks minimize moisture contamination.

Asepsis and Sterility

Research on disease transmission and sources of contamination led to the establishment of sterile practices in the nineteenth century. As mentioned earlier, Lister championed aseptic techniques such as wearing sterile gloves, washing hands, and disinfecting surgical instruments and the operative environment to reduce the incidence of infection. For his pioneering work, Lister is called the "Father of Modern Antisepsis."

Koch's research on the link between microorganisms and disease laid the groundwork for asepsis and sterilization practices that are used today.

Asepsis

Asepsis is the absence of pathogenic microorganisms. To ensure asepsis, sterile compounding personnel must follow aseptic technique during the preparation of CSPs. Aseptic technique is a set of practices designed to not introduce any source of infection into a sterile environment. This aseptic protocol includes appropriate garbing, hand-washing, and gloving procedures. Adhering to aseptic protocol is critical because the patient recipients of CSPs are recovering from infection, surgery, or injury and often cannot mount an effective defense against pathogens introduced via parenteral solutions.

Sterility

Sterility is the absence of all microorganisms. The condition is brought about by **sterilization**, or a process that destroys the microorganisms. When an object such as a medical instrument is sterilized, no need exists to identify the species of microbes on it because sterilization kills even the most resistant microbial life forms present.

Methods of Sterilization Sterilization is required when pharmacies create batches, or large premade stock solutions for use for multiple patients for multiple days. Many types of sterilization exist: heat, dry heat, mechanical, gas, and chemical. Many of these methods may be used in a large hospital setting. Some large university hospital pharmacies may also be responsible for the Central Supply Department—a department involved in the sterilization of surgical instruments. Consequently, pharmacy technicians should be familiar with sterilization methods and their clinical applications.

Heat Sterilization One traditional method for killing microbes is heat sterilization or boiling. Using heat to kill microorganisms is an available, effective, economical, and easily controlled method of sterilization. Boiling kills vegetative forms, many viruses, and fungi in about 10 minutes, but more time is required to kill other microorganisms, such as fungus spores and hepatitis viruses. If the water supply in a home is compromised, then the recommendation is to boil the water before drinking. Automatic dishwashers loosely borrow from the concept of heat sterilization during their drying cycle.

Heat sterilization uses an **autoclave**, a device that generates heat and pressure, to sterilize. When moist heat of 121 °C (or 270 °F) under pressure of 15 psi (pounds per square inch) is applied to instruments, solutions, or powders, most known organisms—including spores and viruses—are killed in about 15 minutes. At home, pressure cookers use the concept of heat and pressure to sterilize vegetables. Heat sterilization is being used less frequently in the hospital setting, partly because of space requirements, equipment expense, and personnel training issues.

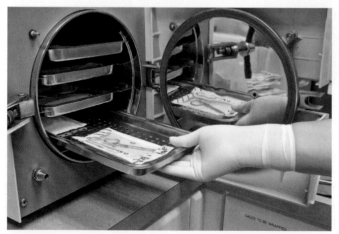

An autoclave generates heat and pressure to sterilize; it kills most known organisms in about 15 minutes.

Dry Heat Sterilization Dry heat, such as direct heat, also destroys all microorganisms. Dry heat is impractical for many substances but is used for the disposal of contaminated objects, which are often incinerated. For proper sterilization using hot, dry air, a temperature of 170 °C must be maintained for nearly two hours. Note that a higher temperature is necessary for dry heat because a heated liquid more readily transfers heat to a cool object.

Mechanical Sterilization Mechanical sterilization is achieved by means of filtration, which is the passage of a liquid or gas through a screenlike material with pores small enough to block microorganisms. This method of sterilization is used for heat-sensitive materials such as culture media (used for growing colonies of bacteria or other microorganisms), enzymes, vaccines, and antibiotic solutions. Filter pore sizes are 0.22 micron for bacteria and 0.01 micron for viruses and some large proteins. Filters may be used in pharmaceutical manufacturing plants as well as in hospital, home healthcare, and long-term care pharmacies. Inline filters used in IV administration sets have been shown to reduce the incidence of infusion-related **phlebitis** (inflammation of the veins). Phlebitis is often caused by microparticulate contamination in IV nutrition preparations as well as select drugs in IV solutions. (For more information on filters, see Chapter 11.)

Gas Sterilization Gas sterilization, which utilizes ethylene oxide, is used for objects that are labile, or subject to destruction by heat. Gas sterilization requires special equipment and aeration of materials after application of the gas. This gas is highly flammable and is used only in large institutions and manufacturing facilities that have adequate equipment to handle the gas. Many prepackaged IV fluids, IV administration sets, and bandages are manufactured and sterilized using this type of sterilization. Ethylene oxide leaves a slight, harmless residue that can be detected as an odor.

Chemical Sterilization Chemical sterilization is the destruction of microorganisms on inanimate objects by chemical means. Few chemicals produce complete sterility, but many reduce microbial numbers to safe levels. A chemical applied to an object or topically to the body for sterilization purposes is known as a **disinfectant**. Iodine, isopropyl alcohol (IPA), and chlorinated bleach are often used as topical or surface disinfectants. Chemical sterilization with sterile 70% IPA is used to clean the work surface of the laminar airflow hood at the beginning of each shift, before each batch, every 30 minutes during continuous compounding periods, after spills, and when surface contamination is known or suspected.

Organizations Overseeing Infection Control

Knowledge of disease transmission and asepsis practices is necessary to understand the importance of infection control. Guidelines and recommendations to prevent infections are developed at both the national level and the local level. At the national level, the Centers for Disease Control and Prevention (CDC) and the United States Pharmacopeia (USP) set guidelines that must be followed by hospitals and healthcare workers. At the local level, a hospital's Infection Control Committee is responsible for implementing these recommendations by developing hospital-specific policies and procedures.

The Centers for Disease Control and Prevention

The **Centers for Disease Control and Prevention (CDC)** is a government agency that provides guidelines and recommendations on infection control. All hospitals must establish infection control policies and oversee their implementation to achieve accreditation by the Joint Commission. Specifically, the CDC publishes reports on the sensitivity and resistance of various bacteria to antibiotics in different regions of the country, providing guidelines on the drug of choice, the dosage, and the duration of treatment for many common infectious illnesses. In addition, the organization also sets guidelines for vaccinations of healthcare workers. This policy has stirred some controversy over whether hospitals can mandate vaccinations for healthcare workers as a condition of their employment—even for those individuals who have no direct patient contact.

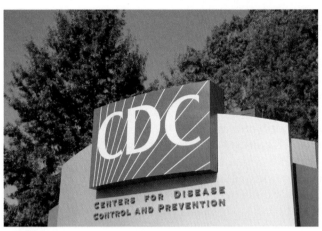

The CDC, based in Atlanta, Georgia, is the government agency that publishes guidelines on infection control to protect both patients and healthcare workers.

Lastly, the CDC publishes and updates guidelines to protect patients and healthcare workers from the transmission of infectious diseases. These guidelines are called Universal Precautions. In fact, the CDC estimates that hospital patients acquire 1.7 million infectious diseases during their stays—a major contributing factor in the death of 99,000 patients each year. Failure of hospitals to adequately train their employees or failure of healthcare personnel to follow proper infection control procedures could produce a high incidence of HAIs, with tragic consequences. (For more information about HAIs, or nosocomial infections, see the section titled "Infection Control Committee.") Some of the infection control procedures outlined in the CDC's guidelines, such as hand hygiene, protective clothing, and vaccinations of personnel, are discussed in the sections below. With the emergence of new, dangerous, or pathogenic strains of bacteria that are resistant to multiple drug therapies, the CDC guidelines outlined below must be strictly followed by all healthcare personnel.

 Safety Note

Sterile compounding personnel who prepare CSPs are required to perform *aseptic hand washing*, a more rigorous hand-washing practice than the guidelines dictated by the CDC. This aseptic hand-washing practice is addressed in the section titled "USP Chapter <797> Standards."

Hand Washing According to the CDC, simple hand washing and hand hygiene are the single most important practices for minimizing touch contamination and reducing the transmission of infectious agents. **Hand washing** is defined as using plain or antiseptic soap and water. To be effective, plain detergent soaps with minimal antimicrobial activity must be used for 20 to 30 seconds, the time needed to rub off the transient skin microorganisms effectively. According to the CDC, the adherence to proper hand-washing technique in the hospital remains less than 50%.

Hand Hygiene **Hand hygiene** is defined as using special alcohol-based rinses, gels, or foams that do not require water. Unless the hands are visibly dirty, the alcohol-based products are preferred because of their superior antimicrobial activity, shorter contact time, quick drying effect, minimal skin irritation, and convenience. Studies of hand hygiene with alcohol-based rubs have demonstrated more effectiveness in reducing microorganisms than antimicrobial or plain soaps. As a result, the transmission of infections within the hospital is minimized.

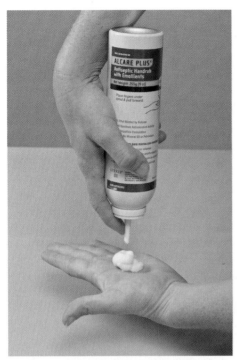

Hand-hygiene practices with alcohol-based foams must be used by healthcare workers and are encouraged for patients and their visitors.

The effectiveness of hand hygiene in infection control may be affected by technique (see Table 10.1), as well as the presence of artificial fingernails and jewelry, which can harbor microorganisms. Hand hygiene is required even if gloves are used or changed. The CDC recommends that every hospital periodically monitor the adherence of staff members to hand-hygiene guidelines. Alcohol-based hand-hygiene products are usually readily available throughout the hospital, including the cafeteria and patient waiting rooms, for use by both healthcare professionals and visitors to minimize the transmission of infection.

Personal Protective Equipment As part of its Universal Precautions, the CDC provides healthcare workers a set of guidelines for the donning of personal protective equipment (PPE). The use of PPE is critical to infection control in a facility, protecting both healthcare workers and others from infectious disease. The donning of PPE must be performed before any contact with a patient and must be removed upon leaving a patient's room. Universal Precautions include the use of a gown or apron to protect clothing and skin; gloves to protect the hands; masks and respirators to protect the mouth, nose, and respiratory tract; goggles to protect the eyes; and face shields to protect the face. The use of these items is dictated by the clinical interaction with the patient.

TABLE 10.1 Hand-Washing and Hand-Hygiene Guidelines

The hand-washing and hand-hygiene guidelines described here are appropriate for infection control procedures in a hospital setting. These procedures are followed by healthcare personnel in several departments, including pharmacy and nursing. *However, it should be noted that special, aseptic hand washing must be performed by personnel preparing sterile products, per USP Chapter <797> guidelines.*

- When washing hands with soap and water, wet hands first with water, apply an amount of product recommended by the manufacturer to hands, and rub hands together vigorously for at least 20 (preferably 30) seconds, covering all surfaces of the hands and fingers. Rinse hands with water and dry thoroughly with a disposable towel. Use the towel to turn off the faucet. Avoid using hot water; repeated exposure to hot water may increase the risk of skin irritation.

- Liquid, bar, or powdered forms of plain soap are acceptable when washing hands with a nonantimicrobial soap and water. When bar soap is used, small bars of soap and soap racks facilitating drainage should be used.

- Dry hands with single-use towels, or air-dry. Multiple-use cloth towels of the hanging or roll type are not recommended for use in healthcare settings because they can transfer infectious agents.

- When disinfecting hands with an alcohol-based hand rub, apply product to the palm of one hand and rub hands together, covering all surfaces of hands and fingers, until hands are dry. Follow the manufacturer's recommendations regarding the volume of product to use.

Source: The Centers for Disease Control and Prevention (CDC), www.cdc.gov

Gown or Apron The gown or apron should be worn over the required uniform or scrubs with the opening in the back. The ties of the gown or apron should be secured.

Masks and Respirators Masks and respirators should be placed over the nose, mouth, and chin and secured to the back of the head using ties or elastic.

Goggles and Face Shields Goggles and face shields should be positioned over the eyes or face and secured to the head with earpieces or elastic.

Gloves The CDC recommends that healthcare workers use gloves, primarily to prevent the transmission of normal or pathogenic skin flora to patients. For most patient care activities, nonsterile gloves are worn. However, sterile gloves must be worn by healthcare practitioners during surgical and other invasive procedures. The donning of gloves is important because aseptic hand washing alone may not prevent the transmission of microorganisms if the hands are heavily contaminated. Personnel who use gloves may be less likely to use correct hand-hygiene practice. For physicians, nurses, and phlebotomists involved in direct patient contact, hand washing and glove use is even more important.

Safety Note

Sterile compounding personnel have different requirements for personal protective equipment. These requirements are dictated by USP Chapter <797> and are discussed in detail in the section titled "USP Chapter <797> Standards."

Gloves are generally made of latex or vinyl; either material appears to offer comparable protection. However, because many healthcare workers and patients may be sensitive to latex, alternative latex-free gloves should be available. Some latex-free gloves are powdered for easier fitting; after their removal, the residual powder may interact with the alcohol-based antiseptic to cause an uncomfortable gritty feel. After glove removal, pharmacy personnel should wash their hands and discard their used gloves in a designated area per hospital procedure. Gloves should never be washed or reused.

Vaccination More than 35,000 individuals die each year as a result of flu complications, with another 200,000 patients hospitalized from contracting the flu virus. In light of those statistics, the CDC recommends that hospital healthcare workers receive an annual flu shot (usually free of charge) to keep those individuals, their family members, and hospitalized patients healthy.

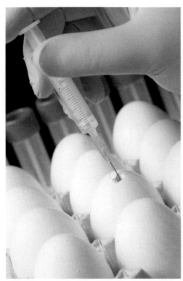

Flu vaccines are created using chicken embryos. These embryos are used to incubate a form of the flu virus that the human body can use to build up immunity against that particular flu strain.

Benefits of the Flu Vaccine For healthcare workers, the flu shot reduces the number of sick days needed. Although many individuals, especially those who are young and healthy, feel as though a flu shot is unnecessary, research has shown that the flu virus can be carried by asymptomatic, healthy individuals and passed on to family members or to hospital patients with whom they have contact. Because many of these hospitalized patients, especially the elderly and young infants, have compromised or weakened immune systems, exposure to the flu virus could be deadly.

A broadscale benefit of the flu shot is a reduction in unnecessary or inappropriate antibiotic use, which can produce drug-resistant organisms. These "superbugs" can cause serious life-threatening infections unresponsive to commercially available antibiotics.

Occasionally, a virulent pathogenic influenza virus can appear and cause a regional epidemic or even a worldwide pandemic. The avian bird flu is an example of a virus that may, in the future, mutate or directly infect humans. In the case of any such outbreak, all healthcare workers should be fully vaccinated to protect themselves and to allow them to provide care for the sick.

Administration of the Flu Vaccine Despite these compelling reasons, studies have shown that only 63% of healthcare workers get an annual flu shot. Flu vaccines are typically 60% to 70% effective during seasons when most circulating influenza viruses are similar to the viruses included in the vaccine. They are not 100% effective because the virus mutates or changes every year. Thus, this year's flu vaccine is often based on the antigenic strains from last year's flu virus. This is why individuals must get a shot every year. The best time to get the vaccination is October or November each year because the immune system can take a few weeks to respond fully to the vaccine. Pharmacy personnel should also be aware that the use of oral or intranasal antiviral drugs may not be as effective as the injectable vaccine.

There are few restrictions for obtaining a flu vaccine. Personnel who have minor illnesses, such as a cold, can be vaccinated. However, healthcare workers who have an acute febrile illness should wait at least 24 hours after the fever has subsided before getting the vaccine. Women who are pregnant can also be vaccinated, but individuals who are hypersensitive to eggs should not receive the flu vaccine. Contrary to popular myth, individuals cannot get the flu from the most common vaccines because these inoculations contain an inactivated (killed) virus. Severe adverse effects are rare.

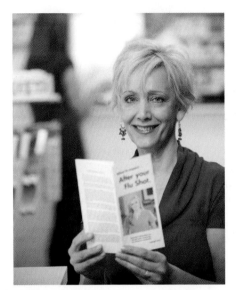

Honest patient information is critical in clearing up misconceptions about the flu vaccine.

 Safety Note

All pharmacy personnel should receive an annual flu vaccine to protect both themselves and their patients from contracting this virus.

Administration of the Nasal Flu Vaccine There is a live, **attenuated virus** present in the nasal flu vaccine marketed as FluMist. This product is indicated for healthy children and adults from ages 2 to 49. According to the Advisory Committee on Immunization Practices (ACIP), the use of the live, attenuated nasal flu vaccine for healthcare workers who care for patients housed in protective environments such as intensive care or cancer patient care units has been a theoretic concern, but transmission of the virus in healthcare settings has not been reported. Because this concern is ongoing, most facilities allow the use of the nasal flu vaccine for healthy healthcare personnel up to age 49 who work in any setting, except those who care for severely immunocompromised patients who require care in an inpatient protective environment.

USP Chapter <797> Standards

The United States Pharmacopeia (USP) publishes guidelines on the preparation of sterile products in a clean room environment using properly trained personnel and protective equipment. For sterile compounding personnel, these guidelines are the primary source of regulations. In 2004, the USP developed the first official and enforceable requirements for sterile compounding to improve the quality standards in the hospital pharmacy. The Joint Commission has adopted these guidelines and evaluates their compliance in hospital pharmacies on future accreditation visits. The original guidelines were modified and updated in 2007 and approved in 2008. Some variance with compliance to the recommendations contained in USP Chapter <797> results from space limitations and hospital size, staffing, and budget; however, most hospital pharmacies strive for full compliance.

The standard, known as **USP Chapter <797>**, focuses on the sterility and stability of a compounded sterile preparation. A **compounded sterile preparation (CSP)** is defined as a sterile product that is prepared outside of the pharmaceutical manufacturer's facility. Sterility refers to the CSP being free from microorganisms, whereas

stability refers to chemical and physical characteristics of the CSP, such as pH, degradation, formation of precipitates (or salts), or unexpected color changes. Both sterility and stability are important considerations in the preparation of a CSP.

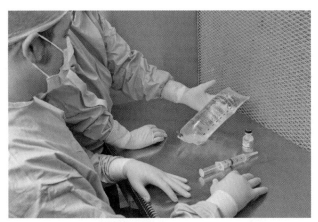
Technicians preparing CSPs must wear personal protective equipment and work in a laminar airflow workbench to ensure sterility of the final product.

As expected, requirements for sterile compounding personnel are more stringent than for healthcare workers who are performing nonsterile compounding (discussed in Chapter 8). Some of these requirements include:

- working in a defined clean-room environment
- monitoring environmental quality specifications
- using special equipment such as a laminar airflow workbench (LAFW)
- performing aseptic hand washing and donning additional garb, such as shoe covers, a hair cover, a face mask, a sterile gown, and sterile gloves
- identifying contamination risk levels of CSPs
- undergoing additional testing and training in principles and practices of aseptic technique
- disinfecting supplies, equipment, and work surfaces

The USP Chapter <797> standards pertain to all personnel—pharmacy technicians and pharmacists—involved in the preparation, storage, and handling of CSPs before administration to the patient. In addition to drugs, CSPs include biologicals, medical imaging diagnostics, nutrients, and radioactive pharmaceuticals. The impact of these standards on the preparation, storage, and handling of total parenteral nutrition (TPN) and hazardous drugs is discussed further in Chapter 11. The USP Chapter <797> standards also apply to all practice settings, including a compounding, nuclear, home health, or long-term healthcare pharmacy, as well as clinics and physicians' offices. If a hospital pharmacy outsources, or sends out, its orders for the preparation of IV additives and/or TPN solutions, then all USP Chapter <797> requirements must be met by the off-site pharmacy.

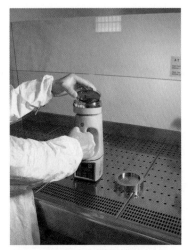
The SAS Air Sampler is a tool for measuring microbial air quality levels in a laminar airflow workbench.

Sterile Compounding Facility A sterile compounding facility is physically designed to minimize contamination. The floor, ceiling, and walls are sealed to provide easy cleaning and to prevent the harboring of microorganisms. The facility is also environmentally controlled by a series of **high-efficiency particulate airflow (HEPA) filter** systems to minimize airborne contamination. The HEPA-filtered heating, ventilation, and air conditioning (HVAC) system of the facility is completely maintained and monitored by the maintenance staff. According to USP Chapter <797>, the air quality must adhere to the **International Organization for Standardization (ISO)** classification system for defining the amount of particulate matter (i.e., potential airborne contamination) allowed in room air where CSPs are prepared. The lower the ISO number is, the less particulate matter is present in the air. Hospital pharmacy labs must conform to the air quality requirements, and workflow patterns must be limited to protect the sterility of the sterile compounding area.

Sterile Compounding Areas As shown in Figure 10.2, the sterile compounding area or IV room is divided into two main areas: the anteroom and the clean room. Personnel are responsible for maintaining the overall cleanliness of these areas. In addition, sterile compounders must follow a routine cleaning schedule of these areas, as outlined in Table 10.2 on the following page.

Anteroom The **anteroom** is where personnel perform aseptic hand washing and garbing procedures, gather the supplies and check for expiration dates and packaging defects, perform calculations, wipe down the surfaces of supplies with an antimicrobial agent, and label the CSP. This is also the area where protective garb is discarded at the completion of the sterile compounding procedure. A small number of supplies used in the sterile compounding procedure are stored in the anteroom, including syringes, needles, and vials. However, cardboard and other materials that have a high potential for shedding should never be stored in this area. The air quality of the anteroom should be maintained at no greater than ISO Class 8.

FIGURE 10.2 Sterile Compounding IV Room Layout

Notice the airflow direction from the high-pressure clean room, through the lower-pressure anteroom, and outward toward the lowest-pressure outer pharmacy area.

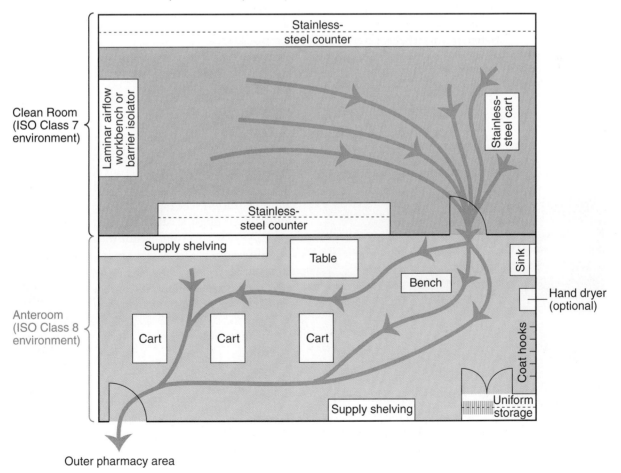

TABLE 10.2 Cleaning in the Sterile Compounding Area

Site	Frequency
LAFWs	At the beginning of each shift, before each batch, every 30 minutes during continuous compounding periods, after spills, and when surface contamination is known or suspected
Counters and easily cleanable work surfaces	Daily
Floors	Daily
Walls	Monthly
Ceilings	Monthly
Storage shelving	Monthly

Clean Room The **clean room**, also known as the *IV room* or *buffer area*, is the inner-most room within the pharmacy and, therefore, is physically segregated from doors and heavy traffic flow to minimize disturbance in airflow. The clean room is the area that houses the laminar airflow hoods used in sterile compounding. Only properly trained and garbed pharmacy personnel have access to this area. The clean room is designed in such a way to maintain an aseptic environment. These design elements include coved and heat-sealed floors and smooth, nonporous walls and ceiling tiles. The temperature and humidity of this room are also maintained at a lower level than surrounding rooms to inhibit the potential for bacterial growth. Finally, a ventilation system pumps HEPA-filtered air in the room to create a positive-pressure environment for sterile compounding. This positive pressure ensures that airflow moves from the high-pressure clean room, through the lower-pressure anteroom, and then outward toward the lowest-pressure outer pharmacy area. The air quality of the clean room should be maintained at no greater than ISO Class 7.

Compounding Equipment and Supplies Only furniture, equipment, and supplies necessary for the preparation of CSPs should be allowed in the defined areas of the compounding area. No long-term storage (i.e., use of IV boxes) is permissible in the clean room. Packaged supplies such as IV bags, administration sets, or syringes should be taken out of their original cartons and cleaned and disinfected with a suitable antimicrobial agent in the anteroom before passage into the clean room area. Similarly, only specific items used for the sterile compounding procedure can be taken into the direct compounding area of the hood.

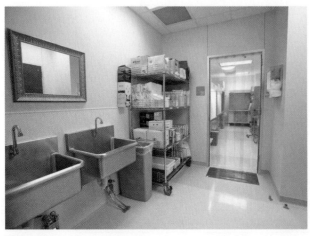

The anteroom is an area where pharmacy technicians stage components and supplies before entering the clean room (seen through the doorway).

Laminar Airflow Hoods Sterile compounding personnel use several types of hoods during the compounding of CSPs. Each type of hood uses HEPA-filtered air to create an ISO Class 5 environment in the **direct compounding area (DCA)** of the hood. An ISO Class 5 environment provides a sterile airflow during the compounding procedure.

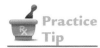

Practice Tip

Pharmacy personnel should be aware that an LAFW is also referred to as a hood.

The two main types of hoods are the horizontal laminar airflow workbench (a positive-pressure LAFW) and the vertical laminar airflow workbench (a negative-pressure LAFW). The horizontal hood is used most frequently in sterile compounding. The vertical hood, which is used to prepare chemotherapy and other hazardous compounds, is typically located away from the horizontal hoods and housed within a negative-pressure room. This negative-pressure environment decreases the risk of employee exposure to dangerous contaminants. In small, rural hospital pharmacies that infrequently prepare hazardous CSPs, the hoods may be located in the same area if a closed-system transfer device (CSTD) is used. This type of transfer device provides a sealed pathway so that hazardous drugs can be safely handled during the compounding procedure. (The CSTD is described in more detail in Chapter 11.)

The specific characteristics and functions of the horizontal and vertical hoods are discussed below.

Safety Note

Sterile compounding personnel should avoid coughing and talking while working in the LAFW to avoid the risk of contamination during sterile product preparation.

Horizontal LAFW A horizontal laminar airflow workbench (LAFW) is a hood used to prepare nonhazardous CSPs. In a horizontal LAFW, room air is pulled into the hood through the prefilter and then through the blower, which forces the air upward, through the HEPA filter, and then horizontally across the work surface toward the worker (see Figure 10.3). As the air passes through the HEPA filter, the filter removes 99.97% of all particles 0.5 micron or larger.

The horizontal LAFW is enclosed on all but one side (the front), and personnel must work at least six inches into the hood to avoid working within the mix of filtered air and room air at the front of the hood. This area, known as the DCA, is the area closest to the hood's HEPA filter and, therefore, receives an uninterrupted flow of sterile air during the compounding process. The air quality of the DCA must be maintained at ISO Class 5 or less to ensure an aseptic area for the preparation of CSPs. Sterile compounding personnel should keep in mind, however, that the risk of contamination from human error or touch still exists in this aseptic area.

FIGURE 10.3
Horizontal Laminar Airflow Workbench

In a horizontal LAFW, room air is drawn into the cabinet, filtered, and forced horizontally across the work surface to prevent contamination during sterile compounding procedures.

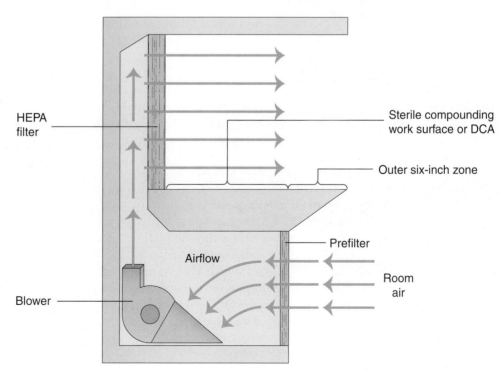

FIGURE 10.4
Overhead View of the Work Surface of a Horizontal Laminar Airflow Hood

Technicians preparing CSPs must work within the direct compounding area to maximize the protective environment of the LAFW.

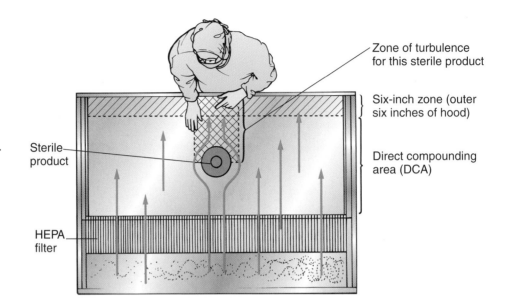

Zone of turbulence for this sterile product

Six-inch zone (outer six inches of hood)

Direct compounding area (DCA)

Sterile product

HEPA filter

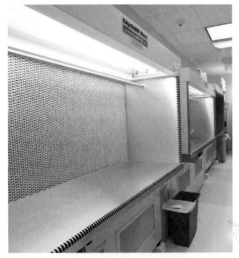

More than one LAFW may be needed in the clean room of a large hospital pharmacy.

To begin sterile compounding procedures, personnel must remove the outer packaging of each supply item while holding the item within the outer six-inch zone of the hood. After discarding the wrappers, workers then place the supply items in designated areas. All small supply items needed for the compounding procedure (ampules, vials, syringes, and so on) are placed within the outer six-inch zone until they are needed. The larger supply items are placed directly within the DCA. The placement of these supplies should not impede the sterile airflow that moves across the work surface and around and over the supplies. Any blockage of airflow, either from the position of supplies or the position of the technician's hands during the compounding procedure, jeopardizes the sterility of the product. The area behind a supply item within the hood, called the *zone of turbulence*, receives an interrupted sterile airflow from the HEPA filter. Consequently, this area is contaminated and should not be used during the compounding procedure. (See Figure 10.4 for an overhead view of the work surface of a horizontal laminar airflow hood.)

Vertical LAFW The **vertical laminar airflow workbench (LAFW)** is a hood used for the preparation of hazardous CSPs, such as chemotherapy drugs. This hood is also known as a Class II biological safety cabinet. In a vertical laminar airflow workbench (see Figure 10.5), the air flows downward through the HEPA filter to the work surface and mixes with room air that enters the prefilter. The air is then forced upward by the blower and through the exhaust HEPA filter to the outside. The front of the hood is partially blocked by a glass shield. The pharmacy technician is often responsible for checking and documenting the status of the operation, a minimum of 12 hourly air exchanges, and HEPA filters for the vertical LAFW.

The technician should wear eye protection, a face mask, and proper apparel—a sterile chemotherapy gown, double sterile gloves, and shoe covers and a hair cover—even when cleaning the vertical laminar airflow hood. The procedures for working with

FIGURE 10.5
Vertical Laminar Airflow Workbench

In a vertical LAFW, room air enters the prefilter and is forced upward through the HEPA filter, then blown downward or vertically from the ceiling toward the work surface, where it is immediately sucked into the air intake grills and drawn away from the worker.

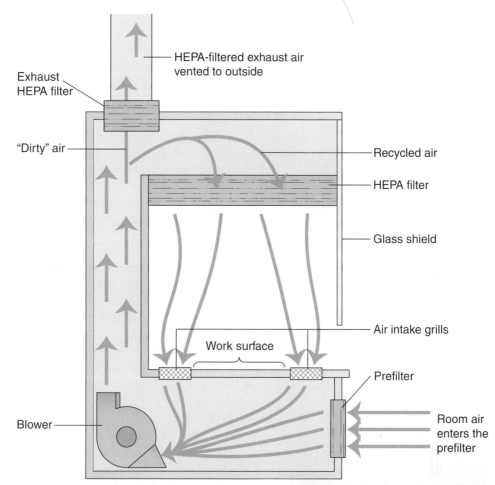

- HEPA-filtered exhaust air vented to outside
- Exhaust HEPA filter
- "Dirty" air
- Recycled air
- HEPA filter
- Glass shield
- Air intake grills
- Work surface
- Prefilter
- Room air enters the prefilter
- Blower

hazardous drugs are designed to protect the hospital pharmacy technician as well as the patient. The preparation, storage, and handling of hazardous drugs are further discussed in Chapter 11.

Maintenance of Both Hoods Horizontal and vertical laminar airflow hoods are regularly cleaned according to USP Chapter <797> guidelines. The hoods' prefilters and HEPA filters require maintenance as well.

Cleaning the Horizontal LAFW The proper cleaning of the horizontal hood is vital to maintaining the sterility of the CSPs. This routine cleaning is an important responsibility of the IV technician and must be documented throughout each shift. The horizontal hood must be cleaned at the beginning of each shift, before each batch compounding session, and every 30 minutes during continuous sterile

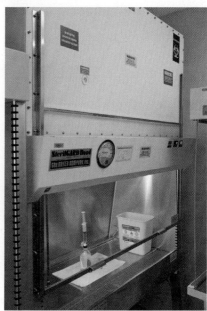

Unlike a horizontal LAFW, a vertical LAFW forces air through an exhaust HEPA filter to the outside. This air movement and a glass shield are present to further protect the healthcare worker.

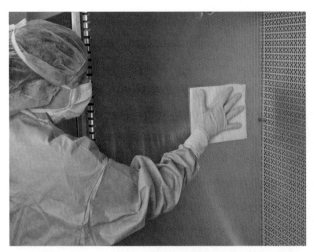

A sterile compounding technician in full protective clothing must clean the entire LAFW before each shift.

Safety Note

During hood cleaning, sterile compounding personnel should never touch the HEPA filter, clean it, or allow fluid to come into contact with the filter. These actions may cause irreparable damage to the HEPA filter.

compounding. The hood also must be cleaned after any spills or suspected contamination. During cleaning, the blower in the laminar airflow hood should remain on, and the technician should be in full protective garb. If the hood is turned off for installation, repair, maintenance, or relocation, then it should be operated for at least 30 minutes before being used to prepare CSPs.

Before cleaning, the sterile compounding technician gathers the necessary supplies in the anteroom, including lint-free, aseptic hood-cleaning wipes, sterile water, and sterile 70% IPA. The entire LAFW, including the clear Plexiglas protective sides, should be cleaned first with sterile water and then with sterile 70% IPA. To protect the integrity of the HEPA filter, these liquid disinfecting agents should be applied to the sterile cleaning wipe rather than directly to the surface of the LAFW.

During the hood-cleaning process, the technician follows a particular sequence, starting with the hood's hang bar and hooks, followed by the hood's ceiling, both sides of the hood, and finally, the work surface (see Figure 10.6). A separate wipe should be used to clean each section of the hood. The cleaning motion depends on the part being cleaned. The top (ceiling) and work surface should be cleaned using overlapping, side-to-side strokes and moving from the innermost part of the work surface to the outer edge of the work surface. The sides should be cleaned using overlapping, down-and-up strokes and moving from the innermost part of the hood to the exterior of the hood. The parts of the hood should be cleaned in the order shown in Figure 10.6—ceiling, back, sides, and work surface—and recorded on a log sheet.

**FIGURE 10.6
Hood-Cleaning Order for a Horizontal LAFW**

The cleaning of a horizontal LAFW is an important responsibility of the pharmacy technician. The sequence and direction of cleaning are important in maintaining a sterile work environment within the hood.

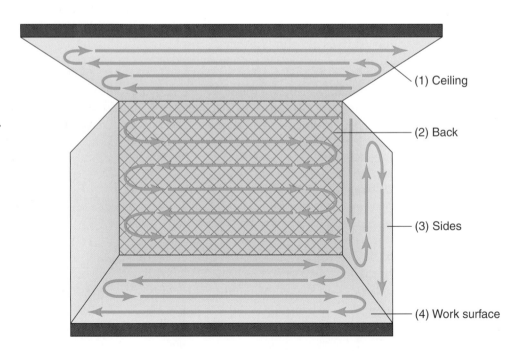

(1) Ceiling

(2) Back

(3) Sides

(4) Work surface

The sterile 70% IPA should remain in contact with the surface for 30 seconds and be fully dry before preparation of a CSP begins. Avoid excessive use of alcohol to disinfect the work surface to avoid buildup of alcohol vapors in the cabinet. Cleaning the work surface with sterile 70% IPA should be repeated after all spills within the LAFW.

Cleaning the Vertical LAFW The proper cleaning of the vertical hood is critical to the sterility of the CSP. Similar to the cleaning of the horizontal hood, the technician first cleans the entire hood with sterile water, followed by the use of 70% IPA. The hood-cleaning process must be completed at intervals prescribed by USP Chapter <797> and documented by sterile compounding personnel. A more thorough, complete decontamination of the hood should be performed at least weekly. The vertical LAFW must be allowed to run continuously during cleaning and decontamination procedures to provide protection to the technician performing the cleaning procedure. In addition, all cleaning procedures should take place at a time when no one else is present in the clean room.

One of the most commonly used vertical hoods is the biological safety cabinet (BSC). The design of the BSC, as well as the type of CSPs prepared in the BSC, necessitates special cleaning procedures. The HEPA filter in the BSC is located in the ceiling of the hood, rather than in the back of the hood as in the horizontal LAFW. Because the HEPA-filtered air flows downward toward the hood's work surface, the cleaning order as well as the direction of the cleaning strokes is different from a horizontal hood. Therefore, the hang bar and hooks should be cleaned first, followed by cleaning the back wall or panel. When cleaning the back panel, technicians should use overlapping side-to-side strokes and move from the area closest to the HEPA filter down toward the work surface. The side walls and glass shield of the BSC should be cleaned using overlapping side-to-side strokes and move from the area closest to the HEPA filter down toward the work surface. The work surface of the BSC should be cleaned using side-to-side strokes and moving from the innermost part of the cabinet toward the outermost edge of the cabinet.

Prefilter and HEPA Filter Maintenance Sterile compounding personnel must replace the hood's prefilter every 30 days and document this process on a checklist located in the anteroom. The HEPA filter, however, is a permanent fixture within the hood and cannot be repaired or replaced. The HEPA filter must be recertified every six months or whenever the hood is moved. This action must also be documented by sterile compounding technicians.

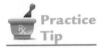
Practice Tip

Pharmacy technicians who prepare sterile products are referred to as IV technicians, sterile compounding technicians, or IV admixture technicians.

Sterile Compounding Personnel Access to the clean room is restricted to those personnel trained to prepare CSPs. Staff members must not wear cosmetics, perfume, hair spray, artificial nails, or nail polish while performing sterile compounding procedures because these substances can flake and compromise the aseptic environment. Any individuals who have certain medical conditions that increase the risk of contamination during the compounding process are also banned from the sterile compounding area. These conditions include respiratory infections, weeping sores, rashes, and sunburn. Lastly, personnel may not have food or beverages in either the anteroom or the clean room and are not allowed to chew gum or engage in horseplay in these areas.

Garbing of Sterile Compounding Personnel The garbing process for sterile compounding personnel follows a strict sequence, moving from the dirtiest or most contaminated item (placing shoe covers on the shoes) to the cleanest item (donning sterile gloves). The sterile gloves must be the cleanest item to avoid microbial touch contamination.

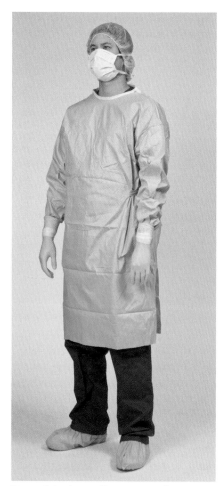

To work in the sterile compounding area, a pharmacy technician must wear full protective clothing to prevent contamination of the CSP.

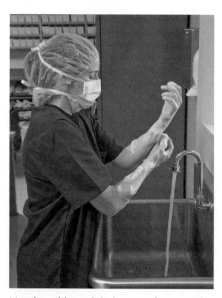

Hand washing minimizes touch contamination and reduces the transmission of disease.

To begin the garbing process, personnel must enter the anteroom and remove all outerwear, such as coats, sweaters, hats, and so on. Compounding technicians must then don lightweight clothing or scrubs before donning protective garb (shoe covers, a hair cover, and a face mask, in that order).

Shoe Covers Disposable shoe covers are placed over the technician's close-toed shoes to keep dirt and other substances from contaminating the floor of the clean room. These shoe covers are removed and discarded upon leaving the anteroom at the completion of sterile compounding procedures in the clean room.

Hair Cover Sterile compounding personnel are required to wear a hair cover or disposable cap. This cap is secured to the head through the use of ties or elastic. Wearing a hair cover avoids contamination of the hood or CSP during sterile compounding procedures.

Face Mask A face mask is worn by technicians to cover the nose and mouth during sterile compounding. This mask is secured to the back of the head with elastic or ties and is used to catch the bacteria contained in the liquid droplets and aerosols that emanate from the nose and mouth. If the sterile compounder has a beard, a beard cover must also be worn to avoid contamination during the procedure.

Aseptic Hand Washing Next, the technicians must perform an aseptic hand washing using an acceptable cleansing agent such as chlorhexidine gluconate. Aseptic hand-washing procedures are rigorous and require personnel to follow a specific cleansing sequence. The cleansing sequence lasts from 2 to 4 minutes and alternates between the left and right hands and forearms. This hand-washing process is completed multiple times during sterile compounding, including upon entering or reentering the sterile compounding area; after a major contamination such as a drug spill; after touch contamination; and after eating, sneezing, coughing, or using the restroom.

Gowning and Gloving The last two procedures before beginning the sterile compounding procedures involve gowning and gloving.

Gowning Personnel must don a sterile, disposable, nonshedding gown available in the anteroom. The gown should be removed from the hanger without touching the floor and should be pulled up the arms and over the shoulders. The gown should be secured by the waist ties and should fit snugly around the wrists.

Safety Note

Pharmacy personnel should *not* use petroleum-based ointments, creams, or lotions before donning sterile gloves as these products may decrease the integrity of the sterile gloves.

Gloving Finally, sterile compounding technicians should don sterile, powder-free gloves. They should inspect the sterile gloves regularly during their shift for tears or punctures and, if found, should immediately replace the sterile gloves with a new pair. In addition, personnel must disinfect the gloves with sterile 70% IPA every time that the gloves touch a nonsterile surface.

Other Garbing Regulations

Personnel should also be aware of USP Chapter <797> guidelines that address specific situations regarding garbing. For example, if a technician leaves the sterile compounding area (to use the restroom, to go to lunch, and so on), then the entire garbing and hand-washing process must be repeated. However, the technician may don the same gown provided that the gown is clean, is turned inside out, and is hung in the anteroom without touching the floor. All garb should be discarded in a designated area of the anteroom at the end of the shift.

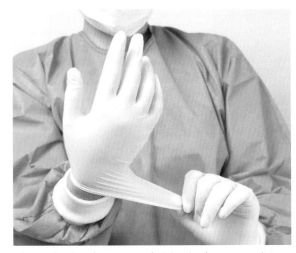

Gloving by the pharmacy technician in the preparation of sterile products provides an additional safeguard to touch contamination.

If a technician is working with hazardous drugs, additional protection such as goggles and a second pair of sterile gloves (known as *double gloving*) is required, and a new gown must be worn each time the clean room area is entered. (For more information on the garbing requirements for compounding hazardous drugs, see Chapter 11.)

Contamination Risk Levels

USP Chapter <797> defines microbial contamination risk levels associated with the preparation of CSPs. These risk levels are based on the probability of microbial, chemical, or physical contamination. As defined in Chapter 8, beyond-use dating (BUD) is the date beyond which a CSP shall not be used or stored. How does a CSP differ from a manufactured sterile product? An IV bag of dextrose and water is a sterile product approved by the FDA, with a manufacturer's **expiration date**, or shelf life. An IV bag of dextrose and water with an antibiotic such as IV penicillin that is compounded in a licensed pharmacy is a CSP with beyond-use dating.

For CSPs, a BUD is a conservative estimate based on contamination risk or specific sterility testing provided by the hospital or manufacturer. Risk levels for CSPs are

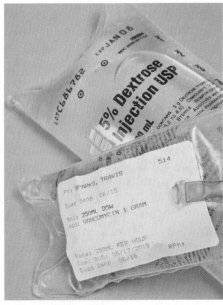

Expiration dating refers to a manufactured product, whereas beyond-use dating, or BUD, refers to a CSP.

defined as low, medium, high, and immediate. Documentation of sterility testing and assignment of beyond-use dating become more comprehensive and restrictive with high-risk CSPs compared with low-risk CSPs.

- Low-risk CSPs include sterile products that have been manipulated using aseptic technique for a single-volume transfer, such as the transfer of a sterile solution withdrawn from an ampule, a vial or bottle, or a bag with a sterile syringe and needle. This level also includes the transfer, measuring, and mixing of a CSP containing three or fewer ingredients.
- Medium-risk CSPs include multiple sterile products combined using automated devices or transferred from multiple sterile containers into a final sterile container such as an IV bag. Unlike low-risk CSPs, those CSPs at this level involve multiple-volume transfers and more complex aseptic technique. An example is a TPN solution containing more than three electrolytes or vitamins.
- High-risk CSPs include products that have been compounded from nonsterile ingredients and sterile products without preservatives or those exposed to inferior air quality. All high-risk CSPs must be sterilized by using a 0.22 micron filter to remove particulate matter, by autoclaving, or by dry heat. The method of sterilization chosen is dependent on the chemical stability of the product. Examples include dissolving nonsterile ingredients into a CSP and filtering before patient use.
- Immediate-use CSPs are any CSPs made outside of a Class 5 ISO, such as those CSPs that might be needed in any emergency situation.

Table 10.3 lists the suggested BUDs of various CSPs by risk level and storage temperature. Some small hospital pharmacies may be involved only in the preparation of low- and medium-risk CSPs. Immediate-use CSPs, such as mixing drugs during a resuscitation code, are exempt from compliance with standards.

TABLE 10.3 Standard Beyond-Use Dating by Risk Level*

Risk Level	Room Temperature	Refrigerator	Freezer
Low	48 hours	14 days	45 days
Medium	30 hours	9 days	45 days
High	24 hours	3 days	45 days

* If reliable scientific testing data are available, then the beyond-use dating can be adjusted.

Training Required to Work with CSPs A pharmacy technician working in the sterile compounding area of a hospital pharmacy clearly holds an important and responsible position and, therefore, must be highly educated and trained. Classroom instruction, interactive learning modules in a laboratory setting, independent assignments, and supervised on-the-job training must be completed before a technician can prepare CSPs. In many hospitals, a technician must work in the hospital pharmacy for one year before training as a sterile compounding technician. Written tests and skills assessments must be passed and documented, usually on an annual basis, to meet USP guidelines and Joint Commission accreditation standards. The technician may be required or encouraged to obtain additional certifications for sterile compounding. With such certifications and experience, the technician may be rewarded in salary for CSP-related responsibilities.

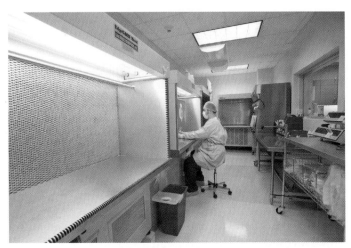

Correct sterile compounding and aseptic technique procedures—performed by highly trained personnel in a clean room environment—are essential to patient health and safety.

In a home healthcare setting, the patient or a caregiver may be responsible for the administration of a CSP. To that end, USP Chapter <797> standards require that a formalized training program be in place to ensure proper understanding and compliance with this complex procedure. Typically, a pharmacist or nurse is responsible for training the patient or caregiver in the proper self-administration of a CSP.

Infection Control Committee

Infection control is the responsibility of all healthcare workers. Patients and employees are only safe from infectious processes when everyone working in the hospital follows good infection control techniques. Within the hospital, the **Infection Control Committee (ICC)** is responsible for implementing CDC and USP guidelines and overseeing the training of all healthcare workers in the facility. The ICC also monitors the incidence of HAIs and the proper use of antibiotics within the hospital. Lastly, the committee plays a major role in ensuring that the hospital is in compliance with the Joint Commission accreditation standards. To gain hospital accreditation (and reimbursement from insurance providers), all of these guidelines and recommendations must be followed carefully.

The ICC is generally made up of physicians, nursing staff, infection control practitioners, quality assurance personnel, and risk management personnel, as well as representatives from microbiology, surgery, central sterilization, and environmental services. A pharmacist with an interest and expertise in antibiotics is also a member of the team. The goal of this interdisciplinary team is to bring together individuals with expertise in different areas of health care.

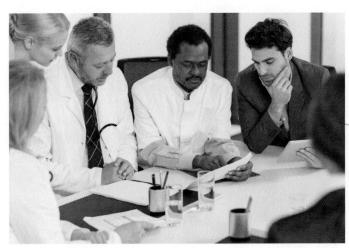

The Infection Control Committee develops infection control procedures within a hospital, including the implementation of measures to control HAIs. This committee typically meets once a month to review infection patterns at the facility.

Role and Responsibilities of the ICC The primary role of the ICC is to prevent, identify, and control **healthcare-associated infections (HAIs)**, as well as infections from the community brought into the hospital. An HAI, also called a *nosocomial infection*, occurs when bacteria, viruses, or fungi found in the hospital from any source cause a patient to develop an infectious disease. Some HAIs are resistant to antibiotic treatment and can be life-threatening. According to the CDC, 2 million patients develop new infections in the hospital each year, or one of every 20 patients hospitalized. These HAIs result in additional costs from an extended hospital stay as well as the increasing use of antibiotics, which can lead to bacterial resistance. More importantly, HAIs may cause patient disability or even death.

Adherence to recommended infection control guidelines can significantly decrease the transmission of infectious agents. The hospital pharmacy technician, especially when preparing CSPs, must rigidly follow guidelines designed to protect the technician as well as the patient recipients of the sterile products.

This committee sets infection control policy and is involved in planning, monitoring, evaluating, updating, and educating healthcare personnel and hospital patients. Some of their responsibilities include:

- surveillance of HAIs
- evaluation of antibiotics and other medications
- investigation of infection outbreaks and infection clusters
- development of infection control procedures for all departments and staff members
- patient education concerning medical waste management

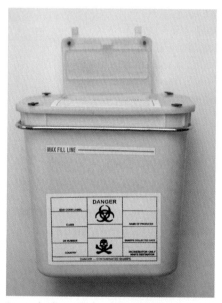

Properly discarded used syringes and needles in a sharps container can minimize disease transmission and needle sticks.

The committee may be involved in evaluating which disinfectant should be used in the surgical operating room or which kind of sterilization is best for medical instruments. If resistance of microorganisms to an antibiotic is increasing, then the committee may review whether the antibiotic is being used inappropriately or in a dosage that is too small. If an outbreak should occur, then the committee investigates to determine the cause of the problem and recommends the necessary education or changes in protocols.

Annual educational programs are conducted for all hospital employees on general infection control guidelines, and mechanisms to update and disseminate new information to staff are designed. Another policy of importance to the pharmacy technician may include the handling and disposal of medical waste, as well as the proper discarding of **sharps** into a special and appropriately labeled container.

In addition to preventing hospital workers from spreading infectious diseases to patients, the hospital is also responsible for preventing workers from contracting infectious diseases from patients. The ICC is responsible for educating all hospital employees about the importance of following necessary procedures to minimize employee exposure. These procedures are adopted from the CDC's Universal Precautions discussed earlier in this chapter.

Implementation of Universal Precautions Because hospital personnel are routinely exposed to blood and bodily fluids (saliva, semen, GI fluid, lymphatic fluid, sebum, mucus, and excrement) that carry bacteria and viruses, a hospital's ICC oversees the implementation and training of personnel in **Universal Precautions**. These guidelines are intended to protect personnel from contracting infections and diseases—such as HIV, tuberculosis (TB), and hepatitis B and C—from their exposure or contact with these fluids. Table 10.4 provides a list of the general guidelines that make up the Universal Precautions. In addition to following Universal Precautions, hospital personnel must be up-to-date on their immunizations before providing patient care.

TABLE 10.4 Universal Precautions

- Universal Precautions apply to all individuals within the hospital.
- Universal Precautions apply to all contact or potential contact with blood, other bodily fluids, or body substances.
- Disposable gloves must be worn when contact with blood or other bodily fluids is anticipated or possible.
- Hands must be washed thoroughly after removing the latex gloves.
- Blood-soaked or contaminated materials, such as gloves, towels, or bandages, must be disposed of in a wastebasket lined with a plastic bag.
- Properly trained custodial personnel must be called if cleanup or removal of contaminated waste is necessary.
- Contaminated materials, such as needles, syringes, swabs, and catheters, must be placed in red plastic containers labeled for disposal of biohazardous materials. Proper institutional procedures generally involve incineration.
- A first-aid kit must be kept on hand in any area in which contact with blood or other bodily fluids is possible. The kit should contain, at minimum, the following items:
  - adhesive bandages for covering small wounds
  - alcohol
  - antiseptic or disinfectant
  - bottle of bleach, which is diluted at the time of use to create a solution containing 1 part bleach to 10 parts water, for use in cleaning up blood spills
  - box of disposable latex gloves
  - disposable towels
  - medical adhesive tape
  - plastic bag or container for contaminated waste disposal
  - sterile gauze for covering large wounds

Universal Precautions are applied more by those healthcare workers with direct patient contact or by those who handle patients' bodily fluids and tissues—such as physicians, nurses, laboratory staff, and respiratory care technicians. Pharmacy personnel generally do not have direct patient contact but should be cautious and cover an open wound or cut before performing their duties. Pharmacists in the community pharmacy and personnel who are working at healthcare fairs are becoming more involved in the administration of vaccines—such as influenza, pneumonia, and shingles—to high-risk patients. Therefore, these healthcare practitioners should be aware of infection control measures discussed in this chapter and should follow Universal Precautions.

Chapter Summary

- The identification of microorganisms as a cause of infectious disease is a surprisingly recent development.
- Bacteria, viruses, fungi, and protozoa are examples of microorganisms that can be harmful.
- Various types of sterilization are available to kill microorganisms on medical instruments, devices, and surfaces.
- The CDC publishes guidelines to minimize the transmission of infectious disease within the hospital environment.
- Proper hand-washing and hand-hygiene practices are the most important ways to minimize touch contamination.
- Certain medical conditions, including respiratory illness, sunburn, weeping sores, and rash, prohibit the pharmacy technician from working in a clean room environment.
- Every healthcare worker should have up-to-date immunizations.

- USP Chapter <797> guidelines provide official and enforceable requirements for improving the quality of CSPs.
- A CSP requires preparation using special aseptic techniques to minimize the risk of contamination.
- The proper use of an LAFW can minimize airborne contamination.
- A vertical LAFW is required for the preparation of hazardous IV drugs.
- A CSP has more restrictive beyond-use dating than a manufactured sterile product or a nonsterile preparation.
- The assignment of BUDs for sterile products depends on contamination risk level and storage conditions.
- The major role of the ICC is the prevention of HAIs.
- Universal Precautions are used to prevent infection when a hospital worker comes into contact with blood or other bodily fluids.

Key Terms

anteroom the area of the sterile compounding lab that is used for hand washing and garbing, staging of components, order entry, CSP labeling, and other high-particulate-generating activities

asepsis the absence of pathogenic microorganisms

attenuated virus a weakened virus contained in some vaccines as opposed to a live or inactive virus

autoclave a device that generates heat and pressure to sterilize objects

bacterium a small, single-celled microorganism that can exist in three main forms, depending on type: spherical (i.e., cocci), rod-shaped (i.e., bacilli), and spiral (i.e., spirochetes)

Centers for Disease Control and Prevention (CDC) a government agency that provides guidelines and recommendations on health care, including infection control

clean room an area that includes the staging areas and the LAFWs; also called the *IV room* or *buffer area*

compounded sterile preparation (CSP) a sterile product that is prepared outside the pharmaceutical manufacturer's facility, typically in a hospital or compounding pharmacy

direct compounding area (DCA) the sterile, compounding work area of the LAFW, in which the concentration of airborne particles is controlled with a HEPA filter providing ISO Class 5 air quality

disinfectant a chemical, such as rubbing alcohol, that is applied to an object or topically to the body for sterilization purposes

epidemic the occurrence of more cases of disease (such as the flu) than expected in a given area or among a specific group of people over a particular period

expiration date the date after which a manufacturer's product should not be used

fungus a single-celled organism similar to human cells that is marked by a rigid cell wall, reproduction by spores, and the absence of chlorophyll; feeds on living organisms (or on dead organic material)

germ theory of disease the idea that microorganisms cause diseases

hand hygiene the use of special dry, alcohol-based rinses, gels, or foams that do not require water

hand washing the use of plain or antiseptic soap and water with appropriate time and technique

healthcare-associated infection (HAI) an infection that a patient acquires as a result of treatment in a healthcare facility; also called a *nosocomial infection*

high-efficiency particulate airflow (HEPA) filter a device used with LAFWs to filter out most particulate matter and to establish an aseptic environment in which to prepare parenteral products

horizontal laminar airflow workbench (LAFW) a type of hood that is used to prepare IV drug admixtures, nutrition solutions, and other parenteral products aseptically

Infection Control Committee (ICC) a hospital committee that provides leadership in relation to infection control policies

International Organization for Standardization (ISO) a classification system to measure the amount of particulate matter in room air; the lower the ISO number, the less particulate matter is present in the air

microbiology the study of microorganisms

microorganism a living microscopic organism or microbe such as a bacterium, fungus, protozoan, or virus

pandemic an epidemic that occurs across several countries and affects a sizable portion of the population in each country

pasteurization a sterilization process designed to kill most bacteria and mold in milk and other liquids

phlebitis an inflammation of the veins often caused by microparticulate contamination

protozoan a single-celled organism that inhabits water and soil

sharp a used needle, which can be a source of infection

spontaneous generation an erroneous belief in the seventeenth century that some forms of life could arise spontaneously from matter; for example, that maggots could arise from decaying flesh

stability the chemical and physical characteristics of the CSP, such as pH, degradation, formation of precipitates (or salts), or unexpected color changes

sterility the absence of all microorganisms

sterilization a process that destroys the microorganisms on a substance

Universal Precautions procedures followed in healthcare settings to prevent infection as a result of exposure to blood or other bodily fluids

USP Chapter <797> guidelines on the sterility and stability of CSPs developed by the United States Pharmacopeia (USP) that have become standards for hospital accreditation

vertical laminar airflow workbench (LAFW) a type of hood that offers additional protection for both the sterile compounding technician and the environment when aseptically compounding toxic chemicals; examples of these types of hoods include a biological safety cabinet and a compounding aseptic containment isolator

virus a minute infectious agent that does not have all of the components of a cell and thus can replicate only within a living host cell

Chapter Review

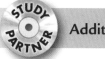

Additional Quiz Questions

Checking Your Understanding

To check your comprehension of this chapter's key concepts, read the following multiple-choice questions and then record your answers on a separate sheet of paper. Write your answers as modeled in these examples: 1d; 2c; 3b; *etc.*

1. A pathogenic microorganism can cause
   a. a heart attack.
   b. an embolism.
   c. a thrombosis.
   d. an infectious disease.

2. The principle of immunization against disease was discovered by
   a. Robert Hooke.
   b. Edward Jenner.
   c. Anton van Leeuwenhoek.
   d. Louis Pasteur.

3. Who was the first individual to demonstrate that microorganisms are present in the air?
   a. Edward Jenner
   b. Joseph Lister
   c. Louis Pasteur
   d. Francesco Redi

4. A small, single-celled microorganism is known as a
   a. bacterium.
   b. protozoan.
   c. virus.
   d. fungus.

5. A virus causes a variety of diseases including
   a. influenza.
   b. strep throat.
   c. malaria.
   d. ringworm.

6. The absence of disease-causing microorganisms is known as
   a. Universal Precautions.
   b. hand hygiene.
   c. asepsis.
   d. mechanical sterilization.

7. What type of sterilization uses an autoclave?
   a. heat
   b. chemical
   c. gas
   d. mechanical

8. Which type of sterilization do IV bags and administration sets undergo during the manufacturing process?
   a. dry heat
   b. mechanical
   c. chemical
   d. gas

9. The most common source of contamination is
   a. touch.
   b. air.
   c. water.
   d. dust.

10. The best way to minimize touch contamination with a CSP is by
    a. not wearing jewelry in the clean room.
    b. hand washing and hand hygiene.
    c. wearing shoe covers.
    d. working in a laminar airflow hood.

11. The laminar airflow hood should be cleaned with 70% IPA
    a. before each shift.
    b. daily.
    c. only after spills.
    d. weekly with change of HEPA filter.

12. Identify the incorrect statement about wearing sterile gloves in the hospital pharmacy.
    a. Sterile gloves are required in the clean room.
    b. Latex-free sterile gloves are available to individuals with latex allergies.
    c. Sterile gloves can be reused if not dirty.
    d. Two pairs of sterile gloves are worn when compounding hazardous drugs.

13. USP Chapter <797> primarily addresses
    a. infection control policies within the hospital.
    b. sensitivity testing for antibiotics to prevent HAIs.
    c. documentation of controlled drugs.
    d. prevention of contamination of CSPs.

14. The primary role of the Infection Control Committee is to
    a. approve antibiotics for the hospital formulary.
    b. purchase antibiotics.
    c. verify correct dosages on all medication orders for antibiotics.
    d. prevent HAIs.

15. Universal Precautions deal with infections by disease-causing microorganisms found in
    a. tap water and other liquid sources.
    b. blood and other bodily fluids.
    c. immediate-use medication vials.
    d. TPN solutions.

Reinforcing Your Learning

To build on your understanding of the topics in this chapter, complete the following enrichment activities.

1. If your instructor can access petri dishes or plates, then experiment with the common sources of contamination, such as touch, air, and water. Incubate the petri dishes or plates overnight at a controlled temperature and check for bacterial growth over the next few days.

2. If you have access to a lab, demonstrate for your instructor correct hand-washing and hand-hygiene techniques. Discuss the pros and cons of soap vs. alcohol use on hands. Which disinfectant should be used on the surface of the LAFW, and how long must it be in contact before the technician begins the sterile compounding process?

3. What is the possible role for each of these members of the Infection Control Committee?
    a. physician
    b. pharmacist
    c. nurse
    d. hospital administrator
    e. representative of the housekeeping staff

Thinking on Your Feet

To gain practice in handling challenging situations in the workplace, consider the following real-world scenarios and then use the guiding questions to help you formulate your responses.

1. The Joint Commission is scheduled for a visit, and the director of pharmacy would like you to review and recommend a policy on pharmacy personnel who come to work with a cold. What written procedures would you implement to reduce and prevent the transmission of viral disease?

2. You receive a medication order for gentamicin 120 mg in 100 mL of D_5W IVPB stat. You have a stock vial of gentamicin with a concentration of 40 mg/mL, with a manufacturer's expiration date of 8/2016.
   a. How many milliliters would be needed to prepare this IVPB?
   b. Is this considered a low-risk, medium-risk, or high-risk CSP?

   c. Besides the drug and IVPB bag, what other equipment do you need to prepare this CSP?
   d. Given that this IVPB was prepared from sterile ingredients in a laminar airflow hood, what beyond-use dating would be appropriate for this CSP?

3. You are randomly selected by a member of the Joint Commission survey team to demonstrate the preparatory procedures you complete (garbing and aseptic hand washing) before entering the clean room. Recite or demonstrate (if garb is available) these procedures in their proper order.

Acquiring Field Knowledge

To expand your knowledge of pharmacy practice, explore the following online activities that focus on research and information retrieval.

Reminder: *As you navigate the Internet, remember to exercise caution and good judgment when evaluating information. A thoughtful review of online text should take into consideration the following factors: the creator and sponsors of the website, the intended audience, the credentials of the authors and contributors, the reliability and validity of the posted information, the frequency of updates to the site, and the ease of navigation for a range of user skill levels.*

1. The importance of sterility of CSPs was demonstrated in the outbreak of infections and death at the New England Compounding Center in 2012. Go to www.paradigmcollege.net/pharmpractice5e/meningitis and www.paradigmcollege.net/pharmpractice5e/compounding. How many total cases were reported to the FDA? What was the primary complication? How many deaths? Were these cases and deaths preventable? What were the causes of the outbreak?

2. On the ASHP website, hover over the Practice & Policy tab and highlight Policy Positions and Guidelines. Click on Medication Therapy and Patient Care and find the ASHP position on the Pharmacist's Role in Antimicrobial Stewardship and Infection Prevention and Control. List eight ways that the pharmacy department can reduce the risk of transmission of infections.

3. Go to www.paradigmcollege.net/pharmpractice5e/immunizations and see what immunizations are recommended for physicians and nurses who elect to work in a hospital.

Sampling the Certification Exam

To provide you with practice for the Certification Exam, read the following questions that have been patterned after the test format and then record your answers on a separate sheet of paper. Write your answers as modeled in these examples: 1d; 2c; 3b; *etc.*

1. What is the name of the set of procedures used to prevent infection caused by exposure to blood or other bodily fluids?
   a. Blood Precautions
   b. Universal Precautions
   c. Sterile Precautions
   d. Aseptic Technique

2. Which ISO class is most appropriate for direct sterile compounding?
   a. ISO Class 8
   b. ISO Class 7
   c. ISO Class 6
   d. ISO Class 5

3. The name for an infection acquired while in the hospital is a/an
   a. healthcare-associated infection.
   b. empirical infection.
   c. aerobic infection.
   d. superinfection.

4. Shingles is caused by a
   a. bacterium.
   b. fungus.
   c. protozoan.
   d. virus.

5. Which of the following activities can best prevent the spread of infection?
   a. hand washing
   b. surface disinfection
   c. sterilization
   d. wearing a face mask

6. Which of the following is *not* considered a disinfectant?
   a. iodine
   b. IPA
   c. chlorinated bleach
   d. sterile water

7. Working under a laminar airflow hood will minimize which type of contamination?
   a. touch
   b. air
   c. water
   d. packaging

8. What is the proper order for cleaning the horizontal LAFW?
   a. hang bar and hooks, ceiling, side, opposite side, work surface
   b. ceiling, hang bar and hooks, side, opposite side, HEPA filter, work surface
   c. work surface, side, opposite side, ceiling, hang bar and hooks
   d. HEPA filter, hang bar and hooks, ceiling, side, opposite side, work surface

9. Which healthcare worker is a candidate for the annual flu vaccine?
   a. an individual who has a history of an adverse reaction to the vaccine
   b. a woman who is pregnant
   c. a person who is allergic to eggs
   d. a patient who has an acute febrile illness

10. Standards for the sterility and stability of CSPs have been developed by the
    a. United States Pharmacopeia.
    b. Centers for Disease Control and Prevention.
    c. Food and Drug Administration.
    d. Drug Enforcement Administration.

Compounding Sterile Products and Hazardous Drugs

11

Learning Objectives

- Identify the role and function of equipment used in intravenous preparation and administration, including syringes, needles, intravenous sets, catheters, infusion pumps, and filters.

- Identify the components of an intravenous administration set.

- Describe common characteristics of intravenous solutions, including pH value, osmolarity and osmolality, tonicity, compatibility, and stability.

- Identify types of intravenous solutions, including large-volume and small-volume parenteral solutions.

- Summarize the steps necessary for aseptic technique in a hospital pharmacy.

- Describe the correct procedure used in preparing compounded sterile preparations from vials and ampules for hazardous and nonhazardous agents.

- Discuss the preparation of total parenteral nutrition.

- Differentiate between expiration dating and beyond-use dating.

- Understand the types of premade parenteral products, including vial-and-bag systems and frozen intravenous solutions, and their handling requirements.

- Calculate intravenous flow rates.

- Discuss the importance of and techniques for preparing, handling, and disposing of hazardous agents.

- Define the purpose and list examples of quality assurance programs in the hospital.

Preview chapter terms and definitions.

Compared with a community pharmacy, a hospital pharmacy carries out unique activities, such as the routine compounding of sterile preparations and the preparing, handling, and disposing of hazardous drugs. A major responsibility of the pharmacy technician is the preparation of these compounded sterile preparations (CSPs) that may contain medications, electrolytes, vitamins, minerals, or nutrition for patients with serious illnesses.

This chapter describes the equipment and aseptic technique used in the preparation of intravenous (IV) products from vials and ampules. **Aseptic technique** refers to the processes and physical preparation methods used by sterile compounding personnel to avoid introducing pathogens, or disease-causing microorganisms, into parenteral products. The preparation of special IV solutions—such as total parenteral nutrition (TPN), frozen antibiotics, and medications available in vial-and-bag systems—is also addressed. Finally, this chapter provides examples for calculating IV flow rates, a skill used by sterile compounding technicians to prepare a 24-hour supply of CSPs for individual patients in designated facilities.

As you learned in Chapter 10, the preparation of all parenteral products must be done in compliance with the sterile compounding and aseptic technique standards established by the United States Pharmacopeia (USP). These standards are included in Chapter <797> of the *USP Pharmacists' Pharmacopeia* and are referred to simply as USP Chapter <797>.

Sterile Supplies for IV Preparation and Administration

A wide variety of supplies is used in the preparation of IV medications in a hospital pharmacy. Most of these supply items are sterile, disposable devices that save the pharmacy preparation time and money and that provide patients with lifesaving sterile products. Disposable supply items that are used to prepare and administer IV products include syringes and needles, IV administration sets, and certain types of filters.

Syringes and Needles

Syringes and needles are used in both the preparation and administration of CSPs. In the hospital pharmacy, sterile compounding technicians use a needle-and-syringe unit for withdrawing or injecting solutions during the preparation of a CSP. These processes may include using a diluent to reconstitute a powdered medication, withdrawing fluid from a vial, or transferring fluid from one container to another. A needle-and-syringe unit is also used by the nursing staff to administer CSPs via **IV push (IVP)** or bolus administration or—more commonly—by IV infusion.

Syringes Syringes are made of glass or plastic. Glass syringes are limited to compounding scenarios in which a drug is incompatible with syringe components or when certain chemotherapy products are prepared. These syringes are expensive to purchase and, when used in sterile compounding, are generally considered to be single-use items. In rare compounding scenarios, such as those requiring preparation of highly concentrated chemotherapy solutions, glass syringes may be reused after sterilization in an autoclave.

Most syringes used in sterile compounding are made of plastic components or polyvinyl chloride (PVC). These syringes offer many advantages. In addition to being less expensive, plastic syringes are supplied by manufacturers in sterile packaging and are disposable.

Parts of a Syringe The main components of a syringe include the syringe tip, the barrel containing the calibration marks, and the rubber-tipped piston plunger (see Figure 11.1). The piston plunger, the inner plunger shaft, and the syringe tip are sterile and must not be touched.

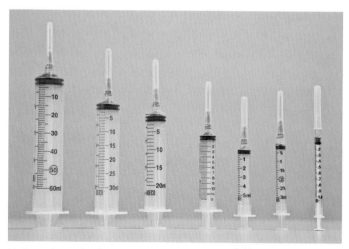

Various sizes of syringes ranging in volume from 60 mL (left) to 1 mL (right) are used in sterile compounding.

FIGURE 11.1
**Syringe
Components**

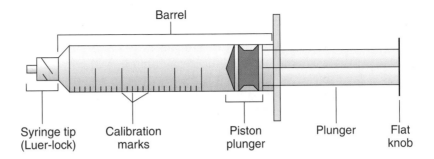

Barrel

Syringe tip
(Luer-lock) Calibration
marks Piston
plunger Plunger Flat
knob

Syringe Selection and Measurement During the sterile compounding process, technicians should select the smallest syringe that is able to hold the desired volume. For the most part, technicians should select a syringe that can be filled at least ¾ full.

A syringe is considered accurate to half of the smallest calibration mark (usually mL or cc) indicated on its barrel. To obtain an accurate measurement, technicians must be mindful of the size of the syringe they are using and the calibration marks on the barrel. Various sizes of syringes deliver significantly different volumes. For example, calibration marks on a 1 mL syringe indicate that each mark is equivalent to $1/100$ of 1 mL, whereas the calibration marks on a 60 mL syringe indicate that each mark is equivalent to 1 mL. To get an accurate dose, technicians should count the number of marks between labeled measurement units. If 10 marks are designated between units, then each mark measures $1/10$ of the unit. If 5 marks are indicated, then each mark measures $1/5$ of the unit. The volume of solution drawn into a syringe is measured at the point of contact between the rubber-tipped piston plunger and the inside of the barrel; this measurement point is often referred to as the *shoulder* of the plunger. The measurement is not read at the tip of the piston plunger.

Needles Needles are made of stainless steel or aluminum and are individually wrapped to maintain their sterility. A needle's size is determined by its length and gauge. Needle lengths range from $3/8$ inch to 6 inches. Needle gauge refers to the diameter of the opening or lumen of the needle and ranges from 31-gauge (smallest bore) to 13-gauge (largest bore). The size of the gauge, or bore, corresponds conversely to the size of the lumen: the larger the gauge number, the smaller the size of the lumen; the smaller the gauge number, the larger the size of the lumen. In the hospital pharmacy, 1-inch and 1½ -inch needles are commonly used, with needle gauges ranging from 16 to 25 (see Figure 11.2).

FIGURE 11.2

**Common
Needle
Lengths and
Gauges Used
in Sterile
Compounding**

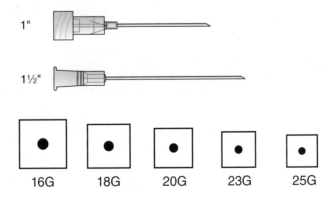

1"

1½"

16G 18G 20G 23G 25G

During sterile compounding, needles are used to inject or withdraw fluid or to puncture containers. They are razor sharp and must be handled carefully. Accidentally touching any part of the sterile needle leads to contamination and requires the disposal of the needle in a sharps container.

Parts of a Needle A needle consists of several parts, including the needle tip, the bevel, the heel, the needle shaft, the lumen, and the needle hub (see Figure 11.3). A needle has a hard plastic cap that covers the needle shaft and tip until the needle is ready to be used. This cap is the only place that can be touched by a technician during the handling of a needle.

Handling of the Needle-and-Syringe Unit As mentioned earlier, a syringe comes from the manufacturer in sterile packaging. Before its use in sterile compounding, the pharmacy technician removes the outer wrapper without touching the syringe tip or blocking airflow around the tip. Using aseptic technique, the technician opens the sterile packaging of the needle, holds the needle by the cap, and uses a twisting motion to attach the needle hub to the syringe tip. Sterile compounding personnel must not touch the sterile parts or critical sites of the syringe or needle during this attachment process (see Figure 11.4). A **critical site** is the part of the supply item that includes any fluid-pathway surface or opening that is at risk for contamination by touch or airflow interruption.

Safety Note

Sterile compounding personnel must not touch the sterile parts of a syringe or needle. Inadvertent touching of these critical sites results in contamination and, consequently, disposal of the needle-and-syringe unit into a sharps container.

FIGURE 11.3
Needle Components

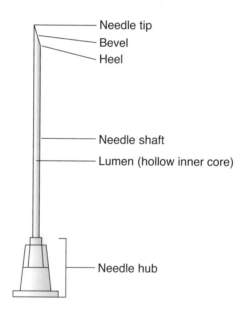

Needle tip

Bevel

Heel

Needle shaft

Lumen (hollow inner core)

Needle hub

FIGURE 11.4
**Critical Areas of a
Needle and Syringe**

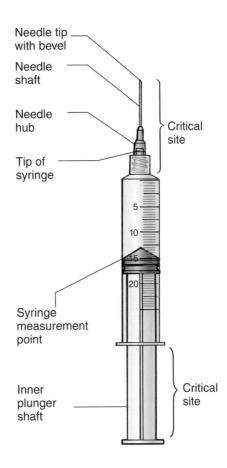

Needle tip
with bevel

Needle
shaft

Critical
site

Needle
hub

Tip of
syringe

5

10

15

20

Syringe
measurement
point

Inner
plunger
shaft

Critical
site

IV Administration Sets

IV medications are compounded in the pharmacy and delivered to the nursing units for patient administration. Administration of these sterile solutions is typically accomplished through the use of an IV administration set. An **IV administration set** is a sterile, disposable device used to deliver IV fluids and injectable medications directly into a patient's vein. Often called *IV tubing* or an *IV set*, an IV administration set comes in a sterile, sealed package with either a clear or an opaque exterior wrapper. A set that has an opaque wrapper shows a diagram of the contents printed on the outer packaging. Healthcare personnel should carefully inspect the IV set package for any exterior tears or other signs of damage. Any damaged or opened packages may result in a loss of sterility and therefore should be discarded. IV sets do not have expiration dates, but they do contain the following legend: "Federal law restricts this device to sale by or on the order of a physician."

An IV set is commonly attached to an IV infusion pump or controller that adjusts the volume and administration rate of the infusion. This type of nondisposable, reusable equipment is often referred to as *durable equipment*.

Components of an IV Set Regardless of manufacturer, IV administration sets have certain basic components. These components include:

- a universal spike adaptor (commonly called a *tubing spike* or *spike*), which pierces the rubber stopper or port of the IV container
- a drip chamber, which allows healthcare personnel to view and count the drops of IV fluid before the solution flows down the tubing

- a roll clamp, which adjusts the flow rate of the IV fluid from the source container into the receiving container or patient
- flexible tubing, which delivers the fluid
- a needle adaptor, which attaches a needle or a catheter to the patient, receiving container, or primary tubing

These IV set components are shown in Figure 11.5.

FIGURE 11.5
Sterile IV Administration Set and Its Components

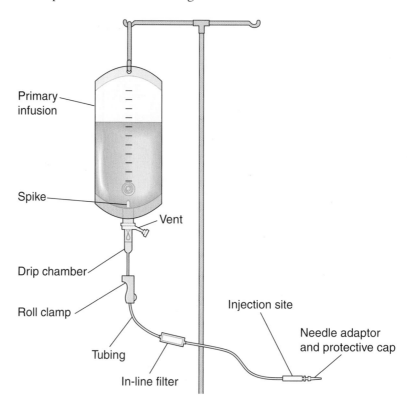

Primary infusion

Spike

Vent

Drip chamber

Roll clamp

Tubing

In-line filter

Injection site

Needle adaptor and protective cap

Universal Spike Adaptor The sharp, plastic **spike** is used to pierce the IV's tubing port. To ensure sterility, the spike is covered with a protective unit, which is removed before insertion into the tubing port. The spike has a rigid area for the healthcare worker to grip during insertion. Some IV sets have an air vent with a bacterial filter cover that is positioned below the spike. This vent allows air to enter the bottle as fluid flows out of it.

Drip Chamber Sitting below the spike is the transparent, hollow drip chamber. The **drip chamber** allows any air bubbles to rise to the top of the IV fluid, thus preventing the air bubbles from entering the tubing and, subsequently, from entering the patient. The drip chamber also allows the attending nurse to set the medication flow or infusion rate by counting the drops.

Drops of fluid fall into the chamber from an opening at the uppermost end, closest to the tip of the spike. The number of drops it takes to make 1 mL identifies an IV set. This calibration is referred to as a **drop set**, also known as the tubing's **drop factor**. The most common IV drop sets are 10, 15, 20, and 60, indicating 10 gtts/mL, 15 gtts/mL, 20 gtts/mL, and 60 gtts/mL, respectively (see Figure 11.6). An opening that provides 10, 15, or 20 gtts/mL is commonly used for adults and is called a *macrodrip set*. An opening that provides 60 gtts/mL is typically used for pediatric patients and for IV medications requiring tight control and is called a *minidrip* or *microdrip set*.

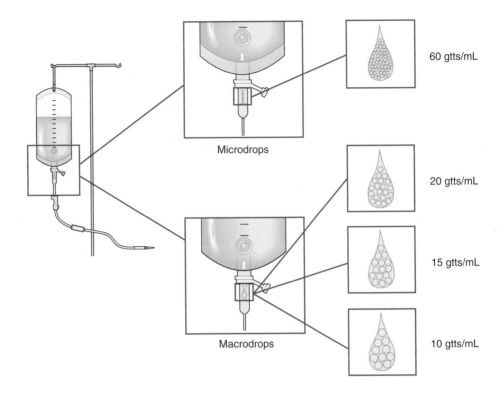

FIGURE 11.6
Microdrip and Macrodrip Drop Sets

Microdrops — 60 gtts/mL

Macrodrops — 20 gtts/mL — 15 gtts/mL — 10 gtts/mL

Roll Clamp A **roll clamp** is a hard, plastic clip that contains a small roller. The clip is loosely attached to the tubing and moves freely along the length of the tubing between the spike adaptor and the needle adaptor, allowing its location to be changed to one that is convenient for the healthcare professional administering the IV medication. When the roller is rolled down toward the needle adaptor, the tubing is constricted, resulting in a reduced flow of fluid. Conversely, when the roller is moved up toward the universal spike adaptor, the tubing opens and increases the flow of fluid. This movement allows healthcare personnel to regulate the IV flow rate.

Safety Note

Healthcare professionals should not use PVC IV sets for nitroglycerin or fat emulsions due to absorption of medication by the PVC tubing. For these medications, personnel should use chlorine-free IV sets made from polyolefin or polybutadiene blends.

Flexible Tubing Most of the length of the **flexible tubing**, or IV tubing, is molded from pliable PVC and other plasticizers. Some drugs, such as the cardiac drugs nitroglycerin and amiodarone, may be absorbed to some extent in the plastic tubing or the IV bag. This absorption reduces the volume delivered intravenously to a patient. In these situations, special types of plastic IV sets are required. For example, Baxter Healthcare Corporation has developed AVIVA containers that are made of non-PVC film and contain no latex or DEHP (di[2-ethylhexyl]phthalate). This system provides a nonabsorbent fluid pathway for IV medication delivery in adults, pediatric patients, and neonates.

Needle Adaptor A **needle adaptor** is usually located at the distal end of the IV set, close to the patient. A needle or catheter may be attached to the adaptor. The adaptor has a standard taper to fit all needles or catheters and is protected by a sterile cover that is removed before connection.

Additional Components of an IV Set Certain IV sets may also have these additional components:

- a flange or a rigid plastic, self-sealing **Y-site injection port**, which allows medication to be added to the IV solution
- an **in-line filter**, which offers protection for the patient against particulates, including bacteria and emboli (see section below titled "Filters")

Preparation of an IV Set The length of IV sets varies, with extensions ranging from 6 to 120 inches. The length of tubing is dependent on the patient's needs, the number of IV lines, and the procedure being performed. Shorter tubing is used in the surgical setting, and longer tubing is used in other areas of the hospital. **Priming** is the action of flushing out the small particles in the tubing's interior lumen before medication administration. This action is accomplished by letting fluid run through the tubing so that all of the air is flushed out. The amount of fluid needed to prime the tubing depends on the length of the set—from 3 mL for the short extension up to 15 mL for longer sets. Widespread use of in-line filters has reduced the need for flushing the line with IV fluid before attaching the set to the patient.

Medication Delivery with an IV Set Nurses typically have the responsibility for administering IV solutions to patients. This procedure involves attaching the IV tubing to the fluid container (commonly, a flexible, vented plastic bag), establishing and maintaining a flow rate, and managing overall regulation of the system during administration of the solution. A **catheter**, or tube, may be implanted in the patient and affixed to the patient's skin with adhesive tape to avoid having to repuncture the patient each time that an infusion is given.

The nurse administering the fluid starts the flow by filling the chamber with fluid from an attached inverted IV container. The chamber sides are squeezed and released to allow fluid to flow into the chamber. The procedure is repeated until an indicated level is reached or approximately half the chamber is full. The nurse then threads the flexible tubing through a pump that is programmed to either constrict or open the tubing to regulate the flow of the CSP from the IV bag, through the tubing, and into the patient at a rate prescribed by the physician.

The IV tubing's injection port, once disinfected with alcohol, is ready for the insertion of a needle and the injection of IV push medication, or the administration of an IVPB medication. IV sets are changed every 24 to 96 hours to minimize the risk of infection.

Fluids and medications are often delivered to a patient via an IV administration set.

Pharmacy Personnel and IV Sets Pharmacy personnel must have a complete understanding of IV sets and their operation due to changes in the scope of pharmacy practice. Pharmacists may now:

- select IV sets that are optimal for the prevention of physical incompatibilities in certain drug–drug or drug–fluid combinations
- serve on cardiopulmonary resuscitation (CPR) or code teams to calculate dosages and drip rates for medications, prepare IV infusions, attach sets, and prepare IV tubing

Other pharmacy personnel may:

- provide in-service training for nurses to familiarize them with the proper use of new IV sets
- use IV sets when transferring fluids between containers while working in a laminar airflow hood
- prime IV sets to prepare chemotherapy CSPs for patient administration

Filters

Filters are used in the IV area of the hospital pharmacy for high-risk CSPs and are also included in many IV administration sets. A **filter** is a device used to remove contaminants such as glass, fibers, and tiny bits of rubber that may have inadvertently entered the CSP during sterile compounding. An IV administration set may have a built-in or in-line filter, which provides a final filtration of the fluid before it enters the patient. A filter occasionally becomes clogged, thus slowing expected flow rates.

Depending on size, final filtration should protect the patient against particulate matter, bacteria, air emboli, and phlebitis. Filters do not remove virus particles or toxins. A 0.5 micron filter is commonly used to prevent large particles from being inadvertently injected into the CSP; however, it is not a sterilizing filter. A 0.22-micron filter is optimal for blocking bacteria and ensuring sterility. Common filter sizes used in IV administration include:

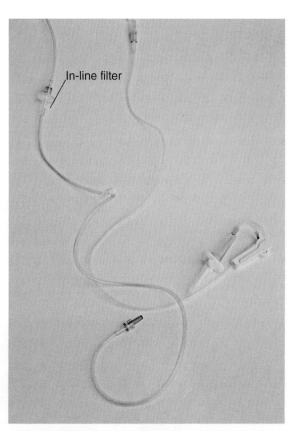

In-line filters vary in size and can minimize the risk of phlebitis or infection.

- 0.5 micron: random path membrane (RPM) filter for removing large particulate matter
- 0.45 micron: in-line filter for IV suspension drug
- 0.22 micron: filter for removing bacteria to produce a sterile solution

IV Solutions

Because the body is primarily an aqueous or water-containing vehicle, most IV preparations introduced into the body are comprised of ingredients added to a sterile water medium or base solution. These ingredients include medications, electrolytes, vitamins, and nutrients. The administration of these CSPs into the blood supply of patients necessitates that these preparations have certain chemical properties or characteristics that do not damage blood cells or vessels or alter the chemical properties of blood. In other words, CSPs must possess chemical characteristics that are similar to blood serum, rendering them safe for patient administration. To that end, pharmacy personnel should have a basic knowledge of these chemical properties to understand the sterile compounding process.

Chemical Properties of IV Solutions

Chemical properties of IV solutions include pH value, osmolarity and osmolality, tonicity, compatibility, and stability. These properties affect the **beyond-use date** of the CSP, or the date and time after which a CSP is no longer sterile, stable, or effective.

pH Value The degree of acidity or alkalinity of a solution is known as its **pH value**. Most high-school chemistry classes teach pH value by using litmus paper to test various solutions. If the litmus paper turns pink when dipped in a solution, then the solution is acidic, meaning its pH is less than 7.0. If the litmus paper turns blue when dipped in a solution, then the solution is alkaline, meaning its pH is more than 7.0. Blood plasma has a pH of 7.4; therefore, it is slightly alkaline. The blood's pH must stay very close to this value for a patient to stay healthy. With that in mind, IV solutions should have a pH that is neutral (or near 7.0) so that they don't adversely affect the pH of the blood.

Osmolarity and Osmolality CSPs also have two other chemical characteristics that must not alter the properties of blood serum: osmolarity and osmolality. **Osmolarity** is a measure of the number of milliosmoles of solute per liter of solution (mOsm/L). With regard to CSPs, osmolarity refers to the osmotic pressure applied by a solution across a cell wall. **Osmotic pressure** is the pressure required to maintain equilibrium, with no net movement of solution across body membranes. **Osmolality** is a measure of the number of milliosmoles of solute per kilogram of solvent. For CSPs, this measurement refers to the number of molecules or ions in a solution. Both osmolarity and osmolality affect the flow of fluid into and out of the body's cells. These cells must be maintained in a state of equilibrium to maintain optimal health.

Generally speaking, an IV preparation must be isoosmotic, meaning the solution should have the same number of particles in solution per unit volume and the same osmotic pressure as blood.

Tonicity **Tonicity** is the manner in which cells or tissues respond to surrounding fluid. The tonicity of a solution can be classified as hypotonic, hypertonic, or isotonic.

Practice Tip

Pharmacy personnel may hear the terms *osmolarity* and *tonicity* used interchangeably. However, these two chemical properties are distinct. Osmolarity is an *absolute measure* of the movement of solutes and fluid through a cell's membrane, whereas tonicity is a *relative measure* of this movement.

Blood plasma has a pH of 7.4 and an osmolarity near 285 mOsm/L. Most IV solutions have a neutral pH and are isotonic (280–310 mOsm/L) or near isotonic, so as not to damage red blood cells.

Safety Note

Patient recipients of hypotonic and hypertonic solutions must be closely monitored for potential risks. Hypotonic solutions may cause a potentially life-threatening electrolyte imbalance. Hypertonic solutions must be administered through a large vein, such as the subclavian vein or superior vena cava, to avoid collapse or destruction of smaller, peripheral veins.

Hypotonic Solution A **hypotonic solution** (or hypoosmolar solution) has a fewer number of dissolved particles than blood cells (less than 280 mOsm/L). Therefore, if cells are subjected to a hypotonic solution, water is drawn into the cells, which causes the cells to swell. An example of a hypotonic solution is 0.45% **sodium chloride** or 1/2 **normal saline (NS)** IV solution.

Hypertonic Solution A **hypertonic solution** (or hyperosmolar solution) has a greater number of dissolved particles than the blood cells themselves (greater than 310 mOsm/L). Consequently, if cells are subjected to a hypertonic solution, water is drawn out of the cells, which causes the cells to shrivel. An example of a hypertonic solution is IV 50% dextrose or 3% sodium chloride.

Isotonic Solution An **isotonic solution** has a similar number of dissolved particles as blood. An isotonic solution is in the range of 280–310 mOsm/L, which is similar to the tonicity of blood (approximately 285 mOsm/L). An example of an isotonic solution is 0.9% sodium chloride (NS).

At times, a pharmacist may need to adjust the tonicity of parenteral preparations to ensure that they are isotonic or nearly isotonic. On occasion, however, hypertonic solutions must be administered to patients. These infusions must be done slowly and cautiously by a nurse or a physician. Some hypertonic solutions, such as a TPN solution, whose osmolarity approaches 900 mOsm/L, must be administered via a central catheter into a larger subclavian vein so that the solution can be sufficiently diluted by the blood.

Safety Note

Sterile compounding personnel prepare CSPs in a manner that ensures that the chemical properties of the components and additives are appropriate for patient administration.

Compatibility With regard to CSPs, **compatibility** is the ability to combine two or more base components or **additives** within a solution, without resulting in changes to the physical or chemical properties of the components or additives.

Stability A final physical characteristic of an IV solution is its stability under various storage conditions. Many IV medications must be refrigerated (or even frozen) after being compounded to maintain their activity. (The preparation and beyond-use dating of these drugs are discussed later in the chapter.) Other IV solutions must be covered with an amber-colored bag to protect the drug from exposure to light. An example of a light-sensitive agent is an IV infusion of the antifungal drug amphotericin B.

Types of IV Solutions

There are multiple IV solutions available in flexible plastic or PVC bags and in various volumes. The vehicles most commonly used for IV infusions are dextrose in water, normal saline, or dextrose in saline solution. The pharmacy technician who compounds sterile preparations in the hospital, home healthcare, or compounding pharmacy setting must become familiar with abbreviations for terms used in medication orders for parenteral solutions (see Table 11.1 on the following page).

TABLE 11.1 Commonly Used IV Products and Abbreviations

Component		Abbreviation
Fluids	2.5% Dextrose in water	$D_{2.5}W$
	5% Dextrose in water	D_5W
	5% Dextrose and lactated Ringer's solution	D_5RL or D_5LR
	10% Dextrose in water	$D_{10}W$
	5% Dextrose and 0.9% Sodium chloride	D_5NS
	2.5% Dextrose and 0.45% Sodium chloride	$D_{2.5}1/2NS$
	5% Dextrose and 0.45% Sodium chloride	$D_51/2NS$
	0.9% Sodium chloride; normal saline	NS
	0.45% Sodium chloride	1/2 NS
	Lactated Ringer's solution	RL or LR
	Sterile water for injection	SW for injection or SWFI
	Bacteriostatic water for injection	BW for injection or BWFI
	Sterile water for irrigation	SW for irrigation
	Normal saline for irrigation	NS for irrigation
Electrolytes	Potassium chloride	KCl
	Potassium phosphate	K phos or KPO_4
	Potassium acetate	K acet
	Sodium phosphate	Na phos or $NaPO_4$
	Sodium chloride	NaCl
Additives	Multivitamin for injection	MVI
	Trace elements (combinations of essential trace elements such as chromium, manganese, and copper)	TE
	Zinc (a trace element)	Zn
	Selenium (a trace element)	Se

FIGURE 11.7
Common
Physician's
Orders for
Parenteral
Solutions

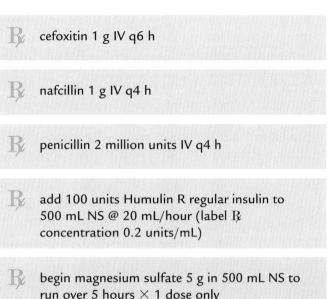

℞ cefoxitin 1 g IV q6 h

℞ nafcillin 1 g IV q4 h

℞ penicillin 2 million units IV q4 h

℞ add 100 units Humulin R regular insulin to
500 mL NS @ 20 mL/hour (label ℞
concentration 0.2 units/mL)

℞ begin magnesium sulfate 5 g in 500 mL NS to
run over 5 hours × 1 dose only

℞ change IV fluids to 0.45 NS with 20 mEq KCl @
125 mL/hour

Sterile compounding technicians typically prepare two types of CSPs for patient administration: large-volume parenterals, which are solutions that are primarily used as a source of hydration for patients, and small-volume parenterals, which are solutions that are "piggybacked" through a primary IV line that contains the IV base solution. These small-volume solutions are commonly antibiotics. Examples of physicians' orders for both types of CSPs are shown in Figure 11.7.

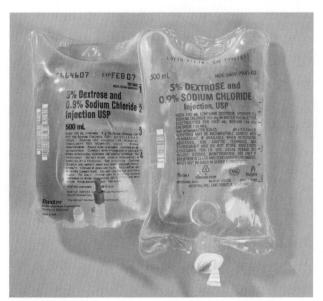

Dextrose 5% in normal saline (0.9%) is a common large-volume parenteral in 500 mL and 1 L sizes.

Large-Volume Parenterals As mentioned earlier, a **large-volume parenteral (LVP)** is used to replenish fluids and to provide drugs, electrolytes, and nutrients such as vitamins, minerals, and glucose to patients. LVPs are commonly available in 250 mL, 500 mL, and 1,000 mL sizes. An LVP usually contains one or more electrolytes that are added to the IV solution. Potassium chloride is the most common additive, but other salts of potassium, as well as magnesium or calcium, can be added based on the requirements of the individual patient. An LVP is administered over a prolonged period that ranges from 1 to 24 hours.

One type of IV solution that contains a specific mixture of electrolytes—called *lactated Ringer's solution*—may be used alone or in combination with a dextrose solution. Examples of the types of medications that may be administered by LVP include TPN solutions, electrolytes, and many chemotherapy drugs.

Small-Volume Parenterals A **small-volume parenteral (SVP)** is a CSP that is dispensed in a minibag and administered to a patient via sterile IV tubing. An SVP typically has a volume of 25 mL, 50 mL, 100 mL, 150 mL, or 250 mL and is typically given intermittently over a short period ranging from 10 minutes to an hour (sometimes longer), based on the frequency ordered by the prescriber. In most cases, a medication is injected into an SVP and the solution is then "piggybacked" through a patient's primary IV line. Some intermittent medications may be mixed in a larger volume of fluid (150 mL, 250 mL, or 500 mL) to obtain a more dilute concentration. Diluting the medication avoids vein irritation (or phlebitis) and patient discomfort.

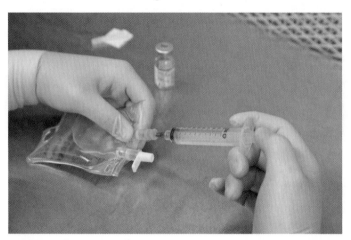

During sterile compounding, a technician injects medication into an IVPB. This minibag will then be attached to a patient's primary IV line for administration.

The majority of SVPs prepared by sterile compounding personnel are **IV piggybacks (IVPBs)**. An IVPB is comprised of a small volume (typically, 50 to 100 mL) of a base solution (such as D_5W) and a medication. The volume of solution needed is dependent on the dose and solubility of the medication. For example, the antibiotic cefazolin is diluted in a 50 mL minibag of D_5W or NS if the dose is less than 1 gram; if the dose is more than 1 gram, the medication is diluted in a 100 mL minibag.

Special SVP solutions that are commonly prepared by the pharmacy technician include frozen IV solutions, premade IVPBs, and vial-and-bag systems, which are discussed later in the chapter.

Preparation of Labels for LVPs and SVPs

When making any sterile IV preparation, including those containing a hazardous agent, a CSP label is generated (see Figure 11.8). The label should contain the following information:

- patient's name and identification number
- room number

FIGURE 11.8
LVP Label and SVP Label

| ****Large-Volume Parenteral**** |
| Memorial Hospital |

| **Pt. Name:** Will Van Ingen | **Room:** Neuro ICU |
| **Pt. ID#:** 8873662 | **Rx#:** 74521 |

Potassium Chloride 30 mEq
Lactated Ringer's 1000 mL
Rate: 40 mL/hr

Expires _____
RPh _____
Tech _____

Keep refrigerated – warm to room temperature before use.

| ****IV Piggyback**** |
| Memorial Hospital |

| **Pt. Name:** Ogard, Christopher | **Room:** 560 |
| **Pt. ID#:** 898372 | **Rx#:** 03127 |

Ampicillin 500 mg
Sodium Chloride 0.9% (NS) 50 mL
Rate: over 20 min

Expires _____
RPh _____
Tech _____

Keep refrigerated – warm to room temperature before use.

- medication name and dose
- base solution and amount
- infusion period (e.g., infuse over 30 minutes)
- flow rate (e.g., 100 mL/hour)
- beyond-use date (or expiration date) and time
- signature or initials of technician and checking pharmacist
- additional information as required by the institution or by state or federal guidelines, including hazardous drug warnings, auxiliary labels, storage requirements, and device-specific or drug-specific information, such as filters

Safety Note

When working in the pharmacy clean room, personnel must be appropriately garbed. Sterile compounding technicians must don shoe covers, a hair cover, a face mask, a sterile gown, and sterile gloves. Additional protection is required for personnel who are preparing hazardous drugs. These safeguards include a chemotherapy gown, chemotherapy gloves, and safety glasses.

Aseptic Preparation of IV Products

Pharmacy personnel compound sterile IV preparations in a form that is ready for patient administration. Sterile preparations include medications stored in single- and multiple-dose vials, ampules, and other containers that must be transferred to an LVP or SVP for patient use. As discussed earlier, sterile devices used to transfer medications include syringes, needles, and IV administration sets.

To be in compliance with USP Chapter <797> guidelines, CSPs must be prepared in an ISO Class 5 laminar airflow hood using correct aseptic technique. A summary of these compounding procedures is listed in Table 11.2. When sterile compounding personnel are working in the hood, they should be free from interruptions to stay mentally focused on following proper aseptic technique during their compounding tasks. Any breach in aseptic technique may lead to product contamination and medication errors.

TABLE 11.2   Summary of Procedures to Maintain Aseptic Technique During Sterile Compounding

1. Remove any outer garments and change into clean scrubs or lightweight clothing. Then remove all jewelry (e.g., watches, rings, bracelets, necklaces).
2. Put on, in sequence, shoe covers, a hair cover, and a face mask. Note that it is important to follow the order of items indicated in this step.
3. Perform an aseptic hand washing for 2–4 minutes using a surgical scrub sponge/brush. This hand-washing procedure should include the hands and arms (up to the elbows).
4. Don a sterile gown.
5. Apply sterile, foamed alcohol to hands and allow them to dry thoroughly.
6. Don sterile gloves.
7. Clean the laminar airflow hood with sterile water first followed by sterile 70% isopropyl alcohol (IPA). The IPA must remain in contact with the surface for 30 seconds before compounding any sterile product.
8. Place only essential materials in the hood—no paper, pens, or labels. Remove the selected syringe(s) from its packaging, aseptically attach a needle, and then discard the waste.
9. Swab needle-penetration closures on vials, injection ports, and other supplies with sterile, 70% IPA.
10. Create the compounded sterile preparation (CSP) by withdrawing the medication from a vial or an ampule and then injecting it into the IV base solution or container.
11. Complete a quality check of the product by inspecting container integrity and by checking the solution for cloudiness, particulates, and appropriate color.
12. Present the CSP, the containers and devices used, and the label to a pharmacist for verification of the product before sending the product to the patient care unit.

Specialized Sterile Compounding Procedures

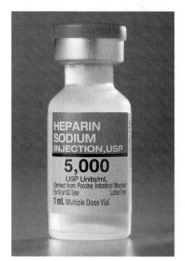

This sealed, sterile, multidose glass vial contains several doses of medication with a preservative.

Because not all parenteral drugs are available in a commercially packaged, ready-to-use form, sterile compounding personnel prepare CSPs for patient use. To do so, personnel must undergo training and testing in several specialized procedures. These procedures include handling medication vials, using ampules, and preparing TPN solutions.

Vials

A **vial** is a sealed, sterile, plastic or glass container that has a hard plastic cap. During sterile compounding, the technician removes this cap to expose a rubber top, which allows the technician to use a needle to access the fluid within. Vials contain a sterile medication in either a liquid or powdered form and are available in sizes ranging from 1 mL to 250 mL.

Types of Vials Vials are available as single-dose vials (SDVs) that do not contain a preservative, and multiple-dose vials (MDVs) that do contain a preservative. The absence of a preservative in an SDV makes this container an ideal medium for microbial growth. Consequently, an SDV is meant for one-time use only and must be used within an hour (under aseptic conditions) or discarded to remain in compliance with USP Chapter <797> guidelines. An MDV, on the other hand, is typically stable for up to 28 days from its initial use, unless otherwise specified from the manufacturer. The technician should mark the beyond-use date on the MDV to ensure that the vial is stored under appropriate conditions and to alert other pharmacy personnel to the medication's expiration date.

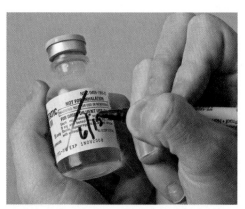

Even though a multiple-dose vial of diluent contains a preservative, it must be discarded after 28 days to avoid the potential for contamination.

Withdrawing Fluid from a Vial To withdraw fluid from a vial, the technician must first disinfect the vial's rubber top by wiping it with sterile 70% isopropyl alcohol (IPA). Next, the technician should use a needle-and-syringe unit to pierce the rubber top. Insertion of the needle must be done carefully. The technician should place the needle bevel on the vial top, with the needle bevel pointing up toward the ceiling. The needle bevel should penetrate the rubber closure at an angle, which is then straightened to 90 degrees so that as additional pressure is applied to the syringe, the bevel heel enters the closure at the same point as the tip. This technique prevents **coring**, or the inadvertent introduction of a small piece of the rubber top into the solution. If coring does occur, the technician must discard the contaminated vial and needle-and-syringe unit and repeat the process with new supplies.

Because a vial is a closed-system container, or a container from which air cannot freely flow in or out, the technician must use a milking technique to release the negative pressure within the vial. To perform this technique for a vial containing liquid medication, the technician must use the needle-and-syringe unit to introduce an amount of air into the vial that is equal to, or slightly less than, the volume of liquid that needs to be withdrawn (see Figure 11.9). For a summary of the steps involved in withdrawing liquid from a vial, refer to Table 11.3.

Safety Note

During sterile compounding in the hood, the technician must hold the vial and syringe so that the airflow to the critical area—which includes the syringe tip, needle, and the vial's rubber top—remains unobstructed.

FIGURE 11.9
Correct Needle Insertion into a Vial

Note the slight bend of the needle during the insertion.

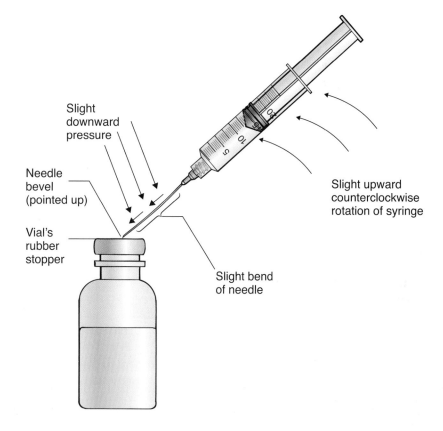

Slight downward pressure

Needle bevel (pointed up)

Vial's rubber stopper

Slight upward counterclockwise rotation of syringe

Slight bend of needle

TABLE 11.3   Using a Syringe to Draw Liquid from a Vial

1. Choose the smallest-gauge sterile needle appropriate for the task. The smaller the needle, the less chance of coring the vial's rubber top and thus introducing particulates into the liquid.

2. Attach the needle to the syringe.

3. Draw into the syringe an amount of air that is equal to the amount of drug to be withdrawn from the vial.

4. Swab the top of the vial with alcohol; allow the alcohol to dry. Puncture the vial's rubber top with the needle bevel up. Then bring the syringe and needle straight up and penetrate the rubber top. Check for coring.

5. Invert the vial with the syringe still inserted, and depress the plunger of the syringe, emptying the air into the vial.

6. Withdraw the necessary volume of liquid from the vial.

7. Withdraw the needle-and-syringe unit from the vial. In the case of a multiple-dose vial, the vial's rubber top closes, sealing the contents of the vial.

8. Inject the liquid medication into an IV base solution, or follow any alternative instructions.

9. To avoid accidental needle sticks, avoid capping the empty syringe at the end of the procedure. If an actual syringe is dispensed, remove and properly dispose of the needle in a sharps container. Then cap the syringe with a sterile syringe cap before sending the medication to the nursing unit. Before patient administration, the nurse will then attach a sterile needle to the syringe.

Reconstituting Powdered Medication in a Vial Many antibiotics, such as cefazolin, are available as lyophilized (or freeze-dried) powder. These powdered medications need to be reconstituted with a **diluent** such as sterile water or NS before being injected into an IV solution. Pharmacy personnel need to read the manufacturer's product package insert or the vial's label to determine the preferred diluents. Once the diluent is selected, personnel must verify the diluent's expiration date before reconstituting the medication.

For a powdered medication, the technician may use a special type of needle called a *vented needle* that allows the diluent to be injected into the vial while simultaneously venting the positive pressure that has built up within the vial. The technician draws up the diluent into the syringe using a regular needle; then removes the regular needle and attaches the vented needle to the syringe. Before proceeding, the technician verifies the volume and dosage of diluent in the syringe and then injects the diluent into the vial.

Various dosages are commercially available in vials that contain inactivated powder. It should be noted that the expiration dates of reconstituted drugs vary. Pharmacy personnel should consult the manufacturer's package insert to determine the expiration date for each reconstituted drug.

Preparing a CSP with a Vial's Contents Once the correct dosage volume has been withdrawn from the vial into a syringe, the technician arranges the vial, filled syringe (with attached, capped needle), and the IV or IVPB base solution on the hood for a pharmacist check. The pharmacist verifies that the technician has drawn up the dose ordered by the physician by checking the drug name and concentration, the base solution type and volume, and the volume that the technician has drawn up into the syringe.

Once the verification check has been completed, the technician repositions the base solution and needle-and-syringe unit in the hood so that the critical components receive uninterrupted airflow from the HEPA filter. After swabbing the injection port of the base solution container, the technician then removes the needle cap and, using using proper aseptic technique, inserts the needle into the injection port. He or she then depresses the flat knob of the plunger until all of the medication has been injected into the base solution. The technician then removes the needle-and-syringe unit and disposes of it in a sharps container. Finally, the technician checks the CSP for leakage and signs of incompatibility—such as flakes, crystallized particles, or a darkening of the solution—and labels the CSP in preparation for delivery to the nursing unit for patient administration.

Ampules

In addition to using medication vials during the sterile compounding process, technicians may also be handling ampules of medication. An **ampule** is a small, hermetically sealed container that has a distinct, elongated neck. Typically made of thin glass, an ampule stores a single dose of sterile medication in either a liquid (most common) or powdered form. Technicians need to be aware that (1) ampules contain no preservatives and (2) some drugs are *only* available as a solution in an ampule because the drugs are incompatible with the rubber or PVC components of vials.

Parts of an Ampule Pharmacy personnel must be familiar with the parts of an ampule to understand the directions on how to open this specialized container. An ampule has a head, neck, shoulder, and body

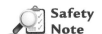

Safety Note

Check the medication package insert to verify which diluent and what volume should be added to the medication vial to make a correct concentration of sterile solution.

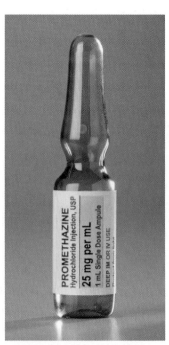

An ampule contains no preservatives. Any unused remaining medication must be discarded, even if you are working in a hood in a clean room environment.

FIGURE 11.10
**Critical Site of
an Ampule**

Pharmacy technicians must not taint the critical site of an ampule through touch contamination or incorrect handling or positioning of the ampule within the hood.

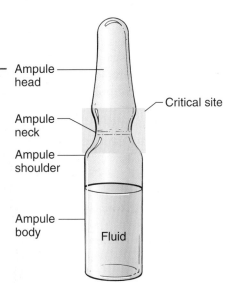

- Ampule head
- Critical site
- Ampule neck
- Ampule shoulder
- Ampule body
- Fluid

(see Figure 11.10). The neck is the critical site of the ampule and must be swabbed with 70% IPA before opening the ampule. Sterile compounding personnel must be careful not to touch the neck and should ensure that airflow around this site remains unobstructed while working in the hood.

Because an ampule is a sealed container, it is typically designed with a break ring. A **break ring** is a scored area on the neck that marks the site where a technician will break the glass to access the ampule's contents. Therefore, the process of opening an ampule has some inherent risks, including contamination of the medication with glass shards, injury to the worker from the breaking of glass, or damage and/or contamination of the hood from the broken glass. Technicians should be aware of these risks and should have sufficient practice in this skill before compounding CSPs.

Opening an Ampule Technicians may use several methods to ensure the safe opening of an ampule. Some workers prefer to place a piece of sterile gauze or a sterile 70% IPA swab over the neck of the ampule while it is being broken (see Figure 11.11). Others slip a small plastic cap called an *ampule breaker* over the head of an ampule to safely open it. Still others prefer to simply use their gloved hands to break an ampule.

FIGURE 11.11
**Opening an
Ampule**

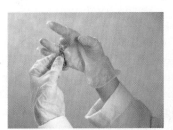

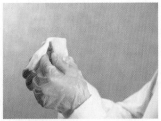

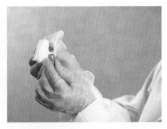

(a) Gently tap the head of the ampule to bring the medication to the body of the ampule.

(b) Wrap a sterile 70% IPA swab around the neck of the ampule.

(c) Using gentle but firm pressure, snap the neck of the ampule away from you.

Before breaking an ampule, the technician must first hold the ampule upright and gently tap or swirl the container to clear the medication contents from the head and neck of the ampule. Next, the worker must clean the neck of the ampule with a sterile 70% IPA swab to remove any microorganisms. Then the technician should hold the body of the ampule in his or her nondominant hand, with the thumb and fingers below the neck of the ampule. With the dominant hand, the technician should grasp the head of the ampule between the thumb and forefinger, placing the fingers above the break ring. The technician should then hold the ampule toward the side of the hood, away from the HEPA filter, and exert a gentle but firm pressure on the break ring to snap the ampule's neck cleanly.

Withdrawing Medication from an Ampule To withdraw medication from an opened ampule, the technician should hold the ampule upright, place the needle bevel (pointing down) of a filter needle or the tip of a filter straw in the corner near the opening, and withdraw the medication. When the ampule is nearly emptied, the technician should tilt the ampule slightly to allow easier access to the remainder of medication. It is required to use a needle equipped with a filter to screen out any tiny glass particles or fibers that may have fallen into the ampule's contents. Filter needles are for one-directional use only, meaning that the needle may only be used to either withdraw fluid from an ampule or inject fluid into an IV or IVPB. The same needle may *not* be used to both withdraw from and inject into a container. The most commonly used filter is a 5-micron filter needle.

Before injecting the contents of a syringe into an IV, the filter needle must be changed to a regular needle to avoid introducing glass or particles into the admixture. If a regular needle is used to withdraw the drug from the ampule, then the needle must be replaced with a filter device before the drug is pushed out of the syringe and into an IV or IVPB. Glass fragment contamination can lead to systemic side effects such as phlebitis (irritation of the veins), especially in pediatric and neonatal patients.

Preparing a CSP with an Ampule's Contents Once the correct dosage volume has been withdrawn from the ampule into a syringe, the technician arranges the ampule, the filled syringe (with attached, capped, regular needle), the used filter needle, and the IV or IVPB base solution on the hood for a pharmacist check. The pharmacist verifies that the technician has drawn up the dose ordered by the physician by checking the drug name and concentration, the base solution type and volume, and the volume that the technician has drawn up into the syringe. Because the drug was withdrawn from an ampule, the pharmacist also verifies that the technician has used both a filter needle and a regular needle to prevent the transfer of glass particles into the CSP.

Once the verification check has been completed, the technician repositions the base solution and needle-and-syringe unit in the hood so that the critical components receive uninterrupted airflow from the HEPA filter. After swabbing the injection port of the base solution container, the technician removes the needle cap and, using proper aseptic technique, inserts the needle into the injection port. He or she then depresses the flat knob of the plunger until all of the medication has been injected into the base solution. The technician then removes the needle-and-syringe unit and disposes of it in a sharps container. Finally, the technician checks the CSP for leakage and signs of incompatibility—such as flakes, crystallized particles, or a darkening of the solution—and labels the CSP in preparation for delivery to the nursing unit for patient administration.

Total Parenteral Nutrition Solutions

Sterile compounding personnel with advanced training and certification may prepare **total parenteral nutrition (TPN)**, or IV solutions that provide long-term nutritional support for a specific patient population. These patients include those who are unconscious or who cannot receive food, water, or medication by mouth (NPO). An NPO designation can be a result of surgery, infection, or inflammation in the GI tract. Many hospitals have special TPN teams comprised of physicians, nurses, dietitians, and pharmacists who specialize in the care of such patients.

TPN solutions are commonly prepared in the hospital but may also be prepared in a home healthcare or compounding pharmacy. The preparation of these solutions may also be outsourced to an off-site pharmacy. Regardless of site, the pharmacy must have a clean room environment.

TPN Components A typical TPN solution contains approximately 15 components, including:

- sterile water for hydration
- dextrose for calories and energy
- amino acids for protein synthesis
- fatty acids for chemical processes and energy
- additives such as electrolytes, vitamins, and minerals for chemical processes
- medication (such as insulin) for treatment of a disease or disorder

Although there are guidelines for typical adult, pediatric, and neonatal daily requirements, the components of a patient's TPN are individualized to the patient, based on laboratory findings and clinical response, and are often changed daily. Specialized order sheets are available to the healthcare team with a list of all common ingredients. Figure 11.12 on the following page is an example of a TPN medication order for an adult patient.

Preparing TPN TPNs are usually prepared in 1,000 mL or 2,000 mL volumes to provide nutritional support for 12 to 24 hours. In small hospital pharmacies, the pharmacy technician may have to perform manual compounding to prepare a TPN solution. In this time-consuming process, the worker prepares the base solution, draws up the various additives into separate syringes, and then injects the additives into the base solution to produce a final TPN preparation per the prescriber's order. For facilities that prepare large volumes of TPN solutions, such as large hospital pharmacies, an **automated compounding device (ACD)** may be used. Some hospital pharmacies may also elect to outsource TPN preparation to an off-site pharmacy that uses an ACD.

At times, an IV fat emulsion (rather than a solution) is prescribed. As you may recall, emulsions are mixtures of two immiscible, or unblendable solutions. These

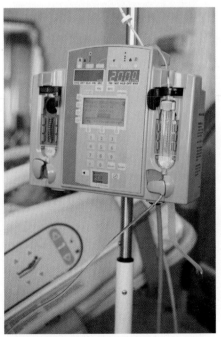

Many medications are administered using an infusion pump at the patient's bedside; the pump accurately controls the rate of fluid delivery.

preparations are oleaginous, or oily. Examples of commercially available parenteral emulsions used for nutritional support are Intralipid and Liposyn II/III. They are administered to patients who cannot or will not feed themselves and who need more calories than can be supplied by maintenance IV solutions or nonlipid-containing TPN solutions. In many cases, the IV fat emulsion is ordered as a component of the TPN solution; this type of TPN is known as a 3-in-1 TPN solution.

Administering TPN The administration of a TPN solution requires the insertion of a **central venous catheter (CVC)**, also called a *central line*, into the subclavian vein of the chest near the clavicle (as opposed to most IVs, which are administered into a peripheral vein in the arm). A large vein is required for TPN administration because of the hyperosmolar or hypertonic concentration of the ingredients and the large amount of fluid (usually 2,000 mL per day) that must be diluted in the bloodstream. The TPN solution, as with most medications, is commonly administered via an infusion pump.

TPN is administered continuously at a rate ordered by the prescriber. The IV tubing includes a special 0.22 micron in-line filter to filter out contaminants and to maintain sterility. Aseptic technique—in both TPN preparation by the pharmacy

FIGURE 11.12 TPN Medication Order

Memorial Hospital Pharmacy

Pt. Name: Sarah Mansfield   **Pt. ID#:** 66734
Room: TCU-07   **Rx#:** 126981

Physician Orders

TOTAL PARENTERAL NUTRITION (TPN) ADULT

Primary Diagnosis: _Multiple Trauma – post MVA_   **Ht:** _181 cm_   **Dosing Wt:** _80 kg_

DOB: _2/11/80_   **Allergies:** _NKDA_

Instructions: This form must be completed for a new order or continuation of PN and faxed to the pharmacy by 2 pm to receive same-day preparation. TPN administration begins at 6 pm daily.

Administration Route: ☒ CVC or PICC   *Note: Proper tip placement of the CVC or PICC must be confirmed prior to PN infusion.*
                ❏ Peripheral IV (PIV) *(Final PN Osmolarity ≤ _____ mOsm/L)*

Monitoring: Daily weights; strict input & output; bedside glucose monitoring every _8_ hours
                  ☒ Na, K, Cl, CO_2, Glucose, BUN, Scr, Mg, PO_4 every _Day_
                  ☒ T. Billi, Alk Phos, AST, ALT, Albumin, Triglycerides, Calcium every _Week_

Base Solution: *Total parenteral nutrition **MUST** be administered through a dedicated infusion port and filtered with a*
Select one   *1.2-micron in-line filter at all times. Discard any unused volume after 24 hours.*

❏ PERIPHERAL 2-in-1	☒ CENTRAL 2-in-1	❏ CENTRAL 3-in-1
Dextrose _____ g	Dextrose 15%	Dextrose _____ g
Amino Acids (*Brand_____*) _____ g	Amino Acids (*Brand Aminosyn*) 3.5%	Amino Acids (*Brand_____*) _____ g
For patients with PIV and established glucose tolerance; provides _____ kcal; maximum rate not to exceed _____ mL/hour.	*For patients with CVC or PICC and established glucose tolerance; provides _____ kcal; maximum rate not to exceed _____ mL/hour.*	Fat Emulsion (*Brand_____*) _____ g
		For patients with CVC or PICC and established glucose/fat emulsion tolerance; provides _____ kcal; maximum rate not to exceed _____ mL/hour.
		Use of additional fat emulsion not required with 3-in-1 base solution.

RATE & VOLUME: _40_ mL/hour for _24_ hours = _960_ mL/day
Must specify

or CYCLIC INFUSION: _____ mL/hour for _____ hours, then _____ mL/hour for _____ hours = _____ mL/day

---

Fat Emulsion (Brand 0) – via PIV or CVC with 2-in-1 base solutions (select caloric density & volume)

❏ 10%   ❏ 20%   Infuse at ____ mL/hour over ____ hours.   Frequency ____

❏ 250 mL   ❏ 500 mL   *(Note: Infusions < 4 or > 12 hours not recommended)*   *Discard any unused volume after 12 hours.*

Additives: (per liter)		Normal Dosages	Additives: (per liter)	
Sodium Chloride	_40_ mEq	*1–2 mEq sodium/kg/day*	**Regular Insulin** _60_ units	
as Acetate	_____ mEq	*pH or CO_2 dependent*	*Recommended if hyperglycemic; start with 1 unit for every 10 g of dextrose.*	
as Phosphate	_____ mmol of PO_4	*Consider if hyperkalemic*		
Potassium Chloride	_20_ mEq	*1–2 mEq potassium/kg/day*		
as Acetate	_____ mEq	*pH or CO_2 dependent*	**Pharmacy Use Only:** Ca/PO_4	
as Phosphate	_12_ mmol of PO_4	*20-40 mmol/day (1 mmol Phos = 1.5 mEq K)*	**Limit Checked** _MKing, RPh_	
Calcium Gluconate	_10_ mEq	*5–15 mEq/day*	*(Note: Some brands of amino acids contain phosphate.)*	
Magnesium Sulfate	_____ mEq	*8–24 mEq/day*		
Adult **Multivitamins**	_10_ mL/day	*Contains vitamin K 160 mcg*		
Adult **Trace Elements**	_5_ mL/day	*Zn __ mg, Cu __ mg, Mn __ mg, Cr __ mcg, Se __ mcg (with normal hepatic function)*		
H_2 **Antagonist**	_____ mg	*____ mg/day with normal renal function*		
Other:				

Physician's Signature _Kumar Singh, MD_   Pager Number: _6-5411_   Date/time: _8/14/2016_

Orders transcribed by: _RMcManus_ Date/time: _8/14/16 11:30 am_ Orders verified by: _MKing, RPh_ Date/time: _8/4/16 2:45 pm_ staff and proper catheter care by the nursing staff—is critical to avoid introducing bacteria directly into the bloodstream. To that end, healthcare personnel must cleanse the catheter site, flush the catheter, and check the catheter site regularly during TPN administration. The tubing is replaced with each new TPN bag (or bottle) to minimize bacterial contamination and infection.

Premade Parenteral Products

The use of premade parenteral products by a hospital pharmacy department benefits not only its personnel but also the nursing staff and the patients they tend. These commercially available products, such as vial-and-bag systems and frozen sterile IV solutions, minimize labor-intensive preparation, contamination, toxicity, and drug wastage.

To prepare these products for patient administration, pharmacy personnel must follow certain handling and labeling requirements. Because these products are not compounded by pharmacy personnel, their expiration dating varies somewhat from standard beyond-use dating (BUD) as defined in USP Chapter <797>. For that reason, personnel should always refer to the manufacturers' recommendations and the pharmacy's Policy and Procedure (P&P) manual for guidance in determining expiration dating for premade parenteral products. The expiration dating is based on scientific studies by the manufacturer and varies with the product, diluent, and storage conditions. The expiration dating can be found on the vial of the medication or in the product package insert.

Vial-and-Bag Systems

A **vial-and-bag system** provides both a single vial of powdered medication with an adaptor and a specified IV solution that acts as the diluent. Just before patient administration, the nurse breaks a small inner seal that separates the powdered medication from the IV solution diluent. This action "activates" the medication which, once it is fully dissolved, is then administered to the patient via an IVPB.

Types of Vial-and-Bag Systems Vial-and-bag systems are marketed under many trade names, such as ADD-Vantage (Hospira) and MINI-BAG Plus (Baxter Healthcare). Only selected products—mostly antibiotics and some chemotherapy agents—are available in vial-and-bag systems. Often, a hospital pharmacy has to purchase more than one delivery system to cover a wider variety of drugs.

Although the vial-and-bag products are assembled by the IV technician in an ISO Class 5 environment, they do not require sterile compounding and, therefore, are not considered CSPs. Because the beyond-use dating guidelines in USP Chapter <797> refer specifically to CSPs, these guidelines do not apply to proprietary vial-and-bag systems. The stability and expiration dating of these products varies with the type and concentration of the drug, the diluent, the storage conditions, and the activation; therefore, the technician is directed to follow the manufacturer's recommendations for handling, storage, and beyond-use dating.

Benefits of Vial-and-Bag Systems Vial-and-bag systems offer a variety of benefits for healthcare personnel. In addition to fewer returns to the pharmacy and less wastage, other advantages are improved safety, efficiency, and cost-effectiveness.

Safety In terms of safety, admixing errors are minimized because doses are standardized, and enhanced labeling and bar coding of both the medication in the vial and the IV solution are provided. In other words, the nurse knows exactly what is in the IV solution. The closed-system sterile packaging also minimizes the risk of contamination. Finally, these devices do not use needles, thus preventing the possibility of inadvertent needle sticks by the pharmacist, technician, or nurse.

Efficiency Vial-and-bag systems are efficient to use because doses are premeasured for rapid reconstitution and easy assembly by the nurse on the patient care unit. There is no need for freezing, thawing, or refrigeration of the solution in the pharmacy or nursing unit because the product is immediately administered to the patient.

Cost-Effectiveness Personnel costs are saved because no admixing is necessary and no additional supply costs—such as for syringes, needles, gauze, and so on—are incurred. These advantages may well outweigh the additional cost per unit.

Assembly and Activation of Vial-and-Bag Systems Each vial-and-bag system differs somewhat in design, but the concept is similar. The vial of drug—which has not been reconstituted—is coupled (with or without an adaptor) with an appropriate volume of IV solution. Depending on the system, many minibags are available in 50 mL, 100 mL, and 250 mL sizes with many diluent options (D_5W, D_5NS, NS, lactated Ringer's, and so on).

Assembly The pharmacy technician is responsible for attaching or assembling a specially designed vial containing the correct drug and dosage to an IVPB bag containing the correct IV solution and volume. This connection process is performed in the hood to maintain the sterility of the solution. The technician is also responsible for proper labeling of the product, including expiration dating.

Activation The nursing staff is responsible for activating the product at the patient's bedside. After scanning the product's bar code, the nurse uses aseptic technique to activate the product just before patient administration. To do so, the nurse breaks a small, internal chamber at the connecting site of the vial and IVPB. This action allows the drug in the vial to mix with the fluid in the bag. Once the medication is mixed, the nurse administers the solution to the patient via sterile IV tubing.

Vial-and-bag systems differ slightly in their activation. Pharmacy personnel may need to complete additional training on these various systems to assist the nursing staff in the various activation techniques.

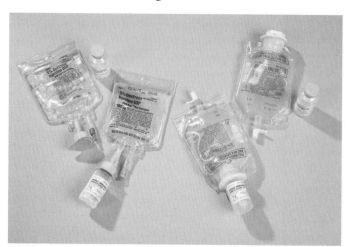

A vial-and-bag delivery system is assembled by the pharmacy technician but activated by the nurse at the patient's bedside. This system is not considered a CSP and, therefore, should be labeled with the manufacturer's recommended expiration dating.

Frozen IV Solutions

Frozen IV solutions are commercially available products and, consequently, are not considered CSPs. Most frozen IV products are antibiotics and are manufactured as SVPs in a premixed frozen state. Hospital pharmacies purchase these frozen products for a number of reasons, including less wastage, longer expiration dates, reduced risk of microbial contamination, and less labor-intensive preparation for pharmacy personnel. These benefits partially offset the higher acquisition cost.

If some products are not commercially available, then the pharmacy technician may be preparing extra CSPs and freezing them for later patient use. In this scenario, the pharmacy department's P&P manual must be followed, and the USP Chapter <797> standards for beyond-use dating must be used. Reconstituted vials of antibiotics have a much shorter half-life than frozen solutions with potentially more wastage and cost.

Handling of Frozen IV Solutions Frozen IV products are kept in the freezer of the hospital pharmacy until a medication order is received. At that time, pharmacy personnel either thaw the product at room temperature or in the refrigerator (if there is sufficient time). The use of a warming bath or microwave to expedite the thawing process ("forced thaw") is *not* recommended. Manufacturers' recommendations for thawing vary among products, so personnel must be sure to check the specific product's label.

After thawing, the technician prepares a patient-specific label with the expiration date. The expiration date varies with the drug and storage conditions. For example, a frozen Ancef antibiotic solution has an expiration date of 48 hours at room temperature, or 30 days if stored in the refrigerator. A Zosyn antibiotic solution has an expiration date of 24 hours at room temperature, or 14 days if stored in the refrigerator. Once thawed, these frozen preparations cannot be refrozen. After preparing the label, the technician affixes the label to the bag and sends the medication to the nursing unit for administration.

Hospital Pharmacy Calculations

Safety Note

Pharmacy personnel must always check and then double-check all calculations.

The pharmacy technician who prepares CSPs in the hospital or home healthcare setting should have a good understanding of certain calculation methods that are commonly used in these environments. These skills include calculations based on IV administration flow rates and determining dosage volumes. In practice, most dosage calculations are done by the pharmacy technician. IV flow rates, however, are typically provided on the medication order by the physician. The technician then uses the ordered IV flow rate to perform a pharmacy calculation that determines days' supply for IVs and IVPBs, and the pharmacist verifies the accuracy of the technician's calculations as a double check.

The calculation and verification process differs for chemotherapy agents, neonatal IV medications, and certain TPN preparations. For these products, the pharmacist typically performs the first set of calculations, which are then verified by another pharmacist. The pharmacy technician then provides the "third-line check" of these calculations.

Determining IV Administration Flow Rates

Sterile compounding personnel are responsible for preparing all of the CSPs needed for all patients for a specified period. This responsibility, called the *daily IV run* or the *batch*, requires personnel to compound a 24-hour supply of CSPs for each patient. In addition to the basic dosage calculations that were presented in Chapter 5, pharmacy technicians are often called upon to perform various IV administration flow rate calculations based on the infusion rate prescribed by the physician. These calculations typically address the following questions:

- What is the infusion rate in mL/hour?
- How long will this bag last?
- What time will the next bag be needed?
- How many bags will be needed for the patient in a 24-hour period?

To answer these questions, technicians need to know the total volume of the LVP and either (1) the infusion rate in milliliters per hour (mL/hr) or (2) the number of hours over which the LVP is to be infused. This information can be found in the physician's medication order or on the CSP. Technicians then perform a series of IV flow rate calculations using either multiplication or division.

To answer the question, *"What is the infusion rate in mL/hr?"* technicians must divide the total volume (TV) by the number of hours (H) over which the CSP is to be administered: $TV/H = x$.

To answer the question, *"How long will this bag last?"* technicians must divide the total volume (TV) by the infusion rate (IR): $TV/IR = x$.

To answer the question, *"What time will the next bag be needed?"* technicians must first divide the total volume (TV) by the infusion rate (IR): $TV/IR = x$. Then they add the number of hours (x) calculated in the previous step to the current standard time.

To answer the question, *"How many bags will be needed for the patient in a 24-hour period?"* technicians must first divide the total volume (TV) by the infusion rate (IR): $TV/IR = x$. Then they divide 24 (the number of hours in a day) by the number of hours calculated in the previous step (x).

Example 1

A physician orders 4000 mL of D$_5$NS to be administered over 24 hours. What is the infusion rate in milliliters per hour?

Begin by identifying the amounts to insert into the equation: $TV/H = x$.

$$TV = 4000 \text{ mL}$$

$$H = 24 \text{ hours}$$

$$4000/24 = 166.67, \text{ rounded up to the nearest whole number}$$

$$x = 167 \text{ mL/hour}$$

Example 2

The prescriber has ordered 500 mg of cefazolin in 50 mL of D_5W to be administered IVPB at 100 mL per hour. How long will it take to administer this medication?

Begin by identifying the amounts to insert into the equation: TV/IR = x.

$$TV = 50 \text{ mL}$$

$$IR = 100 \text{ mL/hr}$$

$$50/100 = 0.5 \text{ (or ½ hour)}$$

$$x = \text{½ hour or 30 minutes}$$

Example 3

You are to prepare 20 mEq of medication in 1000 mL of D_5W to be administered at 125 mL/hr. If the first bag is hung at 10:00 AM, what time will the next bag be needed?

Begin by identifying the amounts to insert into the equation: TV/IR = x.

$$TV = 1000 \text{ mL}$$

$$IR = 125 \text{ mL/hr}$$

$$1000/125 = 8; \text{ one bag will last 8 hours; 8 hours after 10:00 AM is 6:00 PM.}$$

$$x = 6:00 \text{ PM}$$

Example 4

A 1 L IV is running at 250 mL/hour. How many IV bags will be needed in a 24-hour period?

Begin by converting 1 L to 1000 mL, and then identifying the amounts to insert into the equation: TV/IR = x.

$$TV = 1000 \text{ mL}$$

$$IR = 250 \text{ mL/hr}$$

$$1000/250 = 4$$

$$24/4 = 6 \text{ bags will be needed in a 24-hour period.}$$

$$x = 6 \text{ bags}$$

Adding Electrolytes

Many IV fluids used in hospital pharmacy practice contain dissolved mineral salts; such a fluid is known as an **electrolyte solution**. These fluids are so named because they conduct an electrical charge through the solution when connected to electrodes. For example, the compound potassium chloride (abbreviated KCl) breaks down to K+ and Cl– ions in solution. Electrolyte solutions, in addition to being measured in the usual metric units such as milligrams, are also measured in milliequivalents (mEq). Milliequivalents are related to molecular weights, or weights that are based on the atomic weights of common elements.

Compounding LVP solutions typically requires the technician to draw up an additive, such as the electrolyte potassium chloride, and inject it into an IV base solution using correct aseptic technique. When calculating the amount of an additive to add to an IV base solution, technicians must use pharmacy math formulas such as the ratio-proportion method to determine the volume of additive that must be drawn up to provide the prescribed dosage. (For a review of the ratio-proportion method used in pharmacy calculations, see Chapter 5.)

Example 5

You are requested to add 44 mEq of sodium chloride (NaCl) to an IV bag. Sodium chloride is available as a 4 mEq/mL solution. How many milliliters should you add to the bag?

Set up a proportion—comparing the solution that you need to create to the available solution—and solve for the unknown. Review examples in Chapter 5 if you are not sure how to solve a problem using the ratio-proportion method.

$$\frac{x \text{ mL}}{44 \text{ mEq}} = \frac{1 \text{ mL}}{4 \text{ mEq}}$$

$$\frac{(44 \text{ mEq}) \, x \text{ mL}}{44 \text{ mEq}} = \frac{(44 \text{ mEq}) \, 1 \text{ mL}}{4 \text{ mEq}}$$

$$x \text{ mL} = \frac{44 \text{ mL}}{4}$$

$$x = 11 \text{ mL}$$

Hazardous Agents

Pharmacists and pharmacy technicians working in a hospital setting often come in contact with hazardous agents. Unlike other CSPs, hazardous agents require special handling and preparation by pharmacy personnel. These specialized procedures affect the entire compounding process, from garbing and calculations, to compounding and labeling, to administration and disposal of the hazardous products.

Hazardous agents include cytotoxic drugs and antineoplastic drugs. A **cytotoxic drug** is any drug that destroys cancer cells, whereas an **antineoplastic drug** reduces or prevents the growth of cancer cells. Pharmacy personnel should be aware, however, that these two terms are often used interchangeably. Both cytotoxic drugs and antineoplastic drugs are used in chemotherapy and, occasionally, used to treat certain skin conditions. Although the benefit to the patient is greater than the risk of adverse effects, a healthcare worker may be adversely affected by exposure to such an agent in the preparation or administration process.

Before 1980, there were few safety standards for the handling of hazardous drugs. In fact, the use of protective clothing was optional, and most medications were prepared in a horizontal laminar airflow hood or on the nursing unit. In 1979, a study in Finland identified chemotherapy traces in the urine of oncology nurses. This finding was one of the catalysts for research on the effects of chemotherapy exposure in healthcare workers. Several studies in the 1980s demonstrated that nurses had adverse side effects similar to those of their chemotherapy patients who were undergoing drug therapy with hazardous agents. In 1982, pharmacists who handled chemotherapeutic agents were found to have mutagenic changes in their urine. From these findings, as well as other documented cases, the donning of protective clothing and the use of a vertical laminar airflow hood became the accepted norm for the preparation of hazardous drugs.

A 1996 OSHA statement on potential hazards of handling antineoplastic drugs stated that the "preparation, administration, manufacturing, and disposal of hazardous medications may expose hundreds of thousands of workers, principally in healthcare facilities and the pharmaceutical industry, to potentially significant workplace levels of these chemicals." Over the past two decades, several chemotherapy wipe studies have demonstrated persistent contamination in both preparation and patient care areas. USP Chapter <797> safety standards were adopted soon thereafter to address these contamination issues.

Risks of Exposure to Hazardous Agents

The four routes of exposure of personnel to hazardous agents include (1) trauma, (2) inhalation, (3) ingestion, and (4) direct skin contact, illustrated by the following examples:

- *Trauma or injury*: A technician using a syringe to add a drug to an IV bag might accidentally prick himself or herself with the needle or receive a cut from a broken container of the substance.
- *Inhalation of the hazardous substance*: A technician might drop and break a bottle containing a volatile substance or use poor manipulation technique with a multiple-dose vial, thereby releasing a fine mist of the medication from the container and inadvertently inhaling the substance.
- *Ingestion*: A technician might ingest minute powder particles when crushing an oral tablet or cleaning a counting tray.
- *Direct skin contact*: A technician might accidentally spill a medication when pouring it from a large container into a smaller container or flask. Direct contact with some cancer drugs can cause immediate reactions:
  - Asparaginase can cause skin irritation.
  - Doxorubicin can cause tissue death and sloughing if introduced into a skin abrasion.
  - Nitrogen mustards can cause irritation of the eyes, mucous membranes, and skin.
  - Streptozocin is a potential carcinogen if it comes into contact with skin.

With exposure to hazardous agents, healthcare workers may potentially suffer acute, chronic, and long-term health consequences. Acute risks may be from contact resulting in skin rashes or allergic reactions. In women of reproductive age, chronic exposure could result in infertility, miscarriages, or neonates with low birth weight or congenital malformations. Long-term risks with years of chronic exposure may include a higher risk for certain cancers, including skin and bladder cancers and leukemia.

Any woman of reproductive age who routinely works with hazardous agents should have confirmation in writing attesting to an understanding of the risks and the importance of taking additional precautions to prevent pregnancy. A pharmacy worker who is breast-feeding or trying to conceive should notify her supervisor so that extra precautions can be taken to minimize contact with any hazardous substances or a change in work responsibilities is made.

The use of incorrect aseptic technique during the compounding of nonhazardous CSPs may result in contamination and potential infection for the patient recipient. However, the use of incorrect aseptic technique in the preparation of hazardous agents not only poses contamination risks for the patient recipient but also jeopardizes the sterile compounder's own health. The policy and procedures of the department, as well as guidelines and standards from USP Chapter <797>, are designed to help protect the healthcare worker from unnecessary exposure and risks. Innovative closed-system transfer devices (CSTDs) are increasingly being used to prepare and administer hazardous drugs and protect the healthcare worker.

Protective Clothing

USP Chapter <797> dictates the donning of protective clothing when working with hazardous agents. These guidelines are similar to the ones discussed in Chapter 10 for preparing CSPs, but with additional requirements. A disposable, lint-free, impervious, closed-front gown with cuffed sleeves should be worn, as well as a hair cover and shoe covers to reduce the potential for particulate contamination. Other protective clothing includes eye protection, a face mask, and chemotherapy gloves worn over sterile, disposable gloves (a procedure known as *double gloving*).

Double gloving should be done after a thorough washing of the hands. Glove thickness and exposure duration influence glove permeability. All glove sizes should be available so that each worker has a good fit. The first pair of gloves should be tucked under the sleeve cuff of the gown, whereas the second pair should be placed over the top of the cuff. Gloves should be turned inside out as they are removed and must be discarded in designated chemotherapy sharps containers in the clean room.

Before leaving the hazardous drug preparation clean room area, all protective garb must be discarded in specially marked containers. No gowns, gloves, masks, and so on, can be reused (even after a short break), and no contaminated protective clothing can be worn in the general pharmacy area or hospital.

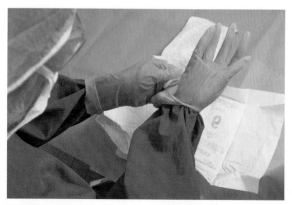

When working with hazardous drugs, pharmacy technicians must use additional precautions such as double gloving and eye shields to protect themselves.

Receipt and Storage of Hazardous Agents

The pharmacy technician must wear gloves not only when preparing hazardous agents, but also when receiving, stocking, inventorying, and disposing of them. Hazardous drugs should be delivered directly to the storage area upon delivery and inventoried. The inventory of these drugs should be separated from other medications to prevent contamination and exposure, as well as to reduce the potential error of pulling a look-alike container from an adjacent shelf or bin. Damaged packages should be inspected in an insulated area, such as a vertical airflow hood. The receipt of broken vials of drugs that have not been reconstituted should be treated as hazardous agent spills, as discussed later in this chapter.

Storage areas, including drug cartons, shelves, bins, counters, and trays, should carry appropriate, brightly colored warning labels ("Caution: Hazardous Agents") and should be designed in such a way as to maximize product recognition and minimize the possibility of falling and breakage. For example, storage shelves should have a barrier at the front; carts should have rims; and hazardous drugs should be stored at eye level or lower. Ideal storage is in a room with frequent air exchanges and negative air pressure to dilute or remove potential airborne contaminants.

Hazardous drugs requiring refrigeration should be stored separately from other drugs, in bins that prevent breakage and contain leakage should it occur. Access to storage areas and work areas for hazardous materials should be limited to specified trained personnel. A list of cytotoxic and otherwise hazardous drugs should be compiled and posted in appropriate locations throughout the workplace. Table 11.4 lists some commonly used cytotoxic and hazardous drugs that have been shown to be cancer-causing agents.

TABLE 11.4 List of Common Carcinogens

Group 1: Carcinogenic to humans	arsenic trioxide, azathioprine, busulfan, chlorambucil, cyclophosphamide, melphalan, semustine, tamoxifen, thiotepa, treosulfan
Group 2A: Probably carcinogenic to humans	azacitidine, carmustine, cisplatin, doxorubicin, etoposide, lomustine, nitrogen mustard, procarbazine, teniposide
Group 2B: Possibly carcinogenic to humans	amsacrine, bleomycin, dacarbazine, daunorubicin mitomycin, mitoxantrone, streptozocin

Data is from the International Agency for Research on Cancer (updated November 2012).

Equipment for Preparing Hazardous Agents

CSPs comprised of hazardous agents should always be prepared using strict aseptic technique under conditions that maximize protection of the healthcare worker. Such agents should be prepared, per USP Chapter <797> guidelines, in either a biological safety cabinet (BSC) or a Compounding Aseptic Containment Isolator (CACI) that provides an ISO Class 5 environment. In large hospitals, these hoods are located in a separate, negative-pressure clean room environment that is designated for the preparation of hazardous medications. For facilities that prepare a small volume of hazardous

CSPs (defined as fewer than five hazardous CSPs per week), the use of a closed-system transfer device (CSTD) within a BSC or a CACI located in a nonnegative pressure room is permitted.

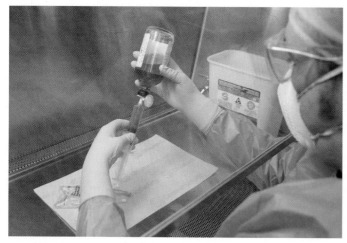

A biological safety cabinet is commonly used to prepare hazardous cancer drugs in the hospital.

Biological Safety Cabinet A **biological safety cabinet (BSC)** is a specialized hood that is used to prepare chemotherapy drugs and other hazardous compounds. Its design allows for HEPA-filtered air to flow downward in a vertical pattern and then outward through small ventilation holes located at the back and sides of the cabinet. This contaminated air is HEPA-filtered again and recirculated into the cabinet or vented to the outside air. In addition to the vertical airflow, the sterile compounder is also protected by a Plexiglas shield at the front of the cabinet. This shield comes down from the top of the cabinet and stops about eight inches from the work surface. The shield's position allows the worker to place his or her hands inside the cabinet while being protected from exposure to hazardous chemicals.

Compounding Aseptic Containment Isolator Similar to a BSC, a **compounding aseptic containment isolator** is a vertical airflow hood that is used in the preparation of hazardous drugs. This type of hood has a fully enclosed cabinet that limits direct exposure to airborne drugs. Sterile compounders place their hands in a pair of fixed gloves located at the front of the cabinet and reach through an inner pass-through window to bring supplies into the direct compounding area of the hood. Like the BSC, this type of hood vents the contaminated air through a HEPA-filtered ventilation system.

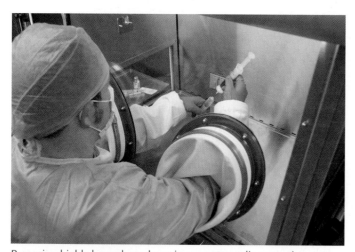

Preparing highly hazardous drugs in a compounding aseptic containment isolator affords the technician additional protection.

Supplies Used in Hazardous Drug Preparation

The process of compounding hazardous drugs involves several specialized supply items in addition to the standard supplies used in nonhazardous drug preparation: a needle-and-syringe unit, IV base solutions, vials, and ampules.

Specialized Supplies Several supplies used in the compounding of chemotherapy drugs include a closed-system transfer device (CSTD), a compounding mat, and a chemotherapy dispensing pin.

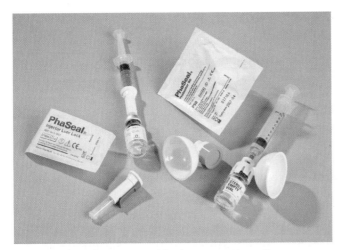

CSTDs such as these are used in the preparation of chemotherapy CSPs.

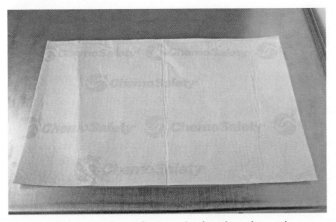

A chemotherapy compounding mat is placed on the work surface of a BSC before beginning chemotherapy compounding.

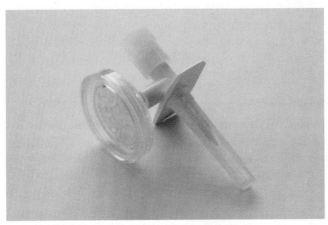

A chemotherapy dispensing pin safely relieves the negative pressure within a drug vial.

Closed-System Transfer Devices Whenever possible, the use of a **closed-system transfer device (CSTD)** is a preferred compounding tool. In general, CSTDs use a double internal needle transfer with dual membranes to provide a tight seal connection. This sealed pathway allows the safe withdrawal of fluid from a vial into a syringe and the safe injection of fluid from a syringe into an IVPB or IV. This design minimizes worker exposure to hazardous agents during the preparation of CSPs. The closed system also avoids pressurization issues with the vial, thus preventing the escape of toxic vapors.

EQUASHIELD and PhaSeal are examples of CSTDs that have met national standards and have shown favorable results in scientific studies. These CSTDs are enclosed and provide fully airtight syringes and vial adaptors that allow for the safe compounding of hazardous drugs. Strict aseptic technique, additional protective clothing, and special preparation and handling procedures must be implemented by pharmacy personnel as well as the nursing staff administering the chemotherapy CSP using a CSTD administration catheter.

Chemotherapy Compounding Mat A **chemotherapy compounding mat** is a thin mat whose one side is made of absorbent material to soak up potential fluid spills within the BSC. The other side of the mat is made of a low-permeability material that prevents fluid from seeping through to the work surface of the hood. This mat is placed by the sterile compounder on the BSC work surface before beginning the compounding procedure.

Chemotherapy Dispensing Pin A **chemotherapy dispensing pin**, or chemo pin, is a small plastic device that has a spike at one end and an adaptor at the other end. In between the two ends is a vent to which a 0.22 micron HEPA filter is attached. This device is used to relieve the negative pressure within a medication vial safely by equalizing the pressure. The built-in HEPA filter traps escaping drug particles or fluid during injection or withdrawal procedures. However, technicians need to be aware that some drug vapors escape the vial.

Hazardous Agents in Vials

Occasionally, sterile compounding personnel are required to prepare hazardous CSPs from a vial. These workers need to be aware that the process of handling a vial during hazardous drug preparation is different from the vial-handling techniques used for nonhazardous drugs. Because of the potential for inadvertent worker exposure to the hazardous agent, the creation of positive pressure within a hazardous drug vial should be avoided, preferably through the use of a CSTD. If a CSTD is unavailable, a vented chemotherapy dispensing pin may be used to safely withdraw fluid from a hazardous drug vial, before injecting the fluid into an IV or IVPB. The chemotherapy dispensing pin may also be used to facilitate the reconstitution of a powder and provide for a safe withdrawal of the solution from the vial since it is a needleless system.

If a CSTD or chemotherapy dispensing pin is not available, the technician may be required to inject a diluent into the vial to reconstitute a powdered hazardous agent. When reconstituting the powder vial, the technician should very slowly inject the diluent into the vial, allowing the excess pressure from the vial to vent into the syringe. When withdrawing the reconstituted drug from the vial, the technician should use negative pressure techniques to ensure that no drug is leaked from the vial or aspirated into the air. This is accomplished by either introducing no air into the vial (i.e., negative pressure) or by introducing a volume of air that is *less than the solution volume* that is to be withdrawn (i.e., relative negative pressure). This negative pressure technique produces a relative negative pressure environment within the vial, thus producing a vacuum and preventing an aspirate when the needle is withdrawn from the rubber closure. After withdrawing the reconstituted drug from the vial, the technician then injects the contents of the syringe into an IV or IVPB.

Excessive air or fluid injected into a hazardous drug vial may build up pressure, causing a bit of the liquid to spray out around the needle, thus increasing the risk of inadvertent exposure to the hazardous drug. It is important that a slight negative pressure be maintained throughout the sterile compounding procedure. To prevent excessive negative pressure, never inject into a hazardous drug vial more than 75% of the volume that you plan to subsequently withdraw from the vial. For example, if you are to withdraw 4 mL of a cytotoxic drug from a multiple-dose vial, then you should inject no more than 3 mL of air (75%) before withdrawing the drug in the syringe. Do not inject a volume of air equal to or greater than the amount of drug to be withdrawn. When adding a diluent such as sterile water for injection or normal saline to a vial, do so slowly, allowing pressure in the vial and syringe to equalize.

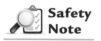

Safety Note

When working with hazardous drugs, sterile compounding personnel should use negative pressure techniques whenever possible. Under no circumstances should a volume of air that is greater than 75% of the volume of the drug withdrawn be injected into the vial.

Hazardous Agents in Ampules

Occasionally, technicians will need to prepare hazardous CSPs from an ampule. As an extra precaution, sterile compounding personnel should use a CSTD and operate in a BSC or CACI. When opening an ampule of a hazardous medication, the technician should gently tap or swirl the container to clear the fluid from the head and neck of the ampule. Next, he or she should sterilize the neck of the ampule with a 70% IPA swab, wrap a pad around the ampule, and hold the body of the ampule in the nondominant hand, pointing the ampule away from the face. Finally, the technician should place the thumb and forefinger of his or her dominant hand on the head of the ampule and gently but firmly break off the top. A 5 micron filter needle should be placed on the syringe to withdraw the solution from the ampule. The fluid should be drawn through the filter needle into the attached syringe. A standard needle is then placed on the syringe before injecting the fluid into an IV or IVPB.

Hazardous Oral Drugs

Hazardous oral drugs may be handled in community, home healthcare, long-term care, and hospital pharmacy settings. During the routine handling of hazardous oral drugs, workers should wear one pair of gloves of good quality and thickness, a gown, and a respirator. The counting and pouring of these drugs (e.g., methotrexate) should be done carefully, and contaminated equipment such as counting trays should be immediately cleaned with detergent and rinsed after each use. Tablet and capsule forms of hazardous materials should not be placed in automated counting or packaging machines.

The hospital pharmacy technician may also need to repackage a hazardous oral agent into unit-dose bubble packaging. When the technician is crushing a hazardous drug in a unit-of-use package, the package should be placed in a small, sealable plastic bag and crushed with a spoon or pestle; the technician should use caution not to break the plastic bag. Compounding involving these drugs should be done in a protected area removed from drafts and traffic.

Radioactive Pharmaceuticals

Radioactive pharmaceuticals are occasionally prepared in a nuclear pharmacy by a specially trained and certified nuclear pharmacy technician. The details of handling, preparation, and disposal of radioactive agents are beyond the scope of this text but can be found in USP Chapter <823>.

Priming, Labeling, and Administering Hazardous Agents

All hazardous CSPs should be primed and labeled according to institutional guidelines. Syringes filled with hazardous agents should never be filled more than ¾ full because overly full syringes have a greater potential for the syringe plunger to become separated from the barrel. If the medication is to be dispensed from the syringe, then the solution should be cleared from the needle and hub and the needle should be replaced with a locking syringe cap. The exterior surface of the prepared syringe should be cleaned with a sterile 70% IPA wipe and then labeled. If the medication is to be added to an IV bag, care should be used to prevent a puncture of the bag.

Priming an IV Administration Set If applicable, an IV administration set should be attached and properly primed. The exterior surface of the administration set and the entire bag should be wiped with sterile 70% IPA and then labeled. The bag should be placed in a sealable plastic bag to capture any potential leakage during transport. Depending on the type of CSP, the nurse may administer the hazardous CSP through either the primed administration set, or through the use of an administration-specific CSTD that is used only on the nursing unit.

The priming of IV administration sets for CSPs containing cytotoxic agents should always be performed in the BSC or CACI in the hospital pharmacy. To prime the IV administration set, the technician should insert the spike of the administration set into the CSP's tubing port. This action allows fluid to run from the CSP through the tubing, thus priming the tubing. The hazardous CSP with an attached, primed administration set is then delivered to the nursing unit in a plastic bag.

Labeling Hazardous Agents All CSPs containing hazardous agents must be properly labeled. These CSP labels must contain the patient's name and room number, the solution name and volume, the drug name(s) and dosage, CSP administration information, and storage requirements. In addition, hazardous agents also require additional labeling that clearly identifies the CSP as a hazardous agent.

Administering Hazardous Agents To administer a hazardous medication, a nurse must wear a mask, gloves, and a special gown. Typically, two nurses check the medication dose and labeling before patient administration. This precautionary measure minimizes drug administration errors. An incorrect dose, especially in a pediatric patient, could prove deadly. Once the administration of the medication is completed, the nurse disposes of his or her garb in a designated hazardous waste container.

Hazardous Agent Spills

In the event of a hazardous agent spill, pharmacy personnel must be aware of the proper cleanup procedures as well as the proper disposal of contaminated drugs and clothing. The goal of the containment of a cytotoxic or hazardous material spill is to ensure that the staff, patients, and visitors are not exposed and that the healthcare environment (both inside and outside the medical facility) is not contaminated.

All spills—small or large—must be addressed immediately. Cleanup and decontamination should be done with a spill kit. Spill kits contain materials to control and clean spills of up to 1000 mL. A commercially available spill kit may be purchased, or one may be assembled with the following contents:

- nonabsorbent, lint-free gown
- two pairs of gloves
- respirator mask
- one pair of goggles
- absorbent towels
- chemo hazard labels
- spill control pillows or towels folded to work as pillows
- scoop and brush (for collecting broken glass)
- plastic disposal bags labeled "Chemo Waste"
- "CAUTION: Chemo Spill" sign

When a spill occurs, a warning sign should be posted outside of and near the location of the spill, so that it will clearly identify the spill area and warn people to stay away from the hazardous area during cleanup. When cleaning spills, personnel must don proper attire—including a gown, double gloves, goggles, and a mask or respirator—and should never use bare hands to handle the hazardous fluids or glass shards. Broken glass should be placed in an appropriate, puncture-proof container. When cleaning up the spill, personnel should start from the edge of the spill and work inward, using absorbent sheets, spill pads, or pillows for the liquids and damp cloths or towels for solids. Use spill pads and water to rinse the area. Detergent should be used to remove residue. The spill area should be wiped down with a detergent solution at least three times to ensure that the hazardous agent has been removed from the spill area.

Spills within the BSC or CACI require additional cleaning steps. The drain trough should be thoroughly cleaned and the cabinet decontaminated according to manufacturer specifications. All contaminated materials from a spill should be sealed in hazardous waste containers and placed in leak-resistant containers. The spill, cleanup, and any personnel exposure must be documented.

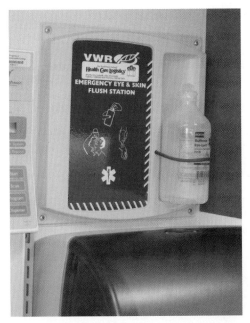

An eyewash station must be located where any parenteral hazardous drugs are being prepared.

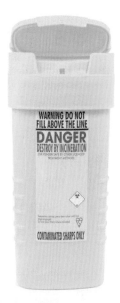

A designated yellow sharps container must be used to dispose of any syringes, needles, or biological waste/spills when working with hazardous drugs.

Procedures in Case of Exposure

Every hazardous substance has a Material Safety Data Sheet (MSDS) outlining specific recommendations on how to handle an exposure (see Figure 11.13 on the following page). If the skin is exposed, the worker should use water to flush the affected area immediately and then thoroughly cleanse the area with soap and water. If the substance comes in contact with the eyes, the worker should flush the eyes with large amounts of water or use an eye-flush kit. Each hospital pharmacy should have an eyewash sink or eye-flush kit close to the clean room in the event of an accidental exposure to a hazardous drug.

The worker should then remove contaminated garments and gloves and dispose of them in specially designated chemotherapy waste containers. No protective clothing should be taken outside the area where the exposure occurred. The worker must also wash his or her hands thoroughly and be sent or escorted to the emergency room. The accidental exposure should be reported to the supervisor, who should notify other staff members to avoid the spread of contamination. An incident report must be completed.

Final Inspection and Delivery to the Patient Care Unit

The medication order, label, compounding procedure, preparation records, and all materials used to make the CSP must be inspected by the pharmacist before being sent to the nursing unit.

Inspection of CSP

The inspection should check for accuracy in the identifications and quantities of ingredients, technique for aseptic mixing and sterilization, packaging, labeling, and physical appearance. The inspection often includes any syringes used to draw up the medication.

FIGURE 11.13

Chemical labeling is changing, as the Occupational Safety and Health Administration (OSHA) phases in the Globally Harmonized System of Classification and Labeling of Chemicals (GHS). Under this international effort to harmonize classification and communication, label contents will change. The familiar MSDS (shown below, on the right) will become the SDS, or Safety Data Sheet (shown below, on the left). Hazard classifications, pictograms, and warning verbiage will change, but the familiar 16-section format will remain. The deadline for full implementation is December 1, 2015. In the interim, pharmacy personnel can expect to see both old (MSDS) and new (SDS) forms from suppliers.

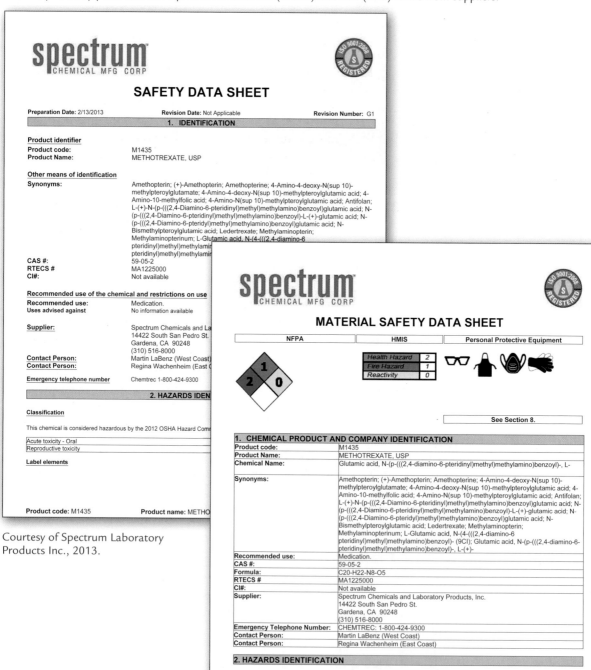

Courtesy of Spectrum Laboratory Products Inc., 2013.

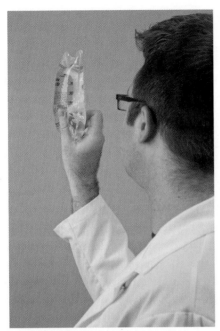

The pharmacist should double-check the technician's calculations and procedures and inspect the prepared IV bag for precipitates.

Occasionally, more than one drug must be added to an IV solution. Once those medications are reconstituted with sterile water, there is the possibility of a physical incompatibility or particulate contamination. If particulate matter is identified, then the preparation cannot be dispensed. The introduction of particles from an incompatible IV solution can cause an embolism, or obstruction in a blood vessel.

If one medication is an acidic salt and the other an alkaline salt, then once the two medications are combined, a solid precipitate may form. For example, if sodium bicarbonate is added to a solution with potassium chloride, then the resulting solution contains potassium bicarbonate and sodium chloride (table salt). A solid precipitate is not desirable, and all final solutions are inspected by the pharmacist and technician against a white or black background to confirm that precipitates are not present.

Most medications today are administered in separate large-volume IVs or small-volume IVPBs, so physical incompatibilities are rare. Some medications may be incompatible when they come in contact with one another in the Y-site plastic tube connector. A useful reference for physical drug incompatibility is the latest edition of *Trissel's Stability of Compounded Formulations*, which is found in most hospital pharmacies.

Delivery and Administration of CSP

The CSP must be delivered to the hospital or nursing unit by such means that its packaging prevents damage, leakage, contamination, or degradation. This is especially important with the transport of hazardous CSPs that are accompanied by primed IV tubing. Proper storage conditions must be met to comply with expiration dating or BUD. If the CSP is prepared and sent off-site (to another hospital), then the medication must be insulated and stored at the appropriate temperature during transit.

The nurse must document the IV administration times in the medication administration record (MAR), which is similar to the documentation required of other administered oral and prn medications. If the CSP is to be administered for later use, then it must be properly labeled and stored in the refrigerator in the pharmacy or nursing unit. As with an oral dose, the nurse scans the patient wristband and then scans the IV label to make sure that the right patient is receiving the right drug at the right strength by the right route and at the right time. (For a discussion of the Five "Rights" [or Five "Rs"] for Patient Drug Administration, see Chapter 12.)

CSP and Manufactured Product Returns

What if a CSP is returned from the nursing unit? The patient may have been discharged, transferred to another hospital, or died, or the physician may have changed the medication order. A CSP can be redispensed only when the pharmacist or technician is certain that it remained sterile and chemically stable during its storage on the nursing unit.

The decision whether to relabel any CSP, commercially available frozen antibiotic, or CSTD is influenced by the storage conditions on the nursing unit. The nursing unit's storage conditions must be in compliance with USP Chapter <797> for the medication to be returned to pharmacy stock or relabeled. Was the CSP stored under refrigeration and, if necessary, protected from light? Is there evidence of compromises in package integrity?

If the CSP storage conditions on the nursing unit are not within USP <797> mandated guidelines, or cannot be adequately determined, the CSP must be discarded according to hospital policy and procedures. Certain CSPs, such as TPN orders, are written with multiple ingredients that are individualized to a specific patient; therefore, it would be difficult to recycle such products even if properly stored on the nursing unit. If a premade, frozen IVPB is stored at room temperature for any length of time, the pharmacist must determine whether it can be relabeled and used with a new expiration date. Extensions in dating can be approved only if they are supported by scientific data. The pharmacist or technician must determine whether the beyond-use (or expiration) dating would occur before the next scheduled dose is administered. If expired, the product must be discarded. If the CSP can be used for another patient, then a new patient-specific label must be generated with an updated beyond-use or expiration date.

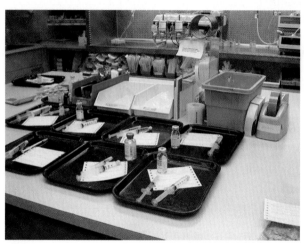

Medication that is prepared by the technician must be reviewed and approved by the pharmacist.

In the case of a proprietary vial-and-bag system that has not been "activated," the vial-and-bag system may be returned to the pharmacy for reuse and relabeling. Depending on the manufacturer's recommendations, once the product has been removed from the sterile packaging, there is a 14 to 30 day shelf life in which to use the product. The manufacturer's product package insert should be consulted for precise expiration dating. Activated doses, however, cannot be relabeled for reuse and must be discarded.

Quality Assurance

A **quality assurance (QA) program** to detect and correct errors is important to ensure quality of care and patient and employee safety and is required for Joint Commission accreditation. QA programs identify problems and try to correct them so that they do not recur. The emphasis on QA programs in the hospital is not to affix blame, but to fix systems. If breakdowns in accuracy or sterility are identified, then existing procedures must be reviewed and all pharmacy personnel may need additional training. A lapse in aseptic technique or policies and procedures in the pharmacy could lead to a serious outbreak of healthcare-associated infections (HAIs), or result in unnecessary and preventable health risks to the employees.

How does the pharmacist or pharmacy technician know whether the sterile CSP that he or she has prepared, labeled, checked, and sent to the nursing unit for patient administration was accurate or free from microorganisms? How do pharmacy personnel know if an ACD used for TPN preparation is injecting the correct components in accurate doses? To address these questions as well as others concerning quality control, each hospital pharmacy must have a QA program outlined in its P&P manual. This section of the manual should offer guidance for pharmacy personnel on ways to avoid medication errors and CSP contamination.

Working in the sterile compounding environment requires comprehensive initial training, experience, certification, and additional on-site training. Following appropriate aseptic technique procedures to minimize microbial contamination of a CSP is important. In the case of working with hazardous agents, use of proper technique may also protect the technician's own health and well-being.

Quality Assurance in Handling Hazardous Agents

Documentation of personnel training for aseptic technique and proper handling of CSPs and hazardous agents is required by USP Chapter <797> guidelines and Joint Commission standards. All personnel in the hospital, including custodial workers, must have proper training in procedures involving identification, containment, collection, segregation, and disposal of cytotoxic and other hazardous drugs. This training must be completed and documented before working with these agents. For hazardous agents, training for pharmacy personnel must cover the following areas:

- safe aseptic manipulation technique
- negative pressure techniques in a BSC or CACI
- correct use of CSTDs
- containment, cleanup, and disposal of breakage or spills
- treatment of personnel for contact and exposure

Training must be repeated and documented every year. For every new hazardous agent (new drug, new investigational drug), an MSDS must be initiated, reviewed with the appropriate staff, and filed for reference. Any organization involved with cytotoxic or other hazardous drugs must have written procedures for proper handling and disposal of such drugs and should provide directions for medical treatment and the procedures for documentation in case of exposure. Environmental and air sampling for hazardous agents must be included in the department's QA program. Government regulations come through the National Institute of Occupational Safety and Health, under the auspices of the CDC.

Table 10.2 in Chapter 10 summarizes the frequency for cleaning of various surfaces and equipment within the sterile compounding area. A quality control procedure for environmental monitoring of the clean room, laminar airflow workbench, buffer area, and anteroom must be in place, in addition to training of all hospital personnel in proper aseptic technique and in the handling of hazardous drugs. As required by USP guidelines and the Joint Commission, sampling of the air, work surfaces, and glove tips should be routinely completed at specified intervals, depending on the contamination risk level of the CSP. Oversight for investigating HAIs is provided by a hospital's Infection Control Committee.

Chapter Summary

- IV infusions are used to deliver parenteral fluids, electrolytes, medications, or nutrients such as lipids, amino acids, sugars, and vitamins.

- Medications for parenteral administration must be prepared in a horizontal or vertical laminar airflow hood using proper aseptic technique and under the supervision of a licensed pharmacist.

- A pharmacy technician must become familiar with various syringes and needles as well as the components of each IV administration set, including the universal spike adaptor, drip chamber, roll clamp, flexible tubing, and needle adaptor.

- Parenteral medications can be administered by bolus injection or by infusion.

- A Y-site injection port allows nursing personnel to add medication to an IV solution.

- An in-line filter in the IV administration set helps to protect the patient against particulate matter, bacteria, air emboli, and phlebitis.

- CSPs have many chemical properties, including pH value, osmolarity, osmolality, tonicity, and stability, that must be understood by the pharmacy technician.

- Many types and volumes of IV solutions such as dextrose in water, NS, and dextrose in NS, may be used as a means of administering parenteral medications.

- Parenteral solutions with or without medications may be administered via IV push, large-volume infusions, or small-volume piggybacked infusions.

- Medications may need to be reconstituted from vials or withdrawn from ampules before adding to the IV solution.

- Special IV solutions prepared or labeled in the pharmacy include TPNs, proprietary vial-and-bag systems, and frozen IV solutions.

- A technician must be able to perform various types of calculations when preparing CSPs.

- Hazardous drugs require special techniques, equipment, and procedures to protect the health of the employee, especially women who are pregnant, breast-feeding, or trying to conceive.

- Accidental spills or exposures require immediate treatment, cleanup, reporting to the supervisor, and the completion of an incident report.

- The pharmacy technician must undergo specific specialized training before working in a sterile compounding environment with parenteral medications and hazardous drugs.

- All parenteral medications must be properly labeled, checked, and physically inspected by the pharmacist before being sent to the nursing unit.

- Unused and returned manufactured parenteral products and CSPs can be used if the beyond-use dating has not been exceeded and if proper storage conditions on the nursing unit can be verified.

- A QA program to detect and correct errors is important to ensure the quality of patient care and patient and employee safety and is required for accreditation.

Key Terms

additive an electrolyte or a medication injected into an LVP or SVP solution for patient administration

ampule a small container made of thin glass that is used as a reservoir for certain single-dose parenteral medications

antineoplastic drug a hazardous agent that reduces or prevents the growth of cancer cells

aseptic technique the manipulation of sterile products and devices in such a way as to avoid contamination by disease-causing organisms

automated compounding device (ACD) a programmable, automated device to make complex IV preparations such as TPNs

beyond-use date the date or time after which a CSP is no longer sterile, stable, or effective

biological safety cabinet (BSC) a vertical laminar airflow hood that is used in the preparation of hazardous compounds, such as chemotherapy CSPs, and is designed to offer protection for the worker during the manipulation of these toxic chemicals

break ring a scored area on the neck of an ampule that marks the site where a technician will break the glass to access the ampule's contents

catheter a device inserted into a vein for direct access to the cardiovascular system

central venous catheter (CVC) a catheter placed into a large vein deep in the body; also called a *central line*

chemotherapy compounding mat a thin mat placed on the BSC work surface to absorb accidental liquid spills during the compounding of chemotherapy drugs

chemotherapy dispensing pin a small plastic device used to relieve the negative pressure within a drug vial safely, while its built-in HEPA filter traps any drug particles or escaping fluid from the vial

closed-system transfer device (CSTD) a small, disposable device that safely draws fluid from a vial into a syringe or injects fluid from a syringe into an IV or IVPB; this device protects the worker from exposure to hazardous drugs

compatibility the ability to combine two more base components or additives within a solution, without resulting in a change to the physical or chemical properties of the components or additives

compounding aseptic containment isolator (CACI) an enclosed vertical laminar airflow hood designed to protect sterile compounding personnel from exposure to hazardous chemicals during compounding procedures

coring an inadvertent introduction of a small piece of the rubber closure into the solution while removing medication from a vial

critical site the part of the supply item that includes any fluid-pathway surface or opening that is at risk for contamination by touch or airflow interruption

cytotoxic drug any drug that destroys cancer cells

diluent a sterile fluid added to a powder to reconstitute, dilute, or dissolve a medication

drip chamber the small, open space just below the spike adaptor where the drops of fluid from the IV bag into the tubing are counted by the nurse to determine the flow rate of the IV solution

drop factor the number of drops that an IV tubing delivers to provide 1 mL; this number may be used by nurses to calculate the IV flow rate when using certain types of primary IV tubing; also called *drop set* or *drip set*

drop set the calibration in drops per milliliter on IV sets

electrolyte solution a solution that contains dissolved mineral salts

filter a device used to remove contaminants such as glass, fibers, rubber cores, and bacteria from IV fluids

flexible tubing the tubing component of a sterile IV administration set that serves as a pathway for IV fluids and parenteral medications during patient administration

hypertonic solution a parenteral solution with a greater number of particles than the number of particles found in blood (greater than 285 mOsm/L); also called a *hyperosmolar solution*, as in a TPN solution

hypotonic solution a parenteral solution with a fewer number of particles than the number of particles found in blood (less than 285 mOsm/L); also called a *hypoosmolar solution*

in-line filter a filter that is connected to, or contained within, an IV administration set; device is used to filter TPN fluid, thus preventing potential precipitates in the solution from being inadvertently administered to a patient

isotonic solution a parenteral solution with an equal number of particles as blood cells (285 mOsm/L); 0.9% normal saline is isotonic

IV administration set a sterile, pyrogen-free, disposable device used to deliver IV fluids to patients

IV piggyback (IVPB) a small-volume IV infusion (50 mL, 100 mL, 250 mL) containing medications

IV push (IVP) the rapid injection of a medication in a syringe into an IV line or catheter in the patient's arm; also called *bolus injection*

large-volume parenteral (LVP) an IV fluid of more than 250 mL that may contain drugs, nutrients, or electrolytes

needle adaptor the end of the tubing (farthest from the universal spike adaptor) to which the needle is attached

normal saline (NS) a sterile solution containing a concentration of 0.9% sodium chloride in water

osmolality a measure of the number of milliosmoles of solute per kilogram of solvent

osmolarity a measure of the milliosmoles of solute per liter of solution (mOsm/L); for example, the osmolarity of blood is 285 mOsm/L; often referred to as *tonicity* for IV solutions

osmotic pressure the pressure required to maintain an equilibrium, with no net movement of solvent

pH value the degree of acidity or alkalinity of a solution; less than 7 is acidic and more than 7 is alkaline; the pH of blood is 7.4

priming the act of running fluid through IV tubing to flush out small particles and expel air from the tubing before medication administration

quality assurance (QA) program a feedback system to improve care by identifying and correcting the cause of a medication error or improper technique

roll clamp the hard, plastic device that provides compression on the tubing, thereby controlling the flow rate of the IV solution

small-volume parenteral (SVP) an IV fluid of 250 mL or less that is commonly piggybacked onto a patient's existing IV line for the infusion of medication

spike the sharp plastic end of IV tubing that is attached to an IV bag of fluid

tonicity the manner in which cells or tissues respond to surrounding fluid

total parenteral nutrition (TPN) an IV solution that provides long-term nutritional support for a specific patient population

vial a sterile medication container made of plastic or glass and sealed with a rubber top

vial-and-bag system a type of SVP in which a specially designed vial and diluent IVPB bag screw or snap together and are activated by the nurse just before patient administration of the medication

Y-site injection port a rigid piece of plastic with one arm terminating in a resealable port that is used to add medication to an IV

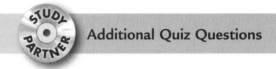
Checking Your Understanding

To check your comprehension of this chapter's key concepts, read the following multiple-choice questions and then record your answers on a separate sheet of paper. Write your answers as modeled in these examples: 1d; 2c; 3b; etc.

1. An example of an isotonic solution is
   a. 0.9% normal saline (NS).
   b. dextrose 50%.
   c. sodium chloride (NaCl) 3%.
   d. 0.45% normal saline (NS).

2. The pH of blood is considered to be slightly
   a. acidic.
   b. alkaline.
   c. neutral.
   d. hypotonic.

3. A vial-and-bag system is activated
   a. by the manufacturer during the assembly of the system.
   b. by pharmacy personnel while stocking the unit-dose cart.
   c. by the nurse at the patient's bedside.
   d. by the pharmacy technician inside a vertical laminar airflow hood.

4. A microdrip IV drop set is typically used for pediatric patients and provides
   a. 10 gtts/mL.
   b. 15 gtts/mL.
   c. 20 gtts/mL.
   d. 60 gtts/mL.

5. What filter size is commonly used to prevent large particles from being inadvertently injected into a CSP?
   a. 0.22 micron filter
   b. 0.45 micron filter
   c. 0.5 micron filter
   d. 7 micron filter

6. The tonicity of a special IV solution, such as a TPN solution, is considered to be
   a. isotonic.
   b. hypertonic.
   c. hypotonic.
   d. hypoosmolar.

7. An IV order is received for D_5W to be infused at a rate of 125 mL/hour. How many 1 L bottles must be prepared for use over the next 48 hours?
   a. two
   b. three
   c. five
   d. six

8. Once activated, a vial-and-bag system's expiration date is
   a. 24 hours.
   b. 48 hours.
   c. 14 days.
   d. determined by the manufacturer's product package insert.

9. To prevent excessive negative pressure, how many milliliters of air should be injected into a vial before drawing up 2 mL of a hazardous drug?
   a. 3 mL
   b. 2 mL
   c. 1.5 mL
   d. 0.75 mL

10. Cytotoxic drugs for IV administration must be prepared
    a. in a vertical laminar airflow hood.
    b. in a horizontal laminar airflow hood.
    c. at the nursing station just before patient administration.
    d. in the nonsterile extemporaneous compounding area.

11. Which additional protective clothing is required when working with hazardous drugs?
    a. a face mask
    b. a hair cover
    c. two pair of gloves (double gloving) and eye protection
    d. shoe covers

12. Which of the following components is *not* part of an IV administration set?
    a. needle adaptor
    b. roll clamp
    c. drip chamber
    d. closed-system transfer device

13. Priming for administration of a chemotherapy CSP should take place
    a. anywhere in the pharmacy before the CSP is sent to the nursing unit.
    b. in the vertical laminar airflow hood.
    c. at the nurse's station before drug administration.
    d. at the patient's bedside before drug administration.

14. Procedures to follow in the case of an accidental exposure to a specific hazardous drug can be found in
    a. USP Chapter <797>.
    b. a pharmacy's P&P manual.
    c. USP Chapter <795>.
    d. the MSDS for that drug.

15. Physical incompatibility data on two or more medications added to an IV solution is best found in
    a. *U.S. Pharmacopoeia.*
    b. *Physician's Desk Reference (PDR).*
    c. *Facts and Comparisons.*
    d. *Trissel's Stability of Compounded Formulations.*

Reinforcing Your Learning

To build on your understanding of the topics in this chapter, complete the following enrichment activities.

1. Pharmacy technicians who work in a hospital pharmacy setting must communicate with other healthcare personnel on a daily basis. Understanding what roles these hospital staff members play in patient health care is essential to effective communication. What duties do each of the following have in IV, TPN, and hazardous drug CSTD therapies?
    a. physician
    b. nurse
    c. pharmacist
    d. pharmacy technician
    e. nutritionist

2. Interview an IV hospital pharmacist or IV pharmacy technician about the applications of milliequivalents into IV admixtures and TPN solutions. Report your findings to the class.

3. Contrast the procedures and protective garb worn in the horizontal and vertical laminar airflow hood areas. If you have access to a laminar airflow hood, demonstrate the cleaning process. If you don't have access, prepare a presentation that addresses the hood-cleaning process. Be sure to include the cleaning products, technique, and frequency of cleaning in your report.

Thinking on Your Feet

To gain practice in handling challenging situations in the workplace, consider the following real-world scenarios and then use the guiding questions to help you formulate your responses.

It is important for a pharmacy technician to read and interpret scientific information from the manufacturer's product insert. Using the following orders below and the reconstitution chart, answer the medication questions.

Minibag Administration Protocol

Agent	Volume	Infusion Rate	Expiration Date
acyclovir (Zovirax)*	≤ 1 g; 50 mL	60 min	24 h RT
imipenem-cilastatin (Primaxin)**	≤ 500 mg; 100 mL NS	60 min	10 h RT
	> 500 mg; 250 mL NS	60 min	48 h REF
oxacillin**	≤ 2 g; 50 mL NS	60 min	96 h RT
	> 2 g; 100 mL NS	60 min	7 day REF
vancomycin (Vancocin)	≤ 250 mg; 50 mL	60 min	96 h RT
	> 250 mg; 100 mL	60 min	
	> 1 g; 250 mL	60 min	

* Do not refrigerate.
** Denotes saline use only.
Note: Prepare each agent in D_5W unless advised otherwise. RT indicates room temperature.
REF indicates refrigeration.

1. acyclovir 1 g q12 h
   a. In what fluid is the drug mixed?
   b. What is the expiration time at room temperature?
   c. Can it be refrigerated?

2. vancomycin 1.5 g q8 h
   a. What size of bag is used?
   b. What is the infusion time?
   c. What is the room temperature expiration?

3. Primaxin 500 mg q6 h × 3 days
   a. In what fluid is the drug mixed?
   b. What size bag is needed?
   c. How many bags are needed?

4. oxacillin 1 g × 5 days
   a. What size bag is needed?
   b. In what fluid is the drug mixed?
   c. If all bags are prepared today, then will the last one expire before the end of therapy?
   d. What is the infusion rate?

5. Solve the following IV rate and administration problems.
   a. A physician orders 3000 mL of 10% dextrose and normal saline ($D_{10}NS$) IV over a 48-hour period. If the IV set delivers 15 gtts/mL, then how many drops must be administered per minute?
   b. A ½ L IV is running at a rate of 100 mL/hour. How long will the bag last?

6. Check a drug reference for guidelines on the reconstitution and stability of the following medications:
   a. 1 g cefazolin sodium for IV infusion in a minibag
   b. amphotericin B 50 mg vial added to an LVP
   c. cyclophosphamide 100 mg added to an LVP

Acquiring Field Knowledge

To expand your knowledge of pharmacy practice, explore the following online activities that focus on research and information retrieval.

Reminder: *As you navigate the Internet, remember to exercise caution and good judgment when evaluating information. A thoughtful review of online text should take into consideration the following factors: the creator and sponsors of the website, the intended audience, the credentials of the authors and contributors, the reliability and validity of the posted information, the frequency of updates to the site, and the ease of navigation for a range of user skill levels.*

1. Visit www.paradigmcollege.net/pharmpractice5e/cancerrisks at the American Society of Health-System Pharmacists (ASHP) website and review the routes of exposure, guidelines on personal protective equipment, and the work practices when handling handling hazardous drugs.

2. Visit www.paradigmcollege.net/pharmpractice5e/hazards. Review the ASHP and NIOSH definitions for hazardous medication and the precautions that personnel should take when working with hazardous drugs in the healthcare setting. Document your findings in a written report.

3. Go to www.paradigmcollege.net/pharmpractice5e/osmolarity and calculate and verify the osmolarity in mOsm/L of the following IV fluid: 1 L of lactated Ringer's solution with 20 mEq of potassium chloride, 10 mEq of calcium chloride, 5 mEq of magnesium sulfate, and 5 mEq of sodium bicarbonate. Is this CSP isotonic, hypertonic, or hypotonic?

4. Go to www.paradigmcollege.net/pharmpractice5e/MSDS and locate an MSDS for cyclophosphamide. List first-aid measures for various exposures to this hazardous drug.

Sampling the Certification Exam

To provide you with practice for the Certification Exam, read the following questions that have been patterned after the test format and then record your answers on a separate sheet of paper. Write your answers as modeled in these examples: 1d; 2c; 3b; etc.

1. Aseptic technique is the process of manipulating sterile products to prevent
   a. introduction of an active ingredient.
   b. introduction of pathogens.
   c. introduction of water.
   d. introduction of asepsis.

2. Which of the following items is necessary to clean up a chemotherapy leak in the hospital?
   a. emergency box
   b. a mop and bucket
   c. spill kit
   d. isopropyl alcohol

3. What is the first thing a pharmacy technician should do when a body area is exposed to a hazardous substance?
   a. Notify the director of pharmacy.
   b. Flush the affected area with water and then thoroughly cleanse the area with soap and water.
   c. Call environmental services for help with cleanup.
   d. Go to the emergency department.

4. What is the most important characteristic of a small-volume parenteral such as acyclovir?
   a. sterility
   b. hypertonicity
   c. alkalinity
   d. hyperosmolarity

5. What part of an ampule is considered the critical area?
   a. rubber top
   b. body
   c. head
   d. neck

6. Which of the following is *not* a component of a TPN solution?
   a. cytotoxic drug
   b. dextrose
   c. additive
   d. amino acid

7. An example of a quality-control measure when mixing a sterile product would be
   a. turning the hood on right before starting to mix.
   b. cleaning all interior working surfaces of the hood with sterile 70% isopropyl alcohol.
   c. turning on the air conditioner to keep the area cool while compounding.
   d. placing all the necessary materials on a shelf behind the hood.

8. Where should doxorubicin, a hazardous substance needing refrigeration, be stored?
   a. next to other refrigerated products on wire racks
   b. separate from other drugs in bins that prevent breakage and contain leakage
   c. in the hood where chemotherapy drugs are compounded
   d. at room temperature as long as the room is air conditioned

9. A filter on an IV set prevents
   a. contamination of the sterile product with viruses.
   b. air in the administration set.
   c. backflow of fluid into the IV bag.
   d. contamination of the IV solution with impurities such as glass shards or rubber cores.

10. Information on how to handle hazardous substances at your facility might be found in a
    a. compounding logbook.
    b. repackaging logbook.
    c. P&P manual.
    d. human resources manual.

Unit

4

Professionalism in the Pharmacy

Medication Safety

**Kimberly Vernachio
PharmD, RPh**

12

Learning Objectives

- Understand the extent of medical and medication errors and their effects on patient health and safety.
- Identify specific categories of medication errors.
- Discuss examples of medication errors commonly seen in pharmacy practice settings.
- Apply a systematic evaluation to search for medication error potential to a pharmacy practice model.

- Define strategies, including the use of automation, for preventing medication errors.
- Identify the common systems available for reporting medication errors.

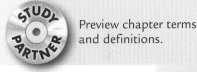

Preview chapter terms and definitions.

The pharmacy technician can play a crucial role in the prevention of medication errors in every pharmacy setting. Identifying, resolving, and preventing medication errors is indeed a team effort that involves prescribers, pharmacy personnel, and the nursing staff. Through categorizing the types of medication errors and their common causes, pharmacy personnel work to establish practices to promote safety throughout the prescription-filling process. For help in defining these practices, pharmacy supervisors also review information from medication error reporting systems. Hospitals, accrediting agencies, and several state boards of pharmacy provide reporting systems to help document medication errors, to study their causes, and to prevent future errors. The Food and Drug Administration (FDA), the United States Pharmacopeia (USP), and the Institute for Safe Medication Practices (ISMP) have developed other medication error reporting systems. The common goal of all of these healthcare initiatives is to protect the health and well-being of patients. In doing so, the costs of healthcare are dramatically lowered. One solution that has clearly been shown to reduce medication errors is the use of automation in both the clinical and pharmacy settings. This chapter will examine the types and causes of medication errors, the strategies that pharmacies can implement to prevent these errors, and the automation technologies that are making a positive impact on medication safety.

Medical Errors

A **medical error** is any circumstance, action, inaction, or decision related to health care that contributes to an unintended health result. A medical error can be as simple as a lab test drawn at the wrong time that returns an inaccurate result or an infection from improper technique, or it can be as serious as a major surgical error that ends in death. A majority of what is known about medical errors comes from information collected in the hospital setting; however, hospital data make up only a part of a much larger picture. Generally, medical errors are difficult to define because the circumstances that can cause them are infinite.

Scope and Impact of Medical Errors

Most health care is administered in outpatient, office-based, or clinic settings. Although medical errors are more difficult to measure in these settings, the number of medical-related lawsuits readily provides a sense of the real scope of medical errors in the United States. Any preventable medical error can cause serious physical injury or death resulting in a major negligence lawsuit.

Several studies have attempted to measure the number and common causes of medical errors. These studies provide estimates on how many people die from medical errors. Examining only medical errors during hospitalization, one study has suggested that as many as 98,000 people in the United States may die each year as a result of medical errors at a cost of more than $29 billion. As the sixth leading cause of death in the United States, there are more deaths from preventable medical errors than from diabetes, Alzheimer's disease, pneumonia, influenza, or kidney disease. Notably, government and private insurers no longer reimburse hospitals for the additional treatment and hospital costs associated with preventable medical errors; hospitals cannot bill the patient for these additional expenses either. Through accreditation and reimbursement, strong incentives exist for a hospital to place a high priority on the prevention of medical errors.

Medication Errors

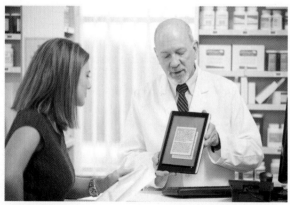

The profession of pharmacy exists to protect the safety of patients from medication errors and adverse effects of drugs. Technological innovations assist the pharmacist and the technician in fulfilling this responsibility.

The National Coordinating Council for Medication Error Reporting and Prevention (NCC MERP) defines a **medication error** as "any preventable event that may cause or lead to inappropriate medication use or patient harm while the medication is in the control of the health care professional, patient, or consumer. Such events may be related to professional practice, health care products, procedures, and systems, including prescribing; order communication; product labeling, packaging, and nomenclature; compounding; dispensing; distribution; administration; education; monitoring; and use."

Scope and Impact of Medication Errors

Medication errors are among the more common types of medical errors. Medication errors include administering or prescribing the wrong drug, providing the wrong dose, or using the wrong route to administer drugs to patients. The information on the effect of medication errors comes mostly from studies done in the hospital setting and is most likely underreported and underestimated.

According to the Institute of Medicine (IOM), more than 1.5 million preventable medication errors cause harm in the United States every year. Deaths from medication-related errors are estimated at about 7,000 annually. In a report issued by the IOM, drug errors cause an estimated 400,000 preventable injuries in hospitals, with twice as many occurring in nursing homes. The IOM estimates that there are more than 500,000 preventable injuries among patients who are eligible for Medicare and are treated in outpatient clinics. The additional healthcare cost to treat hospitalized Medicare patients who suffer a preventable medication error is $1 billion per year.

Far fewer studies of medication errors in community practice exist; however, a few studies give a sense of how large an issue medication errors can be. An estimated 1.7% of all prescriptions dispensed in a community practice setting contain a medication error: In other words, 4 out of 250 prescriptions contain some type of medication error. Although not all medication errors result in harm to a patient, the same study estimated that 65% of the medication errors detected had an adverse effect on the patient's health.[1]

The results of medication errors cannot be easily measured. Lives are lost, and patients are disabled or lose valuable time from work or school. The direct and indirect costs to the healthcare system for errors occurring outside the hospital setting are conservatively estimated to be $3.5 billion annually. These costs are caused by additional hospitalizations (2.4 million extra days), admissions to long-term care, physician visits, and emergency room visits.

On the continuum of healthcare delivery, multiple causes of potential medication errors exist. Pharmacy technicians are an important part of the healthcare team; therefore, they should be constantly on the lookout for possible errors and adopt safety-oriented work practices when dealing with patients. When pharmacy technicians take steps to protect the safety of patients, they become a barrier to adverse patient outcomes. More interdisciplinary communication and automation with the liberal use of bar-code scanning in the community and hospital pharmacy should dramatically reduce the incidence of medication errors.

Patient Response

Most patients benefit from a medication's intended therapeutic response; however, an individual's unique physiological makeup and social circumstances make it impossible to predict which medication errors may cause harm.

Physiological Causes of Medication Errors Each patient's unique response to medication highlights the importance of medication safety. Every person is genetically unique, and the speed at which a body can process medications varies tremendously from person to person. For instance, a patient may lack an enzyme that helps remove or eliminate medications from the body, thus leading to serious harm or even death from an error. Even if a particular problem is caught and corrected before harm occurs, the result is still considered a medication error.

---

[1] Flynn, E. A., et al., "National Observational Study of Prescription Dispensing Accuracy and Safety in 50 Pharmacies." *Journal of American Pharmaceutical Association* 43 (2003): 191–200.

A patient's kidney function also is a physiological cause of medication errors. The kidneys play an important role in excretion, or the process by which drug molecules are removed from the bloodstream. Many patient populations have decreased kidney function because of age or disease. Elderly patients, neonates, and premature babies have diminished kidney function, as well as patients with chronic renal failure, high blood pressure, or diabetes. If a medication dose is not lowered, then the drug could accumulate to toxic levels, causing an adverse reaction and medication error. Consequently, kidney function is one of many factors that the pharmacist must consider before approving and verifying a prescription. A pharmacy technician can assist the pharmacist by updating patients' medical information in the computer database.

When preparing a prescription or medication order, pharmacy technicians must pay special attention to computer software alerts. These alerts include required pharmacist intervention, packaging requirements, inclusion of special medication handouts upon dispensing, and the distribution of clear medication administration directions. This responsibility is especially important in the community pharmacy where patients are responsible for their own compliance when taking the medication at home. Special attention and consideration is made for the young (under age 6) and the elderly (over age 66) due to an increased susceptibility to medication errors and adverse reactions. In many cases, the drug may be contraindicated or dosage may need to be decreased by 25% to 50% or more. In the hospital, special considerations are also made for potential dosage adjustments in neonates including those who were born prematurely.

Social Causes of Medication Errors Patients in the outpatient setting can also contribute to medication errors through incorrect self-administration. As a result, the medication does not work well, does not work at all, or may cause harm. Social causes of medication errors include failure to follow medication therapy instructions because of cost, **noncompliance** (failure to take therapy as the physician instructs), or a misunderstanding of instructions (perhaps because of language or cultural barriers). Patients can contribute to medication errors by doing the following:

- forgetting to take a dose or doses
- taking too many doses
- dosing at the wrong time
- not getting a prescription filled or refilled in a timely manner
- not following directions on dose administration
- terminating the drug regimen too soon

Such social causes may result in an adverse drug reaction or a subtherapeutic—or even toxic—dose. For example, more than 50% of patients on essential long-term medications no longer take their medication after one year. Not taking prescribed medication could result in the progression of a chronic disease. Any of these circumstances could result in lasting harm or death, depending on the drug and the disease being treated. The technician should take note of the refill history when entering an order. If the patient appears to be noncompliant with the prescribed medication, it should be brought to the attention of the pharmacist for a potential counseling intervention. In any event, all of these social circumstances create the potential for medication errors.

Categories of Medication Errors

An exact listing of medication errors is difficult to create because the possible causes of such missteps can often be too numerous to count. However, categorizing errors into types or groups often aids in the identification and prevention of future problems. Classic examples are grouped into the following five major categories:

- An **omission error** occurs when a prescribed dose is due, but not administered.
- A **wrong dose error** occurs when a dose is either above or below the correct amount by more than 5%.
- An **extra dose error** occurs when a patient receives more doses than were prescribed by the physician.
- A **wrong dosage form error** occurs when the dose formulation given to the patient is not the accepted interpretation of the physician's order. Examples include a drug given by mouth for a drug ordered as an intramuscular (IM) injection, an IM-prescribed drug given subcutaneously, or an immediate-release drug dispensed instead of a controlled- or extended-release drug.
- A **wrong time error** occurs when any drug is given 30 minutes or more before or after it was ordered to be administered, up to the time of the next dose. This is a common error in hospitals and nursing homes due to staffing shortages; it does not include **prn** (i.e., as needed) orders.

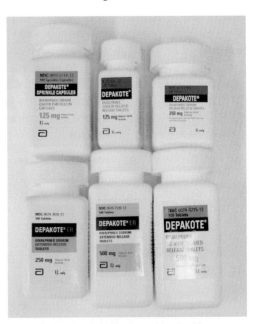

Medication errors can also be categorized according to what caused the failure of the desired result. The purpose of defining errors in this way is to identify clearly what the error was, where it took place, and, through closer examination, what specifically caused it (i.e., the *why*). Such analysis identifies ways to eliminate or reduce future mistakes. Most situations fall into one of three basic classes of failure:

Because of identical names and look-alike packaging, the wrong dosage or formulation of the seizure drug valproic acid may be selected. The technician should carefully check the original prescription and compare NDC numbers to prevent a medication error.

- A **human failure** occurs at an individual level. An example of this type of error includes pulling a medication bottle from the shelf based on memory, without cross-referencing the bottle label with the shelf label and the medication order or prescription or without scanning the National Drug Code (NDC) bar code. As previously discussed, human errors include those made by the patient, such as noncompliance to prescribed drug therapy.
- A **technical failure** results from equipment problems. An example of this type of failure includes the incorrect reconstitution of a medication because of a malfunction of a sterile-water dispenser or the incor-

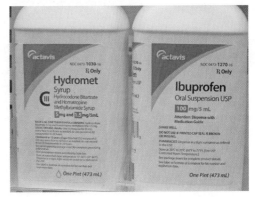

Identical label designs are also a source of confusion and a cause for error when filling a prescription.

rect preparation of a total parenteral solution (TPN) due to a malfunction of the automated compounding device. such as in the mass production of total parenteral nutrition solutions in the hospital pharmacy.

- An **organizational failure** occurs because of a deficiency in organizational rules, policies, or procedures. An example of this type of failure includes a policy or rule requiring the preparing or admixing of parenteral medicines, such as chemotherapy drugs, in an inappropriate setting without proper environmental controls or equipment.

Root-Cause Analysis of Medication Errors

Root-cause analysis is a logical and systematic process used to help identify what, how, and why something happened to prevent recurrence. Using some of the basic principles of root-cause analysis, a person can examine his or her own workflow to determine the potential for error and the type of failure that the potential error may involve. Using this analysis, it is possible to create a list of specific causes. Identifying the potential causes allows a person to take actions to prevent errors and improve patient safety. The actions taken improve the quality of work being done, and thereby boost patient outcomes.

A medication error by handlers and preparers of medications has many causes. Three of the most common causes are an assumption error, a selection error, and a capture error.

- An **assumption error** occurs when an essential piece of information cannot be verified; therefore, an assumption is made. An example of an assumption error that a pharmacy technician might make is misreading a poorly written abbreviation, drug name, or directions on a prescription.
- A **selection error** occurs when two or more options exist, and the wrong option is chosen. An example of a selection error that a pharmacy technician might make is mistakenly using a look-alike or sound-alike drug instead of the prescribed drug or choosing an immediate-release formulation instead of an extended-release drug. Similar manufacturer labels can also lead to a mistaken medication selection.
- A **capture error** occurs when a more practiced behavior automatically takes the place of a less familiar, intended one. In other words, focus on a task is diverted elsewhere and the distraction prevents the person from detecting an error or causes an error to be made. A capture error might occur when taking a phone call in the middle of filling a prescription order and, as a result, dispensing the wrong number of tablets (i.e., the correct number was not double-checked at the conclusion of the phone call), or inadvertently overriding an alert due to a distraction.

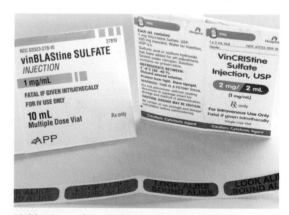

Vinblastine and vincristine are two look-alike, sound-alike chemotherapy medications that can lead to a selection error. For that reason, tall-man lettering is used to emphasize the difference in the similar drug names.

Safety Note

Maintaining focused attention when filling prescriptions is important to avoid errors.

In relation to capture errors, the work habits of the pharmacy technician can determine when and where in the prescription-filling process it is safe to allow focus on a task to be diverted. In other words, when the technician is completing a medication-related task, is there a point in the process at which stopping and answering the telephone is not appropriate? When is it appropriate to allow for such an interruption? Knowing when to allow interruptions and when not to do so is vitally important in maintaining individual safety practices.

Prescription-Filling Process in Community and Hospital Pharmacy Practice

Safety Note

Each person who participates in the filling process has the opportunity to catch and correct a medication error.

A thorough review of potential causes of medication errors in work practices begins with outlining work tasks in a step-by-step manner. Figure 12.1 is an example of a step-by-step prescription-filling process for community and hospital pharmacy practice settings. For the most part, the filling process in both settings is identical; however, in the hospital setting, medications pass through an extra set of hands—the nurse's—before reaching the patient. This extra set of hands provides both another opportunity to prevent medication errors and an additional source of potential medication errors. In the community pharmacy, the technician is often the last check before the delivery of medication to the patient. Automation, if properly implemented and utilized, can greatly diminish medication errors.

Many chain community pharmacies stress and even market how fast prescriptions can be dispensed to gain a competitive advantage. While no one wants to have an unnecessarily long wait to get a prescription filled, it is important that the technician and pharmacist remember that safety cannot be compromised for speed, lest a medication error more likely will result.

FIGURE 12.1
Prescription-Filling Process

Although each step in this process can be a source of medication errors, it is also an opportunity for pharmacy personnel to correct any such mistake.

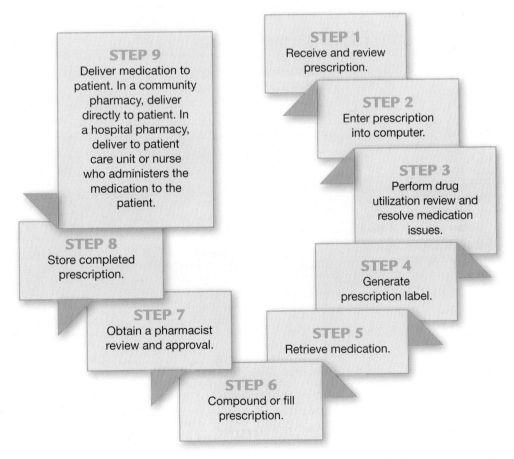

STEP 9
Deliver medication to patient. In a community pharmacy, deliver directly to patient. In a hospital pharmacy, deliver to patient care unit or nurse who administers the medication to the patient.

STEP 1
Receive and review prescription.

STEP 2
Enter prescription into computer.

STEP 3
Perform drug utilization review and resolve medication issues.

STEP 8
Store completed prescription.

STEP 4
Generate prescription label.

STEP 7
Obtain a pharmacist review and approval.

STEP 5
Retrieve medication.

STEP 6
Compound or fill prescription.

Once work practices are broken into individual steps, each step should be reviewed to determine what information is necessary to complete the step and what resources can be used to verify the information. In addition, consideration should be given to the possible errors that might result if information is missed or verification is not performed. Therefore, it is helpful to think of each step in terms of the following three parts:

- information that needs to be obtained or checked
- resources that can be used to verify information
- potential medication errors that would result from a failure to obtain or check the necessary information using the appropriate resources

Step 1: Receive and Review Prescription

Before a new prescription enters the prescription-filling process, an initial check of all key pieces of information is vital. Table 12.1 lists the information needed and the resources used to avoid potential errors in the first step of the prescription-filling

TABLE 12.1   Step 1: Receive and Review Prescription

Information to Check	Resources to Verify Information	Potential Errors Resulting from Failure to Check/Verify Information
Legibility: Can the prescription be read clearly?	Physician, patient, independent reviewer, such as a pharmacist or nurse	Prescription misread
Prescriber Information: Is the prescription valid? Did the prescriber sign the prescription? For narcotic prescriptions, is the prescriber's Drug Enforcement Administration (DEA) number listed? Are the prescriber's name, address, and phone number printed on the prescription?	Physician, pharmacist, nurse	Out-of-date (i.e., invalid) prescription filled; fraudulent prescription filled; patient receives medication intended for another patient
Patient Information: Is all necessary information included? Is this prescription for this patient? Are the patient's name, date of birth, address, phone number, and allergies provided? Does the information match the profile?	Physician, patient, immediate family member, patient profile, pharmacist, nurse	Incorrect patient selected; contraindicated drug dispensed
Medication Information: Is all necessary information included? Are drug name, dose, dosage form, route of administration, refills, directions for use, and dosing schedule included? Is the prescription dated?	Patient, physician, family member, patient profile	Wrong medication dispensed; wrong form or formulation dispensed; wrong dose dispensed; patient administers incorrectly; out-of-date (i.e., invalid) prescription filled

process. A thorough review by the pharmacy technician and pharmacist substantially reduces the chances that an unidentified error will continue throughout the filling process.

Safety Note

Careful review of the prescription or order is very important.

Basic Review of Prescription The first and most basic part of prescription review begins by deciding whether all information involved is clear and legible. Can you read and understand it? Any unclear information should be clarified before any further action is taken.

Verbal Order Precautions Another common cause of error is in the verbal receipt of messages for prescriptions of sound-alike drugs; if the caller did not spell out the name of the drug and the pharmacist (or technician, in some states) is unclear about the correct name, then the order should be clarified before entering it into the computer and filling the prescription. If the nurse calls in the prescription, then the caller is encouraged to read back the order to minimize errors.

There are many occasions when a nurse will leave a voice mail for a new prescription. In some states, the technician is allowed to transcribe a written prescription based on that phone message. In one case, a technician misheard "Pamelor" (an antidepressant) for "Tambocor" (an antiarrhythmic); the error was not discovered for one month. Fortunately, the patient experienced no adverse outcomes. This error might have been prevented by e-prescribing, better knowledge of brand names, or reviewing the profile and calling the nurse back for clarification.

Safety Note

Outdated prescriptions should not be filled.

Safety Note

A prescriber's signature is required for a written prescription to be considered valid.

Validity of Prescription Before considering the details of the information contained in a prescription, determining whether the prescription is, in fact, valid and legal is important. The requirements for a valid prescription may vary from state to state, and every technician should be familiar with the requirements of the state in which he or she practices. Does the prescription contain all of the information necessary to be valid? For example, a prescription is valid only for up to one year (less, in some cases) from the date of its writing. Validity cannot be determined if the prescription is not dated. If it is not determined to be valid, then the prescription should not be filled. If the prescription is for a controlled drug, check to make sure it contains the full and current address of the patient. Does it have a handwritten or electronic signature from the prescriber? In most states, an electronic signature for a controlled drug is not valid.

Detailed Review of Prescription A prescription contains three basic types of information that must be reviewed: prescriber information, patient information, and medication information. In addition, pharmacy personnel must also check for prescribing errors on the prescription.

Prescriber Information Prescriber information should be sufficient to determine whether a licensed and qualified prescriber wrote the prescription. Generally, the physician's contact information should be included. No prescription or medication order is valid without the signature of the prescriber. In the community setting, prescriptions lacking a prescriber signature cannot be filled. (Verbal, fax, and e-prescriptions are exceptions to this rule.) Any verbal prescription order should include all of the information necessary to verify that the caller is, in fact, a valid prescriber or a designated agent of the prescriber. In hospital settings, a physician's signature is still required to validate a prescription; however, orders given verbally are generally honored, provided that a signature is received within a time frame specified per the hospital's policies and procedures.

Patient Information Patient information should include enough detail to ensure that unique individuals can be pinpointed. Full names, addresses, dates of birth, and phone numbers give multiple points to cross-reference and separate patients who might otherwise have similar information (e.g., patients with the same first and last names). Dates of birth and allergy information should always be included because this information helps confirm the appropriateness of the medication. The date of birth is an important identifier and should be placed on each hard copy prescription. Comparing phone numbers may not be as helpful in identifying the patient as the date of birth because many people have home, cellular, and work phone numbers.

Medication Information Medication information should include the drug name, strength, dose, dosage form, route of administration, refills or length of therapy, directions for use, and dosing schedule. The absence of one of these pieces of information opens the way for medication errors, such as dispensing the wrong medication, wrong formulation, or wrong dosage or strength, or filling an invalid prescription.

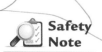
Safety Note

A leading zero should precede values less than one, but no zero should follow a decimal if the value is a whole number.

Prescribing Errors Prescribing errors include the use of poor handwriting, nonstandard abbreviations, confusing look-alike and sound-alike drug names, and "as directed" instructions. An "as directed" instruction does not allow a pharmacist to verify normal recommended dose scheduling or to reinforce the correct dosing regimen to patients. A leading zero should always precede a decimal point (e.g., 0.3). A zero should never follow a decimal (e.g., 3.0) because a tenfold error can occur if the decimal point is not detected. The abbreviations *qd*, *qid*, and *qod* commonly cause medication errors and should be avoided if possible or carefully reviewed with the pharmacist.

Step 2: Enter Prescription into Computer

Table 12.2 lists the information needed and the resources used to avoid potential errors in the second step of the prescription-filling process. In the hospital setting, medication orders are often entered into the computer by the pharmacist; in the community pharmacy setting, the pharmacy technician often enters the prescriptions into the computer database.

Accurate Data Entry Data entry is the act of entering important pieces of information from the prescription or medication order into the computer. The ability to perform this function accurately can make the difference between a patient receiving a correct and appropriate medication and dose and a prescription that potentially causes the patient serious harm or death. With so much at stake, focused concentration on the input of information is important. As each piece of information is entered, the prescription should be compared with choices from the computer menu. Check the brand and generic names of the drugs you are entering and their spellings to determine whether the information on the prescription and in the computer match. Special attention should be paid to dosages, formulations, concentrations, and the increments of

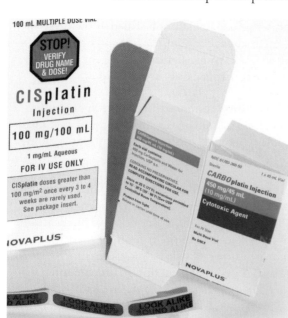

If the technician is not careful or has been distracted, then he or she may select cisplatin instead of carboplatin at the time of computer entry, resulting in a potential medication error.

TABLE 12.2 Step 2: Enter Prescription into Computer

Information to Check	Resources to Verify Information	Potential Errors Resulting from Failure to Check/Verify Information
Are data choices from the computer menu and those on the prescription the same?	Cross-check brand/generic names for identical spelling.	Look-alike or sound-alike drug selection error made
Does the spelling on the prescription match the drug selection options?		
Do the increments of measure on the drug selection options match those on the prescription (e.g., gram vs. milligram vs. microgram)?	Cross-check measure prescribed with drug choices listed.	Patient given incorrect dose
For the dose selected, do available strengths or concentrations match?	Cross-check dose written with available strengths or concentrations on selection menu; cross-check dose or concentrations that use decimals or leading or trailing zeros.	Patient given incorrect dose
Does the dose or concentration have leading or trailing zeros?		
Does it require a decimal?		
Do available forms match the route selected?	Match route to formulation choices (e.g., injection route corresponds to intravenous [IV] or intramuscular [IM] drug; oral route corresponds to capsule, tablet, liquid, or lozenge).	Inappropriate form or formulation selected

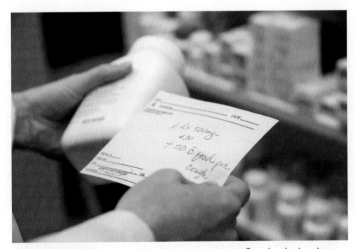

In the hospital pharmacy, it is important to confirm both the drug and the correct route of administration. An IM drug administered as an IV drug is a medication error with potentially serious consequences.

measure. Prescriptions that contain unapproved, error-causing abbreviations must be reviewed with a pharmacist or confirmed with the prescriber.

A common example of an inaccurate computer entry in the community pharmacy setting is a prescription received for a brand name cough and cold remedy that is not carried by the pharmacy, is no longer available, or is not covered by insurance. Most software lists generic equivalents that the technician can choose from to make a substitution. However, because many of these agents contain multiple ingredients, it is often difficult to find an exact generic equivalent. The pharmacist or technician may need to contact the prescriber to recommend a therapeutically equivalent product with similar but not identical ingredients.

Potential Dangers Does the form or formulation match the route of administration? Be aware that certain concentrations or formulations of a given medication may be associated with a particular route of administration. A common example of the potential for mismatching of form or formulation to route of administration is Depo-Medrol and Solu-Medrol. Both are injectable and have similar dosages, depending on the clinical situation. However, Depo-Medrol is for IM administration only and is a cloudy suspension when reconstituted. Solu-Medrol is for IV administration and is a clear solution. A serious and potentially fatal medication error could occur if a suspension was inadvertently administered by the IV route.

Teaspoons vs. Milliliters Mix-ups occasionally occur with the teaspoonful and milliliter dosage amounts. A prescriber may either inadvertently write the wrong instructions on the prescription or the technician might incorrectly enter a dose into the computer. For example, a prescription may be written for 3.5 mL of an antibiotic, but the order is entered as 3.5 teaspoonfuls (or 17.5 mL). If the pharmacist misses the error during the verification process, the patient recipient would receive five times the recommended dose. Therefore, it is recommended to use milliliters for computer entry and labeling to minimize errors.

Formulation Mix-Ups Another mix-up may occur with morphine sulfate. Morphine sulfate is available in a concentrated liquid formulation (20 mg/mL) and a less concentrated liquid (10 mg/5 mL or 2 mg/mL); entering (or selecting) the wrong concentration would result in a tenfold error and cause serious respiratory depression in the patient recipient. Other examples include ointments vs. creams in topical products or solutions vs. suspensions in ophthalmic and otic medications. In some cases, substituting a capsule for a tablet or vice-versa is permissible; if you're unsure, check with the pharmacist.

Precautions with Scheduled Drugs The computer entry of certain Schedule II pain medications is also a potential source of error. OxyContin is the brand name and oxycodone ER is the generic equivalent. By definition, these drugs are commonly prescribed every 8 to 12 hours. Oxycodone is also available as an immediate-release product dosed every 4 to 6 hours; often the two drugs are prescribed together. If the wrong drug is entered into the computer, and the mistake is missed by the pharmacist during the verification process, it is likely that a medication error will occur.

Once the information has been entered in the computer sytem, each data element of the completed entry should be checked against the same data elements on the original prescription before the entry process is finalized. In many chain pharmacies, the original prescription is scanned so the pharmacist can check the technician's entry during the verification process.

Step 3: Perform Drug Utilization Review and Resolve Medication Issues

The risk of medication errors increases with the number of medications, pharmacies, and prescribers that an individual patient uses. One-third of adults in the United States are taking 5 medications per day, others more than 10 per day. The risk of preventable medication errors from drug interactions dramatically increases with the number of drugs someone is taking, especially among elderly patients.

Drug Utilization Review For every prescription, a pharmacist will run a computerized drug utilization review (DUR) of the profile, which should include checks for multiple drug therapy, dosing ranges, existing allergies, pertinent medical diseases, and conditions.

Dosing Ranges and Drug Interactions A DUR should be performed by the pharmacist to check for dosing ranges, drug interactions, or duplication of therapy (see Table 12.3). For pediatric patients, especially those younger than age two, the dosage on the prescription (and entered into the computer) should be checked carefully. Conversely, patients who are older may require a lower dose because of age-related declines in liver and kidney functions and other body changes. If a patient receives an antibiotic prescription for Biaxin, then it may interfere with and increase the risk of toxicity with other drugs, such as blood thinners, or seizure or cholesterol medications. If the pharmacy technician has entered in the computer database that the patient is pregnant, a more careful review of prescriptions must be done by the pharmacist.

Allergy-Related Alerts A DUR often prompts allergy-related questions that need to be addressed by the pharmacist. For example, if the patient is allergic to codeine, then can he or she tolerate hydrocodone, a similar narcotic? Did the patient or his or her caregiver tell the physician about this allergy? Is the patient's allergy a "gastrointestinal upset" rather than a rash, shortness of breath, or another symptom? Has the

Safety Note

Check the patient profile for existing allergies or possible drug interactions.

TABLE 12.3 Step 3: Perform Drug Utilization Review and Resolve Medication Issues

Information to Check	Resources to Verify Information	Potential Errors Resulting from Failure to Check/ Verify Information
Drug Screening: Does the prescribed medication interact with other conditions or medications listed on the profile?	Patient, physician, family member, patient profile, interaction screening program, insurance provider electronic messages, drug information resources (e.g., books, call centers, package inserts, patient information handouts)	Contraindicated drug dispensed; drug–drug or drug–disease interaction occurs
Pediatric Dosing: Are the prescribed dose and frequency of dosing in a pediatric patient consistent with manufacturer recommendations and pharmacy references?	Original prescription, physician, package inserts, electronic database, reference texts, pharmacist experience	Serious overdose (or underdose) leading to side effects, adverse reactions, or treatment failure
Geriatric Dosing: Are the prescribed dose and frequency of dosing in a geriatric patient consistent with manufacturer recommendations and pharmacy references?	Original prescription, physician, package inserts, electronic database, reference texts, pharmacist experience	Serious overdose leading to side effects or adverse reactions

patient received a hydrocodone prescription previously? Similarly, if a child is allergic to penicillin, then there is a chance of cross-sensitivity with other antibiotics. The computer software generally flags allergies, but the pharmacy technician should bring the potential problem to the attention of the pharmacist.

Pharmacist Follow-Up The pharmacist must decide whether to counsel the patient or contact the prescribing physician before approving the filling of this prescription. The computer software also flags duplicate therapy that may lead to serious adverse reactions. For example, is a patient taking both ibuprofen and etodolac? These are similar anti-inflammatory and pain medications that, if taken together for a long period, can lead to a gastric bleed or ulcer.

Step 4: Generate Prescription Label

Table 12.4 lists the information needed and the resources used to avoid potential errors in the fourth step of the prescription-filling process.

Cross-check the label output from the printer with the original prescription to make sure that a typing error or inherent program malfunction did not alter the information. Is the correct patient name on the label? Are the drug, dose, concentration, and route information identical to those indicated in the original prescription? Did the prescription read, for example, "take 1 capsule p.o. q6 h prn," which is the most common direction, or was it written as the less common "take ½ capsule p.o. q6 h prn"?

Step 5: Retrieve Medication

Table 12.5 lists the information needed and the resources used to avoid potential errors in the fifth step of the prescription-filling process.

TABLE 12.4   Step 4: Generate Prescription Label

Information to Check	Resources to Verify Information	Potential Errors Resulting from Failure to Check/ Verify Information
Has the patient information been cross-checked?	Compare label generated with original prescription.	Wrong patient, medication, or dose selected
Are the label and original prescription identical?	Compare label generated with original prescription.	Wrong patient, medication, or dose selected
Are the leading or trailing zeros and unapproved abbreviations correct?	Check with pharmacist or prescriber.	Incorrect dose selected
Do all the data elements match those of the original prescription (e.g., prescriber information, patient information, medication information)?	Use additional information generated on label reference for verification (e.g., brand/generic names; NDC number; manufacturer's name; patient's address, phone number(s), date of birth).	Inappropriate form or formulation selected

TABLE 12.5 Step 5: Retrieve Medication

Information to Check	Resources to Verify Information	Potential Errors Resulting from Failure to Check/ Verify Information
Has the available information on the manufacturer's label been used to verify the medication selection?	Original prescription, shelf- or bin-labeling systems, manufacturers' names, NDC numbers, brand names and generic names, pictographic medication verification references or computer programs	Medication selection error made
Does the brand or generic name on the label match the product container?		
Do the dose strength and form on the label match those indicated on the product container?	Original prescription, shelf- or bin-labeling systems, manufacturers' names, NDC numbers, brand names and generic names, pictographic medication verification references or computer programs	Incorrect dose, form, or formulation selected
Do the NDC numbers and manufacturers' names match those listed on the label?	Bin-labeling systems, NDC numbers, pictographic medication verification references or computer programs	Incorrect dose, form, or formulation selected

Safety Note

Confirm that information entered into the computer matches that of the original prescription.

Safety Practices for Accurate Drug Selection Look-alike labels, similarities in brand or generic names, and similar pill shapes or colors can all contribute to medication errors. Use NDC numbers, drug names, and other information available on manufacturers' labels or patient information handouts to verify that you've selected the correct product. Use both the original prescription and the generated patient information sheet or leaflet when selecting a manufacturer's drug product from the storage shelf.

NDC Numbers Wherever possible, use NDC numbers as a cross-check option because each NDC number is specific to a particular form, packaging, and strength for each medication (see Chapter 3). Therefore, the NDC numbers of two forms of a medication, even at the same strength, do not match (nor do two different strengths of the same form of the same medication). For example, trazodone and tramadol are similar-sounding generic drugs with two distinct indications. Trazone is an antidepressant; tramadol is an analgesic. Selecting one of these medications without checking the NDC number could have serious consequences. Dispensing a drug

Medications with near-identical names and similar manufacturer packaging can lead to a selection medication error; always scan or check the NDC number.

based on appearance could also lead to a medication error. For example, both Fioricet and Fiorinal are dispensed as white tablets. A bar-code scan of the stock bottle would ensure that the correct medication is dispensed.

Heparin Safeguards In the hospital setting, heparin is available in vials of concentrations from 10 units per mL to 10,000 units per mL. The lower concentrations are used to flush or clear an IV or dialysis line or to keep the line open, whereas the higher concentrations are used as blood thinners in adults. Several serious medication errors, including death, have occurred when a nurse inadvertently selected the wrong heparin vial for patient recipients. For that reason, hospitals have developed and implemented policies specifically for the administration of heparin. These policies include additional computer alerts, a nurse-check-nurse system, and the limited availability of certain concentrations as floor stock on the nursing units. Manufacturers, as well, have changed their labeling practices to minimize future adverse events with heparin.

Look-Alike and Sound-Alike Labels Look-alike and sound-alike labeling can lead to medication errors and possible adverse drug reactions, even for over-the-counter (OTC) products. At the request of the FDA, the manufacturer of Maalox voluntarily recalled its products from the market due to consumer confusion around product labeling and proper use. The manufacturer was attempting to increase its market share by **product line extension**—using a brand name to sell various combinations of active ingredients with different indications—leading to consumer selection errors. The manufacturer agreed to change the name of the product, provide educational programs for healthcare professionals and consumers, and add safety monitoring and a reporting program for its products.

Accidental substitution of one drug or pharmaceutical ingredient for another is one of the most serious events that can occur in pharmacy practice. Because differences in potency or toxicity and failure to receive the drug prescribed for treatment or prevention all pose significant risk of harm or possible death to patient recipients, extreme care must be taken not to substitute drugs that have similar names.

In one infamous case, *Troppi vs. Scarf*, a pharmacist accidentally dispensed Nardil, an antidepressant, instead of Norinyl, a contraceptive. The woman who received the incorrect drug gave birth to a child, and the Michigan Court of Appeals held the pharmacist liable not only for the medical expenses incurred in the woman's pregnancy, but also for the costs of raising the child.

Some pharmacies possess a computer-based pill identification program and use a shelf-labeling system to organize inventory. Such identification programs allow the pharmacist or technician to visually verify the medication dispensed with a picture. These sources of information can be used to verify the selection of the correct medication. To prevent similarly labeled drugs or doses from being dispensed, drugs will often be shelved in a non-alphabetical or illogical order so that the technician or pharmacist is less likely to select the wrong stock bottle.

Step 6: Compound or Fill Prescription

Table 12.6 lists the information needed and the resources used to avoid potential errors in the sixth step of the prescription-filling process.

Safety Practices for Accurate Compounding and Filling Calculation and substitution errors are frequent sources of pharmacy-related medication errors in all practice settings. A technician should write out calculations and have a second person check

TABLE 12.6 Step 6: Compound or Fill Prescription

Information to Check	Resources to Verify Information	Potential Errors Resulting from Failure to Check/Verify Information
Have the amount to be dispensed and the increment of measure (e.g., gram, milligram, microgram) been reviewed?	Amount dispensed (count twice), original prescription	Incorrect quantity or incorrect dose dispensed
Does the prescription require a calculation or measurement conversion?	Write out the calculation and conversions; ask another person to review the calculation.	Incorrect dose dispensed
If you are using equipment, has the equipment been calibrated recently?	Equipment (check calibration), pharmacist, patient information handout, package insert	Incorrect dose dispensed
Does the medication dispensed require warning or caution labels?	Pharmacist, patient information handout, package insert	Administration error made by patient

Safety Note

When compounding, do not allow interruptions. Prepare products one at a time.

the answers. Great care should be taken when reading labels and preparing compounded products. Using more than one container of product, preparing more than one product at a time, and paying attention to distractions or interruptions can all contribute to medication errors. Do not allow interruptions or distractions during compounding or filling. If you must stop before filling is complete, then be sure to start over from the beginning.

Equipment Maintenance In addition, all equipment used in the compounding or filling process should be maintained, cleaned, and calibrated on a regular basis. Use of technology presents its own unique potentials for error. In most circumstances, errors caused by technology depend on the user; however, inherent technology malfunctions and program glitches do occur. Therefore, good safety practices should include a check for the accuracy of technology (e.g., computers, scales, robots, infusion pumps, and automated dispensers) used in the prescription-filling process.

This principle is not limited to sophisticated equipment. The act of cleaning counting trays and spatulas on a regular basis is an important part of medication safety. Consider the potential for serious harm to a patient if the residue or dust from an allergy-causing medication contaminated the patient's prescription. For example, penicillin- or sulfa-containing medications should be counted on dedicated counting trays because of the high prevalence of penicillin and sulfa allergies in the general population. If you are dispensing oral hazardous substances, such as methotrexate, then the counting tray must be cleaned to prevent contamination. It is also recommended that you clean the counting tray with isopropyl alcohol after any of these drugs are dispensed.

Auxiliary Labels Caution and warning labels (auxiliary labels) applied to a prescription container are intended to serve as reminders to patients about the most critical aspects of drug handling or administration. In most pharmacy settings with computerized systems, the caution and warning labels are generated with the label and coordinated with more detailed patient information handouts. These labels serve as an ever-present reminder of the most crucial aspects of proper medication administration and should always be included with prescription labeling. Before affixing the auxiliary labels to the prescription vial, technicians should ask the pharmacist which ones to prioritize. Often, as many as six labels are printed or needed, but only three may fit on the vial. In light of that, technicians should ask about the policy at their practice site.

Step 7: Obtain a Pharmacist Review and Approval

Table 12.7 lists the information needed and the resources used to avoid potential errors in the seventh step of the prescription-filling process. (*Note:* The pharmacist must be the one to review and approve the prescription in this step.)

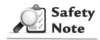

Safety Note

The pharmacist must always check the technician's work.

Responsibilities of the Pharmacist The pharmacist is legally responsible for verifying the accuracy and appropriateness of any prescription or medication order that is filled, but it is not practical for pharmacists to verify each step in the filling process. Rather, a pharmacist verifies the initial computer entry and the quality and integrity of the end product.

Providing all available, useful resources to ensure accurate verification is vital to patient safety. The easiest way to determine what information and resources are important to the verifying pharmacist is to ask whether the information provided with the medication filled allows the pharmacist to retrace the technician's steps in filling the prescription. Can the pharmacist determine whether the prescription is valid, the patient information accurate, and the medication correctly prepared from the information provided with the finished product? For example, the stock bottle of medication should accompany the labeled medication container and original prescription. The information on the label should be compared with the stock bottle and the

TABLE 12.7   Step 7: Obtain a Pharmacist Review and Approval

Information to Check	Resources to Verify Information	Potential Errors Resulting from Failure to Check/Verify Information
Did the pharmacist review the prepared medication?	Original prescription, stock medication bottle or vial, calculations	Invalid or out-of-date prescription filled
Can the pharmacist verify the validity of the prescription using the finished product and the information you provide?	Original prescription	
Can the pharmacist verify the patient information using the finished product and the information you provide?	Original prescription, patient profile, patient, physician or nurse	Wrong patient given medication
Can the pharmacist verify the correctness of the prepared prescription based on the medication information provided?	Physical appearance of prepared medication, calculations and conversions of technician, original manufacturer's container, pictographic medication verification programs, package insert	Medication selection error made; incorrect dose, form, or formulation selected; incorrect medication administered

information on the hard copy of the prescription written by the physician. Scanning the stock bottle's bar code may simplify a portion of this process. The same verification process is needed for a compounded sterile or nonsterile preparation.

Role of the Technician in Verification Process One useful exercise to help the technician become aware of what is needed by a pharmacist is to practice checking a colleague's work. After trading a finished product with another technician, he or she should consider the following questions: Can you retrace the steps taken to fill the prescription? Can you validate all of the key pieces of information? Undertaking this exercise on a regular basis helps highlight bad habits or shortcuts that may open the door for medication errors.

Step 8: Store Completed Prescription

Table 12.8 lists the information needed and the resources used to avoid potential errors in the eighth step of the prescription-filling process.

Proper Storage Conditions Ensuring the integrity of medication is an important part of medication safety. Some medications are sensitive to light, humidity, or temperature. Failure to store medications properly may result in loss of drug potency or effect. In some cases, improper storage of a drug may result in a degraded product that causes serious harm. The following examples illustrate this type of problem:

- Inadvertent freezing of certain types of insulin can result in changes in the formulation and, subsequently, absorption by the body. Once the drug has been thawed and administered, the result is a drug that may demonstrate a different therapeutic effect.
- Improper storage of nitroglycerin—a medication used to treat angina or chest pain—results in a loss of the desired effect. Nitroglycerin molecules adhere to plastics and cotton; therefore, sublingual tablets must be stored in original glass containers under airtight conditions without cotton.
- Overheating of fentanyl patches alters how the drug is released from the patch, resulting in a possible overdose. Patients must be counseled to avoid applying heat to the patch.

TABLE 12.8 Step 8: Store Completed Prescription

Information to Check	Resources to Verify Information	Potential Errors Resulting from Failure to Check/Verify Information
Are storage conditions appropriate for the medication (e.g., humidity, temperature, light exposure)?	Package insert	Medication becomes degraded
Are each patient's medications adequately separated?	Physical review of medications placed in bags, boxes, or bins	Patient receives medication not intended for him or her; patient fails to receive medication (i.e., omission)
Are storage areas kept neat and orderly?	Use of organizational systems (e.g., bins, boxes, bags, alphabetizing, numbering, consolidation)	Patient receives medication not intended for him or her; patient fails to receive medication (i.e., omission)

Because storage temperature can alter medicines, it is important to carefully monitor temperature-controlled equipment. Checking refrigerator and freezer temperatures in the pharmacy or on the nursing unit must be done frequently and be well-documented. Monitoring temperature and keeping a log is often a responsibility assumed by a pharmacy technician; however, any staff member accessing these storage areas should carefully monitor temperature and report any abnormal readings immediately.

Organizational Systems Simple measures—such as well-organized and clearly labeled storage systems—can help keep a patient's medications together and separate from those of other patients. Orderly storage decreases the chances that a patient will receive a prescription intended for someone else or not receive his or her own medication because it was given to another patient. Both scenarios are medication errors, and, depending on the drugs in question, each situation presents the potential to cause serious harm or death if the error goes undetected.

Step 9: Deliver Medication to Patient

Table 12.9 lists the information needed and the resources used to avoid potential errors in the ninth and final step of the prescription-filling process. In a community pharmacy setting, the medication is ultimately received directly by the patient (or a designated representative. In the hospital pharmacy setting, the medication is received

TABLE 12.9   Step 9: Deliver Medication to Patient

Information to Check	Resources to Verify Information	Potential Errors Resulting from Failure to Check/Verify Information
Will the appearance of any of the medications be new to the patient or caregiver?	Prescription label, patient, patient education handouts, patient profile	Administration error made; patient noncompliant with medication instructions
Is the patient receiving medications intended for him or her?	Patient, caregiver, original prescription, patient profile, bar-coding identification system	Patient receives medication not intended for him or her; patient fails to receive medication (i.e., omission)
Does the patient or caregiver understand the instructions for use?	Pharmacist, patient education handouts, drug information resources	Administration error made; patient noncompliant with medication instructions; drug interactions, adverse reactions, degradation of medication occurs because of improper handling or storage
Does the patient or caregiver know what to expect?	Pharmacist, patient education handouts, drug information resources	Side effects and adverse reactions occur; clinical effect not achieved
Are all of the medications prescribed for the patient included?	Consolidation of medications into one bag, bin, or box; use of organizational systems (e.g., bins, boxes, bags, alphabetizing, consolidation)	Patient fails to receive medication (i.e., omission); therapy not completed

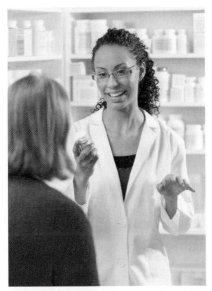

The technician should verify a date of birth or an address to be sure that the correct patient is receiving the correct drug.

by the nurse. In either case, the opportunity exists to verify the prescription information against the knowledge and expectations of the patient or the caregiver.

Verification of Patient Identity In situations where the patient receives the medication directly, it is advisable to confirm the patient's date of birth or address rather than just his or her name. For example, medications for both Richard C. Smith and Richard V. Smith may be in the storage bins; using a date of birth or an address ensures that the correct medication is dispensed to the correct patient.

Explanation of Medication to Patient Once the patient's identity is confirmed, the technician should double-check the number of medications that the patient expects to receive and inquire as to the patient's knowledge of their proper use. If the patient has questions on a medication, the pharmacist should be consulted. Comparing the completed prescription against the information provided by the patient allows the pharmacist a final opportunity to catch potential errors that were unrecognized during the computer entry or filling processes, as well as potential errors resulting from gaps or misunderstandings in the patient's knowledge. In this way, errors—such as receipt of medications into the wrong hands or missing medications (i.e., omission of therapy), as well as drug, dosage form, and administration errors—are caught. Ask basic questions of the patient, such as "Do you know what your medicine is for and how to use it?" Call to the patient's attention the auxiliary warning and caution labels on the medication bottle.

These inquiries may uncover unexpected drug interactions or side effects or indicate a patient in need of counseling by the pharmacist to enhance his or her understanding of correct administration.

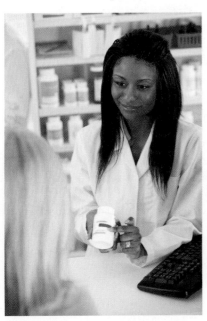

The technician is encouraged to use a "show-and-tell" technique to minimize medication errors. Showing the medication and reviewing the instructions can ensure that the correct drug was dispensed and that the patient understands the labeled directions.

"Show-and-Tell" Technique with Patient In some community pharmacies, a "show-and-tell" technique is employed to prevent medication errors and provide patient education. When a patient comes to the pharmacy to pick up a new prescription, the pharmacy technician or pharmacist opens the vial and shows the drug product to the patient. This added step not only helps the patient identify the drug that he or she will be taking but also provides an extra opportunity for the technician or pharmacist to check that the correct drug product was put into the vial. If the patient notices that a refilled drug looks different from a previously filled drug, then the patient has a chance to point this out and have this discrepancy verified. Often the medication is refilled with a different manufacturer's brand of generic medication, which may look different. When the pharmacist relays this information, the patient will know that the correct medication was dispensed. Medication errors can be caught before they ultimately reach the patient in this final check system.

ISMP's "Tell-Back" System Similar to the "show-and-tell" technique is the recommended program from ISMP called "Tell Back." Studies have demonstrated that patients often leave their physicians' offices with a poor understanding of their health conditions

Safety Note

Pharmacy technicians cannot instruct patients about their medications. If a technician suspects that a patient requires instruction, then the technician should alert the pharmacist.

or recommended treatments. The "tell-back" collaborative questioning approach uses patient-centered, open-ended questions (see Chapter 13) to help determine patient understanding. For example, "Mrs. Rodriguez, you are taking several medications for high blood pressure and cholesterol. I have given you a lot of information on the medication information sheets and MedGuides. It would be helpful for me to hear your understanding of these medications and their side effect profiles." This line of questioning is preferred over the more common, closed-ended questioning such as, "Do you have any questions?" If the pharmacy technician senses a lack of understanding, the pharmacist should be notified and the patient counseled. An educated patient is less likely to make a medication error.

Nursing Unit Delivery of Medication In hospital settings, the medication passes through an extra set of hands (usually a nurse). Adding the caregiver to the medication delivery process provides an additional person to confirm the accuracy and appropriateness of the medication. An additional safeguard that is often implemented by the nursing staff to lower the risk of a medication error is the scanning of the patient's wristband when delivering medication for administration. However, the addition of a new step in the process creates another possibility for a medication error. The task of medication delivery to the nursing station is mainly filled by technicians; therefore, the technician is in the best position to search for potential errors. If unit dose medication carts are returned to the pharmacy with unused, regularly scheduled medication, the pharmacist or pharmacy technician should follow up with the nurses to determine whether an error of omission occurred. Any discrepancies in the automated drug dispensing machines on the nursing unit should be resolved by the nurse with the technician or pharmacist. Upon delivery of the medications to the nursing unit, the technician should determine if the nurse knows about the newly prescribed medications and if the medications delivered were all that were expected.

In the treatment of certain diseases, such as cancer, multiple drug therapy combinations, including investigational medications, are prescribed together because they work in concert to treat the disease. If a particular drug is missing from the drug therapy combination, then treatment is incomplete. Like any omission, incomplete therapy is also a medication error. In addition, many of these drugs are extremely toxic; any dose error could be fatal. Therefore, communication with the nurse or physician when these medications are delivered to the treatment area is also an opportunity to verify that doses prepared are, in fact, correct. All prescriptions and medication orders (and calculations) for chemotherapy and hazardous substances must be checked and double-checked by both the technician and the pharmacist because of the extreme toxicity of these drugs.

Without the cooperative efforts of the pharmacy technician, pharmacist, and nurse to ensure proper medication use, a patient's well-being is not safeguarded, and the best health outcome cannot be achieved.

Medication Error Prevention

Learning to prevent medication errors means carefully examining potential points of failure and using all available resources to verify information or decisions. Keeping in mind that the most common error in dispensing and administration is drug identification, a pharmacy technician becomes a valuable asset in ensuring drug safety, for the pharmacy technician "owns" a substantial portion of the prescription-filling process. A pharmacy technician is often the person who first receives and examines the prescription, enters the data into the computer, and submits the prescription for filling. He or she is also likely to be the last person to handle a medication before it reaches the patient. Consequently, the pharmacy technician often has the most opportunities to prevent medication errors. In addition, pharmacy technicians are also in a position to identify potential sources of errors beyond prescription dispensing because they are the ones who may interact with a patient or nurse when a prescription or medication order comes into or goes out of the pharmacy.

Many medication errors occur during prescribing and administration. Prescriptions often pass first through the hands of a pharmacy technician once they are received from physicians or patients. Prescribers are responsible for ensuring the "five Rs," or five rights (see Figure 12.2). In other words, they must ensure that the prescription is for the right drug, for the right patient, at the right strength, given by the right route, and administered at the right time. Pharmacy practice overlays prescribers' responsibilities and facilitates patient safety and error prevention by processes that verify the following:

Safety Note

Incorrect drug identification is the most common error in dispensing or administration.

- The correct patient is being given the medications, and other associated medications are also correct.
- The correct drug is dispensed (e.g., bupropion SR vs. bupropion XL).
- The correct dose is prepared, whether for a child or an adult, to maintain the correct blood level.
- The correct route of administration is indicated (e.g., oral vs. sublingual).
- The appropriate dosage form is prepared (e.g., oral disintegrating tablets are dispensed for a child instead of oral tablets, and antibiotic suspensions are dispensed for administration to an infant). For a child or an infant, a measuring device should accompany the medication to ensure that a correct dose is given.
- The correct administration times and the correct conditions for administration (e.g., medications that must be taken with or without food) are indicated.

FIGURE 12.2
Five Rs for Patient Drug Administration

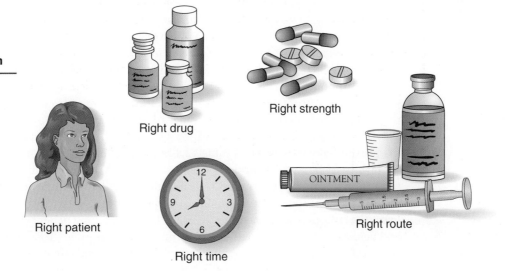

Right drug

Right strength

Right patient

Right time

Right route

Safety Note

The only acceptable number of medication errors is zero.

The Responsibility of Healthcare Professionals

Working in health care means making a commitment to "first do no harm." This means that healthcare workers must put safety first. As discussed in Chapter 1, the profession of pharmacy exists primarily to safeguard the health of the public. Because the effects of potential medication errors on patients cannot be predicted, all professionals working in the healthcare system must focus on treating the patient and

Safety Note

If information is missing from a prescription or medication order, a pharmacy technician must obtain the information from the prescriber. The technician should never make conjectures regarding the missing content.

ensuring the best possible outcome by the safest possible means. As a result, no acceptable medication error exists, and each step in the task of filling medication orders should be reviewed with a 100% error-free goal in mind.

Potential Sources of Errors Although pharmacists are ultimately responsible for the accuracy of the medication-filling process, technicians working in community and hospital pharmacy settings can assist in ensuring safety. For example, through careful listening and observation during a patient or medical staff interaction, a technician can identify potential sources of medication errors on the patient's part and actively prevent any error by notifying the pharmacist. By constant surveillance for potential sources of medication errors, pharmacy technicians become vital assistants to pharmacists and make significant contributions to patient safety beyond the borders of the pharmacy.

Pharmacy technicians can also help to reduce potential medication errors by assuming more routine dispensing tasks in the pharmacy setting. This action allows the pharmacist to spend more time on patient counseling and on taking detailed, accurate medication histories. The importance of the latter task was proven by a study at Northwestern Memorial Hospital in Chicago. The study included a review of medication histories in patients' charts, and the findings were grim. One-third of the patients' charts contained medication errors. More than 85% of the errors originated when hospital personnel took incomplete medication histories upon admission. If pharmacists were given more time for medication history review and could communicate this information to physicians and nurses, the incidence of medication errors would decline.

By following some basic safe-practice guidelines listed in Table 12.10, pharmacists and pharmacy technicians can work together to create a larger margin of safety.

Patient Education

Patients and caregivers must have the basic knowledge needed to administer, handle, and support safe medication use. Pharmacy technicians can encourage patients to ask questions, relay complete medical and allergy history, and check medication labels (both prescription and OTC) carefully for information about how and when medications should be taken. The pharmacy technician should be actively involved in monitoring for potential errors or patient misunderstandings. Although pharmacy technicians cannot counsel patients, they can encourage them to become informed about their conditions and to ask the pharmacist basic questions about the prescribed medications. Patients should understand the 10 key pieces of information about every medication taken, as listed in Table 12.11.

If the patient has prescriptions filled at another pharmacy or via mail order, the technician should attempt to add this information to the computer profile for pharmacist review. However, all patients should be strongly encouraged to use only one pharmacy to lower the risks of serious medication errors. By encouraging patients to ask questions and helping them connect with the pharmacist or appropriate healthcare provider, the technician assists patients in becoming more informed and empowers them to be advocates for their own safety and health. Patients should be encouraged to call their pharmacists if questions on proper medication use arise after leaving the pharmacy.

Innovations to Promote Safety

Many efforts have been made by all healthcare team members to minimize the possibility of medication errors. In addition to e-prescribing, some physicians have adopted a hard copy preprinted prescription in which the drug, dose, schedule,

TABLE 12.10   General Tips for Reducing Medication Errors

General Tips	<ul><li>Always keep the prescription and the label together during the filling process.</li><li>Know the common look-alike and sound-alike drugs, and keep them stored in different areas.</li><li>Keep dangerous or high-alert medications in a separate storage area of the pharmacy.</li><li>Always question illegible handwriting.</li><li>Check that prescriptions and medication orders contain accurate information, including the correctly spelled drug name, strength, appropriate dosing, quantity or duration of therapy, dosage form, and route. Obtain any missing information from the prescriber.</li><li>Use the metric system. A leading zero should always be present in decimal values less than one. (e.g., 0.3).</li><li>Question prescriptions and orders that use uncommon abbreviations. Avoid using abbreviations that have more than one meaning, and verify with the prescriber those abbreviations of which you are unsure.</li><li>Be aware of insulin mistakes. Insulin brands should be clearly separated from one another while stored in the refrigerator. Always educate patients about the proper use of various insulin products at the time of purchase.</li><li>Keep the work area clean and uncluttered. Keep only those drugs that are needed for immediate use close at hand.</li><li>Always verify information at each step of the prescription-filling process.</li><li>Be sure that at least two people compare the label with the original prescription.</li></ul>
Tips for Pharmacists	<ul><li>Check the original prescription, the NDC number, and the drug stock bottle.</li><li>Initial all checked prescriptions.</li><li>Inspect the product in the bottle.</li><li>Cross-reference prescription information with other validating sources.</li><li>Encourage documentation of all medication use, including OTC medications and dietary supplements.</li><li>Document all clarifications on orders.</li><li>Maintain open lines of communication with patients, healthcare providers, and caregivers.</li></ul>
Tips for Technicians	<ul><li>Check the original prescription, the NDC number, and the drug stock bottle.</li><li>Regularly review work habits, and actively look for actions to take that improve safe and accurate prescription filling.</li><li>Verify information with the patient or caregiver when the prescription is received into the pharmacy and when the filled prescription is sent out of the pharmacy.</li><li>Observe, listen to, and report pertinent information that may affect the safety or effectiveness of drug therapy to the pharmacist.</li><li>Keep your work area free of clutter.</li></ul>

TABLE 12.11   Information Patients Must Know About Their Medications

1. Brand and generic names
2. The medication's appearance
3. The purpose of the medication, and the duration of treatment
4. The correct dosage and frequency, and the best time or circumstances to take a dose
5. How to proceed if they miss a dose
6. Medications or foods that interact with the prescribed medication
7. Whether the prescription is in addition to or replaces a current medication
8. Common side effects and how to handle them
9. Special precautions necessary for each particular drug therapy
10. Proper storage for the medication

frequency, amount dispensed, and so on can be circled, thus minimizing transcription or illegible prescription medication errors. This preprinted form may be common with certain specialists such as optometrists or endocrinologists who prescribe a limited number of drugs or medical supplies for their patients. Other innovations in environmental practices; packaging, medication, and label design; and use of automation are reducing medication error incidents.

Workplace Ergonomics The physical setting can make a major contribution to the overall safety of any pharmacy work environment. Adequate space and clean, well-lit conditions are just some of the basics, in addition to adequate staffing. Work shifts of 12 hours or longer by pharmacy staff, physicians, or residents-in-training may correlate directly with a higher incidence of medication errors. Table 12.12 outlines work environment practices that a pharmacy can create to promote safety and to reduce errors.

TABLE 12.12 Workplace Ergonomic Practices to Promote Safety

- Automate and bar code all fill procedures.
- Maintain a clean, organized, and well-lit work area.
- Provide adequate storage areas with clear drug labels on the shelves.
- Encourage prescribers to employ common terminology and only use safe abbreviations.
- Provide adequate computer applications and hardware.

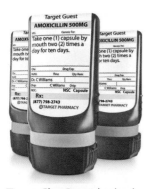

The Target ClearRx packaging is designed to help patients manage their medications by providing information in a clear, easy-to-read format.

Package, Medication, and Label Design To improve medication safety, drug manufacturers and pharmacies have developed innovations in product and packaging designs.

Package Design An innovative package design by Target pharmacies has helped their customers manage their medications more safely. The ClearRx design uses color-coded rings to help patients identify medications intended for them, as opposed to those intended for other family members. In addition, the medication container label is larger and more prominently displayed. A consumer survey indicated a strong preference (85%) for the ClearRx design over conventional labels and medication containers. Consumers felt that the new design improved safety and provided an easier-to-read label featuring better-organized warnings in larger type.

ClearRx won the Gold award from NCC MERP in 2010 in the category, "Solution to a Consumer Problem." That solution includes clear labeling, large font size, an easy-to-use dispenser, and a label magnifier for visually impaired individuals.

Medication Design Many companies are manufacturing formulations with unique colors, shapes, or markings to assist in distinguishing between doses or competitor products. For some products, the markings on the tablet or capsule verify the dose. For other products, different doses of the same medication will have different colors and tablet or capsule identification on the

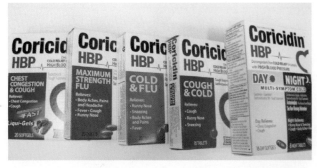

The use of a variety of colors, fonts, and images on a package can help prevent errors by distinguishing among products.

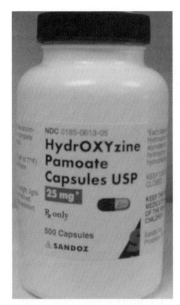

To bring special attention to medication names and prevent errors, tall-man lettering is now used to differentiate between names. In this case, the "OXY" in hydrOXYzine is capitalized to differentiate the packaging from hydrALAZINE.

stock bottle. Still other products may have the middle four numbers of the NDC is either in a larger font or boldface type to minimize selection errors.

Label Design Pharmaceutical manufacturers, with the encouragement of USP's Nomenclature, Safety, and Labeling Expert Committee, are adopting innovations in labeling that should minimize medication errors with their products. USP may recommend "tall man" or enhanced lettering, adding warning statements on the stock labels of high-risk medications, or other labeling changes to better differentiate products and dosages and help reduce medication errors. "Tall man" lettering is often used to distinguish similar medications, such as hydrOXYzine and hydrALAZINE—two products that are available in similar doses.

Use of Automation Many human errors are prevented by using automation. An example of using automation to minimize medication errors in community and hospital pharmacies is the widespread use of electronic technology such as e-prescribing and bar-code scanning.

Electronic Prescribing As discussed in Chapter 6, the electronic transmission of prescriptions (e-prescribing) continues to be increasingly used by physicians to send prescriptions to the community pharmacy. E-prescribing eliminates the problem of illegible prescriptions or sound-alike medications causing a preventable error.

Bar-Coding Technology Many chain pharmacies use bar-coding technology throughout the medication-filling process. The prescription information is entered into the computerized system and verified by the pharmacist; the pharmacy technician then scans the selected stock bottle's NDC number when the drug is selected from stock. The computer automatically compares the scanned bar code against the verified prescription information. If the prescription does not match the NDC code of the selected medication, the system indicates that an incorrect selection has been made. This technology minimizes the chances of selecting the incorrect drug or dose when filling a prescription.

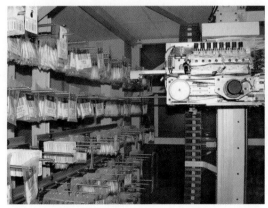

Robot-based medication dispensing increases efficiency and speed of medication delivery without compromising safety. The robot uses bar codes to validate drug selection, significantly reducing the chances of drug selection errors.

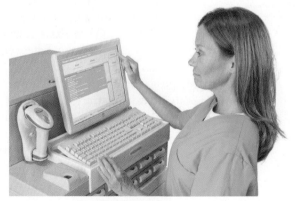

Automated dispensing cabinets are maintained primarily by pharmacy technicians.

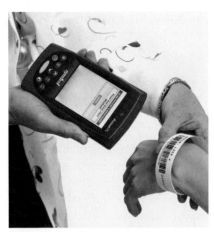
Bar-coding and scanning technologies ensure that the correct patient is receiving the correct medication.

Walgreens also uses bar-coding technology in the final verification by the pharmacist. The computerized database includes images of the physical shape, color, and markings of the medication. The pharmacist can then compare the image on the computer screen against the bar code of the prepared medication to confirm that the appropriate medication was used. At the time of dispensing the medication to the patient, the prescription is scanned one last time to ensure that the right patient is receiving the medication.

Integrated, Automated System Moving from a paper-based system to an integrated, automated system has improved efficiency and allows resources in the hospital to be redeployed to increase patient safety and improve quality of patient care. Automation in the computer order entry, filling, preparation, and administration of medications has dramatically reduced medication errors by more than 50% in several hospital studies.

The physician inputs the medication order directly from a handheld personal digital assistant or PDA. The order is then sent electronically to the pharmacy where it is double-checked for accuracy by the pharmacist. The order is filled by the technician (or robot), checked by the technician and pharmacist, and sent to the nursing unit. The medication is then administered to the patient by the nurse who matches the bar code of the medication with the bar code on the patient wristband. With an **electronic medication administration record (eMAR)**, the administration of a medication is documented electronically by the nurse rather than on paper. The eMAR can minimize medication errors in both hospitals and nursing homes.

The Institute of Medicine encourages the adoption of automation technologies for all medication orders in all hospitals as soon as possible. As discussed in Chapter 9, these technological advances empower the pharmacy technician staff to become more productive; as a result, the pharmacist's time is freed to become more involved in patient care.

Professional Prevention Strategies

In response to several hospital medication errors leading to serious patient injuries or deaths, the American Society of Health-System Pharmacists (ASHP) has developed the Pharmacy Technician Initiative, a partnership with individual state affiliates. The premise of the initiative is that enhanced education and training of pharmacy technicians will improve patient safety and minimize medication errors. To that end, this proposal requires the completion of an ASHP-accredited pharmacy technician training program as well as PTCB certification. These prerequisites would be required for State Board registration and must be completed by technicians before practicing in a hospital pharmacy. Currently, each state has varying requirements on registration, training, and certification for pharmacy technicians. By working with state affiliates, the goal of the ASHP initiative is to encourage state legislation that will result in a more highly qualified workforce in the future.

Personal Prevention Strategies

Pharmacy technicians must take care of themselves as well as their patients. Although refusing to work a long shift or overtime is not always a realistic option, technicians can heed the recommendations of the Healthcare Provider Service Organization (HPSO) to help combat fatigue and, therefore, prevent medication errors. Pharmacy technicians should be mindful of the following lifestyle recommendations:

- Get enough sleep. Experts say that eight hours of sleep a night is best, so go to bed early enough. Avoid staying up until you cannot keep your eyes open any longer; as soon as you feel sleepy, turn out the lights and turn in.
- Exercise regularly. You may feel more tired at first, but regular exercise should eventually help boost your energy level. Plan to do your workout several hours before bedtime so that you are not keyed up when it is time to sleep.
- Take breaks at work. Even when things are busy, take breaks to relax and revitalize yourself, even if it means going outside to clear your head for a couple of minutes. You will not be much help if you cannot think clearly.
- Be wise about food. Eat a well-balanced diet for optimal energy. During your scheduled time, avoid sugar-laden snacks and choose complex carbohydrates for stamina.
- Avoid excessive alcohol. A nightcap at home may relax you at first, but as the alcohol wears off, it disrupts your normal sleep patterns.
- Cut the caffeine. Coffee, tea, and other drinks that contain caffeine do not prevent fatigue; they just hide it. Limit your caffeine intake, especially near bedtime.

If you feel tired on the job, then do not be afraid to ask for help, such as having a colleague double-check your filling, compounding, or dosage calculations.

Medication Error Reporting Systems

If what is not known cannot be fixed, then the first step in the prevention of medication errors is collection of information and identification of problems. Fear of punishment is always a concern when an error arises; as a result, healthcare professionals may decide not to report an error at all, leaving the door open for the same error to occur again. For this reason, anonymous or no-fault systems of reporting have been established. The focus of no-fault reporting is on fixing the problem rather than on assigning blame. In reality, most medication errors are reported internally by the pharmacist and analyzed within the organization rather than reported to a centralized national database.

State Boards of Pharmacy

Several efforts have been made to create a safe and comfortable atmosphere for individuals to report medication errors. Many states have mandatory error-reporting systems, but most officials admit that medical errors are still underreported, mostly because of fear of punishment and liability. State Boards of Pharmacy do not punish pharmacists for errors, as long as a good-faith effort was made to fill the prescription correctly. States such as Florida, Texas, and California have worked to reduce the fear of reporting by passing new regulations that allow pharmacists to document errors and error-prone systems without fear of punishment. Pharmacists in these states, however, need to indicate the steps that are being taken to eliminate weaknesses that might allow such errors to continue.

Nineteen states regulate, require, or recommend a continuous quality improvement (CQI) program to detect, document, and assess medication errors to determine the causes and to develop an appropriate response to prevent future errors. In addition, many legislatures have proposed new laws that protect error reports from subpoena. These error reports must be separate from medical records because all medical records can be subpoenaed, including prescription records.

Error Reporting The task of error reporting is best performed by the pharmacist; however, pharmacy technicians are an integral part of the process of error identification, documentation, and prevention. An understanding of the *what, when, where,* and *why* of error reporting is important for pharmacy technicians, as well as for pharmacists. The final and most important piece of medication error reporting is the delicate task of informing the patient that a medication error has taken place. This is typically the responsibility of the pharmacist. The circumstances leading to the error should be explained completely and honestly. Patients should understand the nature of the error, what (if any) effects the error may have, and how he or she can become actively involved in preventing errors in the future. Generally speaking, people are more likely to forgive an honest error, but rarely accept concealment of the truth. If the medication error will lead to a side effect or adverse drug reaction or impact the disease or illness being treated, the pharmacist must also contact the prescriber.

Joint Commission

Organizations also contribute to error-reporting efforts by creating a centralized site through which all members may channel information safely. A well-established example is the Sentinel Event Policy created by the Joint Commission. A **sentinel event** is an unexpected occurrence involving death, serious physical or psychological injury, or the potential for such occurrences to happen. When a sentinel event is reported, the organization (i.e., hospital, pharmacy, or managed-care company) is expected to analyze the cause of the error (i.e., perform a root-cause analysis), take action to correct the cause, monitor the changes made, and determine whether the cause of the error has been eliminated.

Accreditation and Medication Safety Accreditation of hospitals is dependent on demonstrating an effective medical and medication error–reporting system. The Joint Commission supports the recommendations of the ISMP: (1) the elimination of certain abbreviations and (2) the education of healthcare professionals regarding frequently confused drug names to minimize errors. For example, units of insulin should always be spelled out so that a sloppily written 6U is not confused with 60 units of insulin—a tenfold dosing error that could cause a serious drop in a patient's blood glucose level. Healthcare personnel should also use the abbreviation "mL" rather than the abbreviation "cc." The latter abbreviation is frequently misinterpreted. Students are encouraged to review a list of "error prone" abbreviations at the ISMP website.

The Joint Commission may recommend a safety program to improve communications with physicians and nurses in the ordering, preparation, and dispensing of medications in an effort to minimize medication errors. Other examples are implementation of policies prohibiting the use of nonapproved abbreviations or policies requiring computer checks and balances with sound-alike drugs to ensure that the right drug, in the right dose, is given to the right patient. The survey team is most interested in documenting measurable changes in the implemented safety program.

The Joint Commission's safety-related standards are based on the assumption that, if a preventable medication error occurs, investigating the cause and making necessary corrections in policy or procedure are much more important than fixing blame on an individual. When the cause of the error is identified, a repeat medication error may be prevented in the future. The standards also require that the hospital outline its responsibility to advise a patient about any adverse outcomes of the error.

SPEAK UP Campaign The Joint Commission in concert with the Centers for Medicare & Medicaid Services has also developed an educational series of written brochures and videos as part of its SPEAK UP campaign. This program is designed for consumers to take a more active role in their health care and minimize misunderstandings that may lead to medication errors. SPEAK UP is an acronym that stands for the following:

Speak up if you have questions or concerns. If you still don't understand, ask again. It's your body, and you have a right to know.

Pay attention to the care you get. Always make sure you're getting the right treatments and medications from the right healthcare professionals. Don't assume anything.

Educate yourself about your illness. Learn about the medical tests you get and your treatment plan.

Ask a trusted family member or friend to be your advocate (adviser or supporter).

Know what medications you take and why you take them. Medication errors are the most common healthcare mistakes.

Use a hospital, clinic, surgery center, or other type of healthcare organization that has been carefully checked out. For example, the Joint Commission visits hospitals to see the facilities are meeting the Joint Commission's quality standards.

Participate in all decisions about your treatment. You are the center of the healthcare team.

United States Pharmacopeia

Many professional organizations support patient safety efforts by gathering medical error information and using the data to create tools to support professionals in specific settings or situations. The USP supports two types of reporting systems for the collection of adverse events and medication errors: MEDMARX, an international reporting system developed by Quantros, and ISMP MERP, a national reporting program administered by the ISMP (discussed on the following page).

MEDMARX Reporting System The Internet-based program, used by hospitals and health systems, is known as MEDMARX. **MEDMARX** allows institutions and healthcare professionals to anonymously document, analyze, and track adverse events specific to an institution. Since 1998, MEDMARX has received more than 2 million reports of medication errors from more than 800 hospitals and healthcare systems.

A total of 26,604 medication errors were reported in the most recent MEDMARX report published by USP. Based on this report, 1.4% of these medication errors caused patient harm; seven cases of death were caused or contributed to by a medication error; and more than 60% of these errors occurred during the dispensing process, with pharmacy technicians involved in 38.5% of the occurrences. Major contributing factors to the errors included distraction in the workplace, excessive workload, and inexperience.

The USP has addressed error prevention through medication labeling. For example, the organization established a new labeling standard to improve the safety of neuromuscular blockers in the surgical suites of hospitals. Such drugs now carry the label: "Warning—Paralyzing Agent." For the toxic drug vincristine, administered in the hospital and outpatient cancer clinics, the medication label now reads "For Intravenous Use Only—Fatal if Given by Other Routes." These labeling changes were a direct result of an analysis of voluntary reports of medication errors in MEDMARX.

Institute for Safe Medication Practices

The **Institute for Safe Medication Practices (ISMP)** is a nonprofit healthcare agency whose membership is primarily comprised of physicians, pharmacists, and nurses. The mission of this organization is to understand the causes of medication errors and to provide and communicate time-critical error-reduction strategies to the healthcare community, policymakers, and the public. Unlike the USP, the ISMP does not set standards but focuses on expert analysis and scientific studies to reduce medication errors.

Medication Errors Reporting Program ISMP provides a national voluntary program called the **Medication Errors Reporting Program (ISMP MERP)**. ISMP is a federally certified patient safety organization (PSO), providing legal protection and confidentiality for submitted patient safety data and error reports. This program is designed to allow healthcare professionals to report medication errors directly. The ISMP shares all information and error-prevention strategies with the FDA.

According to the program, medication errors include (1) incorrect drug, strength, or dose; (2) wrong patient; (3) confusion over look-alike and sound-alike drugs or similar packaging; (4) incorrect route of drug administration; (5) calculation or preparation errors; (6) misuse of medical equipment (e.g., infusion pumps, automated controllers, etc.); and (7) errors in prescribing, transcribing, dispensing, administering, or monitoring medications. Reports can be completed online. See Table 12.13 for the type of information collected.

TABLE 12.13 Information Needed for ISMP MERP

1. Describe the error or preventable adverse drug reaction. What went wrong?
2. Was this an actual medication error (that reached the patient), or are you expressing concern about a potential error that was discovered before it reached the patient?
3. If an actual medication error occurred, what was the patient outcome?
4. Specify the practice site (e.g., hospital, private office, retail pharmacy, drug company, long-term care facility, etc.).
5. What are the generic names of all products involved?
6. What are the brand names of all products involved?
7. Describe the dosage form, concentration or strength, and so forth.
8. How was the error discovered or intercepted?
9. Please state your recommendations for error prevention.

Other ISMP Initiatives With valuable input from many professional organizations, the ISMP has also published an extensive checklist of system-based strategies called "ISMP Medication Safety Self Assessment for Community/Ambulatory Pharmacy" to minimize preventable medication errors. The recommendations include:

- adequate pharmacist and technician staffing and training
- appropriate ratios of pharmacists and technicians

- review and verification by pharmacists of all information input by technicians
- review of all medication alerts on dosing and frequency as well as contraindications or warnings about potential drug interactions

This report also emphasizes the importance of a nonpunitive reporting system to minimize future medication errors.

ISMP makes the following recommendations to minimize dispensing errors:

- If possible, the order entry person should differ from the one who fills the order, thus adding an independent validation, or additional checks, to the order-entry process.
- Pharmacy personnel should not prepare prescriptions from the computer-generated label in case an error occurred at order entry; they should use the original (or scanned copy) prescription.
- Pharmacy personnel should keep the original prescription, stock bottle, computer label, and medication container together during the filling process.
- The pharmacist should verify dispensing accuracy by comparing the original prescription to the labeled product, the NDC code on the label, and the manufacturer's stock bottle.

In most pharmacy programs, pharmacists and technicians are taught to check each prescription against the original prescription and medication information sheet at least four times: when the medication is taken from the shelf, during the computer order entry and printing of the label, during the filling of the prescription, and during the verification of the NDC number—both before and after counting the dosage units.

High-alert medications have a high incidence of error in the hospital and community pharmacy settings. High-alert medications include potentially toxic drugs such as chemotherapy agents, digoxin, amiodarone, and warfarin. Due to potential drops in diabetic patients' blood glucose levels, insulins and oral hypoglycemics should also be carefully monitored. The ISMP also publishes a list of common look-alike and sound-alike drugs that often contribute to medication errors—for example, Reminyl vs. Amaryl. Reminyl is used to treat Alzheimer's disease, whereas Amaryl is used to lower blood glucose levels. If these medications are not spelled out or verified during a verbal prescription order, an error could occur. The ISMP stresses awareness of such drugs and promotes adding a medical indication for each drug, as well as encouraging e-prescribing.

ISMP has sponsored national forums on medication errors, recommended the addition of labeling or special hazard warnings on potentially toxic drugs, and encouraged revisions of potentially dangerous prescription writing practices. For example, the organization first promoted the now common practice of using the leading zero in pharmacy calculations. The Joint Commission has adopted many ISMP recommendations, including avoiding the use of common abbreviations, such as "U" or "IU" (spell out), and avoiding the use of the trailing zero when possible (e.g., Lisinopril 5 mg, not 5.0 mg).

ISMP is active in disseminating information to healthcare professionals and consumers, such as e-mail newsletters, journal articles, and video training exercises. In addition, the ISMP has both FDA safety and hazard alerts posted on its website.

Chapter Summary

- Pharmacy technicians play a crucial role in the prevention of medication errors.
- Knowing the potential causes and categories of medication errors is the first step in preventing them from occurring.
- Medication errors may result from physiological and social causes.
- Medication errors can be further categorized as omission, wrong dose, extra dose, wrong dosage form, and wrong time of administration.
- Once errors are identified by root-cause analysis, corrective measures should be put in place, and permanent elimination of the source of error should be the goal.
- Each step of the medication-filling process has the potential to produce a medication error.
- Specific practices, careful work habits, and a clean work environment promote patient safety and decrease illness and injury caused by medication errors.
- Although pharmacy technicians cannot counsel patients concerning their medications,

they can encourage them to ask questions of the pharmacist.
- Helping patients become more informed also empowers them to be advocates for their own safety and health.
- Automation and technological advances including e-prescribing and bar-code scanning can minimize medication errors.
- Medication error prevention must be emphasized by all healthcare team members.
- The pharmacy technician should adopt effective personal prevention strategies to minimize human errors.
- Several medication error reporting systems exist. Pharmacy personnel should be familiar with these outlets and use them to confidentially report errors so that the errors do not occur again.
- The Joint Commission has published an "unapproved abbreviations" list to minimize medication errors.

Key Terms

assumption error an error that occurs when an essential piece of information cannot be verified and is guessed or presumed

capture error an error that occurs when focus on a task is diverted elsewhere and therefore the error goes undetected

electronic medication administration record (eMAR) a computerized patient medical record used to minimize medication errors

extra dose error an error in which more doses are received by a patient than were prescribed by the physician

human failure an error generated by failure that occurs at an individual level

Institute for Safe Medication Practices (ISMP) a nonprofit healthcare agency whose primary mission is to understand the causes of medication errors and to provide time-critical error-reduction strategies to the healthcare community, policymakers, and the public

medical error any circumstance, action, inaction, or decision related to health care that contributes to an unintended health result

medication error any preventable event that may cause or lead to inappropriate medication use or patient harm while the medication is in the control of the healthcare professional, patient, or consumer

Medication Errors Reporting Program (ISMP MERP) a program designed to allow healthcare professionals to report medication errors directly to the Institute for Safe Medication Practices (ISMP)

MEDMARX an Internet-based program of the USP for use by hospitals and healthcare systems for documenting, tracking, and identifying trends for adverse events and medication errors

noncompliance failure to take therapy as the physician instructs; also called *nonadherence*

omission error an error in which a prescribed dose is not given

organizational failure an error generated by failure of organizational rules, policies, or procedures

prn the abbreviation for a common Latin phrase, *pro re nata*, or "in the circumstances." This is commonly used to direct a patient to take medication on an as-needed basis rather than a routinely scheduled dosage.

product line extension a marketing strategy by which a brand name product is brought to market with different combinations of active ingredients and different indications leading to potential consumer errors

root-cause analysis a logical and systematic process used to help identify what, how, and why something happened to prevent recurrence

selection error an error that occurs when two or more options exist and the incorrect option is chosen

sentinel event an unexpected occurrence involving death or serious physical or psychological injury or the potential for such events to occur

technical failure an error generated by failure of equipment

wrong dosage form error an error in which the dosage form or formulation is not the accepted interpretation of the physician order

wrong dose error an error in which the dose is either above or below the correct dose by more than 5%

wrong time error a medication error in which a drug is given 30 minutes or more before or after it was prescribed, up to the time of the next dose, not including as needed orders

Chapter Review

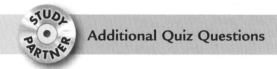

Additional Quiz Questions

Checking Your Understanding

To check your comprehension of this chapter's key concepts, read the following multiple-choice questions and then record your answers on a separate sheet of paper. Write your answers as modeled in these examples: 1d; 2c; 3b; etc.

1. For every 250 prescriptions dispensed in a community pharmacy, how many contain a medication error of some type?
   a. 0
   b. 1
   c. 4
   d. 25

2. Which of the following scenarios is *not* a patient-caused medication error?
   a. The patient took an antibiotic with a meal when instructions said to take it on an empty stomach.
   b. The patient forgot an antibiotic dose yesterday, so he or she took an extra dose today.
   c. The patient did not receive a sufficient quantity of antibiotic suspension from the pharmacy.
   d. The patient took antibiotics left over from the last time that he or she was sick.

3. A wrong dose error occurs when a dose is either above or below the correct amount by more than
   a. 1%.
   b. 3%.
   c. 5%.
   d. 8%.

4. A hospital pharmacy preparing hazardous drugs in a horizontal laminar airflow hood is an example of a(n)
   a. technical error.
   b. human error.
   c. product defect error.
   d. organization error.

5. Filling a prescription with generic buproprion SR when the drug requested was bupropion XL is an example of which type of error?
   a. assumption error
   b. selection error
   c. capture error
   d. omission error

6. When receiving a new prescription, which of the following should a pharmacist or technician avoid doing?
   a. When handwriting is difficult to read, verify all drug information with the pharmacist, appropriate drug references, and/or the prescriber.
   b. Use a trailing zero when the dose written is for a whole number (e.g., 10.0 mg).
   c. Cross-check patient information on the written prescription with the patient.
   d. Verify that the patient has not experienced any new drug allergies and that all profile information is current and correct.

7. Which of the following sources of information is useful to verify that the correct medication has been selected from the shelf to fill the prescription order?
   a. generic and/or brand names on unit stock drug container
   b. NDC number
   c. drug name on original prescription
   d. all of the above

520   **Unit 4** *Professionalism in the Pharmacy*

8. The most important factor in medication error reporting is to
   a. provide the medication at no cost to the patient.
   b. cover up the error from the pharmacist supervisor.
   c. immediately notify the USP.
   d. notify the patient.

9. At a minimum, patients and caregivers should understand 10 key pieces of information about their prescriptions. Which of the following pieces of information is *not* included in those 10 items?
   a. name of the medication
   b. best time to pick up the prescription from the pharmacy
   c. the storage requirements of the medication
   d. medication's pill shape and color

10. A sentinel event is defined by the Joint Commission as
    a. an unexpected occurrence involving death or serious physical or psychological injury, or the potential for the occurrence to happen.
    b. an unexpected outcome as the result of a drug reaction or side effect.
    c. a computer program that monitors medication errors in a hospital pharmacy.
    d. an adverse reaction with a vaccine.

11. Which of the following is an unapproved abbreviation for mL?
    a. cc
    b. mg
    c. mcg
    d. U

12. Identify the incorrect statement. All prescription or medication orders
    a. written as a decimal should have a leading zero.
    b. written as a decimal should have a trailing zero.
    c. written as a whole number should have a trailing zero.
    d. should never use zeros as a leading or trailing number.

13. The recommended abbreviation for the dose of the medication Lantus is
    a. mg.
    b. mL.
    c. IU.
    d. units.

14. To verify that the correct patient is receiving the prescription at pickup, the technician should ask the patient for his or her
    a. social security number.
    b. credit card number.
    c. date of birth or address.
    d. NDC number.

15. To minimize errors during the medication filling process, the technician will scan the bar code of the
    a. prescription number.
    b. medication stock bottle.
    c. patient bracelet.
    d. patient date of birth.

Reinforcing Your Learning

To build on your understanding of the topics in this chapter, complete the following enrichment activities.

1. At a minimum, patients and caregivers should understand 10 key pieces of information about each of their prescriptions. Name five of those items.

2. Table 12.10 outlines activities that a pharmacist can do to reduce errors. Choose one activity and briefly describe how a pharmacy technician can support a pharmacist engaged in this activity to improve patient safety.

3. Using two pairs of drug names that sound alike when spoken out loud, say them to a classmate across the room and see how easily they can be mistaken for each other. Repeat the exercise with other drug names and other students. Challenge students to know the indications of these sound-alike drugs:

   a. Aciphex and Aricept
   b. Celexa and Celebrex
   c. Miralax and Mirapex
   d. Zantac and Zyrtec

Thinking on Your Feet

To gain practice in handling challenging situations in the workplace, consider the following real-world scenarios and then use the guiding questions to help you formulate your responses.

1. Many times, a patient has a question but may hesitate to ask the nurse, pharmacist, or physician because he or she is "so busy." Any time a patient hesitates to ask a question or to understand his or her own condition better, a chance to improve the patient's health or to avoid an adverse event is lost. What could you do or say as a pharmacy technician to help the customer make the connection to the needed information?

2. A distraught patient returns to the pharmacy. A prescription for trazodone was incorrectly filled with a prescription for tramadol. You noticed that you are the technician who entered the prescription incorrectly into the computer database. The patient wants to know how it happened, how your pharmacy will correct the problem, and what incentives you will offer him to keep his business at your pharmacy. How will you respond? How would your classmates respond? If you were the patient, would you be upset? How could you improve this situation?

3. A prescription is received for Bupropion 150 mg XL 1 po q 12 hours #60 with two refills. You enter the prescription into the computer exactly as written, but the pharmacist said you made a medication error. What is the error and how would you resolve it?

Acquiring Field Knowledge

To expand your knowledge of pharmacy practice, explore the following online activities that focus on research and information retrieval.

Reminder: *As you navigate the Internet, remember to exercise caution and good judgment when evaluating information. A thoughtful review of online text should take into consideration the following factors: the creator and sponsors of the website, the intended audience, the credentials of the authors and contributors, the reliability and validity of the posted information, the frequency of updates to the site, and the ease of navigation for a range of user skill levels.*

1. Go to the Institute of Safe Medicine Practices at www.paradigmcollege.net/pharmpractice5e/MERP. Scroll down the home page to the "Report Errors" section. Click on the "Impact of the Medication Errors Reporting Program" (ISMP MERP) link. Read the information and select and record five accomplishments (from 1996 to present day) attributed to the establishment of ISMP MERP. Why should medication errors be reported outside the organization?

2. Conduct an Internet search for "ClearRx." Check the main website to see what label changes were made to improve Target medication vials. Discuss how these changes might improve patient safety.

3. Go to www.paradigmcollege.net/pharmpractice5e/druginfo. Conduct a search for the drugs listed and read the accompanying information. Consider these questions: What might happen if these two drugs were accidentally switched in the pharmacy and given to the patient? Would these mix-ups be life-threatening? Write a summary of your conclusions for each pair of drugs.
   a. hydralazine and hydroxyzine
   b. Adderall and Inderal
   c. bupropion and buspirone
   d. daunorubicin and doxorubicin

Sampling the Certification Exam

To provide you with practice for the Certification Exam, read the following questions that have been patterned after the test format and then record your answers on a separate sheet of paper. Write your answers as modeled in these examples: 1d; 2c; 3b; etc.

1. Which of the following are accurate generic and brand names of the same medication?
   a. clonidine, Klonopin
   b. clonidine, clorazepate
   c. clonazepam, Klonopin
   d. clonazepam, clonidine

2. Which one of the following abbreviations is considered dangerous by the Institute for Safe Medication Practices (ISMP) and should not be used per Joint Commission standards?
   a. t.i.d.
   b. q.d.
   c. mg
   d. PO

3. Checking the temperature of the refrigerators that store medications is an example of
   a. a method to ensure proper storage of medications and avoid waste.
   b. a mechanism to control inventory.
   c. a repackaging requirement.
   d. one of the five rights of filling a prescription.

4. Bar coding of the drug containers of prescription drugs, either unit dose or bulk,
   a. facilitates choosing the right drug for the prescription or medication order.
   b. supplements inventory management required by the DEA.
   c. allows the patient to be assured that the product is FDA-approved.

d. supports the prevention of theft from the pharmacy.

5. Using fentanyl patches with a heating pad may result in
   a. second-degree burns.
   b. a severe maculopapular rash.
   c. an overdose.
   d. a subtherapeutic effect.

6. Which of the following drugs must be kept in its original container to maintain its potency?
   a. nitroglycerin
   b. ferrous sulfate
   c. Viagra
   d. digoxin

7. To minimize patients receiving the wrong medication, what information should the technician ask for and document at the time of prescription drop-off?
   a. age
   b. date of birth
   c. name of spouse
   d. cell phone number

8. The dosing frequency for a prescription for Oxycontin is generally written every
   a. 4 hours.
   b. 6 hours.
   c. 12 hours.
   d. 24 hours.

9. Which of the following is *not* one of the "five rights" of patient drug administration?
   a. right price.
   b. right drug
   c. right patient
   d. right strength

10. The best way to minimize errors between selecting hydroxyzine and hydralazine off the shelf is by the use of
    a. "tall man" lettering.
    b. ClearRx design label.
    c. auxiliary labels.
    d. the "five Rs."

Human Relations and Communications

13

Learning Objectives

- Explain the role of the pharmacy technician as a member of the customer care team in a pharmacy.
- State the primary rule of retail merchandising.
- Identify and discuss desirable personal characteristics of a pharmacy technician.
- Identify the importance of verbal and nonverbal communication skills.
- Provide guidelines for the proper use of the telephone in a pharmacy.
- Identify and resolve linguistic and cultural differences in working with a customer.
- Identify and resolve challenges related to working with a customer who has mental or physical disabilities.
- Define discrimination and harassment, and explain the proper procedures for dealing with these issues.
- Identify examples of professionalism in the pharmacy.
- Explain the importance of managing change and being a team player in the pharmacy.
- Explain the appropriate responses to rude behavior on the part of others in a workplace situation.

- Identify symptoms of drug or alcohol abuse among colleagues and mechanisms to resolve them.
- Define the role of pharmacy personnel in emergency situations in the community.
- Identify appropriate behavior during a robbery using the acronym REACT.
- Identify five strategies for crime prevention in a community pharmacy.
- Define ethics and discuss characteristics of ethical behavior.
- Identify ethical dilemmas that may occur in pharmacy practice.
- Provide examples of corporate integrity in a community pharmacy.
- Identify and discuss the important areas of the regulations of the Health Insurance Portability and Accountability Act (HIPAA).
- Discuss the importance of protecting patient privacy in the pharmacy.

 Preview chapter terms and definitions.

In addition to being an important part of the healthcare system, a community pharmacy is a place of business, and the technician must be sensitive to customer service responsibilities similar to those appropriate in any retail setting. A customer service approach is important in the hospital setting as well, especially when supporting and informing other healthcare providers. This chapter provides examples of first-rate customer service for both retail and hospital pharmacy settings. In all pharmacy practice settings, maintaining patient confidentiality and following federal laws protecting patient privacy are critical.

Personal Service in the Contemporary Pharmacy

Since the Millis Study Commission on Pharmacy report of 1975 and the Hepler and Strand report of 1990, the pharmacy profession has continued to undergo an extensive self-analysis and reevaluation of its duties and goals (see Chapter 1). The upshot of this reexamination of the profession has been an increased emphasis on patient-oriented pharmacy practice, with the provision of more information and counseling regarding medications. The pharmacist is now universally recognized as far more than a dispenser of drugs. His or her duties have expanded to include:

- identifying known allergies, drug interactions, or other contraindications for a given prescription
- verifying that a given medication will not be harmful to a patient, given that patient's age and his or her medical and prescription history
- ensuring that a patient understands what medication he or she is taking, why he or she is taking it, how it should be taken, and when it should be taken
- discussing patient assessment of self-limited illnesses and recommending appropriate over-the-counter (OTC) or dietary supplements to the patient

Just as the pharmacist increasingly plays a more clinical role, so too is the pharmacy technician increasingly expected to be much more than a cash register operator, stock person, or an all-around pharmacy "gofer." Today, the technician is viewed as an important member of the customer service team within the pharmacy.

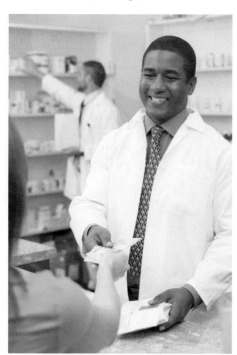

Courteous and attentive assistance makes a good impression on customers and influences their decision to return to your pharmacy.

In the 1960s and 1970s, mass merchandising was an innovative retail marketing strategy, and customers became accustomed to large, impersonal supermarkets, department stores, and pharmacy superstores, with their numbered aisles of merchandise, price tags, and cash registers. In the 1980s, retail merchandisers began to realize that the mass-merchandising model adopted in the 1960s was terribly flawed. Customers missed the days of personal service (i.e., attending to the individual customer's needs) associated with the small, independent neighborhood pharmacy of the past, where everyone affectionately called the pharmacist "Doc."

For this reason, many of the large department store chains reorganized their operations to create separate small operational entities, known as *boutiques*, within their larger stores. They also began extensive training programs to improve the quality of customer service. In pharmacy, a new and welcome emphasis on personal service had also returned.

One mass-marketing research firm conducted an experiment involving bank tellers. In the experiment, a group of tellers was instructed to lightly touch customers on the hand or wrist at some point during each teller transaction. A second control group was instructed to carry out transactions as usual, without this "personal touch." Exit surveys of customer satisfaction were then conducted, with dramatic results.

Although largely unaware that they had been touched during their teller transactions, those customers who had been touched reported a 40% higher satisfaction rate with the overall quality of service of their banks. The lesson to be learned from this research is not that one should make a habit of touching customers; indeed, touching should probably be avoided in most cases. However, a little personal attention pays off. A courteous tone of voice, a smile, eye contact, a listening ear, and a bit of assistance finding merchandise or holding a door can go a long way toward making customers think of the pharmacy in which you work as a pleasant place to visit and do business.

Even if the immediate task is not customer-oriented, the technician should remember the primary rule of retail merchandising: At all times you are representing your company to the patient or customer. Remember that in a pharmacy you are, in a legal sense, an agent of your employer and you enter into a contract to provide care to a patient. Your employer must answer for all of your actions.

Knowledge, Skills, and Qualities of a Pharmacy Technician

A successful pharmacy technician must possess a wide range of knowledge and skills and certain personal characteristics. He or she must have a broad knowledge of pharmacy practice and a dedication to providing a critical healthcare service to customers and patients. In addition, a pharmacy technician must have high ethical standards, an eagerness to learn, a sense of responsibility toward patients and toward the healthcare professionals with whom he or she interacts, a willingness to follow instructions, an eye for detail, manual dexterity, facility in basic mathematics, good research skills, and the ability to perform accurately and calmly in hectic or stressful situations. **Multitasking**, or the ability to work on several projects at the same time, is a useful skill in every pharmacy environment. In addition to these skills and qualities, displaying a professional attitude with good communication and problem-solving abilities are important attributes for a pharmacy technician.

Knowledge of Pharmacy Practice

It is important to get to know the ins and outs of pharmacy practice in your particular facility. Most pharmacies spell out policies in an online or a written manual or during initial job orientation and training, in addition to having some unwritten practices. Be sure you know and understand the practices company management and your supervising pharmacist prefer, and ask questions about unwritten customer service standards and expectations.

Policies and Procedures Many pharmacies, especially within large retail chains and hospitals, have policies and procedures covering a wide range of activities, including technician responsibilities in customer care. A written manual is often necessary in a pharmacy with multiple pharmacists and technicians so that all employees have a clear understanding of their roles and the procedures and customer service standards they are to follow. A **Policy and Procedure (P&P) manual** outlines the roles and responsibilities of staff members as well as the procedures of the facility. The implementation of a P&P manual is particularly important to the smooth operation of large, more complex pharmacies.

Make sure that you are thoroughly familiar with pharmacy guidelines and abide by them in your routine practice. Below are some sample questions that may be addressed in a P&P manual or may be accepted pharmacy practice:

- *Can employees fill their own prescriptions or the prescriptions of family members?* Store or hospital policy may dictate that an employee cannot fill his or her own prescriptions or those belonging to a family member. Violations could result in job termination.
- *What is the store or hospital policy on overtime pay?* In many cases, there many be none approved, even if you have a heavy workload, without the permission of the supervising pharmacist, lead technician, or store manager.
- *Is compensation available if you have to work late?* In some practice settings, you will need to use a time clock to punch in and out, for both your breaks and your shift.
- *Are pharmacy technicians allowed to add auxiliary labels to medication vials?* Some pharmacy practice settings dictate that only the pharmacist can affix auxiliary labels to medication vials.

Although not always written, these guidelines should be learned and followed as you are trained in a particular pharmacy. It may take as long as three months to fully learn the roles and responsibilities of the pharmacy technician in both the community and hospital pharmacy settings. Technicians will be trained to assume different roles in the department to increase scheduling flexibility. As new policies and procedures are implemented, technicians must read and document their understanding of these changes. Deviations from written procedures could have adverse consequences in a legal case involving a medication error.

Other Pharmacy Operations During training, a pharmacy technician will learn how to use the prescription software, the cash register, pricing procedures, and inventory management tools. He or she will also gain an understanding of prescription insurance plans and the processing of claims.

Positive Attitude

Attitude is the overall emotional stance or disposition that a worker adopts toward his or her job duties, customers, coworkers, and employers. Attitude is extremely important in customer relations. In the hospital setting, technicians often conduct their jobs behind the scenes, ordering and stocking items in the pharmacy or nursing unit, retrieving stock for compounding operations, maintaining records, filling prescription or unit-dose carts, preparing compounded sterile preparations in the clean room, and performing general housekeeping tasks to maintain cleanliness in the pharmacy environment. However, in a community pharmacy, the technician is on the front line of customer service. In light of that, the technician must maintain a positive attitude, even on those days that are hectic or understaffed or during times when he or she is feeling ill.

Attitude also means taking pride in your workplace. The technician should provide feedback or offer suggestions to the supervising pharmacist or store manager on ways to improve operations and customer service. Examples may include stocking OTC products, managing customer drop-off or pickup lines, handling insurance issues, ordering from wholesalers, juggling work schedules, and so on. The technician should not criticize management but instead offer thoughtful, constructive solutions. Being an invaluable asset to the overall pharmacy operation can assist you in advancement and in negotiating a pay raise in the future.

Professional Appearance

Appearance is the overall look that an employee has on the job, including dress and grooming. The technician should wear a name tag at all times for easy identification and follow the dress code of the pharmacy, which may be crisp and professional or more relaxed and casual. Proper attire, impeccable grooming, and good personal hygiene are important details to convey a positive, professional atmosphere. Customers hope for a high degree of cleanliness and professionalism in their pharmacies. After all, they are entrusting their health or the health of their loved ones to the pharmacy staff. A pharmacy employee with unkempt hair or a uniform smock thrown over a pair of jeans may make a bad impression. The customer may not consciously register these observations, yet he or she could leave with a vague impression that the pharmacy is not a professional operation.

Attentiveness

Making a personal connection with the customer is important. Greeting patients by name is especially important in a community pharmacy. Patients are far more likely to return to a pharmacy where they have received personal attention than to one where they have not.

Meeting Customers' Needs A pharmacy technician must be sensitive to customer needs. Often a customer is reluctant to ask for help, to avoid imposing on the pharmacy staff member's time. **Triage** customer needs in everyday practice by sorting requests or needs and prioritizing them. In the community pharmacy, many things may be happening at once: You are making a sale; the phone is ringing; a customer is waiting for help in the OTC aisle; and five patients are waiting to pick up prescriptions. Acknowledge the customers by a simple statement such as, "I will be right with you." Then, when attending to their needs, you might say something such as, "Thank you for waiting." Keeping your eye on the customer and meeting his or her needs apply to any retail operation. In other situations, such as a "stat" order in the hospital pharmacy, the order of requests received needs to be ignored in response to a more urgent medical situation.

Empathy

A major emphasis in modern pharmacy is to demonstrate professional caring or empathy toward the patient. Perhaps the patient who comes into your pharmacy has recently lost a loved one, or a loved one has become seriously ill, or the patient may have been recently diagnosed with a serious illness. Perhaps he or she has just been discharged from the hospital or spent the better part of a day or night at the emergency room. Whatever the patient's circumstances, the pharmacy technician should be consistently open and receptive and not make any assumptions so that he or she can live up to the patient's needs to the best of his or her ability.

Helpfulness

Modern chain pharmacies are often large, complex places. When customers enter, the first thing they often do is stand in the middle of the entrance, looking around for the aisle where the product they seek is found. A good employee thus continually scans the surrounding area, noticing customers who are lost or confused and need help.

Once you spot that uncertain look, ask courteously, "May I help you?" Then, after the customer's response, you may have to ask some clarifying questions. If, for example, the customer is looking for aspirin, then he or she may need to know not only where OTC analgesic products are stocked in the store, but also where to locate a specific analgesic (e.g., baby aspirin, aspirin for a migraine, Goody's or BC powders, or an enteric-coated form for those whose stomachs cannot tolerate conventional analgesic dosage forms). If possible, escort the customer to the place where the merchandise is located and then help him or her find it.

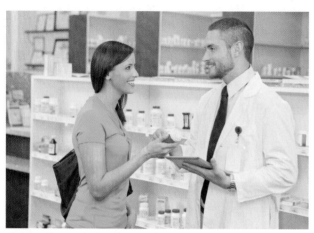
Pharmacists and pharmacy technicians often help customers find products in the retail pharmacy.

In other cases, the customer may want to know whether to take aspirin or another OTC analgesic such as ibuprofen; or he or she may ask whether it is acceptable to take ibuprofen with blood pressure medication. The pharmacy technician can triage or sort out various requests by the customer. Those requests involving product location, availability, or price can be handled by the technician. However, any questions that involve professional judgment or counseling must be referred to the pharmacist. You may say to the customer, "That is a good question; let me have you speak with the pharmacist."

If a customer requests an OTC product outside of the immediate pharmacy department area, then assist him or her by providing the aisle number and location, or page a store manager if you are busy. If a customer requests a specific product that is not in stock, then check with the manager or consult the wholesaler notebook to see whether a special order can be made; if so, let the customer know when the product should be received (usually the next business day) and get his or her name and phone number for a courtesy call. If a product is out of stock, then be sure to apologize to the customer and offer a "rain check." Making an extra effort to provide customer service pays off in long-term dividends and return business for any retail operation.

Insurance Issues Patients (and pharmacy staff) are often confused by myriad insurance issues. Here are some common insurance questions that a technician may encounter in the community pharmacy. (The answers to these questions can be found in Chapter 7.)

- Why isn't this drug covered by my insurance?
- What do you mean my insurance is expired?
- Why isn't my new baby covered on my insurance?
- What do you mean my insurance plan has changed?
- Why is my co-pay $60 for my antibiotic prescription?
- How come my medication costs more this month than last?
- What is a prior authorization, and why do you need it?
- Why do you have to call the physician to clarify my prescription? I am in a hurry!
- What do you mean you cannot fill my narcotic prescription today?
- Why did you give me a 30-day supply when my physician wrote a 90-day supply of my medication?
- What do you mean you do not have my medication in stock?
- Why have you only filled my prescription with a five-day supply?
- What do you mean I am not eligible to use the coupon I received from my doctor's office?

- If I am on Medicare Part D, why can I not use a store or drug discount card?
- I am out of my heart medication and the physician's office is closed. What can I do?
- I forgot my medication and I am on vacation from out-of-state. Can you help me?

Patience

The pharmacy technician must have patience when working with customers. Insurance issues, in particular, can be frustrating for patients—and resolving the issues can be time-consuming for inexperienced pharmacy technicians. It takes time and experience to learn the ins and outs of the various prescription drug insurance plans. If you cannot adequately address the patient's questions or concerns, don't be embarrassed or anxious. Check with a senior technician or the pharmacist to better understand the issue, and how it can be resolved in a reasonable time period.

Good Communication Skills

Communicating effectively takes practice. Once you have the knowledge and vocabulary needed to function effectively in the pharmacy, you can acquire the necessary communication skills with time. Model yourself after someone whom you admire, but keep in mind that some of your coworkers have different roles and thus different communication needs and styles.

The pharmacy technician is the one most accessible to the customer—and is often the final contact with the customer at the time of prescription pickup. Good public relations skills are required. Dealing with the public for an eight-hour shift (or longer) can be difficult and tiring. Therefore, it is common in larger pharmacies to rotate responsibilities so that every two to four hours the technician may have different duties—collecting payments and dealing with the public, entering new prescriptions and refill requests, resolving insurance claims, filling prescriptions, ordering medications, checking inventory, and so on.

The pharmacy technician is often the bearer of bad news when interacting with patients. Take the necessary time to explain why a prescription cannot be filled or can only be partially filled. A pharmacy technician should also alert the patient to a change in the manufacturer of a generic drug (resulting in a different color or shape of the medication) as well as to any medication that is out-of-stock or a partial fill. For the latter situation, the technician should let the patient know when the medication will be in stock and available for pickup. At times, it may be necessary to fill the prescription with two different brands of the same medication; if so, then the patient must be alerted to this change at the time of pickup.

Verbal Communication Skills A pharmacy technician needs good verbal communication skills when receiving prescriptions and also when assisting the patient with an OTC medication. Verbal communication takes practice, and pronouncing medical terms and drug names is one hurdle that you can overcome with study. Listening and asking a coworker to pronounce words for you are the best ways to learn. Repeat difficult words to yourself several times. You may also find it helpful to keep a pocket-sized reference on drug names handy and make notes in it regarding pronunciation and usage.

The technician performs a valuable service by gathering information and relaying it to the pharmacist. Face the patient and speak slowly. Avoid slang expressions that may not be understood or could be misinterpreted by the patient. Be a good listener, and keep the conversation succinct and focused. Rephrase and summarize to make sure you understand the problem correctly. Know your limitations in making recommendations.

Another effective way to gather information from a patient is to ask well-phrased questions that are appropriate to the type of information needed. A **closed-ended question** is asked in a yes-or-no format, such as, "Do you have a headache?" or "Have you tried aspirin?" An **open-ended question** allows the patient to share more information about his or her illness and is more helpful to the pharmacist in recommending the best treatment. Asking the patient open-ended questions such as, "Can you please describe your headache pain for me?" is always preferable.

The heart of verbal communication is, of course, listening. Paying close attention to the words and the voice that you are hearing is important. Maintain eye contact with the person speaking and send the speaker other nonverbal signals indicating that you are genuinely interested in what he or she is saying. Learn to tolerate your own silence. Ask questions to clarify issues and repeat portions of the conversation to confirm that you have correctly heard what was said. Always use a nonjudgmental expression and tone of voice. Never let the patient feel that he or she is imposing or that your time is more valuable than the patient's.

Nonverbal Communication Skills **Nonverbal communication** is easy to understand, and you need only pay attention to the other party to interpret what is being conveyed. As small children, people learn how to interpret nonverbal communication. Facial expression, eye contact, posture, and tone of voice are all methods of communicating without using words. Mannerisms and gestures often indicate agreement or disagreement. The mood of the other party can often be determined through nonverbal communication. Although each individual is unique and may exhibit unusual habits with certain moods, many generalizations can be made regarding nonverbal communication. Simple observation and listening can be effective ways to supplement the verbal portion of what is being communicated.

The following examples demonstrate nonverbal communication in the pharmacy:

Poor: Talk to a patient while filling a prescription or answering the phone.

Better: Ask the patient to wait a moment, complete filling the prescription or place the telephone caller on hold (or have another staff member take the call), and go down to the front counter or private counseling area and talk to the patient. Determine whether you can help the patient, and direct the patient to speak with the pharmacist if necessary.

Poor: Show surprise through an open-mouthed facial expression when a patient shares a diagnosis with you (e.g., human immunodeficiency virus [HIV], gonorrhea, syphilis, or depression).

Better: Be nonjudgmental, with minimal facial expressions, and assist the patient with the information or products that he or she needs. Be empathetic and show genuine concern. Remember that all patient medical information is confidential and protected by law.

Poor: Talk to a patient about an OTC recommendation with your arms crossed, at some distance from the patient.

Better: Move closer to the patient, ask open-ended questions, listen carefully, and be aware of both your body movements and those of the patient. Crossed arms often convey some barrier to communication, such as that you are too busy to be helpful.

Safety Note

The medical information that a patient shares in a discussion with a pharmacy staff member is confidential and protected by law.

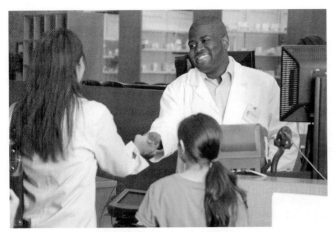
A pharmacy technician should smile and maintain eye contact and a pleasant attitude while talking with patients.

Eye Contact The goodwill that you communicate always comes back to you in one way or another. With that in mind, smile and make eye contact with your customers.

In many cultures, eye contact is often associated with honesty, sincerity, and respect. Eye contact is especially important to older patients and patients who may be hearing impaired. A person who is hearing impaired often learns lipreading to supplement the words that he or she hears. If you speak with your head turned away, then the person may hear you but may not be able to fully interpret what you have said. This is especially important if your pharmacy has a drive-thru window—it is often difficult to communicate over engine and ambient noise. You may need to repeat the customer request—whether it is verifying patient name, date of birth, address, or other information. Remembering to make eye contact ensures that you are looking directly at the person.

Courteous Manner

In every interaction with a customer, use courteous words and phrases. Whenever possible, greet the customer by name. Get to know local and cultural pleasantries and use them to endear your clientele. Be mindful of using good manners and maintain a professional attitude to ensure that your customer has a good experience and will want to come back.

Common Courtesies Begin and end customer interactions, even the briefest ones, with formal courtesies such as "Good afternoon" and "Have a nice day." "Please" and "Thank you" should become a part of your regular vocabulary. Practice courteous speech, as demonstrated in these examples.

Poor: What do you need?
Better: May I help you?

Poor: It's over there.
Better: That item is in aisle three. Follow me, and I'll show you.

Poor: It's $8.39.
Better: That will be $8.39, please.

Poor: Next?
Better: May I help whoever is next? *or* Hello, Mr. Fibich. Are you here to pick up or drop off a prescription?

If a mistake was made in filling the prescription, then apologize immediately and bring it to the attention of the pharmacist according to the policy of the pharmacy. Make eye contact and admit to an honest mistake instead of attempting to cover it up. The pharmacist will then explain to the patient how the mistake occurred and how it will be corrected. If no mistake was made, then the technician should be understanding and address the patient's concerns. If there is a delay in filling the prescription, then apologize to the customer for the inconvenience.

Telephone Courtesies

Customers and healthcare professionals often contact pharmacies by telephone. Customers may be calling in refills, inquiring as to whether a new prescription has been received or filled, asking about the cost of medications, verifying insurance coverage for certain prescriptions, and so on. These are all requests the technician can easily address. The following are some guidelines for using the telephone properly:

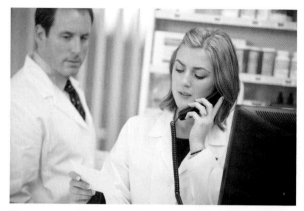

Pharmacy technicians need to be able to communicate effectively over the phone with both customers and healthcare professionals.

- When you answer the phone, identify yourself and the pharmacy as follows: "Good morning, Reinhardt's Pharmacy. My name is Jess. How may I help you?"
- Always begin and close the conversation with a conventional courtesy such as "Good morning" and "Thank you for calling." Stay alert to what the caller is saying and use a natural, conversational voice. You should be friendly but not too familiar with the caller. When speaking to patients who are hard of hearing, speak clearly, pronounce each word distinctly, and be prepared to repeat yourself.
- If the client is calling in a new prescription, you may need to turn over the phone to a pharmacist. In most states, technicians by law are not allowed to take prescriptions over the telephone. Be sure that you are aware of the regulations in your state.
- If the caller has questions about the administration or effects of a medication or about a medical condition, adverse reaction, or drug interaction, place the customer on hold and refer the call to a licensed pharmacist.
- Make sure that any information you provide is accurate. Giving incorrect directions to a customer in need of a prescription can be a life-threatening mistake.
- If the caller is requesting a refill, then politely ask for his or her name, date of birth, or prescription number. After verifying that the prescription can be refilled and dispensed, give the patient an approximate time when it will be ready for pickup, and thank him or her for calling ahead.
- Depending on the regulations in your state and the procedures of your pharmacy, you may be authorized to handle prescription transfers or to provide information related to prescription refills. Follow the procedures outlined by your supervising pharmacist.
- If a customer is calling about a medical emergency or a prescription error, refer the call to your supervising pharmacist.

Sensitivity to Diverse Patient Populations

Be sensitive to the diversity of your pharmacy's patient population. By respecting differences in culture, religion, language, abilities, and other facets, pharmacy personnel can ensure positive interactions with customers and can effectively meet their healthcare needs.

Awareness of Cultural, Religious, Gender, and Ethnic Differences **Culture** is commonly defined as the customs, beliefs, and attitudes that are learned and shared by members of a group. Cultural values influence our behavior and response to medications.

According to studies, cultural differences affect patient attitudes about medical care and treatment. For example, in some Asian countries, mental illness is considered a dishonor to the family; consequently, the number of patients seeking psychiatric care in these countries is small. This stigma continues in several immigrant communities in the United States today.

More and more, we live in a culturally and ethnically diverse society. According to the 2010 U.S. Census, nonwhites make up nearly 30% of the U.S. population, and that number is projected to increase to nearly 50% by 2050. Hispanics make up 16.3% of the population, followed by African Americans at 12.6% and Asians at 4.8%. Within the Asian community are diverse cultural differences among the Chinese, Japanese, Vietnamese, Korean, Filipino, and East Indian populations.

Pharmacies are often located in areas catering to diverse customers. Differences in age, gender, sexual orientation, ethnicity, language, culture, economic status, educational background, and disability will be part of your everyday practice in the pharmacy. With diversity increasing among patient populations in the United States, **cultural sensitivity** is a valuable skill. Cultural competency is defined as awareness, knowledge of, and respect for cultural beliefs that differ from your own. Knowing more about the patient's culture helps you provide higher-quality service and shows customers that you care about them. The pharmacy technician should be sensitive to these issues and try to overcome barriers. What is most important is that every patient feels comfortable and receives the correct information.

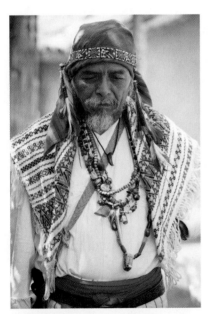

Non-Western medical practices may employ shamans, herbalists, and healers to provide primary care to patients.

Mistrust of Western Medical Practice Considering the complex history of the United States, it is not surprising that many minority cultures do not always accept Western medical practice. For example, African-American communities carry a long tradition of mistrust of conventional medicine, stemming from the brutal legacy of American slavery. Similarly, Native Americans have endured unspeakable hardships at the hands of Western medicine and are often understandably reluctant to seek care. Pharmacy personnel need to be sensitive to these long-standing cultural belief systems.

Reliance on Self-Care Many cultures, especially those that have a history of poverty, have developed a strong reliance on self-care out of necessity. For example, Hispanic patients may rely more on self-care, OTC medications, and dietary supplements and less on physician visits. The African-American population is generally less likely to believe in the benefits of long-term treatments and, therefore, may discontinue their drug therapy before it has run its course. In the Japanese and Vietnamese cultures, patients may self-regulate their medications with lower-than-recommended doses due to their concerns about safety.

Reliance on Herbalists and Healers Healers have a nearly universal presence in indigenous and folk cultures. If you practice in the rural United States, then you may see and hear more about home remedies. Native Americans also place more belief in family and spiritual values than modern Western medicine; for many individuals in this patient population, illness is due to an imbalance in one's life between the natural and supernatural forces. In Mexico, primary care is often provided by traditional healers. The hex on children for the diagnosis of *mal de ojo* or "evil eye" is believed to be broken when a healer passes an egg over the

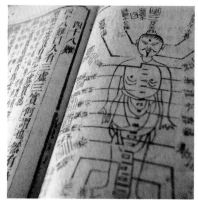

In many non-Western medical traditions, the study of one's internal force, or "Qi," is just as important as any physical ailment.

child's body. Root doctors from the American South use incantations and herbs to restore the body to health. Many patients from the Far East have stronger cultural beliefs in the healing power of herbs rather than prescription medications and Western medical practice. In the Chinese culture, the yin (cold) and yang (hot) energies must be in harmonious balance for the patient to be at optimal health.

Influence of Religion on Medical Care Religious traditions and customs can have a great impact on healthcare practices. For Muslims, the month-long fast of Ramadan may interfere with the need to regularly take prescribed medications. Orthodox Jews or members of certain Islamic sects may prefer a healthcare practitioner of the same sex. Religious faith and prayer have a major impact on health attitudes within many Christian communities.

Gender and Sexuality Concerns Often, people prefer to discuss personal medical issues with pharmacists or technicians of the same gender. For example, some male customers may feel more comfortable discussing questions on condom use or erectile dysfunction drugs with a male technician or pharmacist. Similar issues may arise in the case of a female customer and issues regarding menstruation or menopause. The pharmacy technician should also be understanding of the unique health concerns and needs of the gay, lesbian, bisexual, and transgender populations in the communities they serve. By establishing a comfortable, nonjudgmental environment for the discussion of gender and sexuality issues as they relate to healthcare needs, pharmacy personnel can establish rapport and provide effective treatments for all patients.

Diseases that Disproportionately Affect Ethnic Minorities Certain diseases are on the rise among specific ethnic groups. These health concerns can, in part, be attributed to the unhealthful eating habits of many individuals living in the United States. For example, the incidence of diabetes is much higher among Mexican Americans and Native Americans. The African-American population has a higher incidence of hypertension, stroke, and kidney disease, which can be traced to salt intake. These higher rates are due, in part, to a greater sensitivity to sodium, resulting in blood pressure elevations. As many Asians have adopted a more typical U.S. diet, there is now a higher prevalence of diabetes among this ethnic population.

Communication Strategies for Language Barriers If you cannot understand a customer because of a language difference, then do not speak louder or in a deliberate, slow, and punctuated manner. Simply enunciate your words and avoid using slang terms or abbreviations because the person may not be familiar with them. Apologize courteously for your language deficiency if necessary, and find another store employee who can communicate in the customer's native tongue if possible.

If you have a translator available, summarize the key information that you need to obtain from the patient. Keep sentences short, and repeat the questions using gestures and facial expressions if the patient does not understand. Be patient; give the translator time to formulate thoughts into the client's language; and do not interrupt the exchange. If a translator is not available, then the pharmacist may have counseling sheets that use drawings, diagrams, and clocks made especially for this purpose. Also, be aware the some computer software programs print medication labels and patient information leaflets in different languages.

Accommodations for Mental and Physical Disabilities Patients with visual, hearing, cognitive, and physical deficits require special accommodations by pharmacy personnel.

Visual and Hearing Impairment For patients with visual impairment, the use of large-print or Braille materials is helpful. Customers with hearing impairment benefit from slow, deliberate, short discourse or—if the impairment is severe—from sign language.

Mental and Physical Disabilities Some patients may have varying degrees of mental or physical disabilities. If you are interacting with a mentally disabled patient, you may need to be understanding in obtaining necessary demographic, insurance, and health information. Medication counseling by the pharmacist should be directed at the appropriate level of understanding. For patients with physical disabilities, pharmacy personnel should make every effort to accommodate their needs. These accommodations may include using nonchildproof container lids, providing assistance in obtaining items from shelves, or ensuring their comfort during the medication filling process.

Accommodations for Economic Hardship Hard economic times and rising healthcare costs have made it increasingly difficult for patients to afford medications and other forms of treatment. Many patients may not have prescription drug insurance due to unemployment, part-time employment without benefits, or an inability to pay the high cost of insurance. Pharmacy staff members should be attuned to these patients' needs and offer some cost-saving measures. These measures may include drug or store discount cards (if eligible), store-brand generic products, or—with input from the pharmacist—lower-cost prescriptions. If you have a free clinic or community health center in your area, you might suggest to patients to get a referral to help save some money. (For more information on these cost-saving measures, see Chapter 7.)

Good Problem-Solving Ability

Being a good problem solver for patients or workplace issues is a valuable asset for a pharmacy technician. Problem solving may include following written or unwritten policies and procedures in the pharmacy or resolving potential conflicts with fellow employees, supervisors, or management.

Handling Patient Issues In the community pharmacy setting, in particular, situations may arise that aggravate customers. These situations may include wait times for filling prescriptions, out-of-stock medications, and misunderstanding of prescription insurance coverage. To ease the tension, pharmacy staff members should remain calm and work with patients to solve these problems. For example, if a patient needs an out-of-stock medication, check with your supervising pharmacist and then offer to call neighboring pharmacies to find the medication. If another pharmacy has the medication in stock, arrange for the customer to pick up the prescription at that facility. If there is an insurance problem, offer to call the patient's insurance company to find a resolution or—if you are busy—attempt an insurance override or call the company later and advise the patient of the outcome.

Workplace Issues Pharmacy personnel are members of a healthcare team and, consequently, must work together to provide optimal patient care. To achieve this common goal, technicians must stay focused on their job responsibilities and not be distracted by factors such as conflicts with colleagues, personal health issues, or home concerns. A lack of focus could lead to a serious medication error. With that in mind, technicians should use their problem-solving abilities to resolve conflicts and balance their work lives and home lives. If necessary, technicians should approach their pharmacy supervisor so that appropriate accommodations (decreased workload, leave of absence, etc.) can be implemented without disrupting patient care.

Conflict Resolution Disputes involving duties, hours, pay, and other matters are common occurrences in occupations of all kinds. Try to resolve work-related disputes through rational, calm, private discussion with the parties involved. If you are seeking a pay raise, prepare for the meeting by outlining your career goals, accomplishments, and additional training and certifications that you have received. A reminder of these items may increase the potential for a pay raise. Showing a willingness to take on new responsibilities such as scheduling or training new staff is another way to garner a pay raise. If a pay raise is not possible, you may be able to negotiate for additional fringe benefits, such as health insurance, vacation, or scheduled time off on weekends. Regardless of the outcome, your interactions with your supervisor should always be professional.

Awareness of Discrimination and Harassment The law requires all businesses, pharmacies included, to post information related to workplace discrimination and harassment. **Discrimination** (i.e., preferential treatment or mistreatment) and **harassment** (i.e., mistreatment—sexual or otherwise, particularly if it is of an ongoing or persistent nature) are not only unethical but also illegal.

Discrimination—whether based on age, gender, ethnicity, sexual orientation, or religion—is not tolerated in the workplace. If a facility's hiring or promotion practices fail to follow proper written procedures and guidelines, then the facility may be subject to a lawsuit.

In the past, sexual harassment was defined as unwanted physical contact or as the act of making sexual conduct a condition for advancement, preferential treatment, or other work-related outcomes. However, the Supreme Court has redefined sexual harassment more generally as the creation of an unpleasant or uncomfortable work environment through sexual action, innuendo, or related means. Thus, you do not have to put up with off-color or crude jokes if you do not wish to hear them; be aware that you must not contribute in any way to creating an environment that is uncomfortable for your coworkers. One person's innocent remark, made in the spirit of fun, can be the basis for another person's grounds for a legal action.

If you find yourself the object of discrimination or harassment, first try to resolve the issue with the person or persons involved. Do your best to maintain your composure and to express your discomfort calmly and rationally. If possible, have a witness present to verify your communication. If discrimination or harassment persists, you may need to discuss the matter with a supervisor. If the problem is not resolved, follow up first with store management and then, if necessary, with upper-level management. Most community and hospital pharmacies have written policies and procedures to address such matters; follow the established protocol. If you are unsuccessful, as a last resort, make inquiries regarding the discrimination and harassment laws and procedures in your state.

Levelheadedness

Remaining level-headed when dealing with difficult patients and stressful situations in the pharmacy workplace is certainly beneficial to both customers and to the operation of the facility. In times of crisis, however, this attribute can help organize an appropriate response.

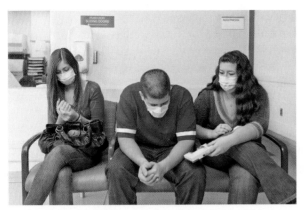

During an outbreak of an easily communicable disease or illness such as the flu, many healthcare facilities may ask patients waiting for treatment to wear masks to avoid spreading contagion to others.

Emergency Preparedness At times of local, regional, or national emergencies or disasters, all pharmacy personnel may be called into action. Your community or hospital pharmacy may be asked by the health department to volunteer and participate in emergency preparedness in your local community. In addition to attending planning meetings, educational programs need to be completed by all staff for the pharmacy to participate fully.

If there is a serious epidemic, what is the plan for your pharmacy? Many personnel may be out sick, and transportation and distribution networks may be seriously compromised. How can your wholesale vendor get medications to you? How can patients from your pharmacy, displaced by floods, tornadoes, or hurricanes, get needed medication? What role can the pharmacy best serve in the community? Can it be a source of information and education for patients? Can the pharmacy share personnel with the department of public health? What type of protective gear will be available, and which personnel will receive vaccines or antiviral medications if dealing with the public? An interested technician could assist in planning and communicating with the health department.

If you have specialized credentials, such as cardiopulmonary resuscitation (CPR) or Advanced Cardiovascular Life Support (ACLS) certification, or experience as an emergency medical technician (EMT) or as a medic in the military, then you could be a valuable asset to your community in the time of a health crisis. **Credentialing** is the process for validating the qualifications of licensed professionals and may define what functions and roles pharmacists and pharmacy technicians can perform. Depending on your training and experience and the extent of the crisis, you may be triaging or screening injuries or illnesses in the field, providing CPR or necessary medications and supplies to medical personnel, or administering vaccines in times of a regional pandemic or epidemic.

Security in the Workplace With money and drugs (especially the latter), the community pharmacy is susceptible to robbery from criminals and addicts. As an employee of a pharmacy, do you know what to do (and not do) during a robbery? Purdue Pharma in conjunction with the National Community Pharmacist Association (NCPA) has developed a crime prevention and training program called RxPatrol. During a robbery, the acronym to remember is REACT:

R = Remain calm, comply, and do not resist.

E = Eyewitness; remember all you can such as age, height, weight, race, gender, body markings, clothing, etc.

A = Activate your panic alarm when safe.

C = Call police; describe the incident and robber and his or her mode and direction of travel.

T = Take charge; lock the door so the robber cannot return, protect the crime scene, keep customers calm, and have them remain in the store as witnesses when police arrive.

Prevention strategies are important to deter potential robberies. Keep an eye on "customers" you do not recognize; many times they may be scoping out the pharmacy.

If you receive a telephone call for a price on a narcotic, say you do not have it, or only have a limited supply. Keep security cameras visible and functional. Post decals at the front door—"This Pharmacy belongs to RxPatrol"—or signs near the pharmacy that read, "Controlled drugs in limited supply in time-release safe." Have more than one panic alarm button, and have an escape plan with your staff. Keep the phone number of your local police precinct readily available.

The RxPatrol website has training videos and a security checklist to help make your pharmacy safer from robbers. There is also a national database of pharmacy robberies. If you have an incident at your pharmacy, you can report it, or you can review the robberies in your geographic area and alert other staff members.

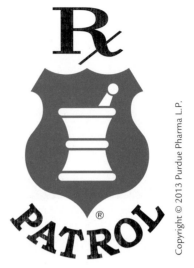

Copyright © 2013 Purdue Pharma L.P.

RxPatrol is a collaborative effort between a pharmacy and law enforcement to track, predict, and prevent crime in the pharmacy setting.

Other Aspects of Professionalism

Other aspects of professionalism include appropriate behavior in the workplace, the ability to be an effective team member, respectful interactions with healthcare professionals, and an understanding of professional boundaries. Ethical behavior is also an important aspect of professionalism and is discussed later in this chapter.

Appropriate Workplace Behavior

Healthcare professionals at all levels are expected to abide by both written laws and ethical guidelines. **Decorum** means proper or polite behavior or that which is in good taste in the pharmacy workplace. Arguing with patients or your supervisor in public is an example of indecorum, or impropriety—a lack of decorum. Another set of social mores to be followed is often referred to as etiquette. **Etiquette**, defined as unwritten rules of behavior, is often recognized most easily when it is not being followed. For example, being disrespectful to a physician, nurse, or colleague is an obvious breach of proper etiquette.

Respect Among Colleagues Respect should be shown to all employees who work in a healthcare facility because each person has an important job to do that contributes to the overall health care provided to the patient. However, additional respect and deference should be shown to those with a high level of medical training and those responsible for managing the facility where you are employed. Intimate personal relationships with coworkers or pharmacists are discouraged in most practice settings. A transfer to another pharmacy may be appropriate if you plan to carry on a relationship with a colleague.

Personal Conduct Personal telephone calls, texting, and visits should be conducted only during breaks. Telling offensive or off-color jokes and making disparaging comments about patients or coworkers is not acceptable or tolerated. When in doubt as to the expected behavior in a situation, be quiet, watch, and learn from someone else in the pharmacy who is a suitable model, and perform your assigned task. If you are not sure, ask questions of the senior pharmacy technician or supervising pharmacist.

Appropriate workplace behavior also demands that you do not let your personal life interfere with your work performance. You must be "on top of your game" to safely and efficiently input, fill, and dispense prescriptions and interact with customers. If you bring your personal problems to the workplace, you may not have the concentration needed to perform your job responsibilities accurately and safely. Intrapersonal issues, such as family obligations, personal health, and the need for more flexible work hours, may cause tension and adversely affect job performance. If you use recreational drugs such as marijuana at home or on the weekend, the effects of the drug can linger in your body and could interfere with your performance at work.

Teamwork

Pharmacy technicians and pharmacists must work together for eight hours or longer each day as a cohesive healthcare team to provide quality care and to process prescriptions for patients efficiently and safely. To work effectively as a team, workers must establish collegial relationships built upon respect for others, an appreciation of their contributions in the workplace, and a willingness to help one another in times of change.

Respecting Differences In any pharmacy, you work with personnel from different age-groups, genders, ethnicities, and religious backgrounds. Personalities differ and sometimes clash. Is someone too talkative or loud, or too quiet and passive? Are some personnel too obsessive and compulsive? Do some seek patient contact and communication whereas others would rather fill prescriptions and minimize patient contact? These differences cannot be allowed to interfere with the work at hand. There must be respect for other personnel, both individually and with regard to their roles in the pharmacy. Unresolved issues should be brought to the attention of the supervising pharmacist privately. Any criticism of an individual's quality of work should be a constructive learning experience. The problem may be simply a typo on a computer entry of the prescription or a more serious error, such as selecting the wrong patient or wrong drug or typing incorrect directions.

Appreciating the Contributions of Colleagues Being aware and appreciative of each team member's contributions to the smooth operation of a pharmacy is important. Staff members should seek out those who are more knowledgeable or skilled to obtain information or to handle a difficult situation. For example, oftentimes pharmacists consult technicians about insurance issues because technicians are well-versed in the nuances of various plans. At other times, technicians rely on the guidance of pharmacists to manage a difficult patient. Recognizing these contributions with common courtesies such as "Thanks for staying late to help out during this busy time" or "Thank you for locating that OTC medication for the customer" can build rapport among team members. You can also build rapport by showing an interest in coworkers' personal lives.

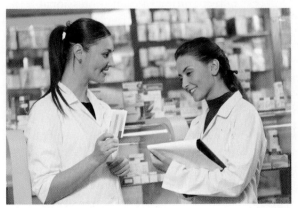
A pharmacy technician may seek guidance from a pharmacist on ways to handle a challenging situation.

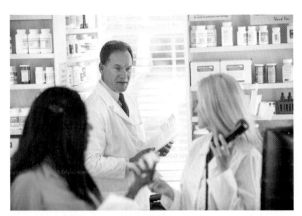
Pharmacy technicians should always interact with other professionals respectfully.

Simple questions such as "Where did you go on vacation?" or "Did you have a fun weekend?" contribute to team building.

Managing Change Teamwork may also mean managing change. By definition, health care is dynamic—always changing. The pharmacy work environment also reflects dynamic change. The change may be in management or a last-minute change in work or vacation schedules, a change in policies and procedures, or a change in insurance plan coverage, not to mention the never-ending changes in drugs—new generics, new formulations, new dosages, and so on. Managing change constructively and being a team player are positive attributes in a pharmacy technician.

Interprofessionalism

Health care is a demanding industry, often requiring long hours and involving stressful, emergency situations. As a result, practitioners in the industry often suffer from fatigue and stress. Sometimes this stress shows itself in unintentionally rude or abrupt behavior toward other professionals and paraprofessionals, including pharmacists, physicians, nurses, medical assistants, administrators, store managers, sales representatives, insurance personnel, and other technicians. For example, busy healthcare professionals may sometimes speak to subordinates in an inappropriate and unprofessional manner. The degree to which you maintain courtesy and respect, even in the face of rudeness, is a measure of your professionalism. If you return rudeness with kindness, then you often find that, immediately or over time, the quality of your interactions improves. If you answer the telephone and someone barks a command at you, then demonstrate your professionalism by attending to the content of the message and not to its tone.

Proper Direct Address Always refer to physicians, chiropractors, osteopathic professionals, and dentists using the title "Doctor." In the presence of patients, refer to the pharmacist as "Doctor" if he or she has a Doctor of Pharmacy degree. Some states have designated all pharmacists as "Doctors" in recognition of their professional experience. When the technician refers to the pharmacist as "Doctor," this raises the level of customer respect not only for the pharmacist but also for the technician, who is the "Doctor's Assistant." Refer to other supervisors using appropriate courtesy titles, such as "Mr., Mrs., or Ms.," plus the last name, or "Sir," "Madam," or "Ma'am." A degree of formality is always in order until you are requested to use more informal modes of address in day-to-day operations.

Professional Restraint New customers also arrive at the pharmacy and speak or inquire about physicians, specialists, and other healthcare professionals. General information and positive recommendations may be given, but opinions on the competence of a particular physician or healthcare provider should not be given out by anyone in the pharmacy. At all times, avoid making disparaging comments about other healthcare providers. If such comments are made and the person's professional reputation is questioned, then that person may sue you for slander.

Professional Boundaries

A pharmacy technician is not trained or licensed to advise customers with regard to medications (including OTC drugs and dietary supplements) and their use. Use common sense to determine whether a given query from a customer exceeds the bounds of common knowledge. As a rule of thumb, refer to a pharmacist any questions involving patient assessment; the proper administration, dosage, uses, or effects of a prescription drug, OTC medication, or dietary supplement; and questions that require a professional opinion or judgment.

Of course, a technician should use common sense while providing customers with information. In the case of OTC medications, sometimes customers need basic information that is readily available on the OTC packaging. For example, a customer might ask for the location of an analgesic or which alternative brands are available or on sale this week, or other routine questions that can be safely answered without referring the customer to the pharmacist.

Do not be afraid of admitting your lack of expertise. Customers appreciate that you are concerned enough to make sure that they receive accurate information. When a question deals with the effects or administration of a medication, ask the customer to wait for a moment while you get someone who can provide an informed and appropriate answer to the question. In some instances, technicians may provide medication-related information when providing refills and when directed to do so by a pharmacist.

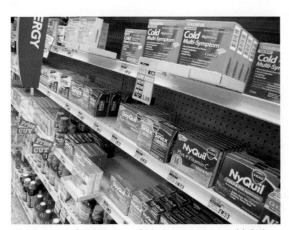

Pharmacy technicians can help customers read labels to compare generic and brand name OTC products.

Personal Ethics

Ethics is the study of standards of conduct and moral judgment that outline the rights and wrongs of human conduct and character. Ethics is a process for reflection and analysis of behavior when the proper course of action is unclear. It is the basis on which to make judgments. In addition, particular individuals, groups, and professions have their own specialized codes of ethics. It is not necessarily inherent to religious belief; even those who subscribe to no religion can have a sense of right and wrong conduct. However, religion often has an influence on personal ethics.

The most important aspect of studying ethics is to internalize a framework or set of guidelines based on high professional standards that guide your decision making and actions. Be aware of a variety of situations you could find yourself in while working in health care, and discuss with your colleagues how to react and behave when faced with them. By thinking through your ethical choices ahead of time, you can avoid the paralyzing quandary of being confronted with questionable circumstances and not knowing what to do.

Everyone faces hundreds of situations in which moral beliefs seem unfounded, uninformed, and anything but a foundation on which to base a decision. Through ethical study, an individual can make decisions using a moral compass and can understand and respect the viewpoints of others. Pharmacy technicians, working side by side with pharmacists, must recognize and adopt the accepted ethical standards of pharmacy practice (see Figure 13.1).

Not all behaviors in pharmacy practice are done solely because of the law. Moral obligations exist that are not legal obligations and vice versa. Using the best-priced option among generic medications, making honest disclosures of prescription wait times, and providing accurate information on out-of-stock situations are examples of these obligations. Laws and regulations governing the practice of pharmacy do not always dictate the proper behavior in every situation.

FIGURE 13.1
Oath of a Pharmacy Technician

Oath of a Pharmacy Technician

I dedicate myself to providing pharmacy technician services of the highest quality to all patients, regardless of situation or circumstance, and I will consider the health and safety of my patients my primary concern.

I will uphold the highest principles of moral, ethical, and legal conduct, and will perform my duties with honesty and integrity.

I will use my knowledge, skills, and abilities to ensure optimal patient treatment outcomes, while always operating within the pharmacy technician's scope of practice.

I will maintain patient confidentiality, promote individual dignity, and treat all patients with respect, compassion, and appreciation for diversity.

I will work closely with pharmacists and other healthcare professionals to ensure that quality pharmaceutical care is dispensed without error.

I will strive to provide excellent customer service and effective communication, supported by an exceptional work ethic, while maintaining absolute accuracy and ensuring patient health and safety.

I will stay informed regarding developments in the field of pharmacy and will maintain professional competency, striving to continually enhance my knowledge, skills, and expertise.

I will participate in the evolution of a pharmaceutical practice that improves patient care, and will actively support organizations that further the profession and support the advancement of pharmacy technicians.

I will respect, value, and support my colleagues; foster a sense of loyalty and duty to the profession of pharmacy; and actively participate as a member of the healthcare team.

I will strive to conduct myself with professionalism and integrity and maintain a full appreciation of the responsibility that the public entrusts to me.

Codes of Behavior

Ethical codes are based on the belief that a relationship of trust exists between a professional (i.e., the pharmacist) or paraprofessional (i.e., the pharmacy technician) and a client (i.e., the patient). There are two reasons for this belief. First, professional service is not standardized; it is unique and personal. These essential qualities cannot be specified in a contract or purchased. Second, the patient often hardly knows what to ask for, let alone how it can be provided. Therefore, the patient is vulnerable to the services provided by the pharmacist and pharmacy technician.

Pharmacy personnel are held to high standards of conduct and must meet selected criteria. First, pharmacists, as highly educated professionals in the practice of pharmacy, hold a specialized body of knowledge, which enables them to perform a highly useful social function. Pharmacy technicians, as paraprofessionals, are also, by extension, held to higher standards of conduct in their everyday practice compared to cashiers or warehouse clerks. Pharmacy technicians who are also certified and/or registered are held to an even higher level of expectations. Technicians, like pharmacists, have a duty to maintain their competence and continually enhance their knowledge.

Second, the attitude one possesses also influences his or her behavior in the workplace. The basic attitude is an unselfish concern for the welfare of others, called altruism. A pharmacy technician must be empathetic because many patients with whom they come in contact on a daily basis feel ill or have serious diseases.

Third, **social sanction** also contributes to an expected code of behavior, just as much as one's attitude or expectation of conduct. Social sanction creates trust between society (i.e., patients), professionals (i.e., pharmacists), and paraprofessionals (i.e., pharmacy technicians). Social sanction is the measure of acceptable behavior of a professional or paraprofessional by those they serve—in this case, the public. The trust that a pharmacist has with society has been transferred more and more by extension to the pharmacy technician. It is important to do what is right for the patient—at times, that may mean giving the patient a few doses of a prescription for a heart or blood pressure medicine at night or on the weekend, even though the patient has no refills remaining.

Codes of ethics regarding professional behavior are often written as formal documents (see Figure 13.1) and supported by professional organizations. These statements provide language to aid in the decision-making process when an ethical issue presents itself in pharmacy practice.

Dilemmas Facing Healthcare Professionals

A code of ethics assists a healthcare professional in choosing the most appropriate course of action to handle an ethical dilemma. An **ethical dilemma** is a situation that calls for a judgment between two or more solutions, not all of which are necessarily wrong. Deciding what action to take when faced with an ethical dilemma in the pharmacy requires considering the circumstances, choosing an action, and justifying the action. To do this, you should ask questions such as:

- What is the dilemma?
- What pharmaceutical alternatives apply?
- What is the best alternative, and can it be justified on moral grounds?

Pharmacy technicians must recognize and accept the ethical standards of pharmacy practice and apply them when working side by side with pharmacists. They must also understand decision-making processes and become personally involved in obtaining facts that are relevant to a dilemma, evaluating the alternatives, and determining the correct solutions. The following scenarios and the ethical dilemmas that they pose are commonly seen in the pharmacy setting:

- You are asked to dispense an OTC emergency contraceptive. You are uncomfortable with meeting that request because you consider the action morally or ethically unsound based on your religious beliefs. Do you have the right to refuse the dispensing of the drug based on your beliefs?
- You receive a legal narcotic prescription from an individual whom you know for certain is selling the drugs on the street. Do you tell the pharmacist and refuse to fill the prescription or contact the physician?
- You are asked to fill narcotic or sedative prescriptions for patients who appear to be physically dependent on the drugs. How would you and the pharmacist proceed to intervene? Do you contact the physician? The police? Is intervention necessary?
- Although the physician wrote a prescription for three tablets a day of a blood pressure medication, after conferring with the patient, you find out that he or she is taking only one tablet a day as directed. You realize that the order is being made for the patient to stockpile the medication and pay a lower co-pay, taking unfair advantage of the insurance company. What steps would you take to work with the pharmacist and physician about this issue?
- You are selling insulin syringes to an out-of-town customer. How would you find out if the patient is using the syringes for the treatment of diabetes or requesting the needles for illegal drug use?
- You are selling OTC pseudoephedrine products to an out-of-state customer. Does he or she have self-limited cold symptoms, or is he or she purchasing the product for an illegal methamphetamine laboratory? For what other reasons might this customer be purchasing this product?

If the pharmacist elects not to fill and dispense the OTC or legal prescription drug (especially at night or on the weekends), what allowances are made for the patient? Will another pharmacist be "on call" to come in and fill the prescription or dispense and sell the OTC product? Will the patient be referred to another local pharmacy? Each community and hospital pharmacy must have policies and procedures in place. Each state has a different law for dealing with such ethical dilemmas, from recognizing the right of the pharmacist to refuse dispensing the medication, to requiring that the pharmacist dispense the medication.

As modern pharmacy practice continues to evolve, new questions will arise that challenge pharmacy personnel in new decision-making deliberations. Advances in medical health, pharmaceutical delivery systems, new medication development, and computerized technologies change how pharmacists and pharmacy technicians conduct their daily work. The answers to such ethical practice questions should certainly come under scrutiny by pharmacy personnel and professional pharmacy organizations. As with any politically, professionally, and emotionally charged topic, a variety of opinions will surface. When those differences occur, the pharmacy technician, whether working in a team or with an individual patient, must learn to respect differing opinions without prejudice.

Corporate Ethics

In addition to a personal code of ethics, many organizations have a Code of Business (or Pharmacy) Conduct policy that all employees agree to maintain. This policy spells out the highest standards of ethical behavior and professional conduct. For example, personnel cannot take even one dose of a prescription medication without a legal prescription or medication order, even for something as simple as a headache. Any unauthorized sale, possession, use, or diversion of controlled drugs would result in termination of employment.

There are also state and federal laws, such as the Red Flags Rule and the False Claims Act, and store policies and agreements in which all employees must agree to avoid any pretense of participation in any fraudulent activity. Pharmacies may be subject to medical identity theft—that is, a person who seeks health care (or retail purchases) using someone else's name, credit card, or insurance information. Examples of medical identity theft include a person submitting an altered or forged driver's license for identification or an individual using a stolen credit card to purchase a large quantity of retail gift cards or to launder cash money. Each healthcare provider is required by federal law to have a policy and a training program in place to help employees spot warning signs or "red flags" to prevent medical identity theft.

Any pharmacy organization that submits claims to a government insurance provider such as Medicare, Medicaid, or Tricare is required by the Department of Health and Human Services to have a training program for all employees on corporate integrity. Any pharmacy organization's billing practices are subject to an annual independent review of compliance. **Compliance** is defined as adherence to a required set of standards, regulations, laws, and practices. The Corporate Integrity Agreement (CIA) is defined as the obligation to report all fraudulent activities under "whistleblower protection." Such activities may occur in the purchasing of pharmaceuticals or the insurance billing and reimbursement policies.

In terms of billing in a community pharmacy practice, all prepared submissions for online adjudication must be accurate. In light of that, a pharmacy technician *cannot*:

- enter or dispense a false prescription
- enter an incorrect days' supply
- backdate an order if a patient's prescriptions has already expired
- dispense a medication and wait to bill the insurance company three days later when insurance for the prescription will be approved
- change a 30-day supply order to a 90-day supply order without documented approval from the medical office (in most states)
- dispense an ordered days' supply of medication (such as 10 days) and change the days' supply to 5 days because the patient's insurance only covers a 5-day supply
- dispense a refill of a drug if the prescription is more than one year old or if a controlled drug prescription is more than six months old
- add a refill and bill insurance if the patient is out of refills without the prescriber's authorization
- accept a store or drug discount card or a manufacturer's coupon from a patient who uses a government insurance program—including Medicare Part D.
- bill insurance for a brand name drug and dispense a generic drug
- dispense a controlled drug unless the prescription is written on security paper and is being used for a legitimate medical purpose.

Pharmacists and technicians are expected to take personal responsibility to fulfill these compliance initiatives. Violations of any of these policies could result in disciplinary action that may include termination. If independent audits demonstrate inaccurate billing, the claim will be denied and the pharmacy will lose both the cost of the drug and the money required to reimburse the government agency for the amount that was submitted. In addition, the pharmacy may be subject to criminal and/or civil monetary penalties if repeated or flagrant fraudulent activity has occurred.

Awareness of Substance Abuse Issues

The abuse of prescription pain medication is the fastest-growing drug problem in the United States. The statistics speak for themselves. According to the Drug Enforcement Administration (DEA), more than 7 million Americans abuse pain and anxiety medications every year, and the numbers are increasing at a fast rate. Prescription pain medicines kill 50 people every day, and send nearly 1,000 more to the emergency room with life-threatening overdoses. In fact, there are more overdoses from legal pain medications than heroin or cocaine. While hydrocodone and oxycontin used to be the recreational prescription drugs of choice, oxymorphone (Opana) is now the preferred drug.

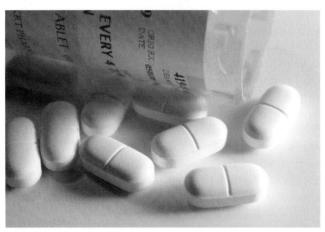

One commonly abused drug is a combination of hydrocodone and acetaminophen.

Certainly drug tolerance and addiction are major reasons for prescription drug abuse. But drug diversion for money, especially in challenging economic times, is also a major cause of abuse. Prescription drugs command a high price on the streets, as shown in these figures: Opana and Oxycontin: $50–$80 per pill; Oxycodone: $12–$40 per pill; Percocet: $10–$15 per pill; and Hydrocodone (Vicodin): $5–$20 per pill. Some Medicare and Medicaid patients give their legal prescriptions for narcotics to drug dealers for cash. National and regional databases will share information about the prescribing and dispensing of these drugs between states to better identify drug seekers.

Drug Abuse and the Healthcare Professional It is estimated that more than 10% of healthcare professionals have a drug or alcohol abuse problem—a statistic that is similar to substance abuse in the general population. Access to controlled drugs offers a temptation to healthcare workers who are drug seekers. For this reason, pharmacies have implemented measures to prevent prescription drug theft, including cameras, tablet-by-tablet inventories, and staff inservice training. Part of that training includes recognizing the signs and symptoms of substance abuse and knowing the course of action to take if you suspect a colleague has a substance abuse problem.

Signs and Symptoms of Substance Abuse Substance abuse is difficult to spot because it is a behavior most people cleverly learn to hide. Possible signs and symptoms include changes in appearance (such as bloodshot eyes) and changes in behavior (such as abrupt mood swings, slurred speech, poor listening skills, belligerence, overconfidence, lying, absenteeism, and forgetfulness). While anyone can have a "bad day," sudden and consistent behavioral changes may indicate a serious problem. The problem may also stem from personal or relationship issues, economics, health issues, stress, or other causative factors.

Course of Action If you are aware that a technician or pharmacist has a problem, you have a legal and ethical responsibility to uphold the law and protect society. There is a natural reluctance to getting involved with a colleague's problems. Anyone would want to avoid retribution or contributing to a technician's termination or a pharmacist's loss of licensure. Encourage your coworker to seek professional drug treatment. By getting help for your colleague, you are protecting not only his or her safety and welfare but that of the other employees and patients. Most state boards of pharmacy have a "Pharmacist Recovery Network" or similar organization to provide assistance and treatment for impaired colleagues who seek help without the risk of losing their license or registration.

Health Insurance Portability and Accountability Act

As discussed in Chapter 2, the **Health Insurance Portability and Accountability Act (HIPAA)** is a comprehensive federal law passed in 1996 to, among other things, protect patients' private health information. All healthcare facilities (including pharmacies in all practice settings) that access, store, maintain, or transmit patient-identifiable medical information must comply with HIPAA regulations. Failure to do so can result in severe civil and criminal penalties. Some states may have more stringent requirements than the federal law; as with controlled drugs, the more stringent policy always takes precedence. For many reasons, only authorized personnel are allowed entrance into the pharmacy—one reason being the safeguarding of patients' private health information. Although HIPAA covers many areas, the following sections are related to security and patient confidentiality.

Patient Identifiers

A pharmacy is required by law to maintain the privacy of **protected health information (PHI)**. Personal health information—printed or spoken—must be protected from unauthorized use and access. Obviously, a physician, nurse, pharmacist, and pharmacy technician have access to medical information to serve the needs of the patient. A pharmacy technician, for example, may be able to identify a medical diagnosis from the medications that are dispensed in the pharmacy (e.g., a patient receiving combination antiretroviral therapy most likely has an HIV infection). However, all healthcare professionals are bound by law and ethics not to disclose this information outside the immediate pharmacy workplace.

To be in compliance, healthcare workers must also remove or conceal from view any information that can identify the patient. Examples of these **patient identifiers** are listed in Table 13.1. In addition, pharmacy personnel must take measures to conceal the medication itself. To the end, an FDA-required Medication Guide should be placed inside the patient's bag or stapled underneath the cover sheet during pickup so that the medication cannot be seen by anyone other than the patient.

A community pharmacy may use PHI to provide and coordinate the treatment, medications, and services that the patient receives. It may also be used to contact the

---

TABLE 13.1 Patient Identifiers

■ Name	■ Health plan identification number
■ Address and zip code	■ Account number
■ Relatives	■ Vehicle identification
■ Employer	■ Certificate or license number
■ Date of birth	■ Uniform resource locater (URL) or Internet protocol (IP) address
■ Telephone number or fax number	■ Fingerprint or voiceprint
■ E-mail address	■ Photo
■ Social security number	
■ Medical record number	

insurer to determine the amount of medication covered by insurance and the resulting co-pay. PHI is occasionally used for quality assurance surveys or in response to a lawsuit. In most legal cases, the lawyer obtains written approvals from the patient to release his or her prescription records, or the pharmacy gets the approval of the patient. PHI may be released without permission in the case of a court order or evidence of a crime or fraudulent activity. All requests for PHI other than by the patient should be directed to the pharmacist.

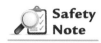

Safety Note

Labels and documents containing patient-related information must be shredded or incinerated for proper disposal.

In the pharmacy, shredding all patient-related information is common practice. Labels, prescription vials, patient profiles, insurance or drug utilization reports, and so on must be discarded appropriately. If not shredded, this information must be discarded in a special designated container (not accessible to the public) that is sealed and mailed for incineration. PHI must never be thrown in the trash. As a technician, be extremely vigilant and sensitive to maintaining patient confidentiality. In addition, be sure to understand the policy and procedures of your pharmacy. If you see potential violations, bring them to the attention of your pharmacist supervisor. Maintaining the privacy and security of health information is an extremely important ethical and legal issue.

Patient Confidentiality

All healthcare professionals must understand the importance of maintaining patient confidentiality. **Confidentiality** may be defined as keeping privileged information about a customer from being disclosed without his or her consent. If a patient cannot trust the pharmacist or pharmacy technician with medical information, then both trust and a good customer may be lost. With that in mind, pharmacy technicians need to be aware of discussing sensitive medical issues in a public setting. They should keep patient communications about medications (including questions that arise at patient pickup or during the location of products in the pharmacy) at a quiet level of discussion. Outside of the immediate pharmacy workplace, such as in the lunch break room, technicians must avoid any discussion of patients and their medications.

Computer screens should be obscured so as to not be visible to the public or unauthorized personnel. A patient may request a private conversation with a pharmacist to discuss a medical issue, and the pharmacist should conduct this discussion quietly and discreetly. When using the telephone, pharmacy personnel should not use speakerphone when talking with a patient about his or her medications and should not leave a message for a patient that divulges any medical or drug information.

Maintaining the security and privacy of a patient's medical information must remain a high priority for the pharmacy technician. Every pharmacy is required to have a written policy on patient confidentiality that must be on display in the pharmacy and provided to patients as a handout. It should be recorded in the patient's profile when a patient receives the policy or any updates. The patient does not have to sign stating he or she received the policy, but the pharmacy must make an effort and any refusal to sign, even if the patient accepts the document, should be recorded.

Security of PHI The issues of security and privacy are closely intertwined with patient confidentiality. *Who* should have access to *what* information inside or outside the pharmacy? How can unnecessary access to patient health information be limited, especially in large organizations such as hospitals, chain pharmacies, research sponsors, or insurance providers?

PHI Sharing Among Healthcare Personnel In the course of diagnosing or treating a patient, the physician and pharmacist (or their agents, on their behalf) may exchange information without restriction or without the expressed written permission of the patient. For example, if a patient was receiving controlled narcotic prescriptions from several physicians, the pharmacist may notify these physicians. In addition, some insurance reimbursement requires diagnostic codes from the physician for select diabetic and respiratory drugs; this information can be provided. In these examples, the permission of the patient is not necessary.

PHI Sharing Among Investigational Drug Personnel How much information about the patient does the sponsor of an investigational drug study (often a pharmaceutical company) need to know? Some—but not all—health information is shared with investigational drug studies. Studies must be designed so that patients cannot be individually identified. A minimum amount of information that directly relates to the study is exchanged with the sponsor according to protocol approved by the Institutional Review Board or Human Use Committee. Investigational drug studies collate medical data so that PHI remains confidential.

PHI Sharing Between Insurance Providers and Employers Another example where limited patient information can be exchanged is within communications between a patient's insurance provider and his or her employer. An insurance company processing a prescription reimbursement has the right to know which drug and dosage was dispensed, but it may not be necessary to share that information with the patient's employer. In the past, insurance companies occasionally shared medical information with an employer, resulting in termination for the employee. No such information is shared with the employer under HIPAA today.

PHI Sharing and Patient Permission Pharmacy personnel must be granted written permission from a patient to share information with family members. In fact, a patient may ask a technician to print his or her annual prescription record (for income tax calculations) but will need written permission from his or her spouse to receive the spousal prescription record. Another example that requires a patient's permission to share information includes the dispensing of birth control pills to a teenager at a family planning clinic. By law, that information cannot be shared with the parents or anyone else without the patient's consent. At times, a pharmacist may need to see a copy of a patient's hospital discharge summary or recent laboratory results. These documents, as well, cannot be viewed without the patient's permission.

Security and Electronic Transmission The electronic transmission of prescriptions and medical and insurance information provides many benefits for both pharmacies and patients, including:

- an increased revenue for the community pharmacy (more prescriptions can be dispensed, reimbursements are paid more rapidly, fewer claims are rejected)
- decreased expenditures in personnel (fewer staff members are needed for billing claims)
- additional time for pharmacists to review patient profiles and offer medication counseling (fewer medication errors)

However, the efficiencies of transmitting medical information electronically must be balanced with the need to maintain security and protect patient confidentiality.

Electronic transmission of data is common in the pharmacy. This transmission involves several parties, including healthcare practitioners, pharmacy personnel, and third-party insurance companies. All such transmissions are protected by state and federal laws. HIPAA sets standards for the electronic submission of patient medical information and provides safeguards to protect the confidentiality of patient information. Other safeguards concerning patient data include limited access of certain healthcare professionals to fields of information and frequent password changes to limit access to patient information. Pharmacy personnel should also keep in mind that patient data privacy laws also extend to e-mail correspondence. Therefore, personnel should avoid sending any e-mails containing patient identifiers in the subject line.

Fax Security Issues The sending of medical or prescription information via fax is a common pharmacy practice, particularly when obtaining a refill authorization from a physician's office. Like other types of electronic submission, a fax must also be carefully monitored. Faxes to and from the pharmacy and medical offices are in an encrypted format. The receipt of faxed information is intended only for personnel of the medical office or pharmacy to which it was sent. This information should be filed or securely disposed of (shredded) after it is has been reviewed. If an inadvertent fax was transmitted to the wrong number, the sender must be notified and the protected information returned or destroyed immediately.

Protection of Proprietary Information You may also need to provide security by protecting your employer's proprietary information from competitors, including prescription volume, pricing issues, or policies and procedures in the pharmacy. If you are not sure, ask a senior pharmacy technician or pharmacist.

Medical records are also considered proprietary. Medical records are owned by the facility that generates them. While a patient and a provider have a right to review and add to them as appropriate, medical records are considered the property of the facility. Although they are considered property, these records are still protected health information and may not be sold or distributed without authorization.

Privacy In addition to HIPAA regulations, the pharmacy technician should be sensitive and respectful of customer privacy regarding health information. Pharmacies sell many products related to private bodily functions and conditions (e.g., condoms and other contraceptives, feminine hygiene and menstrual products, suppositories, hemorrhoid remedies, enemas, adult diapers, catheters, bed pans, scabicides). Customers often are embarrassed to ask about such products and have to work up the nerve to request assistance. Pharmacy technicians need to be approachable and need to provide assistance and information to these customers when possible. For patients who request specific product information that requires expertise or counseling, technicians should refer these patients to the pharmacist. As a pharmacy employee, you are part of the healthcare profession and must adopt a helpful, no-nonsense, professional attitude toward the body and its functions. Responding to an inquiry about such a product with efficiency, courtesy, respect, and a certain degree of nonchalance often relieves your customer's embarrassment and demonstrates your professionalism. Speak in a clear voice, but not so loudly that other customers or employees are privy to your private exchange with the customer. For patients who request specific product information that requires expertise or counseling, technicians should refer these patients to the pharmacist.

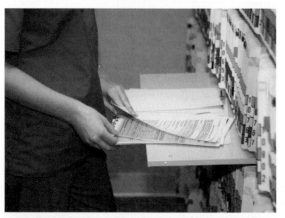

The information contained in both medical and pharmacy records is protected under HIPAA laws.

Privacy and Medication Histories   In addition, often a patient's illness can be determined by his or her medication history. A patient receiving antiviral prescriptions for HIV, antibiotics for gonorrhea, antivirals for herpes, antidepressants, erectile dysfunction drugs, or chemotherapy requires the same amount of privacy as in a physician's office. Many states have specific laws protecting patients with HIV or acquired immunodeficiency syndrome (AIDS).

Privacy and Customer Identification   Privacy should be maintained as you update customer information. If, for example, you are stationed at the pharmacy window and need information for the customer's patient profile, let the customer know why you need the information. Tell the customer, for example, "I need some information for your prescription profile so that we may better serve you. May I ask you a few questions? What is your full name and address? Do you have any medication allergies or health conditions?" You may also need to verify insurance information; most customers are accustomed to presenting a card or proof of insurance regularly at the physician's office and are not upset once the procedure is explained.

When a patient is picking up a prescription, confirm his or her identity and what he or she is picking up. Keep your tone of voice low so as not to broadcast to nearby customers what the patient is receiving. If someone else is picking up a medication, especially for a controlled drug, many pharmacies have a policy of requesting a photo ID such as a driver's license. Many pharmacies now have a separate counseling area for prescription pickup, where the patient can have a higher degree of privacy.

Notice of Privacy Practices   A patient has the right to expect that medical information will be kept confidential. Under HIPAA, each pharmacy is required to have a policy statement that defines patient privacy rights and how patient information will be used and protected by the pharmacy. These policy statements should be explained to all new pharmacy customers at the time that they first visit the pharmacy. To protect the pharmacy's interests, patients may be asked to sign a form to acknowledge and document that they have received the pharmacy's privacy statement, called a **notice of privacy practices**. These signed notices must be kept on file for six years.

This notice also includes the patient's health information rights. Parents can sign for their dependent minor children. Upon request, however, teenage minors may be treated as adults with respect to access and disclosure of health information records. A patient may give written permission to a personal representative to access his or her health information and records. This is a common practice when a son or daughter may help in the care of an elderly adult.

Pharmacy Compliance with HIPAA Regulations   Each pharmacy can develop its own mechanism to implement, communicate, audit, and document compliance with HIPAA regulations. Depending on the size of the pharmacy, formal training programs, with annual refresher courses, may be used. Each pharmacy should have a set of policies and procedures in its manual to cover the HIPAA regulations. Younger pharmacy technicians who are part of Generation Y grew up in the computer and media age and are accustomed to exchanging lots of information with friends. This group must be counseled that breaching confidential information violates legal, regulatory, and ethical principles and is often sufficient reason for immediate termination.

Both state and federal laws govern patient confidentiality. Generally, where conflict exists, the most stringent law is the one that should be followed. The pharmacy technician should know the laws in the state where he or she is practicing; if the technician moves to another state, it is important to learn the regulations and laws of his or her new state.

Chapter Summary

- Community pharmacies are returning to the concept of the small, customer-oriented neighborhood pharmacy of the past.
- Increased emphasis on personal service (i.e., attention to the needs of individual customers) requires the technician to consider carefully all interactions with pharmacy customers.
- Customer service involves professional attire, grooming, and personal hygiene.
- The pharmacy technician should be helpful, understanding, and sensitive to language and cultural differences.
- Skills in both verbal and nonverbal communications are necessary to obtain information and provide good customer service.
- Common courtesy should be used in all telephone communications and conversations with both patients and healthcare professionals.
- Providing customer care to a patient with a mental or physical disability may provide a challenge to the technician.
- A zero-tolerance policy exists with regard to discrimination and harassment in the pharmacy workplace.

- A request for specific medical or pharmacy information should always be referred to a supervising pharmacist.
- Prescription drug abuse continues to be a major problem in health care today.
- During local, regional, or national disasters, or a serious epidemic, an emergency action plan will ensure your pharmacy's ability to assist in managing the crisis.
- It is important that community pharmacy technicians know how to act during a robbery.
- A pharmacy technician must exhibit ethical personal behavior and act in accordance with the pharmacy's corporate code of ethics.
- Ethical dilemmas exist in pharmacy practice and must be resolved following pertinent state laws and policies and procedures of the pharmacy.
- A pharmacy technician must be sensitive to maintaining patient privacy, confidentiality of medical information, and compliance with all state and federal HIPAA regulations.

Key Terms

altruism an unselfish concern for the welfare of others

appearance the overall outward look of an employee on the job, including dress and grooming

attitude the emotional stance or disposition that a worker adopts toward his or her job duties, customers, employer, and coworkers

closed-ended question a question that requires a yes-or-no answer

compliance adherence to a required set of standards, regulations, laws, and practices

confidentiality keeping privileged information about a customer from being disclosed without his or her consent

credentialing the process for validating the qualifications of licensed professionals, such as Basic Life Support (BLS) and ACLS (Advanced Cardiovascular Life Support)

cultural sensitivity an awareness, knowledge of, and respect for cultural beliefs that differ from your own

culture the customs, beliefs, and attitudes that are learned and shared by members of a group

decorum proper or polite behavior that is in good taste

discrimination preferential treatment or mistreatment

ethical dilemma a situation that calls for a judgment between two or more solutions, not all of which are necessarily wrong

ethics the study of standards of conduct and moral judgment that outlines the rights and wrongs of human conduct or character

etiquette unwritten rules of behavior

harassment persistent hostile, unpleasant, and unwelcome mistreatment, whether sexual, verbal, or physical

Health Insurance Portability and Accountability Act (HIPAA) a comprehensive federal law passed in 1996 to protect all patient-identifiable medical information

multitasking the ability to work on several projects at the same time

nonverbal communication communication without words—through facial expression, body language, posture, and tone of voice

notice of privacy practices a written policy of the pharmacy to protect patient confidentiality, as required by HIPAA

open-ended question a question that requires a descriptive answer, not merely yes or no

patient identifiers any demographic information that can identify the patient, such as name, address, phone number, Social Security number, or medical identification number

Policy and Procedure (P&P) manual a book that outlines pharmacy activities, defines the roles and responsibilities of pharmacy personnel, and lists pharmacy practice guidelines to follow

protected health information (PHI) medical information that is protected by HIPAA, such as medical diagnoses, medication profiles, and results of laboratory tests

social sanction the measure of acceptable behavior of a professional or paraprofessional by those they serve

triage the assessment and prioritization by the pharmacist of patients' illnesses or symptoms; outcome may be to recommend an OTC product or to refer the patient to a physician or emergency room; also used to assess and prioritize technician responsibilities within the pharmacy

Chapter Review

Additional Quiz Questions

Checking Your Understanding

To check your comprehension of this chapter's key concepts, read the following multiple-choice questions and then record your answers on a separate sheet of paper. Write your answers as modeled in these examples: 1d; 2c; 3b; etc.

1. The emphasis in retail pharmacy today is on
   a. discount pricing.
   b. customer care.
   c. extensive drug inventory.
   d. expansion of nondrug merchandising.

2. The emotional stance that a worker adopts toward his or her job duties is called
   a. tone.
   b. mood.
   c. attitude.
   d. appearance.

3. Which of the following is the primary rule of retail merchandising?
   a. Always dress and groom yourself neatly.
   b. Respect the customer's privacy.
   c. Explain necessary interactions to the customer.
   d. Be a model representative for your company.

4. Decorum is
   a. proper or polite behavior, or behavior that is in good taste.
   b. dissatisfaction with services provided.
   c. lack of understanding of the options available.
   d. the ability to negotiate for goods and services.

5. The major upward trend in drug abuse is primarily with
   a. cocaine.
   b. heroin.
   c. methamphetamine.
   d. oxymorphone.

6. When asking a customer for information for the patient profile, the pharmacy technician should explain
   a. how and when the prescription should be administered.
   b. why the pharmacy needs this information.
   c. the parts of the label of the prescription.
   d. the differences between the payment policies of various third-party insurance providers.

7. Preferential treatment or mistreatment based on age, gender, ethnicity, or other criteria is known as
   a. harassment.
   b. discrimination.
   c. innuendo.
   d. decorum.

8. When answering the telephone in a retail pharmacy, a person should identify himself or herself and the name of the
   a. supervising pharmacist.
   b. pharmacy.
   c. customer.
   d. prescribing physician.

9. An underage teenager is on a birth control pill. All of the following can review this medical information at the pharmacy except the
   a. parents.
   b. physician.
   c. pharmacist.
   d. pharmacy technician.

10. Protected health information under HIPAA and applicable state laws includes all the following patient information *except*
    a. medication profile.
    b. medical diagnoses.
    c. insurance provider.
    d. laboratory results.

11. Discussing the competency of a local physician with a patient is an example of a breach of
    a. decorum.
    b. credentialing.
    c. etiquette.
    d. confidentiality.

12. Intimate personal relationships within the pharmacy are
    a. encouraged to build teamwork.
    b. discouraged in nearly all cases.
    c. tolerated by management.
    d. approved unless against written policy and procedure.

13. Dispensing a prescription and postdating and billing prescription insurance two days later is a violation of
    a. HIPAA.
    b. corporate ethics.
    c. DEA regulations.
    d. criminal law.

14. The most important nonverbal communication tool in dealing with the elderly or those who are hearing impaired is
    a. maintaining eye contact.
    b. talking in a loud tone of voice.
    c. writing down questions on paper.
    d. crossing your arms during interaction with the patient.

15. If the circumstances require, a patient's prescription information can be shared with all of the following *except*
    a. the patient's employer.
    b. the patient's insurance provider.
    c. the patient's prescriber.
    d. the patient's nurse.

Reinforcing Your Learning

To build on your understanding of the topics in this chapter, complete the following enrichment activities.

1. In a small group, recall your own experiences visiting drugstores or pharmacies. Make a list of problems that you have encountered in pharmacies (e.g., slow service, lack of a comfortable waiting area, lack of a private counseling area, difficulty in finding an item). As a group, brainstorm some ways to solve such problems and to improve customer service.

2. With other students in a small group, brainstorm a list of positive experiences you have had in retail merchandising establishments of all kinds. Using this list, draw up a list of recommendations for making a customer's experience in a pharmacy retail establishment a positive one.

3. Imagine that you are a pharmacy manager who operates a 24-hour facility in a diverse, urban neighborhood with the following demographics:

32%	English-speaking customers
26%	Spanish-speaking customers
16%	Korean-speaking customers
16%	customers who speak other languages (e.g., Thai, Laotian, Hmong, Russian, Latvian, Polish, etc.)
10%	Vietnamese-speaking customers

   With other students, brainstorm a list of steps you might take to meet the needs of the customers whom you serve.

4. Tone of voice can communicate many types of feelings. Consider how to say the following sentences out loud to communicate the feeling listed in parentheses.
   a. I love my job. (Nobody else may love it, but *I* do.)
   b. I love my job. (I more than *like* my job—I love it.)
   c. I love my job. (I may not like anything *else,* but I love my job.)
   d. I love my job. (I don't like my *boss,* but I like my job.)
   e. I love my job. (You have *got* to be kidding me!)

   Try repeating the sentence using your own feelings, and see whether your classmates can interpret your true feelings about your job. Ask yourself whether you know how you sound.

Thinking on Your Feet

To gain practice in handling challenging situations in the workplace, consider the following real-world scenarios and then use the guiding questions to help you formulate your responses.

1. As a class, identify two students to play the roles of a customer and a pharmacy technician. Have them act out some typical interactions in the pharmacy:
   a. a customer demanding to know why insurance will not cover his medication
   b. a customer trying to understand what a "prior authorization" means
   c. a customer seeking advice on an OTC product
   d. a customer registering a complaint

   Demonstrate both open-ended and closed-ended questions. After each scenario, critique the pharmacy technician's response.

2. Have students choose a partner and role-play the following scenarios between a pharmacy technician and a customer:

- a male who is obviously embarrassed asks a female technician for information on condoms;
- a female who is obviously embarrassed asks a male technician for information on feminine hygiene products.

Perform other scenarios with other products until each student has played a role. After each scenario is played out, critique the technician's response. Discuss the kinds of problems that can arise in such situations and how they might be avoided.

3. During your shift, a female patient presents a prescription to you for an abortion pill. Your religious beliefs are strongly "pro-life." How do you resolve this ethical dilemma?

4. The culture of the United States is changing constantly and becoming more diverse. Patients are often influenced by a wide variety of factors in their cultures, religions, and communities. With that in mind, provide a written explanation as to why pharmacy personnel should get to know individual patients, their families, and their cultural beliefs. Include three examples or case illustrations in your explanation.

5. Make a list of all written and typed PHI in the pharmacy. How should unused PHI be discarded?

6. A new customer presents an out-of-state prescription for Oxycontin. You have the drug in stock but you are reluctant to fill the prescription. How will you handle this patient interaction?

Acquiring Field Knowledge

To expand your knowledge of pharmacy practice, explore the following online activities that focus on research and information retrieval.

Reminder: *As you navigate the Internet, remember to exercise caution and good judgment when evaluating information. A thoughtful review of online text should take into consideration the following factors: the creator and sponsors of the website, the intended audience, the credentials of the authors and contributors, the reliability and validity of the posted information, the frequency of updates to the site, and the ease of navigation for a range of user skill levels.*

1. Visit the Keirsey website at www .paradigmcollege.net/pharmpractice5e/ temperament, register (for free), and take the Temperament Sorter II self-evaluation test to discover your personality type.
   a. According to Keirsey Temperament Theory, there are four basic temperament groups that describe human behavior. Keirsey's four temperaments are referred to as Artisans, Guardians, Rationals, and Idealists. What type of person are you?
   b. Were the descriptions of your personality type accurate?
   c. How can knowing your own type and the type of your coworkers assist your communication skills?
   d. Which personality types do you communicate with easily, and which types are more challenging?

2. Today, we have much exposure to various social media. Describe how customer service and patient confidentiality can be positively and negatively impacted by this new technology.

3. A patient asks you if a combination of amitriptyline and alcohol can be fatal. The patient then requests a 90-day supply of medication rather than a 30-day supply from the prescription. Check www .paradigmcollege.net/pharmpractice5e/ amitriptyline and other sources for toxicity and overdose information and write a brief report. How would you handle this delicate situation?

Sampling the Certification Exam

To provide you with practice for the Certification Exam, read the following questions that have been patterned after the test format and then record your answers on a separate sheet of paper. Write your answers as modeled in these examples: 1d; 2c; 3b; etc.

1. Customer service is demonstrated by
   a. smiling and using eye contact when communicating.
   b. pointing to the location of items in the aisle.
   c. not putting the caller on hold when transferring a call.
   d. waiting on as many customers as possible at one time.

2. Which of the following is an example of nonverbal communication?
   a. making eye contact
   b. asking for a patient information update
   c. talking softly
   d. using courtesy titles

3. Which of the following statements about a patient's right to privacy is correct?
   a. The medical record is the property of the facility that generates it, and the information may not be sold or distributed without authorization.
   b. The intellectual property in the medical record is the property of the patient and can only be released with the patient's permission.
   c. The medical record is the property of the patient to remove from the pharmacy.
   d. The patient must get a subpoena to look at his or her own medical records.

4. Which statement regarding a P&P manual is correct?
   a. Technicians should always check their employer's P&P manual to ensure the safe operation of their pharmacy.
   b. State Boards of Pharmacy write the P&P manuals that are used in pharmacies in each state.
   c. Federal law dictates what topics are used included in a P&P manual.
   d. Technicians should always do what the pharmacist tells them, even if it differs from the P&P manual.

5. Taking pride in the workplace is a good example of
   a. attitude.
   b. nonverbal communication.
   c. verbal communication.
   d. listening skills.

6. Unwanted sexual advances in the pharmacy workplace is considered to be
   a. discrimination.
   b. harassment.
   c. ethics violation.
   d. conflict resolution.

7. During a pharmacy robbery, you should do all the following *except*
   a. resist if you are physically able.
   b. remain calm.
   c. be a good eyewitness.
   d. press the panic alarm when safe.

8. According to the DEA, how many individuals die each day as the result of the misuse of prescription pain medications?
   a. 25
   b. 50
   c. 200
   d. 500

9. A patient's private medical and pharmacy information is protected by
   a. USP Chapter <797>.
   b. OBRA 1990.
   c. OSHA.
   d. HIPAA.

10. A former classmate is prescribed a medication for herpes. Under what conditions can you discreetly discuss his or her diagnosis outside of work?
    a. only with your spouse
    b. only with family members
    c. your best friend if he or she promises not to tell
    d. under no circumstances

Your Future in Pharmacy Practice

14

Learning Objectives

- Identify a variety of strategies for successful adaptation to the work environment.
- Define and differentiate the terms *licensure*, *certification*, and *registration*.
- Describe and contrast the format and content of the PTCE and ExCPT certification examinations.
- Explain the criteria for the recertification of pharmacy technicians.
- Discuss the importance of technician involvement in professional organizations and networking with colleagues.

- Make a plan for a successful job search.
- Write a résumé and a cover letter.
- Prepare for and successfully complete an interview.
- Describe the performance review process.
- Discuss some trends for the future of the pharmacy profession and their potential impact on pharmacy technicians.

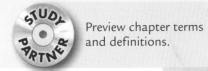

Preview chapter terms and definitions.

The past 50 years have seen dramatic changes in the pharmacy profession, especially as the roles of pharmacists and technicians have expanded and become integral to modern-day practices. Exciting changes are afoot, including an increasing movement toward national and specialty certifications and more formalized training and education of pharmacy technicians. Pharmacy technicians are finding more recognition, placement opportunities, and responsibilities in various employment settings, including community, hospital, managed care, long-term geriatric care, home health, and specialty practices. According to the Bureau of Labor Statistics, the demand for pharmacy technicians is expected to increase 30% by 2018. This chapter presents a useful discussion of these trends and provides information that will better prepare you to become a pharmacy technician.

Pharmacy Practice Preparation

As recognized pharmacy **paraprofessionals**, technicians have taken on an expanded role in the pharmacy practice setting. In addition to assisting the pharmacist—a **professional** with expert knowledge and skills in the preparation and dispensing of medications—technicians now fulfill several responsibilities that formerly belonged to the pharmacist. This shift in responsibilities has allowed the pharmacist to spend more time counseling patients about their medications. Consequently, the education and training for technicians have increased, as have the job performance expectations. Today's pharmacy technicians must be fully prepared to step into the work environment with complete confidence in their knowledge, skills, and problem-solving abilities.

Pharmacy Practice Environment

If you have not worked before or if your work experience has been sporadic, then getting used to your job as a technician might seem like acclimating to life in a foreign country. You have to adjust to a new work culture, different behaviors, unfamiliar customs, and even a new language—the technical jargon of the profession. The following list provides some advice for making your adjustment to the job more comfortable:

- *Attitude*—Do not give in to the temptation to behave in ways that are elitist or superior. Remember that you are part of a healthcare team, and cooperation is extremely important.
- *Reliability*—Health care, like education, is one of those industries in which standards for reliability are very high. You cannot, for example, show up late for work or take days off arbitrarily without good reason and prior supervisor approval. Unreliable employees in the healthcare industry do not keep their jobs for long, so make sure that your employer can always depend on you to arrive at work on time. Staying late does not make up for a tardy arrival. Tardiness can play havoc with other people's work schedules and workloads. Finish dressing, grooming, and eating before you enter your work area.
- *Accuracy and responsibility*—In a pharmacy, you rarely have the leeway to be partially correct. As discussed in Chapter 12, a medication error, even a small one, can have dire consequences for a patient or customer, as well as the pharmacy. Develop work habits to ensure accuracy, and expect to be held responsible for what you do on the job. Work steadily and methodically. Keep your attention focused on the task at hand, and always double-check everything you do.
- *Relationship with your supervisor*—Always show your supervisor a reasonable degree of deference and respect. Ask your supervisor how he or she prefers to be addressed. Be respectful of your supervisor's experience and knowledge. If tensions arise between you and your supervisor, then take positive steps to ease them. Your supervisor has power over your raises, promotions, benefits, and references for future employment. When you disagree with him or her, discuss these differences in private.
- *Personality*—Surprisingly, personality is one of the greatest predictors of job success. Be positive, cooperative, self-confident, and enthusiastic.

Practice Tip

Unreliable employees in the healthcare industry do not keep their jobs for long, so make sure that your employer can always depend on you to arrive at work on time.

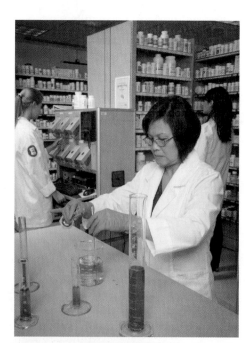

Pharmacy technicians must work methodically and carefully to ensure accuracy in the filling and dispensing of medications.

- *Performance*—Demonstrate that you can get things done and that you put the job first. Employers expect you to devote your full attention to your responsibilities for the entire length of your shift. Rushing through a task because it is close to the end of your shift places patient care at risk. Maintaining attentiveness and accuracy is always important, even close to quitting time.
- *Self-improvement*—Sometimes people are afraid to ask questions because doing so might make them appear less intelligent or less knowledgeable. Nothing could be further from the truth.
- *Dress*—Follow the dress code of the company or institution for which you work.
- *Receptivity*—Listen to the advice of others who have been on the job longer. Accept criticism gracefully. If you make a mistake, then own up to it. If you are criticized unfairly, then adopt a nondefensive tone of voice and explain your view of the matter calmly and rationally. This behavior is key to performing with integrity, an important part of being a professional.
- *Etiquette*—Every workplace has a unique culture. Especially at first, pay close attention to the details of that culture. Pick up on the habits of interaction and communication practiced by other employees, and model the best of these behaviors.
- *Alliances*—In all organizations, two kinds of power systems exist: (1) formal, or organizational, hierarchies and (2) informal collegial relationships, or alliances. Cultivate friendships on the job, but make sure that you are not seen as part of a clique or an exclusive group. Even as a new employee, begin to build power through connections with your colleagues. If a problem or an opportunity arises, then you will probably hear about it first through your allies. If an impending change in the workplace affects you, advance notice may give you the necessary time to plan a strategic response. Most of the big lucky breaks in life come through knowing the right people at the right time. By cultivating alliances, you can control your luck more than you might expect.

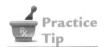
Practice Tip

Do not keep your professional qualifications a secret. Join professional organizations and volunteer to serve on committees within the institution. Aside from building your knowledge of pharmacy practice, these actions make you a valued employee in the workplace.

- *Reputation*—Many people assume that if they work hard and are loyal, they will be rewarded. This is often, but not always, true. Management personnel may be so involved with their own concerns that you remain little more than a face in the crowd. Being pleasant to others helps you to be noticed, as does making helpful or useful suggestions. Do not keep your professional qualifications a secret. Join professional organizations. Volunteer to serve on committees within the institution. Make yourself indispensable to the organization. Be open and flexible to learning new positions, and be proactive, accepting new responsibilities within the pharmacy. When you have won an award or achieved some other success, see that your name is publicized in institutional newsletters, community newspapers, or the publications of professional organizations. Give presentations at professional meetings, civic groups, churches, or synagogues. Write articles for publication in professional journals.
- *Crisis management*—When a crisis occurs, do not overreact. Take time, if you can, to think and then act, and do not keep the crisis a secret from your supervisor.
- *Continuing education*—Pharmacy is a rapidly changing field. Staying current on new drugs, dosage forms, laws, and regulations is important. Accept the idea of continuing education (CE) as a way of life. CE may include reading pharmacy journals and newsletters or attending workshops and professional meetings. You may need to take formal course work or attend CE programs every year to maintain your certification and keep current on the latest trends. Think of your job-related learning as a regular "information workout," as necessary to your employment fitness as aerobic workouts are to your physical fitness.

- *Expertise*—How can you become a person who makes things happen? Become highly knowledgeable about a specialty within your field, such as sterile or nonsterile compounding, hazardous drug preparation, inventory control, and so on. Be the most expert technician that you can be in that area; then move on and master another area. Soon, others will be asking for your advice, and your reputation will grow.
- *Career evaluation*—There will never be a time in your career to coast and relax. Good career opportunities can arise unexpectedly, so make a habit of reviewing your career path and setting goals. Planning lends structure and substance to your career management. Many pharmacy technicians use their experiences as springboards into careers as pharmacists or nurses.

Professional Requirements of Pharmacy Technicians

Just as pharmacists are required to obtain credentials—such as graduating from an accredited pharmacy school, sitting for a licensure examination, and perhaps completing a residency—pharmacy technicians are increasingly asked to acquire education and seek credentials. A **credential** is simply a documented piece of evidence of one's qualifications. Credentials for a pharmacy technician may include licensure and/or certification. This documentation of qualifications is moving the role of technicians forward in the field of pharmacy. Being a pharmacy technician today does not simply mean having a job in a pharmacy; rather, it is a chosen career path in which the technician is a recognized paraprofessional.

As a paraprofessional in health care, technicians have the following specific expectations for job performance: Technicians should be qualified to perform the duties required, use specific knowledge and skill sets, and adhere to a code of ethical conduct.

These expectations are held for all healthcare professionals, elevating their job responsibilities beyond those of an hourly paid employee. Patients come to trust healthcare professionals and paraprofessionals, obliging pharmacy technicians to serve the public good and benefit the lives of patients. Pharmacy technicians may receive on-the-job training at a pharmacy or in the military or may complete a formalized training program at a community college or career school.

Licensure, Registration, and Certification It is important to delineate three terms commonly used to describe the qualifications of pharmacy personnel.

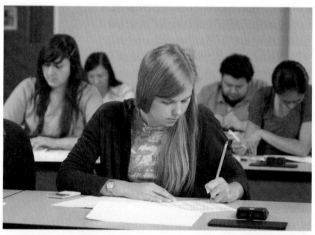

The combination of classroom instruction, hands-on training, and independent study should assist you in passing the necessary exams to become a certified pharmacy technician.

Licensure **Licensure** refers to the granting of a license by the state; it is usually required to work in a particular profession to ensure that the public is not harmed by the incompetence of practitioners. People become licensed through training and/or passing an exam. Licensure is usually renewable and is often dependent on keeping current on knowledge and skills. Pharmacists must be licensed in each state to practice; at this time, licensure is not required for a pharmacy technician.

Registration **Registration** generally means that an individual is required to sign up or register with a state agency, such as the State Board of Pharmacy, before starting to

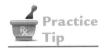
Practice Tip

If you move to another state, you may be required to register in that new state before (or soon after) starting employment.

practice. Registration or annual renewals are often done online for a nominal fee. The initial registration should be completed as soon as possible—often once a credential is earned or when beginning employment. Pharmacists or pharmacy technicians who are not registered, or allow their registration to lapse, cannot work in a pharmacy.

Individuals who wish to register as pharmacy technicians must submit information on where they live and work to the State Board of Pharmacy. It usually does not require additional training or education; registration allows the State Boards to more easily track any individuals with felony, theft, or drug diversion histories. Registration is required in all states but Hawaii, Colorado, Wisconsin, Michigan, Pennsylvania, New York, and the District of Columbia (see Figure 14.1). If you move to another state, you may be required to register in that new state before (or soon after) starting employment.

Certification **Certification** is the process by which a nongovernmental association grants recognition to an individual who has met certain predetermined qualifications specified by that association; unlike licensure, certification is seldom mandatory to practice legally. Unlike licensure and registration, certification is generally valid and transferable to all states.

An increasing number of states recognize national pharmacy technician certification. Some states, such as Arizona, Idaho, Illinois, Iowa, Louisiana, Maryland, Massachusetts, Mississippi, Montana, New Mexico, Oregon, South Carolina, Texas, Utah, Virginia, Washington, West Virginia, and Wyoming, require specific certification for pharmacy technicians.

FIGURE 14.1 States Regulating Pharmacy Technicians

The data represented in this figure is current as of December 31, 2012. For quarterly updates of this information, please visit the website of the Pharmacy Technician Certification Board at www.ptcb.org.

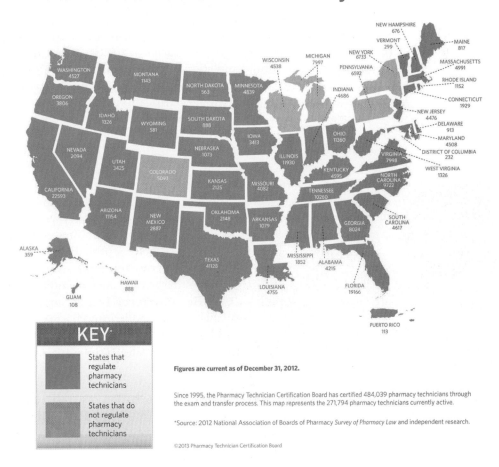

Active PTCB Certified Pharmacy Technicians

Figures are current as of December 31, 2012.

Since 1995, the Pharmacy Technician Certification Board has certified 484,039 pharmacy technicians through the exam and transfer process. This map represents the 271,794 pharmacy technicians currently active.

*Source: 2012 National Association of Boards of Pharmacy *Survey of Pharmacy Law* and independent research.

©2013 Pharmacy Technician Certification Board

Whether required by the state or not, both hospitals and community pharmacies are increasingly calling for technicians to become certified by taking a technician certification exam. Often certification is a requirement for initial employment or strongly encouraged within the first year of employment. The cost of taking the certification exam is commonly reimbursed by the employer. Financial incentives are often in place for technicians to become certified once they are employed. Many states stipulate a maximum ratio of technicians (including pharmacy interns) to pharmacists, which may vary from 2:1 to 4:1; the ratio may be dependent on the number of employed certified pharmacy technicians. Some states may use a higher technician-to-pharmacist ratio if at least one technician is certified.

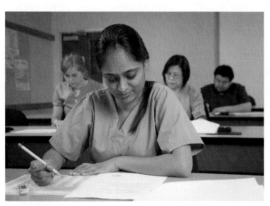

A pharmacy technician student completes an exam in a pharmacy technician education program.

Specialty certifications may be required to practice in certain areas within pharmacy, such as preparing sterile and nonsterile compounds, chemotherapeutic agents, or radioactive agents. The costs of training and examinations are commonly borne by the employer. Such certifications are not required by the state but may be necessary for maintaining accreditation. Such specialty certifications are accompanied by a higher hourly wage.

Pharmacy Technician Education Programs Some states are also beginning to recognize the value of formal technician education programs. For instance, South Carolina now requires completion of an accredited technician education program in addition to certification by the Pharmacy Technician Certification Board (PTCB) and 1,000 hours of work experience to be a certified pharmacy technician.

Many hospital pharmacies have adopted the model curriculum developed by the American Society of Health-System Pharmacists (ASHP) for their technician training programs; the successful completion of the program can also result in certification. Many chain pharmacies have developed in-house technician training programs that prepare technicians for the national certification exam.

The trend is for more standardization of curricular content and experiences within technician training programs. The Pharmacy Technician Workforce Coalition has developed a comprehensive curriculum leading to a two-year Associate of Applied Science (AAS) degree as a standard for technician training. This degree program has the support of the North Carolina Board of Pharmacy and the North Carolina Association of Pharmacists and has been adopted in several community colleges within the state. With these new requirements, technicians are given greater responsibilities—they are even allowed to check the work of other technicians in some practice settings.

All of these developments point to an increase in the presence, responsibilities, and status of the technician within the pharmacy community. As a result, today's employers expect more of (and deliver more to) their technician employees. Two examinations are available for becoming a **Certified Pharmacy Technician (CPhT)**. Practice exams and study guides are also available from the American Pharmacists Association (APhA) and other commercial sources, including Paradigm Publishing's *Certification Exam Review for Pharmacy Technicians, Third Edition*. The PTCB exam has by far the longest track record with more than 450,000 students having taken the exam since 1995.

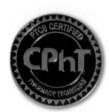

The PTCB-certified CPhT pin indicates that the pharmacy technician candidate has successfully passed the certification exam.

Pharmacy Technician Certification Examination In January 1995, the APhA—along with the ASHP, the Illinois Council of Health-System Pharmacists (ICHP), and the Michigan Pharmacists Association (MPA)—created the PTCB. The mission of the PTCB is to establish and maintain criteria for certification and recertification of pharmacy technicians on a national basis. A nonprofit testing company, the Professional Examination Service (PES), administers the **Pharmacy Technician Certification Examination (PTCE)**, which candidates must pass to become certified and to receive the title of CPhT. Anyone who does not have a felony conviction (or drug violations) and has graduated from high school (or has a general equivalency diploma [GED] or the foreign equivalent) is eligible to apply online and sit for the exam. The candidate must be in good standing with his or her State Board of Pharmacy and follow all PTCB policies including a code of conduct, summarized in Table 14.1.

The goal of the PTCE is to verify the candidate's knowledge and skill base for activities performed by pharmacy technicians under the supervising pharmacist. It is comprehensive in its scope; no specific pharmacy setting or specialty is emphasized. Skills and knowledge from both the community and institutional settings are required to pass this examination, including basic compounding knowledge and skills. No previous education, training, or work experience is required before taking the examination, but experience and/or formal training can greatly assist a candidate in preparing for and passing the examination.

The exam is now taken online by computer-based testing (CBT). The PTCB recommends that individuals taking the examination be familiar with the material in "any of the basic pharmacy technician training manuals." The questions are organized into nine sections, each of which is weighted differently. Table 14.2 on the following page details the content of the examination as specified by the PTCB.

Candidates for certification are given two hours to complete the examination. No electronic devices such as cell phones, personal digital assistants (PDAs), or calculators are allowed. The PTCE is a multiple-choice examination containing approximately 80 questions with four possible choices for each question. A student should answer every question because the final score is based on the total number of questions answered correctly rather than the percentage of correct answers. Educated guesses are encouraged.

Candidates must receive a score of 650 or higher to pass and receive certification. Since its inception, the PTCB reports that 75% of examination takers have passed the test. A technician may retake the examination up to three times if necessary to achieve a passing score; however, an application fee applies each time. The PTCB has three practice exams available that cover pharmacology, calculations, and overall pharmacy practice; these exams may be useful to become familiar with the test format and gain confidence for the certification examination.

Exam for Certification of Pharmacy Technicians The Institute for the Certification of Pharmacy Technicians (ICPT) established the **Exam for Certification of Pharmacy Technicians (ExCPT)** in 2005. This organization is now a part of the National Healthcareer Association (NHA). The stated goal of NHA is "to increase the quality of

---

TABLE 14.1 PTCB Code of Conduct Expectations for Pharmacy Technicians

- Maintain high standards of integrity and conduct
- Accept responsibility for their actions
- Continually seek to improve their performance in the workplace
- Practice with fairness and honesty
- Encourage others to act in an ethical manner consistent with PTCB standards and responsibilities

Source: Pharmacy Technician Certification Board

TABLE 14.2   PTCE Content

Exam Category	Description	Exam Weighting
1. Pharmacology for Technicians	<ul><li>Generic and brand names of medications</li><li>Common indications, doses, side effects, and contraindications</li><li>Drug interactions</li><li>Knowledge of over-the-counter (OTC) drugs, herbals, and dietary supplements</li></ul>	13.75%
2. Pharmacy Law and Regulations	<ul><li>Drug Enforcement Administration (DEA) regulations</li><li>Food and Drug Administration (FDA) recalls</li><li>Infection control standards</li><li>Omnibus Budget Reconciliation Act (OBRA) requirements</li><li>Hazardous drugs</li><li>Health Insurance Portability and Accountability Act (HIPAA)</li><li>Risk Evaluation and Mitigation Strategy (REMS)</li></ul>	12.5%
3. Sterile and Nonsterile Compounding	<ul><li>Infection control (hand washing; personal protective equipment, etc.)</li><li>Handling and disposal requirements</li><li>Beyond-use dating</li><li>Procedures</li><li>Equipment</li><li>Documentation of sterile and nonsterile compounds</li></ul>	8.75%
4. Medication Safety	<ul><li>Error-prevention strategies</li><li>Patient Package Inserts (PPI) and MedGuides</li><li>Pharmacist referrals</li><li>High-risk medications</li><li>Approved labeling</li><li>Abbreviations</li></ul>	12.5%
5. Pharmacy Quality Assurance	<ul><li>Use of National Drug Code (NDC) and bar coding for medication dispensing and inventory control</li><li>Infection control procedures (personal protective equipment, needle recapping, etc.)</li><li>Risk management guidelines</li><li>Customer satisfaction measures</li></ul>	7.5%
6. Medication Order Entry and Fill Process	<ul><li>Intake, interpretation, and data entry</li><li>Calculations</li><li>Filling and dispensing processes</li><li>Labeling</li><li>Packaging requirements</li></ul>	17.5%
7. Pharmacy Inventory Management	<ul><li>Use of NDCs, lot numbers, and expiration dates</li><li>Formulary and approved drug lists</li><li>Ordering, receiving, storage, and removal</li></ul>	8.75%
8. Pharmacy Billing and Reimbursement	<ul><li>Third-party reimbursement policies and plans</li><li>Resolution</li><li>Coordination of benefits</li></ul>	8.75%
9. Pharmacy Information System Usage and Application	<ul><li>Computer applications in the dispensing of prescriptions and medication orders</li><li>E-prescriptions</li></ul>	10.0%

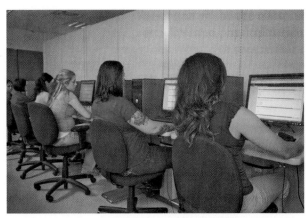

A future pharmacy technician sits for a certification exam, like the PTCE or ExCPT, in a secure environment with other individuals taking similar high-stakes exams.

care and make the healthcare industry better one worker at a time." NHA encourages certification and provides examinations and continuing education for many other paraprofessionals.

The mission of the ExCPT is to recognize pharmacy technicians with the knowledge and skills needed to assist pharmacists to prepare and dispense prescriptions safely, accurately, and efficiently, and to promote high standards of practice. The purpose of the exam is to determine whether an individual has achieved a certain minimum level of competency.

The ExCPT is offered in all 50 states and the District of Columbia and is available to pharmacy technicians from all practice settings. The ExCPT is recognized by several national pharmacy organizations as a valid instrument for pharmacy technician certification. The exam prepares a pharmacy technician to practice in either a community or hospital pharmacy environment.

Eligibility requirements are similar to those for the PTCE. ExCPT is a computer-based online test, consisting of 110 multiple-choice questions from a large test bank, which must be completed within a two-hour time frame. The content for the exam is weighted approximately 25% on regulations and technician duties, 23% on drugs and drug products (Top 200 Rx and Top 100 OTC products), and 52% on the dispensing process. A passing score is 390 out of a possible 500 points. Pharmacy technicians who successfully pass the ExCPT are considered Certified Pharmacy Technicians and receive a certificate that is recognized in most states.

There are math self-assessments, training manuals, and practice tests available at the NHA website to help pharmacy technicians prepare for the exam. The test offers questions that are similar in content and style to those on the ExCPT. Candidates who do not pass the ExCPT are allowed to retake the exam after four weeks.

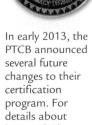

In early 2013, the PTCB announced several future changes to their certification program. For details about how and when those changes will impact certification and recertification requirements between now and 2020, consult your instructor.

Recertification Recertification is required by the PTCB and ExCPT every two years to maintain certification status. To be recertified, you must earn 20 hours of credit in pharmacy-related and approved continuing education; typically one hour of continuing education must come from pharmacy law. Acceptable topics include drug distribution, inventory control, managed health care, drug products, therapeutic issues, patient interaction, communication, interpersonal skills, pharmacy operations, prescription compounding, calculations, pharmacy law, preparation of sterile products, and drug repackaging.

Certificates of participation must be obtained for each CE program. Pharmacy-related continuing education may be provided by professional organization meetings and websites, employers, and professional journals. In some cases, applicable college courses with a grade of C or better may also be eligible for CE credit.

Hierarchy of Pharmacy Technician Positions

Because of expanded recognition of technician credentials, a hierarchy or "career ladder" of pharmacy technician job descriptions has evolved, especially in institutional settings. Although specific job descriptions vary among organizations, many institutions have different levels of technician responsibilities. If certification is not required for an entry-level technician, then it is always required for higher levels. Often, corresponding job titles are Technician I and II or Entry-Level Technician and Technician Specialist or Senior Technician. The difference in responsibility (and reward) grows and expands as the technician moves up the company ladder. For higher levels, added job responsibilities beyond basic competence for an entry-level technician may include these skills:

- prioritization of work
- demonstrated initiative and ability to work independently
- troubleshooting and critical thinking
- supervision of others
- staff training responsibilities
- advanced communication skills (e.g., writing, word processing, and taking refill requests if allowed)
- advanced computer application skills
- advanced calculations
- billing and documentation procedures
- inventory ordering and purchasing

In some cases, nonsterile and sterile compounding and nuclear pharmacy duties may be reserved for higher-level technicians with specialty certifications because of new regulations and standards implemented by the Joint Commission, the United States Pharmacopeia (i.e., USP Chapters <795> and <797>), and other national organizations. Accreditation of specialty pharmacies also may require that all pharmacy staff be trained and certified in specialty practice areas.

Many pharmacy technicians may be hired on a contingency basis (i.e., their performance is reevaluated after three to six months). Applicants with prior hospital experience, formalized training, or certification are considered to be more qualified than other applicants without such experience or training.

Professional Pharmacy Organizations

Being part of a profession means taking an active role in advancing the profession. As paraprofessionals in pharmacy practice, technicians have an obligation and a vested interest to make their views heard in the local, state, and national forums that discuss issues facing their field. The future of the technician role is in the hands of those within the profession. This self-governance, something that is increasing for technicians, is one characteristic of a professional. As the status and role of pharmacy technicians increase, those within the profession should get involved in the decisions and movements affecting it.

Ways to get involved vary widely. Some examples include:

- volunteering to serve on a committee of your local, state, or national pharmacy organization (most of which have technician representation), such as the ASHP, National Association of Boards of Pharmacy (NABP), Pharmacy Technician Certification Board (PTCB), or Pharmacy Technician Educators Council (PTEC).
  - ASHP: The Pharmacy Technician Advisory Group is charged with advising ASHP's staff and Board of Directors about ASHP actions, products, and services pertaining to pharmacy technicians.
  - NABP: Each of the state chapters welcomes technician input and participation.
  - PTCB: The Stakeholder Policy and Certification Councils have opportunities for pharmacy technicians at the national level.

- PTEC: A national professional association of pharmacy technician educators. Members of PTEC include those engaged in the regular training of pharmacy technicians.
■ running for office in your local chapter of the American Association of Pharmacy Technicians (AAPT)
■ applying for membership in the APhA, the National Community Pharmacists Association (NCPA), or the National Pharmacy Technician Association (NPTA)
■ serving on a committee for your state pharmacy association or participating in your state's annual pharmacy legislative day activities
■ attending a national pharmacy technician conference

After attending local, state, or national meetings, report what you learn to your employer and fellow technicians. Learning about and voicing concern for issues facing technicians and taking ownership in decisions made to advance their roles give technicians control over their own destinies. Participating in professional organizations can also provide needed CE credits for recertification.

Current issues that face technicians are standardization of technician training or education, expansion of technician responsibilities to assist with the projected shortages in pharmacy workforces, salary and benefits, and implementation of state requirements for national certification. Contact your local technician organizations and inquire about how you can participate in decisions affecting the future practice of pharmacy in your state.

Job Search

Before you can implement the strategies introduced in the preceding section, you must find the right job. Many people find the prospect of job hunting overwhelming,

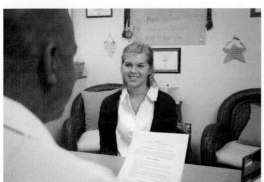

but try to avoid such negative thinking. To help you be successful in your job search, break down the process into the steps identified and explained in this section.

What characteristics do pharmacy and human resources managers look for in a pharmacy technician? First of all, they consider customer service. As discussed in Chapter 13, good communication and interpersonal skills are essential for a pharmacy technician, who interacts with pharmacy coworkers, patients, and other healthcare professionals on a daily basis. The pharmacy technician must also enjoy performing precise work (math calculations, computer prescription entry), where accuracy can be a matter of life or death. Pharmacy technicians must also be able to maintain this accuracy

During the interview, be confident, polite, poised, and enthusiastic, and focus on your strengths.

even in stressful situations or while multitasking. Finally, all employers want dependable employees who show up for work on time and who are willing to be flexible in their work schedules.

Clarifying Career Goals

Finding a job is difficult if you are not sure what you are looking for. Do you want to work in a community pharmacy? Do you want to work in a hospital, a long-term care facility, or a home infusion pharmacy? If you have uncertainties about the setting in

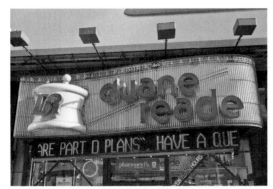

A career awaits you in a variety of settings, including a community pharmacy setting like Duane Reade.

which you wish to work, then arrange to interview pharmacists or technicians who work in these settings.

In addition, do some thinking about what you want out of the job. Are you interested in jobs with opportunities for advancement in management such as a senior pharmacy technician in the hospital or even assistant or store manager in a chain pharmacy? Are you more interested in customer care or prescription dispensing? Do you want to master the preparation of sterile products; the compounding of nonsterile products; or ordering, inventory, and billing? Can you balance your new job with your personal life, child care, and so on? Think about what you want to do; then look for jobs that suit your ambitions. Many programs have career counselors who can help you answer such questions. Check with your instructor or make an appointment to visit and talk to a career counselor. You may also want to use the Internet or the library to obtain more background information.

Establishing a Network

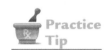
Practice Tip

Today, social media outlets such as Facebook and LinkedIn provide worthwhile online tools for networking.

Tell everyone you know that you are looking for a job. Identify faculty, pharmacists, acquaintances, friends, and relatives who can assist you in your job search. Find individuals within employers' organizations who can provide you with insight into their needs. If you complete any practical on-the-job experiences as part of your schooling, then ask your supervisors and coworkers about anticipated openings. If you perform well as a student-in-training, then you will be viewed as a good potential employee. Even previous graduates of your educational program can provide valuable information about hiring practices. Join state and national professional associations, attend meetings, and network with colleagues and potential employers. Lastly, search online for job opportunities in your geographic area, and join social media sites such as Facebook and LinkedIn for networking.

Identifying and Researching Potential Employers

Your school may have a career placement office. If so, then use the services of that office. Check the classified ads in newspapers. Go to a career library and look up employers in directories. Explore career opportunities posted on websites and job search websites; many local hospitals also have websites that are used to post job vacancies. Contact the state pharmacy and hospital pharmacy association offices or visit their websites for technician position vacancies.

Writing a Good Résumé

Use some of the excellent résumé-writing software now available, or contact a résumé-writing service. A résumé is a brief written summary of what you have to offer an employer. It is a marketing tool, and the product you are selling is yourself. A résumé is an opportunity to present your work experience, your skills, your background, and your education to an employer. Table 14.3 outlines the general topics to be included in a chronological résumé.

TABLE 14.3   The Parts of a Résumé

Heading	Provide your full name, address, and telephone number. Include your zip code in the address, area code in the phone number (and cell phone), and your email address so that a potential employer can contact you.
Education	Provide your high school or college, city, state, degree, major, date of graduation, and additional course work related to the job, to the profession, or to business in general. State your cumulative grade point average (GPA) if it helps to sell you (3.0 or higher). List any honors or recognitions received in high school or college.
Professional Certifications	Provide any professional certifications/licenses, such as your pharmacy technician certification, registration, CPR/First Aid, and so on. You may optionally list your certification or registration number, but it is not required—simply state "available upon request."
Experience	In reverse chronological order, list your work experience, including on-campus and off-campus work. Do not include jobs that would be unimpressive to your employer. Be sure to include cooperative education experience. For each job, indicate your position, employer's name, the location of the employment, the dates employed, and a brief description of your duties. Always list any advancements, promotions, or supervisory responsibilities. Be sure to include any certifications, registrations, or licensures on your résumé.
Skills	If you do not have a lot of relevant work experience, then include a skills section that details the skills that you can use on the job. Doing so is a way of saying, "I'm really capable. I just haven't had much opportunity to show it yet." If you have foreign language or computer software skills, be sure to emphasize them.
Related Activities	Include any activities that show leadership, teamwork, or good communication skills. Include any club or organizational memberships, as well as professional or volunteer community activities that may help sell your skills. Hobbies and interests may be listed to demonstrate your more personal side.
References	State that these are available on request. Speak to former employers about using them as a reference and then have a list of references available when an interview is granted.

Make sure that your résumé follows a consistent, standard format such as the one shown in Figure 14.2 on the following page. Although many employers ask that prospective employees submit their résumés online, you should also have several hard copies available for networking opportunities. Your résumé should be limited to a single page and printed on high-quality 8½ × 11 inch paper. Many special résumé papers are available from stationery and office supply shops; however, ordinary opaque or off-white paper is acceptable. Although printer paper with an unusual color and texture may seem unique and serve to set you apart, it is commonly viewed as unprofessional. Remain conservative when selecting stationery to convey a professional image.

Be sure to check your résumé carefully for errors in spelling, grammar, usage, punctuation, capitalization, and form. No one wants to hire a sloppy technician. Mistakes on your résumé may affect your prospective employer's confidence in the accuracy of your work. Once your résumé is complete, always have another person read through it and check for readability and for errors.

FIGURE 14.2
Sample Résumé

Kelly Nettleton
1700 Beltline Blvd.
My Town, GA 30107
knettleton@emcp.net

Objective: Position as pharmacy technician that makes use of my training in dispensing and compounding medications, ordering and inventory, patient profiling, third-party billing, and other essential functions

Education	Diploma in Health Science—Pharmacy Appalachian Technical College My Town, GA Dean's List	August 201X–May 201X
Certification	(awaiting results) Pharmacy Technician Certification Exam	July 201X
Experience	Clerk Waleska Pharmacy in Tate, GA Duties included serving customers, operating cash register, and stocking inventory.	September 201X to January 201X
	Pharmacy Technician Extern Waleska Pharmacy in Tate, GA Duties included assisting the pharmacist and pharmacy technicians in preparing prescriptions and refills, performing inventory management and control, processing and troubleshooting third-party insurance claims, providing exceptional customer service to patients and healthcare providers, and performing clerical duties (answering telephones, operating the cash register, filing paperwork, and helping to manage workflow)	January 201X to May 201X
	Sales Associate Tommy's Sporting Goods in Canton, GA Duties included serving customers and operating a cash register.	May 201X–September 201X

Skills
　　Pharmacy calculation skills, including conversions, basic formula
　　　　and ratio and proportion methods, and alligation
　　Preparation of aseptic intravenous solutions
　　Proper interpretation of prescriptions and physician's orders
　　Proper interpretation and updating of prescription records
　　Attention to clerical detail
　　Operation of pharmacy computer systems and software
　　Preparation of compounded prescription products
　　Conversational Spanish
　　CPR training

Activities　　Member, National Pharmacy Technician Association

References available on request.

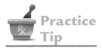

Practice Tip

The cover letter is especially important for online job applications as the employer may not have the time to review all résumés but will scan the letter to screen for qualifications.

Writing a Strong Cover Letter

A cover letter, or letter of application, is the first communication that you send to a prospective employer in response to a job advertisement or posting. This letter can be submitted as a hard copy or, more often, as an online Word or text document or .pdf file. Some employers may use job application software to help screen applications. Applying online is quick, convenient, and saves on travel time and postage costs. The disadvantages of online applications are an increased number of applicants and, occasionally, some fee-based costs at the job search website.

Your résumé should accompany the cover letter. If a hard copy is mailed, the cover letter should be printed on the same kind of paper as the résumé, and both should be placed in a matching business envelope addressed by means of a printer. The letter should be single-spaced, using a block or modified block style. In the block style, all text begins at the left margin. In the modified block style, the sender's address, the complimentary close, and the signature are left-aligned in the center of the paper, and all other parts of the letter begin at the left margin.

The cover letter should highlight your qualifications and call attention to your résumé, preferably in a one-page format (see Table 14.4). The cover letter is especially important for online job applications as the employer may not have the time to review all résumés but will scan the letter to screen for qualifications. A poorly written cover letter detracts from even the most professional résumé. As with your résumé, proofread the cover letter carefully for errors in spelling, grammar, usage, punctuation, capitalization, and form. Address the letter, when possible, to a particular person by name and by title, and make sure to identify the position for which you are applying. Sometimes it takes extra investigation to find out these details, but it shows initiative and professionalism when the letter is addressed to the specific person (with his or her correct degree and title) who is doing the hiring. A letter addressed to "Dear Pharmacy Manager" or "Dear Sir or Madam" does not get the same reception as one addressed to the individual in charge of hiring—for example, the director of pharmacy, pharmacist-in-charge, or the human resources manager.

TABLE 14.4   Suggested Format for Cover Letters

First Paragraph	In your initial paragraph, state why you are writing, what specific position or type of work you are seeking, and how you learned of the opening (e.g., from the placement office, the news media, a friend). If you learned of the opening through someone in your network, then be sure to mention who told you about the position. It may help get the employer's attention.
Second Paragraph	Explain why you are interested in the position, the organization, or the organization's products and services. This may take some investigation, but it shows desire and thoroughness. State how your academic background makes you a qualified candidate for the position. If you have had some practical experience, then point out your specific achievements.
Third Paragraph	Refer the reader to the enclosed or attached résumé: a summary of your qualifications, training, and experience. If specific items on your résumé require an explanation, then tactfully and positively point them out. You can include work experience from outside the pharmacy field, but be sure that it relates to skills that you will use as a technician.
Fourth Paragraph	Indicate your desire for a personal interview and your flexibility as to the time and place. Repeat your telephone number (and cell phone number), as well as the best times to reach you, in the letter. If you use email as a preferred method of communication, then let the employer know that. Close your letter with a statement or question to encourage a response, or take the initiative by indicating a day and date on which you will contact the employer to set up a convenient time for a personal meeting.

FIGURE 14.3
Sample Cover Letter in Block Style

February 1, 201X

James Green, PharmD
Pharmacy Manager
Main Street Community Pharmacy
1500 Main Street
My Town, GA 30107

Dear Dr. Green:

I learned of Main Street Community Pharmacy's need for a pharmacy technician through the placement office at Appalachian Technical College. I was pleased to learn of an opening for a technician at the very pharmacy that my family has frequented for years.

I believe that my education and experience would be an asset to Main Street Community Pharmacy. In May, I graduated from Appalachian Technical College's pharmacy technician training program, and I just took the Pharmacy Technician Certification Examination. I would welcome the opportunity to apply what I have learned to a career with your pharmacy. I bring to the job a number of assets, including a 3.4 grade point average, a commitment to continuing development of my skills as a technician, a willingness to work diligently and accurately, and a desire to be of service.

As you can see from my enclosed résumé, I have experience in the pharmacy setting as well as the retail setting. These positions have required knowledge of business operations and customer service. These skills would certainly lend themselves to your current opening.

I would appreciate an opportunity to discuss the position with you. I will call next week to inquire about a meeting. Thank you for considering my application.

Sincerely,

Kelly Nettleton
1700 Beltline Blvd.
My Town, GA 30107

Enc.: résumé

Pharmacists may have various degrees or titles: Registered Pharmacist (RPh), Bachelor of Science in Pharmacy (BS Pharm), or Doctor of Pharmacy (PharmD). Call the secretary at the employer's office to get the correct spelling (and title if necessary) of the recipient's name. Do not make assumptions. No one likes to receive correspondence with his or her name spelled incorrectly. Figure 14.3 on this page shows a sample cover letter.

Preparing for the Interview

Review your research on the employer and role-play an interview situation. Get plenty of sleep, and eat well on the day before as well as the day of the interview. Find out everything that you can about the company or institution before you go for an interview. Better yet, do this work before you write the cover letter that you send with your résumé. Knowing details about a potential employer can help you assess whether the employer is right for you and can win you points in your cover letter or interview.

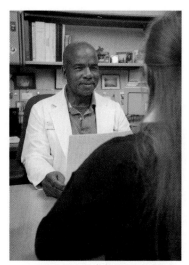

A Pharmacist-In-Charge typically interviews an applicant for a pharmacy technician position.

According to a recent poll reported in *USA Today* from more than 1,900 interviewers, these are the most important factors in how to "blow your interview": not learning about the job or organization (26%), being arrogant (21%), showing up late (15%), not asking any questions (12%), and not speaking professionally (6%). Be cognizant of these pitfalls and come to the interview interested and prepared.

During the interview, follow the guidelines provided in Table 14.5 and be prepared to answer the questions in Table 14.6 on the following page. Rehearse answers to these questions before the interview. Rehearsing out loud can help you identify wording choices and avoid mixing up words during the actual interview. When coming up with answers to such questions, bear in mind the employer's point of view. Imagine what you would want if you were the employer, and then take the initiative during the interview to explain to the employer how you can meet those needs.

Some interviewers pose hypothetical situations and ask for your response, or they may ask you to describe a past experience and how you handled it. These types of questions require you to think on your feet and talk about your problem-solving skills. At the least, be ready to describe a situation or two from your past where you had to deal with a difficult coworker or member of the public. Choose a situation where you were pleased with

---

TABLE 14.5   Guidelines for Job Interviews

1. Find out the exact place and time of the interview. Get directions or information on parking if necessary.
2. Know the full name of the company and its address and the interviewer's full name with its correct pronunciation. Call the employer, if necessary, to get this information.
3. Know something about the company's operations.
4. Pay close attention to your personal appearance. Be sure that your appearance reflects good hygiene and that your clothing and shoes are clean, neat, and appropriate for the job.
5. Bring to the interview your résumé and the names, addresses, and telephone numbers of people who have agreed to provide references.
6. Arrive 10 to 15 minutes before the scheduled time for the interview.
7. Be courteous to the receptionist, if one is present, and to other employees. Any person with whom you meet or speak may be in a position to influence your employment.
8. Greet the interviewer and call him or her by name. Introduce yourself at once. Shake hands only if the interviewer offers to do so. Remain standing until invited to sit down.
9. Be confident, polite, poised, and enthusiastic.
10. Look the interviewer in the eye.
11. Speak clearly and loudly enough to be understood. Be positive and concise in your comments. Do not exaggerate, but remember that an interview is not an occasion for modesty.
12. Focus on your strengths. Be prepared to enumerate these qualities, using specific examples to support the claims that you make about yourself.
13. Do not hesitate to ask about the specific duties associated with the job. Show keen interest as the interviewer tells you about these responsibilities.
14. Avoid bringing up salary requirements until the employer broaches the subject.
15. Do not chew gum or smoke.
16. Do not criticize former employers, coworkers, or working conditions.
17. At the close of the interview, thank the interviewer for his or her time and for the opportunity to learn about the company.

TABLE 14.6 Interview Questions

1. Why did you apply for a job with this company?

2. What part of the job interests you most and why?

3. What do you know about this company?

4. What are your qualifications?

5. What did you like the most and the least about your work experience? (*Note:* Explaining what you liked least should be done in as positive a manner as possible. For example, you might say that you wish that the job had provided more opportunity for learning about this or that and then explain that you made up the deficiency by studying on your own. Such an answer indicates your desire to learn and grow and does not cast your former employer in an unduly negative light.)

6. Why did you leave your previous job? (Avoid negative responses. Find a positive reason for leaving, such as returning to school or pursuing an opportunity.)

7. What would you like to be doing in five years? How much money would you like to be making? (Keep your answer reasonable, and show that you have ambitions consistent with the employer's needs.)

8. What are your weak points? (Say something positive such as, "I am an extremely conscientious person. Sometimes I worry too much about whether I have done something absolutely correctly, but that can also be a positive trait.")

9. Why do you think that you are qualified for this position?

10. Would you mind working on the weekends or putting in overtime? How do you feel about traveling?

11. Do you prefer working with others or by yourself? Do you prefer a quiet or a noisy environment?

12. If you could have any job you wanted, then what would you choose, and why?

13. What information would you like to share about yourself?

14. What are your hobbies and interests?

15. Why did you attend the college that you attended?

16. Why did you choose this field of study?

17. What courses did you like best? What courses did you like least? (State your responses to both questions in positive ways.)

18. Do you plan to continue your education?

19. What have you learned from your mistakes?

20. What motivates you to put forth your greatest efforts?

how you responded, and describe the measures you took to improve the end result. Interviewers should not ask you questions about your religion, marital status, or if you have or plan to have children. You are not obligated to answer questions such as these. If the opportunity arises toward the end of the interview, then be sure to ask any questions that you may have—such as typical work schedule, weekends, vacation, benefits, and so on.

After the interview, follow up with a note thanking the interviewer for seeing you and (within an appropriate time) follow up with a telephone call. Be persistent but not pushy. If you did not get the position, then thank the employer for the opportunity to interview and request that the company keep your cover letter and résumé on file for consideration of future positions.

Performance Reviews

Congratulations, you got the job! Your orientation will include self-study on the computer of pertinent policies and procedures specific to your organization. If you are not certified yet, your organization may pay you for classes, travel costs, and the application fee for the examination. In many large organizations, your performance is under review by your supervisors for the first three to six months. You will be evaluated in many different areas such as:

- customer service and phone etiquette
- computer skills
- pharmacy policy and procedures
- attendance and tardiness
- claims processing
- completion of assignments, teamwork, and communications
- improvement in learning and job skills
- motivation and self-direction

These or similar job responsibilities, skills, and competencies would be evaluated on some sort of scale similar to exceeding, meeting, or falling short of expectations. It is common to self-evaluate your performance, and for a supervisor to independently evaluate your performance. You would meet with your supervisor on a quarterly, semi-annual, or annual basis per policy to compare evaluations. Hopefully, you

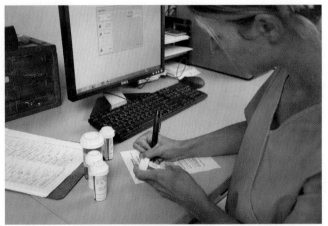

One duty of a pharmacy technician is to reconcile a patient's home medications.

will meet or exceed expectations, but if there are areas that need improvement, you may need to focus on those areas before your next review. You may elect to write down a personal goal or two you hope to achieve in the upcoming months. You and your supervisor often both sign your review for documentation of the meeting and future reference.

Industry Awareness

Pharmacy is continuing to evolve alongside our ever-changing society. Rising healthcare spending will drive demand, creating more jobs for technicians and pharmacists alike. The implementation of the new healthcare law in the United States brings with it untold changes across the healthcare professions, while the development of electronic pharmacy processes is well under way. At the same time, changing demographics and new innovations point to a rapidly shifting landscape for pharmacists, technicians, and patients. It is important for pharmacy technicians to watch the trends of today that will affect the profession for decades to come.

Trends in Healthcare Costs

The United States spends a higher percentage of its gross national product (GNP) on health care than any other country in the world. However, the United States is not among the leaders in average life span: This may be because of risky health behavior (poor diet, lack of exercise, smoking, excessive alcohol consumption, and so on) and the fact that millions of citizens have been without health insurance.

In 2010, the United States spent more than $2.6 trillion on health care, or 17.6% of the gross domestic product (GDP). According to a study by the Kaiser Family Foundation, the average annual health insurance premium for family coverage in 2011 was $15,073.

Health insurance has been increasingly unaffordable for many Americans, especially for those individuals who are out of work, are working only part-time, or have preexisting health conditions. Many businesses are reluctant to hire because of high cost of employer-sponsored health insurance. These higher costs have contributed to many jobs being outsourced overseas. Because of the Affordable Care Act, more uninsured Americans will become insured in 2014 and beyond. The impact on pharmacy will be more new and refill prescriptions dispensed by pharmacy technicians and more need for counseling and monitoring by pharmacists.

According to the Center for Medicare and Medicaid Services (CMS), the annual rate of health spending for the next decade is projected to be 5.8%. That is 1.1% higher than the optimistically projected growth in the GDP. By 2020, healthcare spending is projected to reach $4.64 trillion, accounting for more than one-fifth of the GDP.

This increase in healthcare costs could result in higher taxes, higher insurance premiums, or significant reductions in government programs such as defense, education, or social programs. The passage of recent legislation to initiate government health programs to cover senior citizens and the uninsured accounts for a portion of this expected increase. The long-term impact of Medicare Part D and the Affordable Care Act—coupled with an aging population and budgetary shortfalls—is unknown.

According to the IMS National Prescription Audit, the annual cost of prescription drugs was $307 billion in 2011. By comparison, the annual cost in 1990 was just more than $40 billion. That's a 700% increase in just 20 years! According to the Department of Health and Human Services, the projected drug cost will be $458 billion by 2019—a 100% increase from 2008.

With an aging population and more at-risk patients becoming eligible for insurance programs, prescription volume and drug spending will continue to increase over the next decade and will represent 11% of the nation's GDP, according to economists at the CMS. These cost increases will occur despite the dispensing of more generic drugs and insurance controls such as tiered pricing and prior authorizations.

As patients spend more on health care in the United States, employers who offer health insurance as a benefit pay more and thus experience greater drains on their

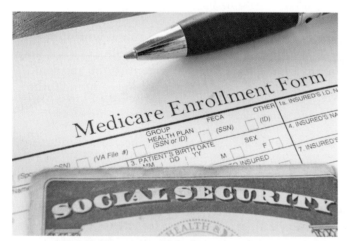

Eligible patients must complete a Medicare Enrollment Form to enroll in the program and receive benefits.

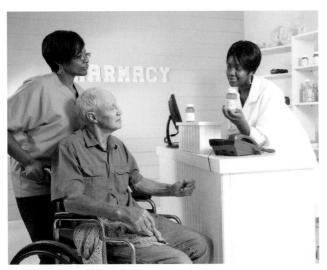

Demand for pharmacy technicians is expected to continue to grow during the next decade because of the increased pharmaceutical needs of a larger elderly population.

bottom lines. As they ask employees to share in the financial burden of these increased costs, patients themselves are becoming more sensitive to the costs of health care and prescription drugs. The trend for employers and individuals alike is for more consumer-driven health insurance plans with higher deductibles to cope, at least partially, with rising healthcare costs and insurance premiums.

An increasing number of prescriptions dispensed translates to an increase in workforce; both pharmacists and pharmacy technicians will be required to meet this need. In addition, pharmacists will be expected to play a more prominent role in controlling drug costs through more effective counseling of patients as well as monitoring disease outcomes with the most cost-effective therapies.

Trends in Pharmacy Practice

One of the wonderful things about a career in pharmacy is that it is a dynamic profession, changing continually. Consider how different the average community pharmacy of today is from the druggist's shop at the turn of the century, in which premanufactured medicines were novelties and rows of bottled tonics and elixirs vied for customers' attention along with open barrels of hard candies. Undoubtedly, the profession will change as much or more in the next 30 years as it did in the past 100 years. Some of these anticipated developments in pharmacy practice are discussed below.

Growing Workforce Needs As the volume of prescriptions rises and reliance on drug therapy increases, the need for qualified personnel in the pharmacy profession continues to grow. The number of prescriptions filled today is more than 4.2 billion per year, and some estimate that this volume will double over the next 5 to 15 years. Consequently, the need for pharmacists to handle this increased workload is expected to double as well. By 2020, up to 400,000 pharmacists may be needed to handle the increased prescription volume. The number of pharmacists, however, is expected to increase only 30% (from less than 200,000 to 260,000) over that same period. Therefore, the need for well-trained, qualified technicians to bridge the gap between the workload and the available personnel will be critical.

Mail-Order Pharmacies The number of mail-order pharmacies increased throughout the 1990s as plan sponsors continued to embrace its use, based on claims of cost savings. To contain rising healthcare costs, many employers mandate mail order or provide financial incentives to participate. Few studies, however, have proven a cost savings. Recent studies on patient satisfaction indicate a preference for local pharmacies by a wide margin over mail-order pharmacies. The co-payments are slightly higher at a local pharmacy, but the personalized customer service is worth the extra cost to many patients.

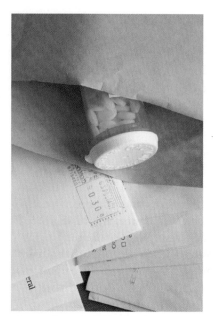

The number of mail-order pharmacies increased in the 1990s.

Until recently, mail order had been the fastest growing distribution channel almost every year. Since 2007, mail-order pharmacies have averaged annual growth of only 1.2% vs. 9.9% for chain pharmacies. In 2011, there were 792 million prescriptions dispensed from mail-order pharmacies. Mail order now represents more than 18% of all U.S. prescription sales with more than $20 billion in annual sales.

The typical patient who uses mail order is at or near retirement age and needs several medications for the many chronic illnesses of aging. Mail order may be especially useful to those patients who are sick and homebound, or do not drive. A mail-order pharmacy is typically a warehouse operation, using the latest automation, with the capacity to dispense 1,000 or more prescriptions per hour, 24 hours a day. (Large national mail-order pharmacies have the capacity to fill 2 million prescriptions per week.) Personnel needs for both pharmacists and pharmacy technicians will expand to oversee these operations and meet the expected growth in this area of practice.

Managed Care Managed care has been applying fiscal constraints to the healthcare system since the early 1990s. Because of its increased emphasis on primary and preventive care and on cost-effective medical services, managed care has revolutionized the healthcare system. As such, the practice of pharmacy has felt the squeeze. Pharmacy is increasingly called upon to provide the most appropriate drug therapy at the lowest possible cost. Technicians will find new opportunities available in support roles with pharmacists who work closely with programs and efforts to encourage smart but inexpensive drug use. These new responsibilities may include gathering data and preparing documentation for pharmacist review, including medication reconciliation, collection/compilation of patients' laboratory results, and patient compliance information. The nature of this work may differ greatly in its day-to-day, hands-on time with drug products. Increased communication, writing, and computer application skills will be necessary for technicians specializing in managed-care settings.

Geriatrics As the population of the United States ages, the volume of dispensing medications will increase. The aging of the population, especially among baby boomers, will place great financial burdens on the healthcare system as a whole and on pharmacy in particular, leading inevitably to political decisions that will affect the workload and workplace of the pharmacist and the technician. According to a 2010 Prudential Research Report, the average cost of a semiprivate room in a nursing home is well over $200 per day with wide geographic variation; in an assisted living facility, with less nursing care, the daily cost is approximately 50% less.

In addition, with Medicare Part D drug insurance, senior citizens now have some coverage for prescription costs. Although this is good news, the Medicare Part D program (and other drug insurance programs) is complex and can be confusing to a population that already finds navigating the Internet and the healthcare system difficult. The concepts of deductibles, co-payments, donut holes, prior authorization, tiered pricing, etc. are confusing to anyone. Pharmacists and technicians will increasingly provide services to the population of older adults in the community pharmacy, as well as in the nursing home and the home healthcare setting.

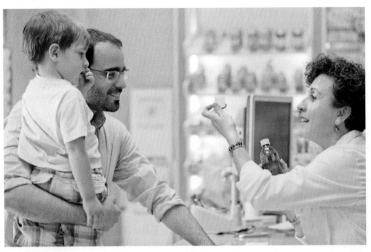
A pharmacist counsels a father on how to give his son the proper dose of medication.

Home Health Care The home health-care industry is one of the most rapidly growing of all industries in the developed world. The reasons behind this growth include reduced cost (compared with hospital care), improvements in technology that make home health care more practical, and the preference of individuals to remain under treatment at home rather than in institutions. Examples may include home total parenteral nutrition (TPN) therapy, HIV/AIDS therapy, cancer chemotherapy, hospice care, home antibiotic infusions, and biogenetic treatments for autoimmune diseases. The average cost of home health care is now more than $200 per day—almost the same as a semi-private room in a nursing home. The growth of the home healthcare industry shows no signs of abating; therefore, in the future, more pharmacists and technicians will find themselves servicing this industry.

Expanding Clinical Applications The pharmaceutical care movement continues to grow. In the future, more of the pharmacy professional's time and energies will be given to educational and counseling functions. For instance, more pharmacies offer specialty services in education and management for patients who have diabetes or asthma. Pharmacists can also improve patient compliance to drug therapy. Research studies have demonstrated that only 50% of patients are taking their medications as prescribed and obtaining the necessary refills. If a patient does not take the prescribed medication(s), then his or her health condition or disease is not controlled. In fact, studies estimate an excess of 125,000 deaths at a cost of $300 billion per year because of noncompliance to medication. Many of these deaths may be prevented or at least delayed with effective counseling and better compliance to therapy.

Pharmacists are commonly administering vaccinations in their communities. Managed care pharmacists may specialize in areas such as anticoagulation control and cholesterol management of patients with high risk for heart disease. In the hospital, pharmacists may specialize in TPN, pharmacokinetics, infectious disease, neonatology, and so on. Home healthcare pharmacists may specialize in pain management for hospice patients. This growth in clinical applications by the pharmacist requires increasing support by pharmacy technicians in the routine functions of medication preparation and dispensing.

Changing Roles and Responsibilities for Pharmacy Technicians Some states are already experimenting with allowing trained technicians to check the work of other technicians. Other states allow pharmacy technicians to accept new prescriptions from a physician's office or operate in a telepharmacy. A telepharmacy uses state-of-the-art telecommunications to provide pharmacy services to patients at a distance. (See page 585 for more information on telepharmacies.) In the future, you can expect technicians to be given greater responsibilities; more technicians will become specialized in particular areas of service, such as sterile and nonsterile compounding and diabetes education. Technicians could find themselves working more on a one-on-one basis with patients to help them choose and use a glucose meter or a blood pressure monitor.

New Medicines and Drug Development Technologies Every day, new medicines come to market, many involving new drug development technologies such as genetic engineering. To work in pharmacy is to be at the front line when new medications are introduced to combat AIDS, cancer, heart disease, cystic fibrosis, and other challenging diseases. Automation in every facet of drug distribution will play an increasingly important role in the profession. What the future holds is anyone's guess, but the one certainty is that new dosage forms, delivery mechanisms, and technologies will continue to evolve and emerge.

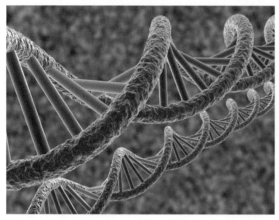

Emerging technology may soon allow for innovative medications based on genetic information.

Innovative New Dosage Forms and Drug Delivery Mechanisms New dosage forms and drug delivery mechanisms are not introduced as often as new drugs, but the pace of innovation is increasing rapidly. In the past few years, such innovations as additional transdermal medications, ocular inserts, long-acting medications lasting more than a month, liposomes, and monoclonal antibodies have been introduced. Newer biotechnological cancer therapies will target the cancer cells without harming normal cells and causing adverse side effects. Biotechnological therapies will continue to be prescribed for patients with rheumatoid arthritis, resulting in dramatic pain relief.

In the near future, a wearable intravenous (IV) infusion pump may be combined with a continuous sensory meter, creating, in effect, an artificial pancreas. The pharmaceutical industry will continue to manufacture innovative injectable diabetic medications in both vials and pens to help control the blood glucose levels of an ever-increasing patient population. In fact, checking blood glucose levels noninvasively with lasers or administering insulin injections without needles may be commonplace within the next five years as technologies continue to advance.

Use of Automation As you have already learned, automation will continue to improve the efficiency and safety of medication dispensing and will help to bridge the manpower gap. Many community and hospital pharmacies will invest in automated robotic dispensing systems as the costs decrease. The use of bar-code scanning technologies—to verify, fill, dispense, and administer medications and monitor inventory—will continue to grow and improve the quality and safety of health care in our pharmacies and hospitals. Automated controllers for making labor-intensive TPN solutions and widespread use of programmable IV infusion pumps all result in fewer dosing and administration errors.

The use of e-prescriptions and adoption of interdisciplinary electronic medical records will continue to increase over the next decade. This electronic documentation will certainly have a positive impact on medication errors attributed to poor handwriting and transcription. E-prescribing alone increased from 326 million prescriptions in 2010 to 570 million in 2011.

A successful telepharmacy pilot project in North Dakota is being adopted in many areas without close proximity to a pharmacy. These telepharmacies are staffed by pharmacy technicians (or nurses) predominantly in rural areas. The technician uses a remote camera to send the following information to an off-site pharmacist: the original prescription, computer-generated label, stock bottle, and the patient medication vial/bottle/tube. After approval, the patient has a mandatory private consultation with a pharmacist through real-time video and audio.

Shifting Roles As the pace of work in pharmacies around the country increases, the demands on pharmacists for more direct patient care, drug therapy assessment, and cognitive duties will also expand. Pharmacists will place more emphasis on medication counseling and monitoring for adverse reactions and drug interactions as well as consulting with prescribers. The goal would be to prescribe the most cost-effective medication for the medical condition and to dispense the prescription or medication order without error. Technicians must step in to manage the routine workflow and prescription processing systems in the community and hospital pharmacies to keep up with these new demands on the pharmacists' time. Employment opportunities for pharmacy technicians look extremely good, especially for technicians who are certified or who have formal training or previous experience. For those technicians with previous experience, several innovative positions are rapidly developing, including:

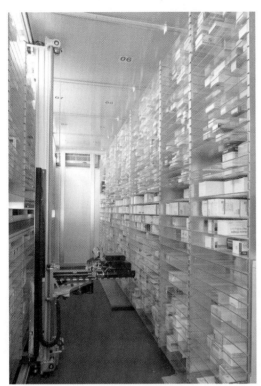

The increased use of automation technology helps pharmacy personnel provide services more efficiently and safely.

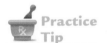

Practice Tip

The use of barcode scanning and automated e-prescriptions has greatly improved patient safety.

- nuclear pharmacy technician
- pharmacy distribution center supervisor
- pharmacy benefits manager
- sterile compounding technician
- nonsterile compounding technician
- medication reconciliation pharmacy technician
- pharmacy informatics technician
- quality assurance pharmacy technician
- lead pharmacy technician/supervisor
- pharmacy technician instructor or program director

Chapter Summary

- Preparing to work in an institutional or community-based pharmacy requires serious thought about one's attitude, reliability, accuracy, responsibility, personal appearance, organizational skills, and ability to relate to others.
- Society holds the pharmacy technician, as a paraprofessional, to a strict code of ethics.
- Technicians will have increasing opportunities for job advancement as requirements for certification and training increase.
- Certification for pharmacy technicians is offered through the Pharmacy Technician Certification Board (PTCB) and the Institute for the Certification of Pharmacy Technicians (ICPT).
- More states are requiring national certification and a standardized formal education for pharmacy technicians.
- Specialty certifications and experience may be required in select areas of pharmacy practice.
- A hierarchy of pharmacy technician positions has evolved to reflect specialization, training, and credentials.

- Active involvement in professional organizations is important for establishing a network of colleagues and for professional advancement.
- Clarifying your career goals, networking, and researching the job market are crucial first steps to starting your career.
- Writing a comprehensive, attractive résumé and cover letter is an important part of a carefully planned job search.
- Preparing for a job interview is integral to obtaining a desirable pharmacy technician position.
- Total healthcare and prescription costs will increase as a part of the U.S. gross domestic product over the next decade.
- Several trends will have an impact on the role of pharmacy technicians in the workplace, including an aging patient population, the use of automation, and the changing role of the pharmacist.
- The short- and long-term occupational outlooks for pharmacy technicians are promising.

Key Terms

certification the process by which a professional organization grants recognition to an individual who has met certain predetermined qualifications

Certified Pharmacy Technician (CPhT) a pharmacy technician who has passed the Pharmacy Technician Certification Examination (PTCE) or Exam for Certification of Pharmacy Technicians (ExCPT)

credential a documented piece of evidence of one's qualifications

Exam for Certification of Pharmacy Technicians (ExCPT) an examination developed by the Institute for the Certification of Pharmacy Technicians (ICPT) that technicians must pass to be certified and receive the title of CPhT

licensure the granting of a license by the state, usually to work in a profession, to protect the public

paraprofessional a trained person who assists a professional person

Pharmacy Technician Certification Examination (PTCE) an examination developed by the Pharmacy Technician Certification Board (PTCB) that technicians must pass to be certified and receive the title of CPhT

professional an individual with recognized expertise in a field who is expected to use his or her knowledge and skills to benefit others and to operate ethically with some autonomy

recertification the periodic updating of certification

registration mandatory signing up or registering with the State Board of Pharmacy before
starting to practice

Chapter Review

 Additional Quiz Questions

Checking Your Understanding

*To check your comprehension of this chapter's key concepts, read the following multiple-choice questions and then
record your answers on a separate sheet of paper. Write your answers as modeled in these examples: 1d; 2c; 3b; etc.*

1. An organization that certifies pharmacy
   technicians is the
   a. Pharmacy Technician Certification
      Board (PTCB).
   b. American Pharmaceutical Association.
   c. Food and Drug Administration.
   d. State Board of Pharmacy.

2. The format for the PTCE and ExCPT
   examinations is
   a. essay.
   b. multiple choice.
   c. true or false.
   d. on-site laboratory assessment.

3. According to the Bureau of Labor Statistics,
   the need for pharmacy technicians within
   the next few years will
   a. increase.
   b. decrease.
   c. remain the same.
   d. depend on State Board of Pharmacy
      regulations.

4. Which of the following items is *not* a
   requirement for a candidate taking the
   pharmacy technician certification exam?
   a. 18 years of age or older
   b. a high school diploma or GED
   c. 50 hours of work experience in a
      community or hospital pharmacy
   d. no felony convictions

5. Once a technician becomes certified (i.e., a
   CPhT), he or she must become recertified
   every
   a. six months.
   b. year.
   c. two years.
   d. five years.

6. Which category of the PTCE carries the
   highest weighted percentage?
   a. Pharmacology for Technicians
   b. Medication Safety
   c. Pharmacy Laws and Regulations
   d. Medication Order Entry and Fill Process

7. A standard résumé typically does *not*
   provide
   a. the job objective.
   b. the applicant's employment history.
   c. the applicant's name, address, and
      telephone number.
   d. the names, addresses, and telephone
      numbers of references.

8. A candidate without a great deal of
   work experience can compensate for this
   deficiency by emphasizing the
   a. employment history section of the
      résumé.
   b. references section of the résumé.
   c. job objective section of the résumé.
   d. skills section of the résumé.

9. The cover letter sent with a résumé should highlight your
   a. qualifications.
   b. personality.
   c. network of connections.
   d. need for the job.

10. How will the increasing geriatric patient population affect the job responsibilities of pharmacy technicians?
    a. Technicians will be needed to focus on patient compliance to drug therapy.
    b. Technicians will be needed to consult with prescribers about the specific medication needs of patients.
    c. Technicians will need to become familiar with Medicare Part D to assist these patients in gaining needed information about this drug coverage program.
    d. Because of a shortage of pharmacists, technicians will be needed to counsel patients.

11. Which of the following statements about pharmacy technician certification is correct?
    a. Certification is granted by a governmental body.
    b. Certification is mandatory in all states.
    c. Certification is transferrable to all states.
    d. Certification requires college course work.

12. Since its inception, the passing rate for the PTCB certification exam is approximately
    a. 25%.
    b. 50%.
    c. 75%.
    d. 90%.

13. Studies have demonstrated that the *most important* part of preparing for a job interview is to
    a. be on time.
    b. learn as much as you can about the job and responsibilities.
    c. ask a lot of questions, especially about salary and benefits.
    d. wear professional attire.

14. Within the next decade, prescription costs alone are projected to consume what percent of the gross domestic product (GDP) in the United States?
    a. 11%
    b. 17.6%
    c. 20%
    d. 26.2%

15. What is the estimated number of excessive deaths due to noncompliance to prescribed medication?
    a. 50,000
    b. 125,000
    c. 140,000
    d. 175,000

Reinforcing Your Learning

To build on your understanding of the topics in this chapter, complete the following enrichment activities.

1. Compile a list of three potential employers of pharmacy technicians in each of the following areas in your state: community pharmacy, hospital pharmacy, long-term care, and home infusion. Each list should include the name of the employer, the address, the telephone number, an email address, and a contact person. Collect the lists prepared by the students in your class to make a master list.

2. Choose one potential employer of pharmacy technicians and find more information about the employer. Write a brief report providing information that might be of interest to a potential employee of this pharmacy or institution. Write a résumé and cover letter that you might use to apply for a job as a pharmacy technician.

3. Practice role-playing an interview situation with other students in your class. Use the interview questions supplied in this chapter. Develop or update your résumé. Share your résumé with another student. Ask that student to critique and identify your strengths, based on your résumé.

Thinking on Your Feet

To gain practice in handling challenging situations in the workplace, consider the following real-world scenarios and then use the guiding questions to help you formulate your responses.

1. You live in a northern border state. A patient without prescription drug insurance is trying to make ends meet and asks about purchasing drugs from a mail-order pharmacy in Canada. How can you assure the patient that the pharmacy and drugs are legitimate? What resources would you recommend?

2. During an interview, the interviewer asks you to describe your strengths and weaknesses. How would you respond? How could you strengthen the weaknesses you identified?

3. You are planning to enroll in pharmacy school next year. During the interview for a pharmacy technician position, the interviewer asks you to discuss your long-term goals. How would you respond? If you answer honestly, might it jeopardize your chances? Do you say you are making a long-term commitment to the tech position, or do you say your career goals may change in the future?

4. During "open enrollment," an elderly relative requests your assistance in selecting a Medicare Part D prescription insurance plan. Go to the Medicare website (www .paradigmcollege.net/pharmpractice5e/ prescriptionplan) and enter the prescription information. Determine what prescription plan would be best for your relative and calculate its monthly cost.

Acquiring Field Knowledge

To expand your knowledge of pharmacy practice, explore the following online activities that focus on research and information retrieval.

> **Reminder:** *As you navigate the Internet, remember to exercise caution and good judgment when evaluating information. A thoughtful review of online text should take into consideration the following factors: the creator and sponsors of the website, the intended audience, the credentials of the authors and contributors, the reliability and valididty of the posted information, the frequency of updates to the site, and the ease of navigation for a range of user skill levels.*

1. As a certified pharmacy technician, you are required to complete continuing education courses. One source is the website www .paradigmcollege.net/pharmpractice5e/ CEcredits. Select and complete a CE course of your choosing and submit a short written summary. Identify other online sites for CE for pharmacy technicians.

2. Go to the websites or write a letter to the PTCB (www.paradigmcollege .net/pharmpractice5e/PTCEcertexam) or ICPT (www.paradigmcollege.net/ pharmpractice5e/ExCPTcertexam)

reviewing or requesting the information needed to take their certification exam. Check their mission statements and affiliations with professional organizations. Which organization do you prefer, and why?

3. Search the Web for the American Association of Pharmacy Technicians (AAPT) at www.paradigmcollege.net/ pharmpractice5e/jobs. Go to the Career Center and look for jobs in your state. Sign up for job alerts.

4. Go to your local state pharmacist association website and seek available pharmacy technician job opportunities. Check out available online and in-person CE programs at your state pharmacist association website.

5. Patients may elect to receive medications from online pharmacies. Go to www.para digmcollege.net/pharmpractice5e/VIPPS and investigate VIPPS. What is VIPPS? Identify four criteria to become a VIPPS pharmacy.

Sampling the Certification Exam

To provide you with practice for the Certification Exam, read the following questions that have been patterned after the test format and then record your answers on a separate sheet of paper. Write your answers as modeled in these examples: 1d; 2c; 3b; etc.

1. By definition, a certified pharmacy technician is considered a
   a. professional.
   b. paraprofessional.
   c. clerk.
   d. cashier.

2. While all the following qualities are important, one of the greatest predictors of job success is your
   a. attitude.
   b. personality.
   c. sense of responsibility.
   d. reliability.

3. Within 30 days of working in a pharmacy, most states require you to register with the
   a. FDA.
   b. USP.
   c. State Board of Pharmacy.
   d. state pharmacy association.

4. For the pharmacy technician, proper credentialing is accomplished through
   a. licensure.
   b. continuing education.
   c. registration.
   d. certification.

5. The trend in technician training programs is
   a. less standardization and more experiences.
   b. more standardization and fewer experiences.
   c. more standardization and more experiences.
   d. all didactic coursework with experiences postcertification.

6. Misspellings on your résumé may negatively reflect on your
   a. accuracy.
   b. reliability.
   c. communication skills.
   d. ability to work on a team.

7. Within the next decade, total healthcare spending will consume what percent of gross domestic product (GDP) in the United States?
   a. 10%
   b. 20%
   c. 30%
   d. 40%

8. The number of prescriptions projected to be filled annually over the next 5 to 15 years in retail pharmacies is
   a. 1.9 billion.
   b. 2.4 billion.
   c. 4.2 billion.
   d. 8.4 billion.

9. Prescription coverage for seniors over age 65 is covered under which Medicare plan?
   a. Part A
   b. Part B
   c. Part C
   d. Part D

10. By 2020, what will be the projected shortage of pharmacists in the United States?
    a. 55,000
    b. 98,000
    c. 140,000
    d. 200,000

Appendix A
Most Commonly Prescribed Drugs

This table presents the most commonly prescribed drugs in the United States. The drugs are listed by their generic names.

Generic Name	Pronunciation	Classification	Brand Name
acetaminophen/ codeine	a-seat-a-MIN-oh-fen/ KOE-deen	opioid analgesic	Tylenol/ codeine
acyclovir	ay-SYE-kloe-veer	antiviral	Zovirax
albuterol	al-BYOO-ter-ole	beta-2 agonist	Ventolin HFA
albuterol (nebulizer solution)	al-BYOO-ter-ole	beta-2 agonist	AccuNeb
albuterol HFA	al-BYOO-ter-ole	beta-2 agonist	Pro-Air HFA
alendronate	a-LEN-droe-nate	bisphosphonate	Fosamax
allopurinol	al-o-PURE-i-nole	antigout agent xanthine oxidase inhibitor	Zyloprim
alprazolam	al-PRAY-zoe-lam	benzodiazepine	Xanax
amitriptyline	a-mee-TRIP-ti-leen	antidepressant tricyclic	Elavil
amlodipine	am-LOE-di-peen	antianginal calcium channel blocker	Norvasc
amoxicillin	a-moks-i-SIL-in	antibiotic penicillin	Amoxil
amoxicillin ER	a-moks-i-SIL-in	antibiotic penicillin	Moxatag
aripiprazole	ay-ri-PIP-ra-zole	antipsychotic	Abilify
aspirin (EC)	AS-pir-in	antiplatelet	Bayer Aspirin EC
atenolol	a-TEN-oh-lole	beta blocker	Tenormin
atorvastatin	a-TORE-va-sta-tin	antilipemic	Lipitor
azithromycin	az-ith-ro-MYE-sin	antibiotic macrolide	Zithromax, Z-Pak
baclofen	BAK-loe-fen	skeletal muscle relaxant	Lioresal
benazepril	ben-AY-ze-pril	ACE inhibitor	Lotensin
benzonatate	ben-ZO-na-tate	antitussive	Tessalon

Generic Name	Pronunciation	Classification	Brand Name
bisoprolol-hydrochlorothiazide	bis-OH-proe-lol hye-droe-klor-oh-THYE-a-side	beta blocker/diuretic	Ziac
budesonide/formoterol	byoo-DES-oh-nide/for-MOH-te-rol	beta-2 agonist/corticosteroid	Symbicort
buprenorphine/naloxone	byoo-pre-NOR-feen/nal-OKS-own	opioid analgesic	Suboxone
bupropion	byoo-PROE-pee-on	antidepressant	Budeprion, Wellbutrin, Zyban
bupropion SR	byoo-PROE-pee-on	antidepressant	Budeprion SR, Wellbutrin SR
bupropion XL	byoo-PROE-pee-on	antidepressant	Budeprion XL, Wellbutrin XL
butalbital acetamino-phen-caffeine	byoo-TAL-bi-tal a-seat-a-MIN-oh-fen KAF-een	barbiturate	Fioricet, Esgic Plus
carisoprodol	kar-eye-so-PROE-dole	skeletal muscle relaxant	Soma
carvedilol	kar-ve-DI-lole	beta blocker	Coreg
cefdinir	SEF-di-ner	antibiotic cephalosporin	Omnicef
celecoxib	sele-KOKS-ib	NSAID	Celebrex
cephalexin	sef-a-LEKS-in	antibiotic cephalosporin	Keflex
chlorhexidine gluconate	klor-HEKS-i-deen GLOO-ko-nate	antiseptic	Peridex
ciprofloxacin	sip-roe-FLOX-a-sin	antibiotic quinolone	Cipro
citalopram	sye-TAL-oh-pram	antidepressant SSRI	Celexa
clarithromycin	kla-RITH-roh-my-sin	antibiotic macrolide	Biaxin
clobetasol	kloe-BAY-ta-sol	corticosteroid	Temovate, Olux
clonazepam	kloe-NAZ-e-pam	benzodiazepine	Klonopin
clonidine	KLON-i-dine	alpha-2 adrenergic agonist	Catapres
clopidogrel	kloe-PID-oh-grel	antiplatelet agent	Plavix
clotrimazole-betamethasone	kloe-TRIM-a-zole bay-ta-METH-a-sone	antifungal/corticosteroid	Lotrisone
colchicine	KOL-chi-seen	antigout	Colcrys
cyclobenzaprine	sye-kloe-BEN-za-preen	skeletal muscle relaxant	Flexeril
dextroamphetamine-amphetamine	deks-troe-am-FET-a-min am-FET-a-meen	stimulant	Adderall

Generic Name	Pronunciation	Classification	Brand Name
dextroamphetamine-amphetamine XR	deks-troe-am-FET-a-meen am-FET-a-meen	stimulant	Adderall XR
diazepam	dye-AZ-e-pam	benzodiazepine	Valium
diclofenac	dye-KLOE-fen-ak	NSAID	Cataflam
dicyclomine	dye-SYE-kloe-meen	anticholinergic	Bentyl
digoxin	di-JOKS-in	antiarrhythmic	Lanoxin
diltiazem CD	dil-TYE-a-zem	antianginal calcium channel blocker	Cardizem CD
divalproex	dye-VAL-pro-ex	anticonvulsant	Depakote
donepezil	doh-NEP-e-zil	acetylcholinesterase inhibitor	Aricept
doxazosin	doks-AY-zoe-sin	alpha-1 blocker	Cardura
doxycycline	doks-i-SYE-kleen	antibiotic tetracycline	Vibramycin
duloxetine	doo-LOKS-e-teen	antidepressant SSRI	Cymbalta
dutasteride	do-TAS-teer-ide	5-alpha-reductase inhibitor	Avodart
enalapril	e-NAL-a-pril	ACE inhibitor	Vasotec
escitalopram	es-sye-TAL-oh-pram	antidepressant SSRI	Lexapro
esomeprazole	es-oh-MEP-rah-zole	proton pump inhibitor	Nexium
estradiol	es-tra-DYE-ole	estrogen	Estrace, Climara, Femring
estrogens (conjugated)	ES-troe-jenz	estrogen	Premarin
eszopiclone	es-zoe-PIK-lone	hypnotic	Lunesta
ethinyl estradiol-drospirenone	ETH-in-yl es-tra-DYE-ole droh-SPYE-re-none	contraceptive	Ocella, Yaz
ethinyl estradiol-etonogestrel	ETH-in-yl es-tra-DYE-ole et-noe-JES-trel	contraceptive	NuvaRing
ethinyl estradiol-levonorgestrel	ETH-in-yl es-tra-DYE-ole LE-voe-nor-jes-trel	contraceptive	Aviane
ethinyl estradiol–norethindrone and ferrous fumerate	ETH-in-yl es-tra-DYE-ole nor-eth-IN-drone	contraceptive	Loestrin 24 FE
ethinyl estradiol-norgestimate	ETH-in-yl es-tra-DYE-ole nor-JES-ti-mate	contraceptive	Tri-Sprintec, Ortho Tri-cyclen Lo, Sprintec, TriNessa
ezetimibe	ez-ET-i-mibe	antilipemic	Zetia

Generic Name	Pronunciation	Classification	Brand Name
ezetimibe-simvastatin	ez-ET-i-mibe SIM-va-stat-in	antilipemic	Vytorin
famotidine	fa-MOE-ti-dine	H₂ antagonist	Pepcid
fenofibrate	fen-oh-FYE-brate	antilipemic	TriCor
fenofibric acid	fen-oh-FYE-brik AS-id	antilipemic	Trilipix
fentanyl (transdermal)	FEN-ta-nil	opioid analgesic	Duragesic
ferrous sulfate	FER-us SUL-fate	iron supplement	Feosol, Slow FE
fexofenadine	feks-oh-FEN-a-deen	antihistamine H₁ antagonist	Allegra
finasteride	fi-NAS-teer-ide	5-alpha-reductase inhibitor	Proscar
fluconazole	floo-KOE-na-zole	antifungal	Diflucan
fluoxetine	floo-OKS-e-teen	antidepressant SSRI	Prozac
fluticasone (HFA)	floo-TIK-a-sone	corticosteroid	Flovent
fluticasone (nasal spray)	floo-TIK-a-sone	corticosteroid	Flonase
fluticasone/salmeterol	floo-TIK-a-sone/sal-ME-ter-ole	beta-2 agonist/ corticosteroid	Advair
folic acid	FOE-lik AS-id	vitamin	Folate
furosemide	fyoor-OH-se-mide	diuretic	Lasix
gabapentin	GA-ba-pen-tin	anticonvulsant	Neurontin
glimepiride	GLYE-me-pye-ride	antidiabetic sulfonylurea	Amaryl
glipizide	GLIP-i-zide	antidiabetic sulfonylurea	Glucotrol
glipizide ER	GLIP-i-zide	antidiabetic sulfonylurea	Glucotrol XL
glipizide XL	GLIP-i-zide	antidiabetic sulfonylurea	Glucotrol XL
glyburide	GLYE-byoor-ide	antidiabetic sulfonylurea	DiaBeta, Glynase
glyburide/metformin	GLYE-byoor-ride/met-FOR-man	antidiabetic biguanide/sulfonylurea	Glucovance
guaifenesin/codeine	gwy-a-FEN-e-sin/KOE-deen	antitussive	Cheratussin AC
hydralazine	hye-DRAL-a-zen	vasodilator	Apresoline
hydrochlorothiazide	hye-droe-klor-oh-THYE-a-side	diuretic	Microzide
hydrocodone/ acetaminophen	hye-droe-KOE-done/ a-seat-a-MIN-oh-fen	opioid analgesic	Lortab, Vicodin, Norco

Generic Name	Pronunciation	Classification	Brand Name
hydroxyzine	hy-DROKS-i-zeen	H$_1$ antagonist	Vistaril, Atarax
ibandronate	eye-BAN-droh-nate	bisphosphonate derivative	Boniva
ibuprofen	eye-byoo-PROE-fen	NSAID	Advil, Motrin
insulin aspart	IN-soo-lin AS-part	antidiabetic	NovoLog
insulin glargine	IN-soo-lin GLAR-jeen	antidiabetic	Lantus
insulin lispro	IN-soo-lin LYE-sproe	antidiabetic	Humalog
ipratropium-albuterol	i-pra-TROE-pee-um al-BYOO-ter-ole	anticholinergic beta-2 agonist	Combivent
irbesartan	ir-be-SAR-tan	angiotensin II receptor blocker	Avapro
isosorbide	eye-soe-SOR-bide	antianginal vasodilator	Imdur
lamotrigine	la-MOE-tri-jeen	anticonvulsant	Lamictal
latanoprost	la-TA-noe-prost	antiglaucoma prostaglandin	Xalatan
levetiracetam	lee-va-tyre-RA-se-tam	anticonvulsant	Keppra
levothyroxine	lee-voe-thye-ROKS-een	thyroid hormone replacement	Synthroid, Levoxyl
lisdexamfetamine	les-dex-am-FET-a-meen	stimulant	Vyvanse
lisinopril	lyse-IN-oh-pril	ACE inhibitor	Prinivil, Zestril
lisinopril-hydrochlorothiazide	lyse-IN-o-pril hye-droe-klor-oh-THYE-a-side	ACE inhibitor/diuretic	Prinzide, Zestoretic
lorazepam	lor-AZE-pam	benzodiazepine	Ativan
losartan	loe-SAR-tan	angiotensin II receptor blocker	Cozaar
losartan-hydrochlorothiazide	loe-SAR-tan hye-droe-klor-oh-THYE-a-side	angiotensin II receptor blocker	Hyzaar
lovastatin	LOE-va-sta-tin	antilipemic agent	Mevacor
meclizine	MEK-li-zeen	antiemetic H$_1$ antagonist	Antivert
meloxicam	mel-OKS-a-kam	NSAID	Mobic
memantine	me-MAN-tine	N-Methyl-D-Aspartate receptor agonist	Namenda
metformin	met-FOR-min	antidiabetic biguanide	Glucophage
methocarbamol	meth-oh-KAR-ba-mole	skeletal muscle relaxant	Robaxin
methotrexate	meth-oh-TREKS-ate	antineoplastic	Rheumatrex
methylphenidate	meth-il-FEN-i-date	stimulant	Concerta
methylprednisolone	meth-il-pred-NIS-o-lone	corticosteroid	Medrol
metoclopramide	met-oh-KLOE-pra-mide	antiemetic	Reglan
metoprolol (succinate)	me-toe-PROE-lole	beta blocker	Toprol XL

Generic Name	Pronunciation	Classification	Brand Name
metoprolol (tartrate)	me-toe-PROE-lole	antianginal	Lopressor
metronidazole	met-roe-NYE-da-zole	antibiotic and amebicide	Flagyl
mirtazapine	mir-TAZ-a-peen	antidepressant	Remeron
mometasone	moe-MET-a-sone	corticosteroid	Nasonex
montelukast	mon-te-LOO-kast	leukotriene receptor agonist	Singulair
moxifloxacin	moks-i-FLOKS-a-sin	antibiotic quinolone	Vigamox
nabumetone	na-BYOO-me-tone	NSAID	Relafen
naproxen	na-PROKS-en	NSAID	Aleve, Anaprox
nebivolol	ne-BIV-oh-lole	beta blocker	Bystolic
niacin	NYE-a-sin	antilipemic	Niaspan
nifedipine ER	nye-FED-i-peen	antianginal calcium channel blocker	Adalat, Procardia
nitroglycerin	nye-tro-GLIS-er-in	antianginal vasodilator	Minitran, Nitro-Dur
nortriptyline	nor-TRIP-ti-leen	tricyclic antidepressant	Pamelor
nystatin (topical)	nye-STAT-in	antifungal	Nystop
olanzapine	oh-LANZ-a-peen	antipsychotic	Zyprexa
olmesartan	ole-me-SAR-tan	angiotensin II receptor blocker	Benicar
omega-3 acid	oh-MEG-a three AS-id	antilipemic	Lovaza
omeprazole	oh-MEP-ra-zole	proton pump inhibitor	Prilosec
oxycodone ER	oks-i-KOE-done	opioid analgesic	OxyContin
oxycodone-acetaminophen	oks-i-KOE-done a-seat-a-MIN-oh-fen	opioid analgesic	Percocet, Tylox
pantoprazole	pan-TOE-pra-zole	proton pump inhibitor	Protonix
paroxetine	pa-ROKS-e-teen	antidepressant SSRI	Paxil
phenazopyridine	fen-az-oh-PEER-i-deen	urinary analgesic	Pyridium, Azo-Standard
phentermine	FEN-ter-meen	anorexiant	Adipex-P
pioglitazone	pye-oh-GLI-ta-zone	antidiabetic thiazolidine	Actos
polyethylene glycol	pol-i-ETH-i-leen GLY-col	laxative	MiraLAX
potassium chloride	poe-TASS-e-um KLOR-ide	electrolyte supplement	Klor-Con
potassium chloride ER	poe-TASS-e-um-KLOR-ide	electrolyte supplement	K-Dur, Klor-Con M
pravastatin	prav-a-STAT-in	antilipemic agent	Pravachol
prednisolone	pred-NISS-oh-lone	corticosteroid	Orapred, Pediapred

Generic Name	Pronunciation	Classification	Brand Name
pregabalin	pre-GAB-a-lin	analgesic anticonvulsant	Lyrica
promethazine	pro-METH-a-zeen	antiemetic	Phenergan
promethazine-codeine	pro-METH-a-zeen KOE-deen	opioid analgesic	Phenergan/codeine
propranolol	proe-PRAN-oh-lol	beta blocker	Inderal
quetiapine	kwe-TYE-a-peen	antipsychotic	Seroquel
quinapril	KWIN-a-pril	ACE inhibitor	Accupril
rabeprazole	ra-BEP-ra-zole	proton pump inhibitor	AcipHex
raloxifene	ral-OKS-i-feen	estrogen receptor modulator	Evista
ramipril	RA-mi-pril	ACE inhibitor	Altace
ranitidine	ra-NI-ti-deen	H_2 antagonist	Zantac
risperidone	ris-PER-i-done	antipsychotic	Risperdal
rosuvastatin	roe-soo-va-STAT-in	antilipemic	Crestor
sertraline	SER-tra-leen	antidepressant SSRI	Zoloft
sildenafil	sil-DEN-a-fil	phosphodiesterase-5-enzyme inhibitor	Viagra
simvastatin	sim-va-STAT-in	antilipemic	Zocor
sitagliptin	sit-a-GLIP-tin	antidiabetic DPP-4 inhibitor	Januvia
spironolactone	speer-on-oh-LAK-tone	diuretic	Aldactone
sumatriptan	soo-ma-TRIP-tan	serotonin 5-HT 1 receptor agonist	Imitrex
tadalafil	tah-DA-la-fil	phosphodiesterase-5 enzyme inhibitor	Cialis
tamsulosin	tam-SOO-loe-sin	alpha-1 blocker	Flomax
temazepam	te-MAZ-e-pam	benzodiazepine	Restoril
terazosin	ter-AY-zoe-sin	alpha-1 blocker	Hytrin
tiotropium	ty-oh-TRO-pee-um	anticholinergic	Spiriva
tizanidine	tye-ZAN-i-deen	alpha-2 adrenergic agonist	Zanaflex
tolterodine LA	tole-TER-oh-deen	anticholinergic	Detrol LA
topiramate	toe-PIE-ruh-mate	anticonvulsant	Topamax
tramadol	TRA-ma-dole	opioid analgesic	Ultram
trazodone	TRAZ-oh-done	antidepressant SSRI	Desyrel
triamcinolone	try-am-SIN-oh-lone	corticosteroid	Kenalog

Generic Name	Pronunciation	Classification	Brand Name
triamterene-hydrochlorothiazide	try-AM-ter-en hye-droe-klor-oh-THYE-a-side	diuretic	Dyazide, Maxzide
trimethoprim-sulfamethoxazole	try-METH-oh-prim sul-fa-meth-OKS-a-zole	antibiotic sulfa	Bactrim
valacyclovir	val-ay-SYE-kloe-veer	antiviral	Valtrex
valsartan	val-SAR-tan	angiotensin II receptor blocker	Diovan
valsartan-hydrochlorothiazide	val-SAR-tan hye-droe-klor-oh-THYE-a-side	angiotensin II blocker/diuretic	Diovan/HCT
venlafaxine XR	ven-la-FAX-een	antidepressant SSRI	Effexor XR
warfarin	WAR-far-in	anticoagulant	Coumadin
zolpidem	zole-PI-dem	hypnotic	Ambien
zolpidem CR	zole-PI-dem	hypnotic	Ambien CR

Appendix B

Top Drugs Administered in Hospitals

This table contains the most commonly administered drugs in hospitals in the United States. The drugs are listed by their generic names.

Generic Name	Category	Brand Name
adenosine	antiarrhythmic	Adenocard
atorvastatin	lipid-lowering agent	Lipitor
azithromycin	antibacterial	Zithromax
bevacizumab	monoclonal antibody	Avastin
bivalirudin	anticoagulant	Angiomax
bovine thrombin	coagulant	Thrombin-JMI
caspofungin	antifungal	Cancidas
cetuximab	monoclonal antibody	Erbitux
clopidogrel	antiplatelet	Plavix
daptomycin	cyclic lipopeptide	Cubicin
darbepoetin alfa	renal disease	Aranesp
desflurane	anesthetic	Suprane
docetaxel	plant alkaloid	Taxotere
enoxaparin	heparin	Lovenox
epoetin alfa	colony-stimulating factor	Procrit
eptifibatide	glycoprotein antagonist	Integrilin
esomeprazole	proton pump inhibitor	Nexium
filgrastim	colony-stimulating factor	Neupogen
fluticasone-salmeterol	anti-asthma	Advair Diskus
gemcitabine	antineoplastic agent	Gemzar
imipenem-cilastatin	carbapenem	Primaxin
immune globulin	hepatitis	Gamunex
infliximab	monoclonal antibody	Remicade
levofloxacin	quinolone	Levaquin
linezolid	antibiotic	Zyvox

Top Drugs Administered in Hospitals (continued)

Generic Name	Category	Brand Name
morphine	analgesic	MS Contin
nicardipine	calcium channel blocker	Cardene
olanzapine	antipsychotic	Zyprexa
oxaliplatin	alkylating agent	Eloxatin
palivizumab	monoclonal antibody	Synagis
pantoprazole	proton pump inhibitor	Protonix
pegfilgrastim	colony-stimulating factor	Neulasta
piperacillan-tazobactam	penicillin	Zosyn
propofol	anesthetic	Diprivan
quetiapine	antipsychotic	Seroquel
risperidone	antipsychotic	Risperdal
rituximab	monoclonal antibody	Rituxan
sevoflurane	anesthetic	Ultane
simvastatin	lipid-lowering agent	Zocor
sodium chloride	electrolyte	(none)
trastuzumab	monoclonal antibody	Herceptin
vancomycin	antibiotic	Vancocin
zoledronic acid	bisphosphonate	Zometa

Abbreviation	Meaning
A-B-C	
aaa	apply to affected area
ac; a.c.; AC	before meals
ad; a.d.; AD	right ear
AM; a.m.	morning
APAP	acetaminophen; Tylenol
as; a.s.; AS	left ear
ASA	aspirin
au; a.u.; AU	both ears; each ear
b.i.d.; BID	twice daily
BUD	beyond-use date
°C	degrees centigrade; temperature in degrees centigrade
Ca^{++}	calcium
Cap	capsule
CSP	compounded sterile preparation
D-E-F	
D_5; D_5W; D5W	dextrose 5% in water
D_5 ¼; D5 1/4	dextrose 5% in ¼ normal saline; dextrose 5% in 0.225% sodium chloride
D_5 ⅓; D5 1/3	dextrose 5% in ⅓ normal saline; dextrose 5% in 0.33% sodium chloride
D_5 ½; D5 1/2	dextrose 5% in ½ normal saline; dextrose 5% in 0.45% sodium chloride
D_5LR; D5LR	dextrose 5% in lactated Ringer's solution
D_5NS; D5NS	dextrose 5% in normal saline; dextrose 5% in 0.9% sodium chloride
DAW	dispense as written
DC; d/c	discontinue
D/C	discharge
DCA	direct compounding area
Dig	digoxin
disp	dispense
EC	enteric-coated
Elix	elixir
eMAR	electronic medication administration record
EPO	epoetin alfa; erythropoietin
ER; XR; XL	extended-release
°F	degrees Fahrenheit; temperature in degrees Fahrenheit
$FeSO_4$	ferrous sulfate; iron

Abbreviation	Meaning
G-H-I	
g, G	gram
gr	grain
gtt; gtts	drop; drops
h; hr	hour
HC	hydrocortisone
HCTZ	hydrochlorothiazide
HIPAA	Health Insurance Portability and Accountability Act
HMO	Health Maintenance Organization
HRT	hormone replacement therapy
h.s.; HS	bedtime
IBU	ibuprofen; Motrin
IM	intramuscular
Inj	injection
IPA	isopropyl alcohol
ISDN	isosorbide dinitrate
ISMO	isosorbide mononitrate
IV	intravenous
IVF	intravenous fluid
IVP	intravenous push
IVPB	intravenous piggyback
J-K-L	
K; K+	potassium
KCl	potassium chloride
kg	kilogram
L	liter
LAFW	laminar airflow workbench; hood
lb	pound
LD	loading dose
LVP	large-volume parenteral
M-N-O	
Mag; Mg; MAG	magnesium
MAR	medication administration record
mcg; µg*	microgram
MDI	metered-dose inhaler
MDV	multiple-dose vial

Abbreviation	Meaning
mEq	milliequivalent
mg	milligram
MgSO$_4$†	magnesium sulfate; magnesium
mL	milliliter
mL/hr	milliliters per hour
mL/min	milliliters per minute
MOM; M.O.M.	milk of magnesia
M.S.†	morphine sulfate
MU†; mu	million units
MVI; MVI-12	multiple vitamin injection; multivitamins for parenteral administration
Na$^+$	sodium
NaCl	sodium chloride; salt
NDC	National Drug Code
NF; non-form	nonformulary
NPO	nothing by mouth
NR; d.n.r.	no refills; do not repeat
NS	normal saline; 0.9% sodium chloride
½ NS	one-half normal saline; 0.45% sodium chloride
¼ NS	one-quarter normal saline; 0.225% sodium chloride
NSAID	nonsteroidal anti-inflammatory drug
NTG	nitroglycerin
od; o.d.; OD	right eye
ODT	orally disintegrating tablet
OPTH; OPHTH; Opth	ophthalmic
os; o.s.; OS	left eye
OTC	over the counter; no prescription required
ou; o.u.; OU	both eyes; each eye
oz	ounce
P-Q-R	
p.c.; PC	after meals
PCA	patient-controlled anesthesia
PCN	penicillin
PHI	protected health information
PM; p.m.	afternoon; evening
PO	orally; by mouth
PPE	personal protective equipment

Abbreviation	Meaning
PPI	proton pump inhibitor
PR	per rectum; rectally
PRN; p.r.n.	as needed; as occasion requires
PV	per vagina; vaginally
PVC	polyvinyl chloride
q	every
q.h.; qhour	every hour
q2h	every 2 hours
q4h	every 4 hours
q6h	every 6 hours
q8h	every 8 hours
q12h	every 12 hours
q24h	every 24 hours
q48h	every 48 hours
QA	quality assurance
QAM; qam	every morning
qDay; QD†	every day
q.i.d.; QID	four times daily
QOD; Q other day; Q.O. Day	every other day
QPM; qpm	every evening
qs; qsad	quantity sufficient; a sufficient quantity to make
QTY; qty	quantity
qwk; qweek	every week
Rx	prescription; pharmacy; medication; drug; recipe; take
S-T	
sig	write on label; signa; directions
SL; sub-L	sublingual
SMZ-TMP	sulfamethoxazole and trimethoprim; Bactrim
SR	sustained-release
SS; ss	one-half
SSRI	selective serotonin reuptake inhibitor

Abbreviation	Meaning
Stat	immediately; now
Sub-Q; SC; SQ; sq	subcutaneous
SUPP; Supp	suppository
susp	suspension
SVP	small-volume parenteral
SW	sterile water
SWFI	sterile water for injection
Tab	tablet
TBSP; tbsp	tablespoon; tablespoonful; 15 mL
TDS	transdermal delivery system
t.i.d.; TID	three times daily
t.i.w.; TIW	three times a week
TKO; TKVO; KO; KVO	to keep open; to keep vein open; keep open; keep vein open (a slow IV flow rate)
TPN	total parenteral nutrition
TSP; tsp	teaspoon; teaspoonful; 5 mL
U-V-W	
ung	ointment
ut dict	as directed
VAG; vag	vagina; vaginally
Vanco	vancomycin
VO; V.O.; V/O	verbal order
w/o	without
X-Y-Z	
Zn	zinc
Z-Pak	azithromycin; Zithromax

† Please note that this abbreviation is on the Joint Commission's Official "Do Not Use" List of Abbreviations. However, you may occasionally encounter its use in your practice. If you see this abbreviation on a medication order, alert the pharmacist who will, in turn, clarify the order with the prescriber.

* Please note that this abbreviation is being considered for possible future inclusion in the Joint Commission's Official "Do Not Use" List of Abbreviations.

Glossary

A

abbreviated new drug application (aNDA) the process by which applicants must scientifically demonstrate to the FDA that their generic product is bioequivalent to or performs in the same way as the innovator drug

accreditation the status achieved by a hospital, community college, college, or university that meets quality standards and fulfills the requirements designated by the accrediting organization

active ingredient the biochemically active component of the drug that exerts a desired therapeutic effect

addiction compulsive and uncontrollable use of controlled substances, especially narcotics

additive an electrolyte or medication injected into an LVP or SVP solution for patient administration

admitting order a medication order written by a physician on admission of a patient to the hospital; may or may not include a medication order

adulterated product a product that differs in drug strength, quality, and purity

adulteration the process of corrupting or tainting drug products by the addition of foreign, impure, or inferior substances that may be toxic

adverse drug reaction (ADR) an unexpected negative consequence from taking a particular drug

aerosol a pressurized container with a propellant that is used to administer a drug through oral inhalation into the lungs

alchemy the European practice during the Middle Ages that combined elements of chemistry, metallurgy, physics, and medicine with astrology, mysticism, and spiritualism to turn a common item into something special or extraordinary; an example would be the transmutation of a base metal into silver or gold

allergy a hypersensitivity to a specific substance, manifested in a physiological disorder

alligation the compounding of two or more products to obtain a desired concentration

altruism an unselfish concern for the welfare of others

ampule a small container made of thin glass that is used as a reservoir for certain single-dose parenteral medications

anabolic steroid a synthetic, performance-enhancing drug that mimics the human hormone testosterone; because of abuse by athletes, this drug has been reclassified by the DEA as a controlled substance

anteroom the area of the sterile compounding lab that is used for hand washing and garbing, staging of components, order entry, CSP labeling, and other high-particulate-generating activities

antibiotic a chemical substance that is used in the treatment of bacterial infectious diseases and has the ability to either kill or inhibit the growth of certain harmful microorganisms

antibody the part of the immune system that neutralizes antigens or foreign substances in the body

anticipatory compounding the preparation of excess product (besides an individual compound prescription) in reasonable quantities; these preparations must be labeled with lot numbers

antineoplastic drug a hazardous agent that reduces or prevents the growth of cancer cells

apothecary a shop in which medicines were compounded by skilled artisans using herbs and other natural ingredients

apothecary system a weight-based measurement system developed by the Romans

appearance the overall outward look of an employee on the job, including dress and grooming

Arabic system a mathematical system using numbers, fractions, and decimals

aromatic water a solution of water containing oils or other substances that has a pungent, and usually pleasing, smell and is easily released into the air

asepsis the absence of pathogenic microorganisms

aseptic technique the manipulation of sterile products and devices in such a way as to avoid contamination by disease-causing organisms

assumption error an error that occurs when an essential piece of information cannot be verified and is guessed or presumed

attenuated virus a weakened virus contained in some vaccines as opposed to a live or inactive virus

attitude the emotional stance or disposition that a worker adopts toward his or her job duties, customers, employer, and coworkers

audit a challenge on a reimbursement from a PBM or insurance provider on a prescription claim that has been previously processed

autoclave a device that generates heat and pressure to sterilize objects

automated compounding device (ACD) a programmable, automated device to make complex IV preparations such as TPNs

automated medication dispensing system (AMDS) a secure, locked storage cabinet of designated drugs on a nursing unit whose software can track the dispensing and administration of each dose of medication to each patient

auxiliary label a supplementary label added to a medication container at the discretion of the pharmacist that provides additional directions

average wholesale price (AWP) the average price that wholesalers charge the pharmacy for a drug

avoirdupois system a system of measurement that originated in France and is used for common measurements in the United States; units of measure include the foot, mile, grain, pound, and ounce

B

bactericidal having the ability to destroy bacteria

bacterium a small, single-celled microorganism that can exist in three main forms, depending on type: spherical (i.e., cocci), rod-shaped (i.e., bacilli), and spiral (i.e., spirochetes)

bar-code point-of-care (BPOC) the use of automation scanning by a nurse at a patient's bedside to minimize medication administration errors

beyond-use dating the documentation of the date after which a compounded preparation expires and should no longer be used

bioavailability the time it takes for a generic drug to reach the bloodstream in healthy volunteers

bioequivalent a generic drug that delivers approximately the same amount of active ingredients into a healthy volunteer's bloodstream in the same amount of time as the innovator or brand name drug

biological safety cabinet (BSC) a vertical laminar airflow hood that is used in the preparation of hazardous compounds, such as chemotherapy CSPs, and is designed to offer protection for the worker during the manipulation of these toxic chemicals

biotechnology the field of study that combines the sciences of biology, chemistry, and immunology to produce synthetic, unique drugs with specific therapeutic effects

black box warning a warning statement required by the FDA indicating a serious or even life-threatening adverse reaction from a drug; the warning statement is on the product package insert (PPI) for the pharmacy staff and in the MedGuide for consumers

blending the act of combining two substances using techniques such as spatulation, sifting, and tumbling

body surface area (BSA) a measurement related to a patient's weight and height, expressed in meters squared (m^2), and used to calculate patient-specific dosages of medications

botany a branch of biology dealing with plant life

brand name the name under which the manufacturer markets a drug; also called *trade name*

brand name medically necessary a designation on the prescription by the physician indicating that a generic substitution by the pharmacist is not allowed; commonly seen on prescriptions for thyroid medication; often abbreviated as "brand necessary"

break ring a scored area on the neck of an ampule that marks the site where a technician will break the glass to access the ampule's contents

buccal route of administration a transmucosal route of administration in which a drug is placed between the gum and the inner lining of the cheek

burden of proof the obligation of a person or party filing a lawsuit to provide evidence to prove a case

C

cannula the barrel of a syringe or bore area inside the syringe that correlates with the volume of solution

caplet a hybrid solid dosage formulation sharing characteristics of both a tablet and a capsule

capsule the dosage form containing powder, liquid, or granules in a gelatin covering

capture error an error that occurs when focus on a task is diverted elsewhere and therefore the error goes undetected

cart fill list a printout of all unit dose profiles for all patients

catheter a device inserted into a vein for direct access to the cardiovascular system

Celsius temperature scale the temperature scale that uses 0 °C as the temperature at which water freezes at sea level and 100 °C as the temperature at which it boils

Centers for Disease Control and Prevention (CDC) a government agency that provides guidelines and recommendations on health care, including infection control

central venous catheter (CVC) a catheter placed into a large vein deep in the body; also called a *central line*

certificate of medical necessity form to be completed and signed by the prescriber for Medicare Part B insurance payment for diabetic supplies

certification a voluntary process by which a nongovernmental organization recognizes an individual who has met predetermined qualifications specified by that organization; a pharmacy technician may become certified by the Pharmacy Technician Certification Board (PTCB)

Certified Pharmacy Technician (CPhT) a pharmacy technician who has passed the Pharmacy Technician Certification Examination (PTCE) or Exam for Certification of Pharmacy Technicians (ExCPT)

chain pharmacy a community pharmacy that consists of several similar pharmacies in the region (or nation) that are corporately owned

charge-back a rejection of a prescription claim by a PBM or an insurance provider that must be investigated and resolved

chemotherapy compounding mat a thin mat placed on the BSC work surface to absorb accidental liquid spills during the compounding of chemotherapy drugs

chemotherapy dispensing pin a small plastic device used to relieve the negative pressure within a drug vial safely, while its built-in HEPA filter traps any drug particles or escaping fluid from the vial

chewable tablet a solid oral dosage form meant to be chewed that is readily absorbed; commonly prescribed for school-age children

child-resistant container a medication container with a special lid that cannot be opened by 80% of children under age 5 but can be opened by 90% of adults; a container designed to prevent child access to reduce the number of accidental poisonings

civil law the areas of the law that concern U.S. citizens and the crimes they commit against one another

Class III prescription balance a two-pan balance used to weigh material (120 g or less) with a sensitivity rating of +/–6 mg; also called a *Class A prescription balance*

clean room an area that includes the staging areas and the LAFWs; also called the *IV room* or *buffer area*

closed-ended question a question that requires a yes-or-no answer

closed-system transfer device (CSTD) a small disposable device that safely draws fluid from a vial into a syringe or injects fluid from a syringe into an IV or IVPB; this device protects the worker from exposure to hazardous drugs

coinsurance a percentage-based insurance plan in which the patient must pay a certain percentage of the prescription price

colloid the dispersion of ultrafine particles in a liquid formulation

comminution the act of reducing a substance to small, fine particles using techniques such as trituration, levigation, and pulverization

common law the system of precedents established by decisions in cases throughout legal history

community pharmacy any independent, chain, or franchise pharmacy that dispenses prescription medications to outpatients; also called a *retail pharmacy*

compatibility the ability to combine two more base components or additives within a solution, without resulting in a change to the physical or chemical properties of the components or additives

compliance adherence to a required set of standards, regulations, laws, and practices

compounded preparation a patient-specific medication prepared on-site by the technician, under the direct supervision of the pharmacist, from individual ingredients

compounded sterile preparation (CSP) a sterile product that is prepared outside the pharmaceutical manufacturer's facility, typically in a hospital or compounding pharmacy

compounding the process of preparing a medication for an individual patient from bulk ingredients according to a prescription by a licensed prescriber

compounding aseptic containment isolator (CACI) an enclosed vertical laminar airflow hood designed to protect sterile compounding personnel from exposure to hazardous chemicals during compounding procedures

compounding log a printout of the prescription for a specific patient, including the amounts or weights of all ingredients and instructions for compounding; used by the technician to prepare a compounded medication for a patient

compounding pharmacy a pharmacy that specializes in the compounding of nonsterile (and sometimes sterile) preparations that are not commercially available

compression tablet a tablet consisting of an active ingredient and an inactive ingredient (diluent, binder, disintegrant, or lubricating agent) that is manufactured by means of great pressure

computer an electronic device for inputting, storing, processing, and/or outputting information

computerized prescriber order entry (CPOE) the process of having a prescriber use a handheld device at a patient's bedside to enter and send medication orders to the pharmacy

confidentiality keeping privileged information about a customer from being disclosed without his or her consent

conjunctival route of administration the placement of sterile ophthalmic medications in the conjunctival sac of the eye(s)

continuous quality improvement (CQI) a process of written procedures designed to identify problems and recommend solutions

controlled-release (CR) formulation a dosage form that is formulated to release medication over a long duration

controlled substance a drug with potential for abuse; organized into five schedules that specify the way the drug must be stored, dispensed, recorded, and inventoried

Controlled Substances Act (CSA) laws created to combat and control drug abuse

coordination of benefits (COB) online billing of both a primary and a secondary insurer

co-payment (co-pay) the amount that the patient is to pay for each prescription as determined by insurance

coring an inadvertent introduction of a small piece of the rubber closure into the solution while removing medication from a vial

counterbalance a two-pan balance used for weighing material up to 5 kg with a sensitivity rating of +/-100 mg

crash cart a mobile cart that holds necessary drugs for an emergency CPR code

cream a cosmetically acceptable oil-in-water (O/W) emulsion for topical use on the skin

credential a documented piece of evidence of one's qualifications

credentialing the process for validating the qualifications of licensed professionals, such as Basic Life Support (BLS) and ACLS (Advanced Cardiovascular Life Support)

credit card a method of online payment that is a type of loan, either paid totally at the end of the month or partially with a finance charge added

critical site the part of the supply item that includes any fluid-pathway surface or opening that is at risk for contamination by touch or airflow interruption

cultural sensitivity an awareness, knowledge of, and respect for cultural beliefs that differ from your own

culture the customs, beliefs, and attitudes that are learned and shared by members of a group

cytotoxic drug any drug that destroys cancer cells

D

daily order a medication order written by a physician to continue treatment; similar to a refill of medication

database management system (DBMS) application that allows one to enter, retrieve, and query records

days' supply the duration of time (number of days) a dispensed medication will last a patient; required on drug claims submitted for online insurance billing

DEA number an identification number assigned by the Drug Enforcement Administration (DEA) to identify someone authorized to handle or prescribe controlled substances within the United States

debit card a method of online cash payment that instantly deducts the cost of the purchase from the customer's bank account

decimal any number that can be written in decimal notation using the integers 0 through 9 and a point (.) to divide the "ones" place from the "tenths" place (e.g., 10.25 is equal to 10¼)

decorum proper or polite behavior that is in good taste

deductible an amount that must be paid by the insured before the insurance company considers paying its portion of a medical or drug cost

defendant one who defends against accusations brought forward in a lawsuit

delayed-release (DR) formulation a dosage form, such as an enteric-coated aspirin tablet, that contains a special coating designed to delay absorption of the medication and to resist breakdown by acidic gastric fluids

denominator the number on the bottom part of a fraction that represents the whole

deoxyribonucleic acid (DNA) the helix-shaped molecule that carries the genetic code

destructive agent a drug that kills bacteria, fungi, viruses, or even normal or cancer cells

diagnostic agent a chemical containing radioactive isotopes used to diagnose and treat disease

dietary supplement a category of nonprescription drugs that includes vitamins, minerals, and herbs that is not regulated by the FDA

digital electronic analytical balance a single-pan balance that is more accurate than Class III balances or counterbalances; it has a capacity of 100 g and sensitivity as low as +/–2 mg

diluent a sterile fluid added to a powder to reconstitute, dilute, or dissolve a medication

diluent powder an inactive ingredient that is added to the active drug in compounding a tablet or capsule

direct compounding area (DCA) the sterile compounding work area of the LAFW, in which the concentration of airborne particles is controlled with a HEPA filter providing ISO Class 5 air quality

director of pharmacy the chief executive officer of the hospital pharmacy department

discharge order an order written by a physician that provides take-home instructions, including prescribed medications and doses, for a discharged patient

discount a reduced price

discrimination preferential treatment or mistreatment

discus a device that contains nonaerosolized powder used for inhalation

disinfectant a chemical, such as rubbing alcohol, that is applied to an object or topically to the body for sterilization purposes

dispense as written (DAW) a notation identical to "brand name medically necessary"; indicates on a prescription that a brand name drug is necessary or that a generic substitution is not allowed; DAW2 is often used to indicate patient preference for a brand name drug

dispersion a liquid dosage form in which undissolved ingredients are mixed throughout a liquid vehicle

donut hole insurance coverage gap in Medicare Part D programs by which the patient must pay a higher portion of the cost of the medication; to be phased out by 2019

dosage form the physical manifestation of a drug (for example, a capsule or a tablet)

drip chamber the small, open space just below the spike adaptor where the drops of fluid from the IV bag into the tubing are counted by the nurse to determine the flow rate of the IV solution

drop factor the number of drops that an IV tubing delivers to provide 1 mL; this number may be used by nurses to calculate the IV flow rate when using certain types of primary IV tubing; also called *drop set* or *drip set*

drop set the calibration in drops per milliliter on IV sets

dropper a device used to accurately measure medication dosage for infants

drug any substance taken into or applied to the body for the purpose of altering the body's biochemical functions and thus its physiological processes

drug delivery system a design feature of the dosage form that affects the delivery of the drug; such a system may protect the stomach or delay the release of the active drug

Drug Enforcement Administration (DEA) the branch of the U.S. Justice Department that is responsible for regulating the sale and use of drugs with abuse potential

drug formulary a list of approved medications for use within the hospital; this list is approved by the P&T Committee

drug recall the process of withdrawing a drug from the market by the FDA or the drug manufacturer for serious adverse effects or other defects in the product

drug seeker one who requests early refills on medications or gets prescriptions from multiple physicians or multiple pharmacies for controlled substances to obtain more than the typically prescribed amount of medication

drug tolerance a situation that occurs when the body requires higher doses of a drug to produce the same therapeutic effect

drug utilization review (DUR) a procedure built into pharmacy software designed to help pharmacists check for potential medication errors in dosage, drug interactions, allergies, and so on

dual co-pay insurance coverage in which a patient pays one co-pay for brand name drugs and a lower co-pay for generic drugs

dumb terminal a computer device that contains a keyboard and a monitor but does not contain its own storage and processing capabilities

durable medical equipment (DME) medical equipment such as hospital beds, wheelchairs, canes, or crutches that may be covered under Medicare Part B insurance

E

e-prescriptions prescriptions that are transmitted via electronic means

effervescent salts granular salts that release gas and dispense active ingredients into solution when placed in water

electrolyte solution a solution that contains dissolved mineral salts

electronic medication administration record (eMAR) a computerized patient medical record used to minimize medication errors

elixir a clear, sweetened, flavored solution containing water and ethanol

embolism a blockage of a blood vessel from a blood clot or inadvertent injection of an air bubble

emulsion the dispersion of a liquid in another liquid varying in viscosity

enema a solution, such as a Fleet enema, to be administered into the rectum to evacuate colon contents

enteric-coated tablet (ECT) a tablet coating designed to resist destruction by the acidic pH of the gastric fluids and to delay the release of the active ingredient

epidemic the occurrence of more cases of disease (such as the flu) than expected in a given area or among a specific group of people over a particular period

estrogen replacement therapy (ERT) treatment consisting of some combination of female hormones

ethical dilemma a situation that calls for a judgment between two or more solutions, not all of which are necessarily wrong

ethics the study of standards of conduct and moral judgment that outlines the rights and wrongs of human conduct or character

etiquette unwritten rules of behavior

Exam for Certification of Pharmacy Technicians (ExCPT) an examination developed by the Institute for the Certification of Pharmacy Technicians (ICPT) that technicians must pass to be certified and receive the title of CPhT

excipient an inert or inactive ingredient that forms a vehicle for a drug

expiration date the date after which a manufacturer's product should not be used

extended-release (XL) formulation a tablet or capsule designed to reduce frequency of dosing compared with immediate-release and most sustained-release formulations

extra dose error an error in which more doses are received by a patient than were prescribed by the physician

extract a potent dosage form derived from animal or plant sources from which most or all the solvent has been evaporated to produce a powder, an ointment-like form, or a solid

F

Fahrenheit temperature scale the temperature scale that uses 32 °F as the temperature at which water freezes at sea level and 212 °F as the temperature at which it boils

FDA Online Orange Book an online reference that provides information on the generic and therapeutic equivalence of drugs that may have many different brand names or generic manufacturer sources

film-coated tablet (FCT) a tablet coated with a thin outer layer that prevents serious GI side effects

filter a device used to remove contaminants such as glass, fibers, rubber cores, and bacteria from IV fluids

Flex card a medical and prescription insurance credit card

flexible tubing the tubing component of a sterile IV administration set that serves as a pathway for IV fluids and parenteral medications during patient administration

floor stock medications stocked in a secured area on each patient care unit

fluidextract a liquid dosage form prepared by extraction from plant sources and commonly used in the formulation of syrups

Food and Drug Administration (FDA) the agency of the federal government that is responsible for ensuring the safety and efficacy of food and drugs prepared for the market

forceps an instrument used to pick up small objects, such as pharmacy weights

formulary a list of drugs that has been preapproved for use by a committee of healthcare professionals; used in hospitals, in managed care, and by many insurance providers; also called a *pharmacopeia* or *dispensatory*

four Ds of negligence four areas of negligence, which include duty, dereliction, damages, and direct cause; the plaintiff in a negligence or malpractice lawsuit must produce evidence that proves that the defendant committed a breach of responsibility and that this breach led to personal injury of the plaintiff

fraction a portion of a whole that is represented as a ratio

franchise pharmacy a pharmacy that is part of a small chain of professional community pharmacies that dispense and prepare medications but are independently owned; sometimes called an *apothecary*

fungus a single-celled organism similar to human cells that is marked by a rigid cell wall, reproduction by spores, and the absence of chlorophyll; feeds on living organisms (or on dead organic material)

G

gel a dispersion containing fine particles for topical use on the skin

generic drug a drug that contains the same active ingredients as the brand name product and delivers the same amount of medication to the body in the same way and in the same duration of time; a drug that is not protected by a patent

generic name a common name that is given to a drug regardless of brand name; sometimes denotes a drug that is not protected by a trademark; for example, acetaminophen is the generic drug name for Tylenol

genetic engineering process of using DNA biotechnology to create a variety of drugs

genome the entire DNA in an organism, including its genes

geometric dilution method a process that uses a mortar and pestle to gradually combine several drugs and inactive ingredients

germ theory of disease the idea that microorganisms cause diseases

glycerogelatin a topical preparation made with gelatin, glycerin, water, and medicinal substances

good compounding practices (GCPs) USP standards in many areas of practice to ensure high-quality compounded preparations

good manufacturing practices (GMPs) general principles and guidelines used during the manufacturing process to ensure a quality product

graduated cylinder a flask used for measuring liquids

grain a dry weight unit of measurement in the apothecary system (for example, 5 grains [5 gr] of aspirin are equivalent to approximately 325 mg)

gram the metric system's base unit for measuring weight

granules a dosage form larger than powders that is formed by adding very small amounts of liquid to powders

gross profit the difference between the purchase price and the selling price; also called *markup*

H

hand hygiene the use of special dry, alcohol-based rinses, gels, or foams that do not require water

hand washing the use of plain or antiseptic soap and water with appropriate time and technique

harassment persistent hostile, unpleasant, and unwelcome mistreatment, whether sexual, verbal, or physical

health insurance coverage of incurred medical costs such as physician and emergency room visits, laboratory costs, and hospitalization

Health Insurance Portability and Accountability Act (HIPAA) a comprehensive federal law passed in 1996 to protect all patient-identifiable medical information

health maintenance organization (HMO) an organization that provides health insurance using a managed-care model

healthcare-associated infection (HAI) an infection that a patient acquires as a result of treatment in a healthcare facility; also called a *nosocomial infection*

herbal medicine the use of natural plant products to maintain health by preventing or curing certain illnesses

high-efficiency particulate airflow (HEPA) filter a device used with LAFWs to filter out most particulate matter and to establish an aseptic environment in which to prepare parenteral products

home health care the delivery of medical, nursing, and pharmaceutical services and supplies to patients at home

home healthcare pharmacy a pharmacy that prepares and dispenses drugs and medical supplies directly to the home of the patient

homeopathic medications a class of drugs in which very small dilutions of natural drugs are taken to stimulate the body's immune system

horizontal laminar airflow workbench (LAFW) a type of hood that is used to prepare IV drug admixtures, nutrition solutions, and other parenteral products aseptically

hormone replacement therapy (HRT) therapy consisting of some combination of estrogen and progestin (female) and androgen (male) hormones

hospice care home healthcare services typically involving pain management of a terminally ill patient

hospital pharmacy an institutional pharmacy that dispenses and prepares drugs and provides clinical services in a hospital setting

household system a system of measurement based on the apothecary system; units of measure include the ounce, pound, drop, teaspoon, tablespoon, and cup

human failure an error generated by failure that occurs at an individual level

hypertonic solution a parenteral solution with a greater number of particles than the number of particles found in blood (greater than 285 mOsm/L); also called a *hyperosmolar solution*, as in a TPN solution

hypotonic solution a parenteral solution with a fewer number of particles than the number of particles found in blood (less than 285 mOsm/L); also called a *hypoosmolar solution*

I

in-line filter a filter that is connected to, or contained within, an IV administration set; device is used to filter TPN fluid, thus preventing potential precipitates in the solution from being inadvertently administered to a patient

independent pharmacy a community pharmacy that is privately owned by a pharmacist

inert ingredient an inactive chemical—such as a filler, preservative, coloring, or flavoring—that is added to one or more active ingredients to improve drug formulations while causing little or no physiological effect; also called an *inactive ingredient*

Infection Control Committee (ICC) a hospital committee that provides leadership in relation to infection control policies

informed consent a document that states, in easily understandable terms, the purpose and risks of the drug research

inhalation route of administration the administration of a drug by inhalation into the lungs; also called *intrarespiratory route of administration*

injection the administration of a parenteral medication into the bloodstream, muscle, or skin

inpatient drug distribution system a pharmacy system to deliver all types of drugs to a patient in the hospital setting; commonly includes unit dose, repackaged medication, floor stock, and IV admixture and TPN services

inscription the part of the prescription listing the medication or medications prescribed, including the drug names, strengths, and amounts

Institute for Safe Medication Practices (ISMP) a nonprofit healthcare agency whose primary mission is to understand the causes of medication errors and to provide time-critical, error-reduction strategies to the healthcare community, policymakers, and the public

institutional pharmacy a pharmacy that is organized under a corporate structure, following specific rules and regulations for accreditation

Institutional Review Board (IRB) a committee of the hospital that ensures that appropriate protection is provided to patients using investigational drugs; sometimes called the *Human Use Committee*

insulin pen a portable device in which the dose of insulin can be easily dialed up before administration

International Organization for Standardization (ISO) a classification system to measure the amount of particulate matter in room air; the lower the ISO number, the less particulate matter is present in the air

intranasal route of administration the placement of sprays or solutions into the nose

intrauterine device (IUD) a device that delivers medication to prevent conception

intravenous (IV) admixture service a centralized pharmacy service that prepares IV and TPN solutions in a sterile, clean room work environment

intravenous (IV) infusion the process of injecting fluid or medication into the veins, usually over a prolonged period

inventory the entire stock of products on hand for sale at a given time

inventory turnover rate the amount of time the average drug inventory will be replaced during a 12-month period; most pharmacies replace inventory every two to four weeks

inventory value the total value of the entire stock of products on hand for sale on a given day

investigational drug a drug used in clinical trials that has not yet been approved by the FDA for use in the general population, or a drug used for non-approved indications

investigational new drug application (INDA) process by which a manufacturer submits research results from animal studies to the FDA to gain approval to gather data and investigate a new drug in humans

irrigating solution any solution used for cleansing or bathing an area of the body, such as the eyes or ears

isotonic solution a parenteral solution with an equal number of particles as blood cells (285 mOsm/L); 0.9% normal saline is isotonic

IV administration set a sterile, pyrogen-free, disposable device used to deliver IV fluids to patients

IV bolus injection an injection in which a drug is administered intravenously all at once; also called *IV push (IVP)*

IV infusion an infusion in which a drug is administered intravenously slowly over a given period

IV piggyback (IVPB) a small-volume IV infusion (50 mL, 100 mL, 250 mL) containing medications

IV push (IVP) the rapid injection of a medication in a syringe into an IV line or catheter in the patient's arm; also called *IV bolus injection*

J

jelly a gel that contains a higher proportion of water in combination with a drug substance, as well as a thickening agent

Joint Commission an independent, not-for-profit organization that sets the standards by which safety and quality of health care are measured and accredits hospitals according to those standards

just-in-time (JIT) purchasing frequent purchasing in quantities that just meet supply needs until the next ordering time

L

large-volume parenteral (LVP) an IV fluid of more than 250 mL that may contain drugs, nutrients, or electrolytes

law a rule that is designed to protect the public and usually enforced through local, state, or federal governments

law of agency and contracts the general principle that allows an employee to enter into contracts on the employer's behalf

leading zero a zero that is placed in the ones place in a number less than zero that is being represented by a decimal value

legend drug a drug that requires a prescription; labeled "Rx only" on medication stock bottle

levigation a process usually used to reduce the particle size of a solid during the preparation of an ointment

licensure the process by which a state board grants permission to an individual to engage in a given occupation upon finding that the applicant has attained the minimum degree of necessary competency to safeguard the public; all pharmacists must be licensed to practice by their state boards of pharmacy

liniment a medicated topical preparation, such as BENGAY, that is applied to the skin

liquid any free-flowing fluid that is commonly used to dissolve solids

liter the metric system's base unit for measuring volume

localized effect the site-specific application of a drug

long-term care facility an institution that provides care for geriatric and disabled patients; includes extended-care facility (ECF) and skilled-care facility (SCF)

lotion a liquid for topical application that contains insoluble dispersed solids or immiscible liquids

lozenge a medication in a sweet-tasting formulation that is absorbed in the mouth; also called a *troche*

M

magma a milklike liquid colloidal dispersion, such as milk of magnesia, in which particles remain distinct, in a two-phase system

mail-order pharmacy a large-volume, centralized pharmacy operation that uses automation to fill and mail prescriptions to a patient

malpractice a form of negligence in which the standard of care was not met and was a direct cause of injury

managed care a type of health insurance system that emphasizes keeping the patient healthy or diseases controlled to reduce healthcare costs

manufactured products products prepared off-site by a large-scale drug manufacturer

markup the difference between the purchase price and the selling price; also called *gross profit*

master control record a recipe for a compound preparation that lists the name, strength, dosage form, ingredients and their quantities, mixing instructions, and beyond-use dating; many recipes available from PCCA

Material Safety Data Sheet (MSDS) a document that contains important information on hazards and flammability of chemicals used in compounding and procedures for treatment of accidental ingestion or exposure

MedGuide written patient information mandated by the FDA for select high-risk drugs; also called a *patient medication guide*

Medicaid a state government health insurance program for low-income and disabled citizens

medical chart a legal document that contains a patient's demographics and room number as well as all orders written by the healthcare team

medical error any circumstance, action, inaction, or decision related to health care that contributes to an unintended health result

Medicare Part D a voluntary insurance program that provides partial coverage of prescriptions primarily for patients who are eligible for Medicare

medication administration record (MAR) a form in the patient's medical chart used by nurses to document the administration times of all drugs

medication container label a label containing the dosage directions from the prescriber, affixed to the container of the dispensed medication; the pharmacy technician may use this copy to select the correct stock drug bottle and to fill the prescription

medication error any preventable event that may cause or lead to inappropriate medication use or patient harm while the medication is in the control of the healthcare professional, patient, or consumer

Medication Errors Reporting Program (ISMP MERP) a program designed to allow healthcare professionals to report medication errors directly to the Institute for Safe Medication Practices (ISMP)

medication information sheet a leaflet printed from the prescription software and provided to patients on each medication dispensed; the technician may use this copy to select the correct stock drug bottle and fill the prescription

medication order a prescription written in the hospital setting

medication special a single-dose preparation not commercially available that is repackaged and made for a particular patient

MEDMARX an Internet-based program of the USP for use by hospitals and healthcare systems for documenting, tracking, and identifying trends for adverse events and medication errors

MedWatch a voluntary program run by the FDA for reporting serious adverse events, product problems, or medication errors; serves as a clearinghouse to provide information on safety alerts for drugs, biologics, dietary supplements, and medical devices as well as drug recalls

meniscus the moon-shaped or concave appearance of a liquid in a graduated cylinder; used during the measurement process

meter the metric system's base unit for measuring length

metered-dose inhaler (MDI) a device used to administer a drug in the form of compressed gas through the mouth and into the lungs

metric system a measurement system based on subdivisions and multiples of 10; made up of three basic units: meter, gram, and liter

microbiology the study of microorganisms

microemulsion a clear formulation, such as Haley's M-O, that contains one liquid of tiny droplets dispersed in another liquid

microorganism a living microscopic organism or microbe such as a bacterium, fungus, protozoan, or virus

military time a measure of time based on a 24-hour clock in which midnight is 0000, noon is 1200, and the minute before midnight is 2359; also called *24-hour time* or *international time*

misbranded product a product whose label includes false statements about the identity or ingredients of the container's contents

mortar and pestle equipment used for mixing and grinding pharmaceutical ingredients

multiple compression tablet (MCT) a tablet formulation on top of a tablet or a tablet within a tablet, produced by multiple compressions in manufacturing

multitasking the ability to work on several projects at the same time

N

National Association of Boards of Pharmacy (NABP) an organization that represents the practice of pharmacy in each state and develops pharmacist licensure exams

National Drug Code (NDC) a 10- or 11-character code that is assigned by the FDA to each drug product; each code is unique and identifies the manufacturer or distributor, the drug formulation, and the size and type of packaging

nebulizer a device used to deliver medication in a fine-mist form to the lungs; often used in treating asthma

needle a thin, hollow transfer device used with a syringe to inject drugs into the body or withdraw fluids such as blood from the body

needle adaptor the end of the tubing (farthest from the universal spike adaptor) to which the needle is attached

negligence a tort for not providing the minimum standard of care

new drug application (NDA) the process through which drug sponsors formally propose that the FDA approve a new pharmaceutical for sale and marketing in the United States

noncompliance failure to take therapy as the physician instructs; also called *nonadherence*

nondurable medical supplies consumable, disposable items that can only be used by one patient for a specific purpose

nonsterile compounding the preparation of a medication, in an appropriate quantity and dosage form, from several pharmaceutical ingredients in response to a prescription written by a physician; sometimes called *extemporaneous compounding*

nonverbal communication communication without words—through facial expression, body language, posture, and tone of voice

nonvolumetric glassware a beaker or flask that is not calibrated and cannot be used to accurately measure liquids; its use is limited to store, contain, and mix liquids with other bulk ingredients

normal saline (NS) a sterile solution containing a concentration of 0.9% sodium chloride in water

notice of privacy practices a written policy of the pharmacy to protect patient confidentiality, as required by HIPAA

NPI number a unique National Provider Identifier for any healthcare provider involved in writing prescriptions or billing insurance for any healthcare-related service

nuclear pharmacy a specialized practice that compounds and dispenses sterile radioactive pharmaceuticals to diagnose or treat disease

numerator the number on the upper part of a fraction that represents the part of the whole

O

Occupational Safety and Health Administration (OSHA) an agency of the Department of Labor whose primary mission is to ensure the safety and health of U.S. workers by setting and enforcing regulations and standards

ocular route of administration the placement of sterile ophthalmic medications into the eye

oil-in-water (O/W) emulsion an emulsion containing a small amount of oil dispersed in water, as in a cream

ointment a semisolid emulsion for topical use on the skin

ointment slab a flat, hard, nonabsorbent surface used for mixing compounds; also called a *compounding slab*

omission error an error in which a prescribed dose is not given

online adjudication real-time insurance claims processing via wireless telecommunications

open-ended question a question that requires a descriptive answer, not merely *yes* or *no*

oral disintegrating tablet (ODT) a solid oral dosage form designed to dissolve quickly on the tongue for oral absorption and ease of administration without water

oral route of administration the administration of medication through swallowing for absorption along the GI tract into systemic circulation

oral syringe a needleless device used for administering medication to pediatric or older adult patients unable to swallow tablets or capsules

organizational failure an error generated by failure of organizational rules, policies, or procedures

orphan drug a medication approved by the FDA to treat rare diseases

osmolality a measure of the number of milliosmoles of solute per kilogram of solvent

osmolarity a measure of the milliosmoles of solute per liter of solution (mOsm/L); for example, the osmolarity of blood is 285 mOsm/L; often called *tonicity* for IV solutions

osmotic pressure the pressure required to maintain an equilibrium, with no net movement of solvent

osmotic pressure system a drug delivery system in which the drug is slowly "pushed out" into the bloodstream

otic route of administration the placement of solutions or suspensions into the ear

out of stock (OOS) a medication not in stock in the pharmacy; a drug that must be specially ordered from a drug wholesaler

over-the-counter (OTC) drug a medication that the FDA has approved for sale without a prescription; also called a *nonprescription drug*

P

pandemic an epidemic that occurs across several countries and affects a sizable portion of the population in each country

paraprofessional a trained person who assists a professional person

parenteral route of administration the injection or infusion of fluids and/or medications into the body, bypassing the GI tract

parenteral solution a product that is prepared in a sterile environment for administration by injection

partial fill a supply dispensed to hold the patient until a new supply is received from the wholesaler; this practice is due to an insufficient inventory in the pharmacy, which prevents completely filling the prescription

paste a water-in-oil (W/O) emulsion containing more solid material than an ointment

pasteurization a sterilization process designed to kill most bacteria and mold in milk and other liquids

patent drug another name for an over-the-counter (OTC) medication

pathophysiology the study of disease and illnesses affecting the normal function of the body

patient identifiers any demographic information that can identify the patient, such as name, address, phone number, Social Security number, or medical identification number

patient profile a record kept by the pharmacy that lists a patient's identifying information, insurance information, medical and prescription history, and prescription preferences

patient-controlled analgesia (PCA) infusion device a device controlled by a patient to deliver small doses of medication for chronic pain relief

percent the number or ratio per 100

percentage of error the acceptable range of variation above and below the target measurement; used in compounding and manufacturing

perpetual inventory record a record that accounts for each unit of Schedule II drug dispensed or received

pH value the degree of acidity or alkalinity of a solution; less than 7 is acidic and more than 7 is alkaline; the pH of blood is 7.4

pharmaceutical alternative drug product a drug product that has the same active therapeutic ingredient but contains different salts or different dosage forms; cannot be substituted without prescriber authorization

pharmaceutical care a philosophy of care that expanded the pharmacist's role to include appropriate medication use to achieve positive outcomes with prescribed drug therapy

pharmaceutical elegance the physical appearance of the final compounded preparation

pharmaceutical weights measures of various sizes made of polished brass, often used with a two-pan prescription balance; available in both metric and apothecary weights

pharmaceutically equivalent drug product a drug product that contains the same amount of active ingredient in the same dosage form and meets the same *USP–NF* compendial standards (i.e., strength, quality, purity, and identity); can be substituted without contacting the prescriber

pharmaceutics the study of the release characteristics of specific drug dosage forms

pharmacist one who is licensed to prepare and dispense medications, counsel patients, and monitor outcomes pursuant to a prescription from a licensed healthcare professional

pharmacodynamic agent a drug that alters body functions in a desired way

pharmacogenomics a field of study that examines the relationship between an individual's genes and his or her body's response to drugs

pharmacognosy the study of medicinal functions of natural products of animal, plant, or mineral origins

pharmacokinetics the study of how drugs are absorbed into the bloodstream, circulated in tissues throughout the body, inactivated, and eliminated from the body

pharmacology the scientific study of drugs and their mechanisms of action

pharmacopeia a listing of drugs; also called a *formulary* or *dispensatory*

Pharmacy and Therapeutics (P&T) Committee a committee of the hospital that reviews, approves, and revises the hospital's formulary of drugs and maintains the drug use policies of the hospital

pharmacy benefits manager (PBM) a company that administers drug benefits for many insurance companies

Pharmacy Compounding Accreditation Board (PCAB) an organization that provides quality and safety standards for a compounding pharmacy through voluntary accreditation

pharmacy technician an individual working in a pharmacy who, under the supervision of a licensed pharmacist, assists in activities not requiring the professional judgment of a pharmacist; also called a *pharmacy tech* or *tech*

Pharmacy Technician Certification Examination (PTCE) an examination developed by the Pharmacy Technician Certification Board (PTCB) that technicians must pass to be certified and receive the title of CPhT

phlebitis an inflammation of a vein from the administration of drugs

physical dependence a state in which abruptly terminating a drug produces physical withdrawal symptoms such as restlessness, anxiety, insomnia, diarrhea, vomiting, and goose bumps

pick station an area of the inpatient pharmacy that houses frequently prescribed formulary drugs in commercially available unit dose packaging, thus allowing efficient medication cart filling

pipette a long, thin, calibrated hollow tube used for measuring small volumes of liquids

plaintiff one who files a lawsuit for the courts to decide

plaster a solid or semisolid, medicated or nonmedicated preparation that adheres to the skin

Policy & Procedure (P&P) manual a written, step-by-step set of instructions for pharmacists and technicians alike on all operations within the pharmacy department

posting the process of reconciling the invoice and updating inventory at time of receipt

powder volume (pv) the amount of space occupied by a freeze-dried medication in a sterile vial, used for reconstitution; equal to the difference between the final volume (fv) and the volume of the diluting ingredient, or the diluent volume (dv)

powders fine particles of medication used in tablets and capsules

preferred drug list a formulary provided by an insurance company that indicates preferred prescription generic and brand name drugs and their corresponding co-pays

prescription an order written by a qualified, licensed practitioner for a medication to be filled by a pharmacist to treat a patient's medical condition

prescription drug a drug that requires a prescription from a licensed provider for a valid medical purpose; also called a *legend drug*

prescription record a computer-generated version of the compounding log that documents the compounding recipe for a specific prescription and patient

prime vendor purchasing an agreement made by a pharmacy for a specified percentage or dollar amount of purchases

priming the act of running fluid through IV tubing to flush out small particles and expel air from the tubing before medication administration

prior authorization (PA) approval for coverage of a high-cost medication or a medication not on the insurer's approved formulary, obtained after a prescriber calls the insurer to justify the use of the drug; must be obtained before the drug is dispensed by the pharmacy to be covered by insurance

private insurance coverage for medical or prescription costs provided by an employer or purchased by an individual

prn the abbreviation for a common Latin phrase, *pro re nata*, or "in the circumstances"; commonly used to direct a patient to take medication on an as-needed basis rather than a routinely scheduled dosage

product line extension a marketing strategy by which a brand name product is brought to market with different combinations of active ingredients and different indications leading to potential consumer errors

product package insert (PPI) scientific information supplied to the pharmacist and technician by the manufacturer with all prescription drug products; the information must be approved by the FDA

professional an individual with recognized expertise in a field who is expected to use his or her knowledge and skills to benefit others and to operate ethically with some autonomy

professional standards guidelines of acceptable behavior and performance established by professional associations

profit the amount of revenue received that exceeds the expense of the sold product, services, and overhead

prophylactic agent a drug used to prevent disease

proportion a comparison of equal ratios; the product of the means equals the product of the extremes

protected health information (PHI) medical information that is protected by HIPAA, such as medical diagnoses, medication profiles, and results of laboratory tests

protozoan a single-celled organism that inhabits water and soil

psychological dependence a state in which taking a drug produces a sense of well-being and, consequently, the abrupt termination of the drug may create anxiety withdrawal symptoms

pulverization the process of reducing particle size, especially by using a solvent

punch method a method for filling capsules in which the body of a capsule is repeatedly punched into a cake of medication until the capsule is full

purchasing the ordering of products for use or sale by the pharmacy

pyrogen a fever-producing by-product of microbial metabolism

Q

quality assurance (QA) program a feedback system to improve care by identifying and correcting the cause of a medication error or improper technique

R

radiopharmaceutical a drug containing radioactive ingredients, often used for diagnostic or therapeutic purposes

rapid-dissolving tablet (RDT) a tablet that disintegrates rapidly (within 30 seconds) on the tongue

ratio a comparison of numeric values

reasonable doubt the standard of proof or evidence that the plaintiff must provide in a case involving crimes against the local, state, or federal government

receipt a printout that is a proof of purchase

receiving a series of procedures for accepting the delivery of products to the pharmacy from a wholesaler or centralized warehouse

recertification the periodic updating of certification

reciprocation the administrative process for relicensure of pharmacists in another state

rectal route of administration the delivery of medication via the rectum

refill an approval by the prescriber to dispense the prescribed medication again without the need for a new prescription order

registration the process of being enrolled on a list created by the state board of pharmacy; most state boards require pharmacy technicians to register with their state of practice

regulation a written rule and procedure that exists to carry out a law of the state or federal government

regulatory law the system of rules and regulations established by governmental bodies

remote computer a minicomputer or a mainframe that stores and processes data sent from a dumb terminal

repackaging control log a form used in the pharmacy when drugs are repackaged from manufacturer stock bottles to unit doses; the log contains the name of the drug, dose, quantity, manufacturer lot number, expiration date, and the initials of the pharmacy technician and pharmacist

ribonucleic acid (RNA) an important component of the genetic code that arranges amino acids into proteins

risk evaluation and mitigation strategy (REMS) a requirement by the FDA that procedures be developed by drug manufacturers to ensure that the benefits of selected high-risk drugs on the market outweigh their risks

roll clamp the hard, plastic device that provides compression on the tubing, thereby controlling the flow rate of the IV solution

Roman system a mathematical system in which numerals are expressed in either capital letters or lowercase letters

root-cause analysis a logical and systematic process used to help identify what, how, and why something happened to prevent recurrence

route of administration a way of getting a drug onto or into the body, such as orally, topically, or parenterally

S

schedule a listing of controlled substances categorized by the DEA according to their potential for abuse and physical or psychological dependence

Schedule II drug administration record a manual or electronic form on the patient care unit to account for each dose of each Schedule II narcotic administered to a patient

Schedule V drug a medication with a low potential for abuse and a limited potential for creating physical or psychological dependence; available in most states without a prescription

selection error an error that occurs when two or more options exist and the incorrect option is chosen

semisynthetic drug a drug that contains both natural and synthetic components

sentinel event an unexpected occurrence involving death or serious physical or psychological injury or the potential for such events to occur

sharps any needle, lancet, scalpel blade, or other medical equipment that could cause a cut or puncture

sifting a process used to blend powders through the use of a sieve

signa ("sig") the part of the prescription that indicates the directions for the patient to follow when taking the medication

small-volume parenteral (SVP) an IV fluid of 250 mL or less that is commonly piggybacked onto a patient's existing IV line for infusion of medication

smart terminal a computer that contains its own storage and processing capabilities

smurfing a practice that occurs when a patient is paid cash by an individual to illegally purchase pseudoephedrine from more than one pharmacy

social sanction the measure of acceptable behavior of a professional or paraprofessional by those they serve

solute an ingredient dissolved in a solution or dispersed in a suspension

solution a liquid dosage form in which the active ingredients are completely dissolved in a liquid vehicle

solvent the vehicle that makes up the greater part of a solution

spacer device a device commonly prescribed for children and older adults to assist in the administration of drugs from MDIs; medication can be inhaled at will rather than through timed, coordinated breathing movements

spatula a stainless steel, plastic, or hard rubber instrument used for transferring or mixing solid pharmaceutical ingredients

spatulation a process used to blend ingredients; often used in the preparation of creams and ointments

specific gravity the ratio of the weight of a substance compared to an equal volume of water when both have the same temperature

spike the sharp plastic end of IV tubing that is attached to an IV bag of fluid

spirit an alcoholic or hydroalcoholic solution containing volatile, aromatic ingredients

spontaneous generation an erroneous belief in the seventeenth century that some forms of life could arise spontaneously from matter; for example, that maggots could arise from decaying flesh

spray the dosage form that consists of a container with a valve assembly that, when activated, emits a fine dispersion of liquid, solid, or gaseous material

stability the extent to which a compounded product retains the same physical and chemical properties and characteristics it possessed at the time of preparation

standard a set of criteria to measure product quality or professional performance against a norm

standard of care the usual and customary level of practice in the community

standing order a preapproved list of instructions, including specific medications and doses, commonly written after surgery or a procedure

stat order a medication order that is to be filled and sent to the patient care unit immediately

state boards of pharmacy governing bodies responsible for the regulation of the practice of pharmacy within the states

statutory law a law passed by a legislative body at either the federal, state, or local level

sterile compounding the preparation of a parenteral product in the hospital, home healthcare, nuclear, or community pharmacy setting; an example is an intravenous antibiotic or an ophthalmic solution

sterility the absence of all microorganisms

sterilization a process that destroys the microorganisms on a substance

sublingual route of administration oral administration in which a drug is placed under the tongue and is rapidly absorbed into the bloodstream

subscription the part of the prescription that lists instructions to the pharmacist about dispensing the medication, including information about compounding or packaging instructions, labeling instructions, refill information, and information about the appropriateness of dispensing drug equivalencies

sugar-coated tablet (SCT) a tablet coated with an outside layer of sugar that protects the medication and improves both appearance and flavor

suppository a solid formulation containing a drug for rectal or vaginal administration

suspension the dispersion of a solid in a liquid

sustained-release (SR) formulation an extended-release dosage form that allows less frequent dosing than an immediate-release dosage form

synthesized drug a drug created artificially in the laboratory but in imitation of a naturally occurring drug

synthetic drug a drug that has been created from a series of chemical reactions to produce a specific pharmacological effect

syringe a device used to inject a parenteral solution into the bloodstream, muscle, or under the skin

syrup an aqueous solution thickened with a large amount of sugar (generally sucrose) or a sugar substitute such as sorbitol or propylene glycol

systemic effect the distribution of a drug throughout the body by absorption into the bloodstream

T

tablet the solid dosage form produced by compression and containing one or more active and inactive ingredients

tablet splitter a device used to manually split or score tablets

tamper-resistant prescription pad (TRPP) a paper pad that is specifically designed to prevent copying, erasure, or alteration

targeted drug delivery system technology to deliver high concentrations of drugs to the diseased organ rather than expose the whole body to adverse side effects; commonly designed for cancer chemotherapy

technical failure an error generated by failure of equipment

therapeutic agent a drug that prevents, cures, diagnoses, or relieves symptoms of a disease

therapeutic effect the desired pharmacological action of a drug on the body

therapeutics the study of applying pharmacology to the treatment of illness and disease states

tiered co-pay insurance coverage in which the patient has an escalating cost or co-pay, depending on whether the filled prescription is a generic drug, a preferred brand name drug, or a nonpreferred brand name drug

tincture an alcoholic or hydroalcoholic solution of extractions from plants

tonicity the manner in which cells or tissues respond to surrounding fluid

topical route of administration the administration of a drug on the skin or any mucous membrane such as the eyes, nose, ears, lungs, vagina, urethra, or rectum; usually administered directly to the surface of the skin

tort the legal term for personal injuries that one citizen commits against another in a lawsuit

total parenteral nutrition (TPN) a specially formulated parenteral solution that provides nutritional needs intravenously to a patient who cannot or will not eat

traditional Eastern medicine herbal-based treatments based on ancient East Indian or Asian philosophies that blend various healing modalities to bring balance and harmony to the body

traditional Western medicine medical treatment by a licensed professional who identifies the cause of an illness by physical examination and then treats the illness with various natural and synthetic medicinal products or drugs

transdermal dosage form a formulation designed to deliver a continuous supply of drug into the bloodstream by absorption through the skin via a patch or disk

transmucosal route of administration the absorption of drugs across any mucous membrane of the body including the mouth, eyes, ears, nose, rectum, vagina, and urethra

triage the assessment and prioritization by the pharmacist of patients' illnesses or symptoms; outcome may be to recommend an OTC product, or refer patient to a physician or emergency room; also used to assess and prioritize technician responsibilities within the pharmacy

Tricare a federal government health insurance program for active and retired military personnel and their dependents

trituration the process of rubbing, grinding, or pulverizing a substance to create fine particles, generally by means of a mortar and pestle

troche a small, circular lozenge that contains active medication

tumbling a process used to combine powders by placing them in a bag or container and shaking it

U

uninsured patients with no insurance who must pay out-of-pocket for medical and/or prescription costs

unit dose a dosage unit that is individually labeled and packaged by the manufacturer in sealed foil and considered tamper-proof

unit dose cart a movable storage unit that contains individual patient drawers of medication for all patients on a given nursing unit

unit dose label directions for use on a patient-specific medication order

unit of use a fixed number of dose units in a stock drug container, usually consisting of a month's supply of tablets or capsules, or 30 tablets or capsules

United States Pharmacopeia (USP) the independent, scientific organization responsible for setting official quality standards for all drugs sold in the United States as well as standards for practice

United States Pharmacopeia–National Formulary (USP–NF) a drug reference that contains standards for medicines, dosage forms, drug substances, excipients or inactive substances, medical devices, and dietary supplements

Universal Precautions procedures followed in healthcare settings to prevent infection as a result of exposure to blood or other bodily fluids

urethral route of administration the administration of a drug by insertion into the urethra

USP Chapter <795> a chapter of the *United States Pharmacopeia* that contains national standards for pharmacies formulating nonsterile preparations

USP Chapter <797> guidelines on the sterility and stability of CSPs developed by the United States Pharmacopeia (USP) that have become standards for hospital accreditation

usual and customary charges the total cost of dispensing a prescription to the general public; a pharmacy cannot bill government insurance programs more than the usual and customary charge

V

vaccine a substance introduced into the body to produce immunity to disease

Vaccine Adverse Event Reporting System (VAERS) a postmarketing surveillance system operated by the FDA and CDC that collects information on adverse events that occur after immunization

vaginal route of administration the administration of a drug by application of a cream or insertion of a tablet into the vagina

vertical laminar airflow workbench (LAFW) a type of hood that offers additional protection for both the sterile compounding technician and the environment when aseptically compounding toxic chemicals; examples of these types of hoods include a biological safety cabinet and a compounding aseptic containment isolator

vial a sterile medication container made of plastic or glass and sealed with a rubber top

vial-and-bag system a type of SVP in which a specially designed vial and diluent IVPB bag screw or snap together and are activated by the nurse just before patient administration of the medication

virus a minute infectious agent that does not have all of the components of a cell and thus can replicate only within a living host cell

viscosity the thickness and flow characteristics of a fluid

volumetric measurement a calibrated graduated cylinder or pipette that accurately measures liquids

W

water-in-oil (W/O) emulsion an emulsion containing a small amount of water dispersed in an oil, such as an ointment

wax matrix system a reservoir-controlled release drug delivery system using osmotic pressure or an ion exchange resin

weighing boat a plastic container used to weigh large quantities of chemicals

weighing paper a special paper that is placed on a weighing balance pan to avoid contact between pharmaceutical ingredients and the balance tray; also called *powder paper*

wholesaler purchasing the ordering of drugs and supplies from a local or regional vendor who delivers the product to the pharmacy on a daily basis

workers' compensation insurance provided for a patient with a medical injury from a job-related accident; also called *workers' comp*

wrong dosage form error an error in which the dosage form or formulation is not the accepted interpretation of the physician order

wrong dose error an error in which the dose is either above or below the correct dose by more than 5%

wrong time error a medication error in which a drug is given 30 minutes or more before or after it was prescribed, up to the time of the next dose, not including as-needed orders

Y

Y-site injection port a rigid piece of plastic with one arm terminating in a resealable port that is used to add medication to an IV

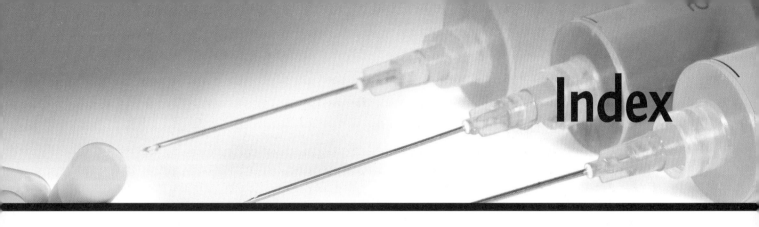

Index

Note: The letters accompanying certain page numbers have the following meanings: "*f*" indicates a figure; "*p*" indicates a photo; "*t*" indicates a table.

negligence
- defined, 54
- four Ds of, 54

new drug application (NDA), 36–37, 85–86

Nexium, 86t

Next Choice, 259

nicotine gum, 118, 123, 123t

nifedipine, 97, 97t

nitroglycerin
- ointment form, 129
- patch, 145
- route of administration, 108, 121
- storing, 123

NKA (no known allergies), 226

NKMA (no known medication allergies), 226

nonaerosolized inhaler, 131

non-child resistant containers, 237

noncompliance, 488

nondurable medical equipment, 260

nonformulary drug, 360
- purchasing for hospital pharmacy, 367–368

nonprescription sales
- dietary supplements, 259
- medical supplies, 260–264
- over-the-counter drugs, 254–259

nonsterile compounding
- accreditation, 318–319
- attire for, 319–320
- beyond-use dating, 317–318
- comminution and blending, 332–334, 333f, 333p
- defined, 311
- documentation of, 320–322
  - of calculation, 322
  - compounding log, 321, 322f
  - master control record, 320–321, 320f, 338f, 341f
- equipment for, 323–331
- general facility requirements, 314–315
- laws and standards for, 312–319
- possible scenarios for, 311–312
- process of
  - final check by pharmacist, 345–346
  - labeling and cleanup, 344–345
  - patient counseling by pharmacist, 346
  - reimbursement for, 346
  - selecting medication containers, 343–344
  - steps in, 344t
- product inventory
  - beyond-use dating, 317–318
  - bulk ingredients, 315–316
  - controlled substances, 317
- references for, 347
- role of technician in, 312
- specific formulations
  - capsules, 336–338
  - hormone formulations, 342
  - ointments, creams and lotions, 340–342
  - powders, 334–335
  - solutions, 338
  - suppositories, 342–343
  - suspensions, 339–340
  - tablets, 335–336
  - troche, 336
- techniques for mixing, 331–334
- USP Chapter <795>, 314

nonsteroidal anti-inflammatory drugs (NSAIDs), allergy to, 227

nonverbal communication, 532–533

nonvolumetric glassware, 330

no refills permitted, 213

normal saline, 131, 443, 444t

nosocomial infection, 423–424

notice of privacy practices, 553

Novolin, 254

NPI number, 204
- processing prescriptions and, 228

NSAIDs, 90t

nuclear medicine, 83

nuclear pharmacy, 13–14

nuclear pharmacy technician (NPT), 23

numerator, 169

numeric systems, 165

nursing unit drug administration/documentation
- floor stock, 383–384
- medication administration record, 385–387
- narcotics, 384–385
- as step in prescription filling process, 506

nystatin, 118

O

Occupational Safety and Health Administration (OSHA), 34
- responsibilities of, 49

ocular route of drug administration, 119

oil-in-water (O/W) emulsion, 127

ointment mill, 330

ointments
- advantages and disadvantages of, 129
- characteristics of, 126–127, 126p, 127p, 340
- compounding, 340–341
- dispensing and administration of, 129

ointment slab, 330

omega-3 fatty acids, 260t

omeprazole, 255t

omission error, 489

Omnibus Budget Reconciliation Act (OBRA-90), 42–43

ondansetron, 111

online adjudication, 291

open-ended questions, 532

ophthalmics
- advantages and disadvantages of, 121
- characteristics of, 119
- dispensing and administration of, 123–124, 124f

opium, 75, 75p

oral disintegrating tablet (ODT), 111

oral dosage forms
- capsules, 111
- liquids, 112–114
- powders and effervescent salts, 112
- preparing to dispense, 233–234
- tablets, 109–111

oral route of administration, 108–117
- advantages and disadvantages of, 114–116
- dispensing and administration of, 116–117
- dosage forms, 108–114

oral syringe, 117, 117p, 329

oral transmucosal fentanyl citrate (OTFC), 118, 123

OraQuick, 263

organizational failure, in medication errors, 490

Orphan Drug Act, 40–41

orphan drugs, 40–41

osmolality, 442

osmolarity, 442

osmotic pressure, 442

osmotic pressure system, 144

otic route of drug administration, 119

otics
- advantages and disadvantages of, 122
- characteristics of, 119
- dispensing and administration of, 124, 125f
- solutions and master control record for, 338, 338f

ounce, 161, 162t
- conversion issues, 164

out-of-stock (OOS) medications, 232, 273

over-the-counter drugs, 254–259
- benefits of, 255
- common OTC and indications, 254–255, 255t
- consumer precautions, 256
- containing pseudoephedrine and ephedrine, 257–259
- defined, 254
- as drug class, 79
- emergency contraception, 259
- FDA and labeling of, 47
- increased use of, 255
- label for, 79, 79p, 255–256
- prescriptions for, 255
- role of pharmacy personnel and, 256
- Schedule V drugs, 257

ovulation cycle kit, 263

oxaprozin, 110

oxymetazoline, 255t

S

safety, medication
    medical errors, 486
    medication errors, 486–491
    prescription-filing process and, 491–506
    preventing medication errors, 506–513
St. John's wort, 260t
salicylic acid, 127, 128
Salk, Jonas, 73
saw palmetto, 6, 260t
Schedule I drugs, 38, 39t
Schedule II drug administration record, 384, 385f
Schedule II drugs, 38, 39t
    automated inventory systems, 384–385
    data entry precaution for, 496
    emergency dispensing of, 217
    inventory control procedures, 275–278, 368
    partial fill, 215–216
    preparing to dispense, 234
    prescription requirements, 215
    refills, 215–216
    signature for, 215
    state boards of pharmacy and, 51
    storage of, 231
    time period for filling, 215
    transfer warning on label, 238
Schedule III drugs, 38, 39t
    anabolic steroids as, 42
    automated inventory systems, 384–385
    inventory control procedures, 275–276
    preparing to dispense, 234
    refills, 216–217
    state boards of pharmacy and, 51
    storage of, 231
    transfer warning on label, 238
Schedule IV drugs, 38, 39t
    automated inventory systems, 384–385
    inventory control procedures, 275–276
    preparing to dispense, 234
    refills, 216–217
    storage of, 231
    transfer warning on label, 238
Schedule V drugs, 38, 39t
    inventory control procedures, 275–276
    record of sale, 257
    refills, 217
    restrictions and requirements for sale of, 257
    state boards of pharmacy and, 51
    storage of, 231
    transfer warning on label, 238
Scientific era for pharmacists, 15
scruple, 161, 162t

Secundum Artem: Current & Practical Compounding Information for the Pharmacist, 347
selection error, 490
semisynthetic drugs, 76
sentinel event, 514
sharps, disposal of, 278–279, 424, 424p
shoe covers, 420
show-and-tell technique, 505
side effects, listed on product package insert (PPI), 88–89
sifting, 332
signa, 204t, 206
Sildenafil, 90t
single-dose vials (SDVs), 448
smallpox, 71, 401, 404
small-volume parenterals (SVPs), 446–447
smart terminal, 264
smurfing, 258
social sanction, 545
sodium sulfacetamide, 119
solute, 112
    compounding solutions, 338
solutions
    characteristics of, 112
    common, 112
    compounding, 338
    gel-forming, 121
    irrigating, 118, 128
    less common, 113
    parenteral, 132
solvent, 112
    compounding solutions, 338
somatotropin, 75
Sotret, 93
spacer device, 132
Spanish flu, 404
spatula, 330
spatulation, 332
SPEAK UP campaign, 515
specific gravity, 188–189
spike, 437, 438
spirit, 113
spontaneous generation, 400–401
spray, 119
stability, product, 317, 412
    IV solutions, 443
Stability of Compounded Formulations, 98
standard of care, 35, 54
standards, drug, 35
standing order, 372
state boards of pharmacy, 50–51
    medication error reporting, 513–514
    preventive measure for controlled substance abuse, 220
statins, 41
stat order, 372
statutory laws, 36
sterile compounding, 23. *See also* compounded sterile preparation (CSP)
    beyond-use dating, 317–318
    overview of, 310–311

specialized procedures
    ampules, 450–452
    total parenteral nutrition solutions, 452–455
    vials, 448–450
    USP Chapter <797>, 314, 411–423
sterile supplies, for IV preparation and administration, 434–441
sterile water for injection, 131
sterility, 406
sterilization
    chemical, 407
    defined, 406
    dry heat, 407
    gas, 407
    heat, 406
    mechanical, 407
steroids, anabolic, 42
Strand, Linda, 16
Strattera, 90t
streptomycin, 75
subcutaneous route
    characteristics of, 133–134
    dispensing and administration of, 139–141
    insulin administration, 140–141
    needles, 139
sublingual medication
    advantages and disadvantages of, 121
    characteristics of, 118
    dispensing and administration of, 123
sublingual route of administration, 118
Suboxone, 93, 94, 223
subscription, 204t, 205, 205f
substance abuse
    course of action, 548–549
    healthcare professionals and, 548
    signs and symptoms of, 548
Subutex, 93, 94
sugar-coated tablet (SCT), 110
sulfa antibiotics, 75
    allergy to, 227
suppositories, 120p
    advantages and disadvantages of, 122
    characteristics of, 119–120
    compounding, 342–343
    dispensing and administration of, 125, 126t
Surescripts, 209, 211
suspensions, 113
    compounding, 339–340
sustained-release (SR) formulation, 143
synthesized drugs, 75–76
synthetic drugs, 75
syringes
    accuracy and, 435
    glass, 136, 434
    handling of needle-and-syringe unit, 436, 437f
    home disposal of, 279
    hypodermic, 136, 136p

Photo Credits

4 Wikipedia/Public Domain; **5** *top*, Wikipedia/Illustration from the Vienna Dioscurides/Public Domain; *bottom*, Wikipedia/Lithograph by Pierre Roche Vigneron/Public Domain; **6** © iStockphoto/AntiMartina; **8** © Shutterstock/Iakov Filimonov; **9** © iStockphoto/jcarillet; **10** IMS Health, 2012; **11** © iStockphoto/nano; **12** © iStockphoto/3bugsmom; **13** Photograph provided courtesy of Kara Duncan Weatherman, PharmD, BCNP, Purdue University Nuclear Pharmacy Programs. Copyright (2008) Purdue University; **14** © iStockphoto/HultonArchive; **15** © iStockphoto/stevecoleimages; **17** © iStockphoto/sjlocke; **18** © Paradigm Publishing; **19** *top*, © iStockphoto/sshepard; *bottom*, Courtesy of American Association of Colleges of Pharmacy; **21** © Paradigm Publishing; **22** © George Brainard; **23** © Paradigm Publishing; **24** © iStockphoto/bowdenimages; **34** Wikipedia/United States Department of Justice/Public Domain; **36** Wikipedia/Chromolithograph by Hughes Lithographers, Chicago/Public Domain; **37** © Paradigm Publishing; **40** © iStockphoto/cglade; iStockphoto/monpierre **41** Courtesy of Robert Anderson; **42** Wikipedia/Kevin Rushforth; **44** © Shutterstock/mangostock; **46** Courtesy of Robert Anderson; **48** © Paradigm Publishing; **49** © Paradigm Publishing; **51** Courtesy of Robert Anderson; **53** © iStockphoto/Neustockimages; **56** Used with permission of The United States Pharmacopeial Convention (USP); **70** © Paradigm Publishing; **71** © iStockphoto/gchutka; **72** *top*, © iStockphoto/MarkHatfield; *bottom*, © iStockphoto/photomak; **73** © iStockphoto/FrankRitchie; **75** © iStockphoto/mafoto; **76** *top*, © iStockphoto/smartstock; *bottom*, © Humalog is a registered trademark of Eli Lilly and Company; **77** © Paradigm Publishing; **78** Mallinckrodt LLC; **79** © Paradigm Publishing; **80** Courtesy of Robert Anderson; **81** Used with permission of The United States Pharmacopeial Convention (USP). The Dietary Supplement Verification Program certification mark is a registered trademark of USP; **82** © iStockphoto/monkeybusinessimages; **83** © iStockphoto/fluxfoto; **85** © Paradigm Publishing; **88** *top*, © Pfizer Inc. Used with permission; *bottom*, Courtesy of Tova Wiegand-Green; **89** © George Brainard; **92** U.S. Food and Drug Administration; **93** Courtesy of Robert Anderson; **108** © Shutterstock/IDAL; **110** © Paradigm Publishing; **111** © Paradigm Publishing; **112** © iStockphoto/ruizluquepaz; **113** © Paradigm Publishing; **115** © Paradigm Publishing; **116** iStockphoto/WellfordT; **117** Courtesy of Tova Wiegand-Green; **118** © George Brainard; **120** Courtesy of Tova Wiegand-Green; **121** © Shutterstock/BW Folsom; **124** © Paradigm Publishing; **125** © Paradigm Publishing; **126** © Shutterstock/Kesu; **127** Courtesy of Tova Wiegand-Green; **130** *top*, © iStockphoto/leschnyhan; *bottom*, © Paradigm Publishing; **131** *top*, Courtesy of Tova Wiegand-Green; *bottom*, © iStockphoto/ladyminnie; **132** © iStockphoto/xavigm; **133** © Paradigm Publishing; **134** © iStockphoto/CreativeI; **136** © Paradigm Publishing; **137** *top*, © iStockphoto/Sean_Warren; *bottom*, © Paradigm Publishing; **138** *top*, © iStockphoto/smartstock; *bottom*, © Shutterstock/Rob Byron; **139** © Paradigm Publishing; **140** © Paradigm Publishing; **141** *top*, Courtesy of Robert Anderson; *bottom*, © Paradigm Publishing; **144** © Paradigm Publishing; **145** Wikipedia/Public Domain; **146** © iStockphoto/Eduardo Luzzatti; **158** © iStockphoto/Spanic; **160** © Paradigm Publishing; **162** © Paradigm Publishing; **166** © iStockphoto/malerapaso; **170** © Paradigm Publishing; **180** © Paradigm Publishing; **185** Courtesy of Apothecary Products, Inc.; **200** Courtesy of Robert Anderson; **201** *top*, Parata Systems, LLC; *bottom*, © iStockphoto/youngvet; **202** *top*, Copyright Eli Lilly and Company. All Rights Reserved. Used with Permission. Strattera is a trademark of Eli Lilly and Company; *bottom*, © iStockphoto/kzenon; **203** © George Brainard; **205** © Paradigm Publishing; **207** © Paradigm Publishing; **209** © George Brainard; **210** © Paradigm Publishing; **211** © iStockphoto/katalinamas; **212** © Paradigm Publishing; **216** *top*, © Shutterstock/Scott Rothstein; *bottom*, © Paradigm Publishing; **220**

Photo Micro Format, Inc.; **222** © iStockphoto/sjlocke; **224** © Paradigm Publishing; **226** © Paradigm Publishing; **227** © Paradigm Publishing; **229** © iStockphoto/Syldavia; **230** *Middle,* Courtesy of Robert Anderson; *bottom,* © Copyright Eli Lilly and Company. All Rights Reserved. Used with Permission. Cymbalta is a trademark of Eli Lilly and Company.; **231** Courtesy of Robert Anderson; **232** Courtesy of Robert Anderson; **233** © iStockphoto/uchar; **234** *top,* Courtesy of Tova Wiegand-Green; *bottom,* © iStockphoto/art-4-art; **235** Courtesy of Robert Anderson; **236** *top,* Courtesy of Robert Anderson; *bottom,* Courtesy of Apothecary Products, Inc.; **238** © Paradigm Publishing; **239** © Paradigm Publishing; **240** *top,* Courtesy of Tova Wiegand-Green; *bottom,* © iStockphoto/stevecoleimages; **241** © Paradigm Publishing; **242** © Paradigm Publishing; **254** Courtesy of Robert Anderson; **255** © Paradigm Publishing; **256** © iStock/leaf; **257** © Shutterstock/Cheryl Casey; **258** *top,* Courtesy of Robert Anderson; *bottom,* © Paradigm Publishing; **259** *top,* Courtesy of Robert Anderson; *bottom,* © Paradigm Publishing; **261** Courtesy of Robert Anderson; **262** © Paradigm Publishing; **263** Courtesy of Robert Anderson; **265** © Paradigm Publishing; **266** Courtesy of Robert Anderson; **267** © iStock/Deklofenak; **268** *top,* Courtesy of Robert Anderson; *bottom,* Eyecon® model 9400 shown courtesy of Avery Weigh-Tronix.; **269** *top,* Parata Systems, LLC; *bottom,* Courtesy of Robert Anderson; **272** © iStock/sjlocke; **274** © Food and Drug Administration; **275** © iStock/SWInsider; **276** Public Domain; **277** *top,* Courtesy of Robert Anderson; *bottom,* © Paradigm Publishing; **279** *top,* Courtesy of Apothecary Products, Inc.; *bottom,* Courtesy of Robert Anderson; **283** © iStock/spxChrome; **284** *top,* Statistics courtesy of the IMS Institute for Healthcare Informatics; *bottom,* © iStock/stevecoleimages; **287** © iStock/lisafx; **288** © iStock/BrianAJackson; **290** © Paradigm Publishing; **292** Photo courtesy of Bausch & Lomb Incorporated; **310** *top,* © iStockphoto/duncan1890; *bottom,* © George Brainard; **311** *top,* © Paradigm Publishing; *bottom,* © iStockphoto/narxx; **312** © Paradigm Publishing; **313** Courtesy of Robert Anderson; **314** Courtesy of Lisa McCartney; **316** Courtesy of Lisa McCartney; **317** Courtesy of Robert Anderson; **319** *top,* Courtesy of the Pharmacy Compounding Accreditation Board (PCAB); *bottom,* © iStockphoto/kadmy; **320** Screen capture courtesy of PK Software's CompounderLab™. CompounderLab is a trademark of PCCA.; **322** © Paradigm Publishing; **323** iStockphoto/DenGuy; **324** Courtesy of Tova Wiegand-Green; **325** *top,* Courtesy of Tova Wiegand-Green; *bottom,* © George Brainard; **327** © Paradigm Publishing; **328** © Paradigm Publishing; **329** *top left,* © Shutterstock/fotohunter; *top right,* © Shutterstock/Kimberly Hall; *bottom,* Courtesy of Tova Wiegand-Green; **330** *top,* Courtesy of Lisa McCartney; *middle,* © George Brainard; *bottom,* Courtesy of Tova Wiegand-Green; **331** *top,* Courtesy of Robert Anderson; *bottom,* Provided courtesy of Topi-CLICK. Topi-CLICK is a registered trademark. For more information about this product, visit www.Topi-Click.com.; **333** Courtesy of Tova Wiegand-Green; **334** Courtesy of Robert Anderson; **336** © Paradigm Publishing; **337** *top,* © George Brainard; *bottom,* Courtesy of Torpac, Inc. (photographer: Eric Hobaichan); **338** Courtesy of Loyd V. Allen, Jr., PhD; **341** Courtesy of Loyd V. Allen, Jr., PhD; **343** *top,* Courtesy of Tova Wiegand-Green; *bottom,* © Paradigm Publishing; **345** © iStockphoto/YinYang; **346** © iStockphoto/energyy; **358** Courtesy of Lisa McCartney; **359** © Ghislain & Marie Davide de Lossy, cultura, Jupiterimages; **361** Courtesy of Lisa McCartney; **362** Courtesy of Lisa McCartney; **365** © George Brainard; **366** Courtesy of Lisa McCartney; **367** Courtesy of McKesson Provider Technologies, Inc.; **368** Photo by: © Spacesaver Corporation; **369** © Paradigm Publishing; **370** Courtesy of Lisa McCartney; **371** Courtesy of Lisa McCartney; **372** © Paradigm Publishing; **373** © iStockphoto/YanC; **375** *top,* Courtesy of McKesson Provider Technologies, Inc; *bottom,* © George Brainard; **377** *top,* Copyright 2013 Medi-Dose, Inc. All Rights Reserved. Used with Permission.; *bottom,* © Paradigm Publishing; **378** © Paradigm Publishing; **379** Courtesy of Lisa McCartney; **380** Courtesy of McKesson Provider Technologies, Inc.; **381** © Paradigm Publishing; **382** Courtesy of Tova Wiegand-Green; **383** Courtesy of McKesson Provider Technologies, Inc.; **385** © Paradigm Publishing; **386** *top,* © Paradigm Publishing; *bottom,* Photo courtesy of McKesson Corp.; © 2004 Bard Wrisley; **387** Courtesy of McKesson Provider Technologies, Inc.; **400** *top,* © Paradigm Publishing; *bottom,* © iStockphoto/sitox; **401** © Visual Art Library (London), Alamy; **402** *top,* Courtesy of the National Library of Medicine; *bottom,* © Paradigm Publishing; **403,** *middle,* BSIP/Superstock; *bottom,* Cultura Limited/SuperStock; **404** © Shutterstock/lynea; **405** Courtesy of the Centers for Disease Control and Prevention/James Gathany; **406** © iStockphoto/DenGuy; **408** © iStockphoto/sshepard; **409** © Paradigm Publishing; **410** © iStockphoto/dra_schwartz; **411** © iStockphoto/sjlocke; **412** *top,* © Paradigm Publishing; *bottom,* Bioscience International, Inc.; **413** © Paradigm Publishing; **414** © Paradigm Publishing; **415** © Paradigm Publishing; **416** © Paradigm Publishing; **417** © Paradigm Publishing; **418** © Paradigm Publishing; **420** © Paradigm Publishing; **421** *top,* © Shutterstock/IMAGE LAGOON; *bottom,* © Paradigm Publishing; **423** *top,* © Paradigm Publishing; *bottom,* © iStockphoto/Geber86; **424** © iStockphoto/RapidEye; **434** © Paradigm Publishing; **435** © Paradigm Publishing; **436** © Paradigm Publishing; **437** © Paradigm Publishing; **438** © Paradigm Publishing; **439** © Paradigm Publishing, **440** © iStockphoto/annedde; **441** © Paradigm Publishing; **442** © iStockphoto/Eraxion; **445** © Paradigm Publishing; **446** © Paradigm Publishing; **448** *top,* © Paradigm Publishing; *bottom,* © George Brainard; © Paradigm Publishing; **449** © Paradigm Publishing; **450** © Paradigm Publishing; **451** © Paradigm Publishing; **453** © iStockphoto/nazdravie; **454** © Paradigm Publishing; **456** © Paradigm Publishing; **462** © Paradigm Publishing; **464** © Paradigm Publishing; **465** © Paradigm Publishing; **469** *top left,* © Paradigm Publishing; *top right,* © Shutterstock/Rihardzz; *bottom,* © George Brainard; **470** Courtesy of Spectrum Laboratory Products Inc., 2013; **472** Courtesy of Tova Wiegand-Green; **486** © iStockphoto/sjlocke; **489** Courtesy of Robert Anderson; **490** © Paradigm Publishing; **491** © Paradigm Publishing; **491** © Paradigm Publishing; **494** © Paradigm Publishing; **495** iStockphoto/sjlocke; **499** Courtesy of Robert Anderson; **505** *top,* iStockphoto/YinYang; *bottom,* iStockphoto/sjlocke; **507** © Paradigm Publishing; **510** *top,* © Target Corporation. Used with permission.; *bottom,* Courtesy of Robert Anderson; **511** *top,* Courtesy of Robert Anderson; *bottom left,* Courtesy of Tova Wiegand-Green; *bottom right,* Courtesy of McKesson Provider Technologies, Inc.; **512** Courtesy of McKesson Provider Technologies, Inc.; **526** © iStockphoto/asiseeit; **530** © iStockphoto/asiseeit; **533** © iStockphoto/asiseeit; **534** © iStockphoto/sjlocke; **535** © iStockphoto/MickyWiswedel; **536** © iStockphoto/4X-image; **539** © iStockphoto/nano; **540** Copyright © 2013 Purdue Pharma L.P.; **541** © iStockphoto/kadmy; **542** © iStockphoto/sjlocke; **543** © iStockphoto/sjlocke; **544** © Paradigm Publishing; **547** © iStockphoto/dptulk; **552** © iStockphoto/spxChrome; **562** © Paradigm Publishing; **564** © Paradigm Publishing; **565** © 2013 Pharmacy Technician Certification Board; **566** *top,* © Paradigm Publishing; *bottom,* © 2012 Pharmacy Technician Certification Board; **569** © Paradigm Publishing; **571** © Paradigm Publishing; **572** © iStockphoto/omada; **574** © Paradigm Publishing; **576** © Paradigm Publishing; **577** © Paradigm Publishing; **579** © Paradigm Publishing; **580** © iStockphoto/zimmytws; **581** © iStockphoto/fstop123; **582** © iStockphoto/hillwoman2; **583** © iStockphoto/katalinamasQ; **584** © Shutterstock/dencg; **585** © iStockphoto/clu